AF676287

COMPLEXITY IN STRUCTURE AND FUNCTION OF THE LUNG

LUNG BIOLOGY IN HEALTH AND DISEASE

Executive Editor

Claude Lenfant
Director, National Heart, Lung and Blood Institute
National Institutes of Health
Bethesda, Maryland

1. Immunologic and Infectious Reactions in the Lung, *edited by Charles H. Kirkpatrick and Herbert Y. Reynolds*
2. The Biochemical Basis of Pulmonary Function, *edited by Ronald G. Crystal*
3. Bioengineering Aspects of the Lung, *edited by John B. West*
4. Metabolic Functions of the Lung, *edited by Y. S. Bakhle and John R. Vane*
5. Respiratory Defense Mechanisms (in two parts), *edited by Joseph D. Brain, Donald F. Proctor, and Lynne M. Reid*
6. Development of the Lung, *edited by W. Alan Hodson*
7. Lung Water and Solute Exchange, *edited by Norman C. Staub*
8. Extrapulmonary Manifestations of Respiratory Disease, *edited by Eugene Debs Robin*
9. Chronic Obstructive Pulmonary Disease, *edited by Thomas L. Petty*
10. Pathogenesis and Therapy of Lung Cancer, *edited by Curtis C. Harris*
11. Genetic Determinants of Pulmonary Disease, *edited by Stephen D. Litwin*
12. The Lung in the Transition Between Health and Disease, *edited by Peter T. Macklem and Solbert Permutt*
13. Evolution of Respiratory Processes: A Comparative Approach, *edited by Stephen C. Wood and Claude Lenfant*
14. Pulmonary Vascular Diseases, *edited by Kenneth M. Moser*
15. Physiology and Pharmacology of the Airways, *edited by Jay A. Nadel*
16. Diagnostic Techniques in Pulmonary Disease (in two parts), *edited by Marvin A. Sackner*
17. Regulation of Breathing (in two parts), *edited by Thomas F. Hornbein*
18. Occupational Lung Diseases: Research Approaches and Methods, *edited by Hans Weill and Margaret Turner-Warwick*
19. Immunopharmacology of the Lung, *edited by Harold H. Newball*
20. Sarcoidosis and Other Granulomatous Diseases of the Lung, *edited by Barry L. Fanburg*

21. Sleep and Breathing, *edited by Nicholas A. Saunders and Colin E. Sullivan*
22. *Pneumocystis carinii* Pneumonia: Pathogenesis, Diagnosis, and Treatment, *edited by Lowell S. Young*
23. Pulmonary Nuclear Medicine: Techniques in Diagnosis of Lung Disease, *edited by Harold L. Atkins*
24. Acute Respiratory Failure, *edited by Warren M. Zapol and Konrad J. Falke*
25. Gas Mixing and Distribution in the Lung, *edited by Ludwig A. Engel and Manuel Paiva*
26. High-Frequency Ventilation in Intensive Care and During Surgery, *edited by Graziano Carlon and William S. Howland*
27. Pulmonary Development: Transition from Intrauterine to Extrauterine Life, *edited by George H. Nelson*
28. Chronic Obstructive Pulmonary Disease: Second Edition, Revised and Expanded, *edited by Thomas L. Petty*
29. The Thorax (in two parts), *edited by Charis Roussos and Peter T. Macklem*
30. The Pleura in Health and Disease, *edited by Jacques Chrétien, Jean Bignon, and Albert Hirsch*
31. Drug Therapy for Asthma: Research and Clinical Practice, *edited by John W. Jenne and Shirley Murphy*
32. Pulmonary Endothelium in Health and Disease, *edited by Una S. Ryan*
33. The Airways: Neural Control in Health and Disease, *edited by Michael A. Kaliner and Peter J. Barnes*
34. Pathophysiology and Treatment of Inhalation Injuries, *edited by Jacob Loke*
35. Respiratory Function of the Upper Airway, *edited by Oommen P. Mathew and Giuseppe Sant'Ambrogio*
36. Chronic Obstructive Pulmonary Disease: A Behavioral Perspective, *edited by A. John McSweeny and Igor Grant*
37. Biology of Lung Cancer: Diagnosis and Treatment, *edited by Steven T. Rosen, James L. Mulshine, Frank Cuttitta, and Paul G. Abrams*
38. Pulmonary Vascular Physiology and Pathophysiology, *edited by E. Kenneth Weir and John T. Reeves*
39. Comparative Pulmonary Physiology: Current Concepts, *edited by Stephen C. Wood*
40. Respiratory Physiology: An Analytical Approach, *edited by H. K. Chang and Manuel Paiva*
41. Lung Cell Biology, *edited by Donald Massaro*
42. Heart–Lung Interactions in Health and Disease, *edited by Steven M. Scharf and Sharon S. Cassidy*
43. Clinical Epidemiology of Chronic Obstructive Pulmonary Disease, *edited by Michael J. Hensley and Nicholas A. Saunders*
44. Surgical Pathology of Lung Neoplasms, *edited by Alberto M. Marchevsky*
45. The Lung in Rheumatic Diseases, *edited by Grant W. Cannon and Guy A. Zimmerman*

46. Diagnostic Imaging of the Lung, *edited by Charles E. Putman*
47. Models of Lung Disease: Microscopy and Structural Methods, *edited by Joan Gil*
48. Electron Microscopy of the Lung, *edited by Dean E. Schraufnagel*
49. Asthma: Its Pathology and Treatment, *edited by Michael A. Kaliner, Peter J. Barnes, and Carl G. A. Persson*
50. Acute Respiratory Failure: Second Edition, *edited by Warren M. Zapol and Francois Lemaire*
51. Lung Disease in the Tropics, *edited by Om P. Sharma*
52. Exercise: Pulmonary Physiology and Pathophysiology, *edited by Brian J. Whipp and Karlman Wasserman*
53. Developmental Neurobiology of Breathing, *edited by Gabriel G. Haddad and Jay P. Farber*
54. Mediators of Pulmonary Inflammation, *edited by Michael A. Bray and Wayne H. Anderson*
55. The Airway Epithelium, *edited by Stephen G. Farmer and Douglas Hay*
56. Physiological Adaptations in Vertebrates: Respiration, Circulation, and Metabolism, *edited by Stephen C. Wood, Roy E. Weber, Alan R. Hargens, and Ronald W. Millard*
57. The Bronchial Circulation, *edited by John Butler*
58. Lung Cancer Differentiation: Implications for Diagnosis and Treatment, *edited by Samuel D. Bernal and Paul J. Hesketh*
59. Pulmonary Complications of Systemic Disease, *edited by John F. Murray*
60. Lung Vascular Injury: Molecular and Cellular Response, *edited by Arnold Johnson and Thomas J. Ferro*
61. Cytokines of the Lung, *edited by Jason Kelley*
62. The Mast Cell in Health and Disease, *edited by Michael A. Kaliner and Dean D. Metcalfe*
63. Pulmonary Disease in the Elderly Patient, *edited by Donald A. Mahler*
64. Cystic Fibrosis, *edited by Pamela B. Davis*
65. Signal Transduction in Lung Cells, *edited by Jerome S. Brody, David M. Center, and Vsevolod A. Tkachuk*
66. Tuberculosis: A Comprehensive International Approach, *edited by Lee B. Reichman and Earl S. Hershfield*
67. Pharmacology of the Respiratory Tract: Experimental and Clinical Research, *edited by K. Fan Chung and Peter J. Barnes*
68. Prevention of Respiratory Diseases, *edited by Albert Hirsch, Marcel Goldberg, Jean-Pierre Martin, and Roland Masse*
69. *Pneumocystis carinii* Pneumonia: Second Edition, Revised and Expanded, *edited by Peter D. Walzer*
70. Fluid and Solute Transport in the Airspaces of the Lungs, *edited by Richard M. Effros and H. K. Chang*
71. Sleep and Breathing: Second Edition, Revised and Expanded, *edited by Nicholas A. Saunders and Colin E. Sullivan*
72. Airway Secretion: Physiological Bases for the Control of Mucous Hypersecretion, *edited by Tamotsu Takishima and Sanae Shimura*

73. Sarcoidosis and Other Granulomatous Disorders, *edited by D. Geraint James*
74. Epidemiology of Lung Cancer, *edited by Jonathan M. Samet*
75. Pulmonary Embolism, *edited by Mario Morpurgo*
76. Sports and Exercise Medicine, *edited by Stephen C. Wood and Robert C. Roach*
77. Endotoxin and the Lungs, *edited by Kenneth L. Brigham*
78. The Mesothelial Cell and Mesothelioma, *edited by Marie-Claude Jaurand and Jean Bignon*
79. Regulation of Breathing: Second Edition, Revised and Expanded, *edited by Jerome A. Dempsey and Allan I. Pack*
80. Pulmonary Fibrosis, *edited by Sem Hin Phan and Roger S. Thrall*
81. Long-Term Oxygen Therapy: Scientific Basis and Clinical Application, *edited by Walter J. O'Donohue, Jr.*
82. Ventral Brainstem Mechanisms and Control of Respiration and Blood Pressure, *edited by C. Ovid Trouth, Richard M. Millis, Heidrun F. Kiwull-Schöne, and Marianne E. Schläfke*
83. A History of Breathing Physiology, *edited by Donald F. Proctor*
84. Surfactant Therapy for Lung Disease, *edited by Bengt Robertson and H. William Taeusch*
85. The Thorax: Second Edition, Revised and Expanded (in three parts), *edited by Charis Roussos*
86. Severe Asthma: Pathogenesis and Clinical Management, *edited by Stanley J. Szefler and Donald Y. M. Leung*
87. *Mycobacterium avium*–Complex Infection: Progress in Research and Treatment, *edited by Joyce A. Korvick and Constance A. Benson*
88. Alpha 1–Antitrypsin Deficiency: Biology • Pathogenesis • Clinical Manifestations • Therapy, *edited by Ronald G. Crystal*
89. Adhesion Molecules and the Lung, *edited by Peter A. Ward and Joseph C. Fantone*
90. Respiratory Sensation, *edited by Lewis Adams and Abraham Guz*
91. Pulmonary Rehabilitation, *edited by Alfred P. Fishman*
92. Acute Respiratory Failure in Chronic Obstructive Pulmonary Disease, *edited by Jean-Philippe Derenne, William A. Whitelaw, and Thomas Similowski*
93. Environmental Impact on the Airways: From Injury to Repair, *edited by Jacques Chrétien and Daniel Dusser*
94. Inhalation Aerosols: Physical and Biological Basis for Therapy, *edited by Anthony J. Hickey*
95. Tissue Oxygen Deprivation: From Molecular to Integrated Function, *edited by Gabriel G. Haddad and George Lister*
96. The Genetics of Asthma, *edited by Stephen B. Liggett and Deborah A. Meyers*
97. Inhaled Glucocorticoids in Asthma: Mechanisms and Clinical Actions, *edited by Robert P. Schleimer, William W. Busse, and Paul M. O'Byrne*
98. Nitric Oxide and the Lung, *edited by Warren M. Zapol and Kenneth D. Bloch*

99. Primary Pulmonary Hypertension, *edited by Lewis J. Rubin and Stuart Rich*
100. Lung Growth and Development, *edited by John A. McDonald*
101. Parasitic Lung Diseases, *edited by Adel A. F. Mahmoud*
102. Lung Macrophages and Dendritic Cells in Health and Disease, *edited by Mary F. Lipscomb and Stephen W. Russell*
103. Pulmonary and Cardiac Imaging, *edited by Caroline Chiles and Charles E. Putman*
104. Gene Therapy for Diseases of the Lung, *edited by Kenneth L. Brigham*
105. Oxygen, Gene Expression, and Cellular Function, *edited by Linda Biadasz Clerch and Donald J. Massaro*
106. $Beta_2$-Agonists in Asthma Treatment, *edited by Romain Pauwels and Paul M. O'Byrne*
107. Inhalation Delivery of Therapeutic Peptides and Proteins, *edited by Akwete Lex Adjei and Pramod K. Gupta*
108. Asthma in the Elderly, *edited by Robert A. Barbee and John W. Bloom*
109. Treatment of the Hospitalized Cystic Fibrosis Patient, *edited by David M. Orenstein and Robert C. Stern*
110. Asthma and Immunological Diseases in Pregnancy and Early Infancy, *edited by Michael Schatz, Robert S. Zeiger, and Henry N. Claman*
111. Dyspnea, *edited by Donald A. Mahler*
112. Proinflammatory and Antiinflammatory Peptides, *edited by Sami I. Said*
113. Self-Management of Asthma, *edited by Harry Kotses and Andrew Harver*
114. Eicosanoids, Aspirin, and Asthma, *edited by Andrew Szczeklik, Ryszard J. Gryglewski, and John R. Vane*
115. Fatal Asthma, *edited by Albert L. Sheffer*
116. Pulmonary Edema, *edited by Michael A. Matthay and David H. Ingbar*
117. Inflammatory Mechanisms in Asthma, *edited by Stephen T. Holgate and William W. Busse*
118. Physiological Basis of Ventilatory Support, *edited by John J. Marini and Arthur S. Slutsky*
119. Human Immunodeficiency Virus and the Lung, *edited by Mark J. Rosen and James M. Beck*
120. Five-Lipoxygenase Products in Asthma, *edited by Jeffrey M. Drazen, Sven-Erik Dahlén, and Tak H. Lee*
121. Complexity in Structure and Function of the Lung, *edited by Michael P. Hlastala and H. Thomas Robertson*
122. Biology of Lung Cancer, *edited by Madeleine A. Kane and Paul A. Bunn, Jr.*

ADDITIONAL VOLUMES IN PREPARATION

Rhinitis, *edited by Robert M. Naclerio, Stephen R. Durham, and Niels Mygind*

Lung Tumors, *edited by Christian Brambilla and Elisabeth Brambilla*

Air Pollutants and the Respiratory Tract, *edited by David L. Swift and Michael Foster*

Interleukin-5: From Molecule to Drug Target for Asthma [TBC], *edited by Colin J. Sanderson*

The Lung at Depth, *edited by Claes Lundgren and John N. Miller*

Diagnostic Pulmonary Pathology, *edited by Philip T. Cagle*

Immunotherapy of Asthma, *edited by Jean Bousquet and Hans Yssel*

Viral Infections of the Lung, *edited by Raphael Dolin and Peter F. Wright*

Pediatric Asthma, *edited by Shirley J. Murphy, H. William Kelly, and Bennie C. McWilliams*

LAM and Other Diseases Characterized by Smooth Muscle Proliferation, *edited by Joel Moss*

GERD and Airway Disease, *edited by Mark R. Stein*

Control of Breathing in Health and Disease, *edited by Murray D. Altose and Yoshikazu Kawakami*

Neurobiology of Sleep and Circadian Rhythms, *edited by Fred Turek and Phyllis Zee*

Multimodality Treatment of Lung Cancer, *edited by Arthur T. Skarin*

Cytokines in Pulmonary Infectious Disease, *edited by Steven Nelson and Thomas Martin*

Exercise-Induced Asthma, *edited by E. Regis McFadden, Jr.*

Asthma's Impact on Society: The Social and Economic Burden, *edited by Kevin B. Weiss, A. Sonia Buist, and Sean D. Sullivan*

The opinions expressed in these volumes do not necessarily represent the views of the National Institutes of Health.

COMPLEXITY IN STRUCTURE AND FUNCTION OF THE LUNG

Edited by

Michael P. Hlastala
H. Thomas Robertson

University of Washington
Seattle, Washington

MARCEL DEKKER

MARCEL DEKKER, INC. NEW YORK • BASEL • HONG KONG

ISBN: 0-8247-9879-1

This book is printed on acid-free paper.

Headquarters
Marcel Dekker, Inc.
270 Madison Avenue, New York, NY 10016
tel: 212-696-9000; fax: 212-685-4540

Eastern Hemisphere Distribution
Marcel Dekker AG
Hutgasse 4, Postfach 812, CH-4001 Basel, Switzerland
tel: 44-61-261-8482; fax: 44-61-261-8896

World Wide Web
http://www.dekker.com

The publisher offers discounts on this book when ordered in bulk quantities. For more information, write to Special Sales/Professional Marketing at the headquarters address above.

Copyright © 1998 by Marcel Dekker, Inc. All Rights Reserved.

Neither this book nor any part may be reproduced or transmitted in any form or by any means, electronic or mechanical, including photocopying, microfilming, and recording, or by any information storage and retrieval system, without permission in writing from the publisher.

Current printing (last digit)
10 9 8 7 6 5 4 3 2 1

PRINTED IN THE UNITED STATES OF AMERICA

INTRODUCTION

> I think with your friend, that it has been of late too much the mode to slight the learning of the ancients.
>
> Benjamin Franklin (1773)

This statement, taken from a letter written by Benjamin Franklin to his friend William Browning, applies very much to the content of this book, which is concerned with integrative physiological approaches. Of course, physiological approaches and studies are very old; indeed, they can be traced to the emergence of medicine in Egypt in 3000 BC. Modern concepts of respiratory physiology, the subject of this book, began to develop about 400 years ago, and are tied to the great names of Leonardo da Vinci, Vesalius, Serventus, and Harvey, among others. Claude Bernard is unquestionably seen as the founder of integrative physiology with the development of the concept of the "milieu interieur."

Are we today forgetting the ideas of these great scientists, each of whom was ahead of his time? I do not believe so. The fast pace of today's discoveries undoubtedly rests on what we learned from the ancients!

N. P. Adelon—perhaps a modest researcher, but certainly a noted professor of medicine at the University of Paris—was the author of a multipart treatise (2nd ed, 1831) titled *Physiologie de l'Homme*. One of the volumes has a section on the function of respiration, with a truly fascinating description: "de l'organe de la respiration proprement dit, du Poumon." Allow me to quote some key statements (translated in footnote):

> D'après l'idée générale que nous avons donnée du poumon, cet organe doit être une espèce de sac, dans l'interieur duquel l'air est reçu. . . .

> Mais cette forme, que nous assignons au poumon, n'est vraie que pour les animaux les plus simples . . .

> Par exemple, dans la salamandre, cet organe consiste: 1) en un canal ouvert au fond de la bouche; 2) en un sac qui fait suite à ce canal, et qui, formant une cavité unique . . .
>
> Chez l'homme, le poumon . . . est une cavité . . . résultant des mille et mille ramifications de ce canal.

Although naive, these statements explain the evolutionary complexity of the structure of the lung and, consequently, of its function.

In their Preface, the editors of this volume, Michael P. Hlastala and H. Thomas Robertson, explain the rationale for their effort very well: we have here a structurally very complex organ but yet with an homogeneous, perhaps simple, respiratory function. Unless the most sophisticated researchers of today understand this, they will not be successful in unlocking the mysteries of this function at the molecular level. Without giving it a name, Claude Bernard introduced the concept of integrative physiology. This concept has greatly evolved to include molecular approaches as a subset of physiology.

Much has been learned about the respiratory function of the lungs, but probably much more needs to be investigated. This volume, which gathers experts with great achievements and reputations, brings to the reader a state-of-the-art knowledge and also paves the way for further discoveries. I am greatly indebted to my friend Mike Hlastala and his colleague Tom Robertson for their development and realization of this volume and for giving me the privilege of including it in the Lung Biology in Health and Disease series.

Claude Lenfant, M.D.
Bethesda, Maryland

"According to the general idea we have given of the lung, this organ must be a type of sac, within which air is received. . . . "

"But this shape, that we give to the lung, is only true for the simplest animals. . . "

"For example, in the salamander, this organ consists of 1) an open canal at the back of the mouth; 2) a sac that follows this canal, forming a single cavity. . . "

"In man, the lung . . . is a cavity . . . resulting from thousands and thousands of ramifications of the canal."

PREFACE

For the lung, perhaps more than any other organ, simple models have proven exceptionally fruitful in the process of investigation. Our textbooks are filled with analogies of springs and dashpots, sluices and waterfalls, gravitational gradients, and bubbles. When the simplest analogies failed to precisely represent observed properties, the inclusion of two or three compartments with different parameters usually sufficed to smooth over discrepancies between predictions and observations. While these old simplifications remain essential teaching tools, a puzzling new reality has emerged for all contemporary investigators working in pulmonary physiology: we have come to recognize that a "balloon on a straw"* bears little resemblance to the very complex and heterogeneous structure of the lung. Yet the gas-exchange properties of the normal lung are remarkably homogeneous. The challenge for explanation lies within the scope of classical physiology: to describe how these heterogeneous elements function together to produce the remarkably homogeneous physiological properties of the lung (the same properties that made the simple models so very successful).

This book was envisioned as a state-of-the-art description of the complexity observed in the normal lung as viewed from the vantage points of pulmonary mechanics, circulation, airways, and gas exchange. Gathering and editing the contributions of our authors has been an exciting task for us. They bring to this volume a remarkable breadth and depth of expertise in pulmonary physiology. The chapters have validated our belief that despite the many exciting developments in molecular biology of the lung, there are unique scale-dependent properties of the organ elucidated only by integrative physiological approaches. It is also important to note that as new insights are gained from the integrative perspective, questions will be volleyed back to the molecular biologists to investigate the ontogeny of these integrated properties.

This volume owes its genesis to Dr. Claude Lenfant. While he has enthusiastically supported investigation of the molecular biology of the lung, he continues to encourage the role of the integrative physiologist to translate the observed

*This wry description of classical physiological models was contributed by Dr. Jim Butler.

into an understanding of the complex behavior of living organisms. We also want to acknowledge the effective administrative support provided by Sandra Beberman and Connie Casella at Marcel Dekker, Inc., and the cheerful and tireless logistical support of Lorna Roach at the University of Washington.

Michael P. Hlastala
H. Thomas Robertson

CONTRIBUTORS

Hans Bachofen, M.D. Professor, Pulmonary Division, Department of Medicine, University of Berne, Inselspital, Berne, Switzerland

Akhil Bidani, M.D., Ph.D. Professor of Physiology, Biophysics, and Medicine; and Director, Division of Pulmonary and Critical Care Medicine, Department of Internal Medicine, University of Texas Medical Branch, Galveston, Texas

Aladin M. Boriek, Ph.D. Assistant Professor of Medicine and Physiology, Department of Medicine, Baylor College of Medicine, Houston, Texas

Robert Brown, M.D., M.Ph. Associate Professor, Department of Anesthesiology and Critical Care Medicine; Division of Physiology, Department of Environmental Health Sciences; and Department of Radiology, Johns Hopkins School of Hygiene and Public Health, Baltimore, Maryland

James P. Butler, Ph.D. Lecturer on Physiology, Physiology Program, Department of Environmental Health, Harvard School of Public Health, Boston, Massachusetts

Chantal Darquenne, Ph.D. Assistant Research Physiologist, Department of Medicine, University of California, San Diego, La Jolla, California

Christopher A. Dawson, Ph.D. Professor of Physiology and Research Physiologist, Department of Physiology, Medical College of Wisconsin and Zablocki Veterans Affairs Medical Center, Milwaukee, Wisconsin

Karen B. Domino, M.D. Associate Professor, Department of Anesthesiology, University of Washington School of Medicine, Seattle, Washington

Jeffrey J. Fredberg, Ph.D. Professor of Bioengineering and Physiology, Physiology Program, Department of Environmental Health, Harvard School of Public Health, Boston, Massachusetts

Steven C. George, M.D., Ph.D. Assistant Professor, Chemical and Biochemical Engineering and Materials Science, University of California, Irvine, Irvine, California

Robb W. Glenny, M.D. Associate Professor, Division of Pulmonary and Critical Care Medicine, Department of Medicine, and Department of Physiology and Biophysics, University of Washington School of Medicine, Seattle, Washington

Michael P. Hlastala, Ph.D. Professor of Physiology and Biophysics, and Professor of Medicine, Division of Pulmonary and Critical Care Medicine, Department of Medicine, University of Washington School of Medicine, Seattle, Washington

Eric A. Hoffman, Ph.D. Professor, Department of Radiology, University of Iowa College of Medicine, Iowa City, Iowa

Susan R. Hopkins, M.D., Ph.D. Assistant Adjunct Professor, Department of Medicine, University of California, San Diego, La Jolla, California

Donald E. Ingber, M.D., Ph.D. Associate Professor, Department of Pathology, Harvard Medical School, Boston, Massachusetts

Gary S. Krenz, Ph.D. Associate Professor, Department of Mathematics, Statistics, and Computer Science, Marquette University, Milwaukee, Wisconsin

Stephen J. Lai-Fook, Ph.D. Professor of Biomedical Engineering and Physiology, Center for Biomedical Engineering, University of Kentucky, Lexington, Kentucky

John H. Linehan, Ph.D. Rose Eannelli-Bagozzi Professor and Chair, Department of Biomedical Engineering, Marquette University, Milwaukee, Wisconsin

Stephen H. Loring, M.D. Associate Professor of Anesthesia, Harvard Medical School, and Scientific Director of Respiratory Therapy, Beth Israel Deaconess Medical Center, Boston, Massachusetts

Wayne A. Mitzner, Ph.D. Professor, Division of Physiology, Department of Environmental Health Sciences, Johns Hopkins School of Hygiene and Public Health, Baltimore, Maryland

Lynne E. Olson, Ph.D. Professor, Department of Veterinary Sciences, Ohio State University, Columbus, Ohio

Manuel Paiva, Ph.D. Professor, Biomedical Physics Laboratory, Université Libre de Bruxelles, Brussels, Belgium

Fred Possmayer, Ph.D. Professor, Department of Obstetrics and Gynecology and Department of Biochemistry, MRC Group in Fetal and Neonatal Health and Development, University of Western Ontario, London, Ontario, Canada

Edward M. Postlethwait, Ph.D. Associate Professor, Division of Pulmonary and Critical Care Medicine, Departments of Internal Medicine, Pathology, and Pharmacology and Toxicology, University of Texas Medical Branch, Galveston, Texas

Frank L. Powell, Ph.D. Professor, Department of Medicine, University of California, San Diego, La Jolla, California

Robert G. Presson, Jr., M.D. Associate Professor, Department of Anesthesia, Indiana University School of Medicine, Indianapolis, Indiana

H. Thomas Robertson, M.D. Professor of Medicine, Division of Pulmonary and Critical Care Medicine, Department of Medicine, University of Washington School of Medicine, Seattle, Washington

Joseph R. Rodarte, M.D. Professor, Section of Pulmonary and Critical Care, Department of Medicine, Baylor College of Medicine, Houston, Texas

Samuel Schürch, Ph.D. Professor, Department of Physiology and Biophysics, University of Calgary, Calgary, Alberta, Canada

Jennifer E. Souders, M.D. Research Scientist, Division of Pulmonary and Critical Care Medicine, Department of Medicine, and Clinical Assistant Professor, Department of Anesthesiology, University of Washington School of Medicine, Seattle, Washington

Dimitrije Stamenović, Ph.D. Associate Professor, Department of Biomedical Engineering, Boston University, Boston, Massachusetts

Erik R. Swenson, M.D. Associate Professor, Department of Medicine, University of Washington School of Medicine, Seattle, Washington

José G. Venegas, Ph.D. Assistant Professor of Anesthesia (Bioengineering), Department of Anesthesia, Harvard Medical School, Boston, Massachusetts

Wiltz W. Wagner, Jr., Ph.D. V. K. Stoelting Professor of Anesthesiology, Indiana University School of Medicine, Indianapolis, Indiana

Ning Wang, Sc.D. Assistant Professor of Physiology and Cell Biology, Department of Environmental Health, Harvard School of Public Health, Boston, Massachusetts

Ping M. Wang, Ph.D. Senior Research Analyst, Center for Biomedical Engineering, University of Kentucky, Lexington, Kentucky

Theodore A. Wilson, Ph.D. Professor, Department of Aerospace Engineering and Mechanics, University of Minnesota, Minneapolis, Minnesota

CONTENTS

Part One

MECHANICAL PROPERTIES

1

Heterogeneity in Airways

ROBERT BROWN and WAYNE A. MITZNER

Johns Hopkins School of Hygiene and Public Health
Baltimore, Maryland

I. Introduction

A. Relevance to Complexity

Airflow through the airway tree allows gas exchange to occur in the alveoli. Several diseases lead to obstruction of flow, causing both difficulty in breathing and impaired gas exchange. Although these disease processes never occur uniformly across all airways, assessment rarely includes more than a measure of the average obstruction of all airways in series and parallel. The reasons for such a limited global assessment are the inability to assess regional disease and the difficulty in evaluating the complex relations between local and global obstruction. Although the ultimate goal is to interpret the functional consequences of this interaction between local disease and total lung function, in this chapter, only the regional variability in airway size and responsiveness under a variety of conditions is described. Once the magnitude of the airway heterogeneity is better understood, then the complexity of its interaction with lung function can be better analyzed.

B. In Vitro and In Vivo Heterogeneity

There is little systematic information on the extent of heterogeneity in baseline airway size or airway responses to relevant stimuli. However, all airways do not respond the same. When such variability is seen in vitro, it is generally ascribed to various factors related to the experimental method required to set up the quasiphysiological environment for the desired protocols. In the search for the airway response, there is often an implicit assumption that the variability in the responses is related to how the measurements are made. That is, the normal variability that might exist among similar airways is viewed as more artifact than signal. In this chapter, however, we present evidence that this so-called artifact is often of comparable magnitude to the signal.

When the in vivo lung is challenged with agonists that constrict the airway smooth muscle, the airway lumen narrows and measurements of airway resistance increase. By assuming specific flow properties, such measurements can be related to how much the airway lumen has actually decreased. For example, if the flow were laminar and if the resistance increased fourfold, one could conclude that the *average* airway lumen area decreased by 50%. Given the fact that resistance is only a single number, one cannot say much more. However, it seems reasonable to expect that some airways might have decreased by 51% and others by 49%. Is it reasonable to expect some to decrease by 40% and others by 60%, or by 30% and 70%, and so on? There has been little evidence in the literature to address this question. Not only does one need information on the responsiveness of similar size airways across the lung, but also one requires information on the responsiveness of the increasingly smaller airways further along the airway pathway. These requirements demand that the sample size of measured airways be sufficiently large. Computed tomography (CT) is the only method currently available that allows such measurements in sufficient number. Figure 1 shows a typical high-resolution CT (HRCT) scan of a dog lung with airways relaxed with atropine and after contraction with methacholine. Scans were also done at low and high transpulmonary pressure (Ptp). This figure illustrates the capability of this technique. Accurate quantification of airway size can be made in airways as small as 2 mm (1).

In several CT studies, we have obtained considerable data that bear on this heterogeneity question. These studies have examined the long-term stability of airway size, the difference between intravenous and aerosol challenge, and the effect of lung inflation. Results from each of these studies are discussed herein. Overall, these findings show that there is a marked degree of heterogeneity in the in vivo responses of individual airways. In addition, more recent results demonstrate that airways are capable of a remarkable degree of distortion in the axial direction, suggesting that heterogeneity can even occur within a single airway branch.

C. General Methodologic Approaches

Most of the experimental results presented in the following sections were done in anesthetized dogs using high-resolution CT. Animals were not sacrificed at the end of each experiment and consequently could be studied on multiple occa-

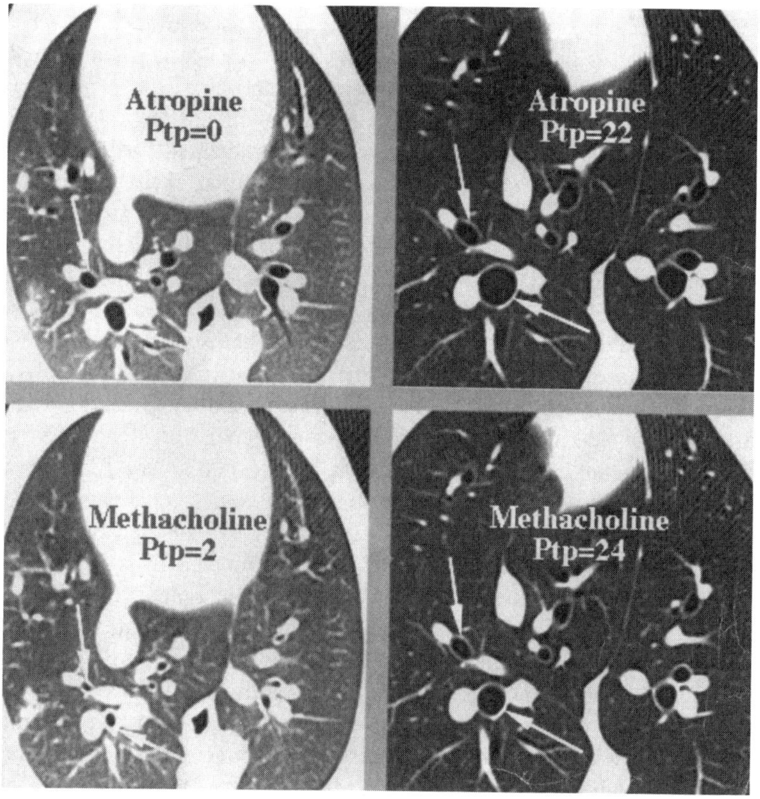

Figure 1 Representative high-resolution CT scan showing same airways under four different experimental conditions: airways relaxed with atropine or contracted with methacholine, each at low and high transpulmonary pressure (Ptp). Two individual airways in each condition are indicated by arrows.

sions. In one block of 45 sequential scans (spaced 1 mm apart), we can typically measure about 15 individual airways. Accuracy and variability of the software program to measure known areas has been previously documented (2). Additional specific details of the experimental methods can be found in the cited papers.

D. Outline of Experiments

In the remainder of this chapter, we describe a series of experimental results in the dog and human that help to define and document the degree of complexity inherent in the airway tree. Using a method that allows measurement of individual segments of this tree, we can quantify the heterogeneity of individual airways in response to agonist challenge and lung inflation. Although the mechanisms underlying this heterogeneity remain poorly understood, it is clear that the existence of such widespread heterogeneity in the airway tree produces a complexity in the lung that must have substantive impact on lung function. Local narrowing of airway segments must lead to increased airflow in other regions. This phenomenon could lead to altered regional shear stress on the epithelium, to altered particle deposition, and to altered airway water balance, all processes that may impact on the development of lung disease.

We first describe experiments that document extensive variability in the baseline size of airways. We quantify this variability over extended periods of time. These results demonstrate that, even in the baseline state, there is an enormous variability in local airway tone and that this tone shows substantial variability on a week to week or month to month time period. We then define how this variability impacts on responses to exogenous agonist challenges. Airway responsivity plays an important role in both testing pulmonary function and in determining how the lung behaves with immunological challenge. Results demonstrate a wide variability in responsiveness of individual airways, not only within animals but also between animals. This is followed by a study of the impact of lung inflation on the airway size at baseline and on the responsiveness to agonist challenge. The global airway response to lung inflation has been shown to be different in asthmatic subjects. However, there is little published data that can be used to interpret how actual responses of individual airways impact on this important clinical observation. Results contained herein demonstrate a significant heterogeneity in the response to lung inflation, with some airways even showing a narrowing at high lung volume. We then report new findings on the extent of airway contraction along the axis of the airway. This last observation, showing that even large airways can reach closure over a local region as short as 5 mm, adds a new complexity to the interpretation of pulmonary function. Finally, we present additional new results from measurements of individual airways in human subjects. These human studies clearly demonstrate that the heterogeneity demonstrated in canine airways in vivo is also manifested in human airways. Thus, interpretations of the complexity that can be gleaned from analysis of the more complete experimental results in the dog may have direct application in humans.

II. Heterogeneity in Baseline Airway Diameters Over Extended Periods of Time

During clinical or experimental studies in which protocols are repeated or changed, one normally waits for a return to baseline before starting the subsequent protocols. There is an implicit assumption in this practice that there exists a “normal” airway size on which multiple comparisons can be based. Indeed, when there is a failure to return to baseline, serious interpretive problems must be addressed. But what determines the normal baseline size? We know that many variables might alter this, with vagal tone being one of the most important. In vivo airways never operate in a completely relaxed condition. In the normal dog, for example, average baseline airway tone is sufficient to reduce airway area to only about 50% of the fully relaxed size at functional residual capacity (FRC). However, there is enormous variability in airway tone in individual airways, varying from 5%–100% of the totally relaxed airway area (see Section V).

Given such a high and variable level of normal baseline tone, one might reasonably ask, how much does this vary from hour to hour, day to day, or month to month? We do know that, at least for time periods on the order of experimental protocols in anesthetized animals (several hours), baseline size is reasonably stable. There is little information on day to day variability, but, in one report, we present data on changes in baseline airway size on multiple occasions over about a 1-year time period (3).

In that study, five anesthetized dogs were studied at FRC. After stopping the ventilator, HRCT images were acquired 30 seconds later. The same 13 to 16 airways, ranging in size from 2.1 to 14.0 mm in diameter, were matched and measured in each dog during the study interval. The dogs were studied between five and eight times over a time span ranging between 5 and 15 months. Although the study period varied in length among dogs, there was considerable temporal overlap among the dogs. To assess potential location-dependent differences, we used the following nomenclature to identify each airway: R and L (right and left); U and L (upper and lower), MSB (main stem bronchus). When multiple airways were measured on the same scan, the airways were numbered sequentially in the caudal to apex direction. Overall variability of airway size data were analyzed by linear regression with the coefficients of variation (CV) of each airway being the dependent variable and mean airway diameter being the independent variables. The mean airway sizes and their standard deviations for each dog were analyzed for between dog variability by one-way analysis of variance with Bonferroni correction for multiple pairwise comparisons. A level of $p < 0.05$ was considered significant.

Figure 2 shows the baseline size of the individual airways in each of five dogs at the time points measured. All individual airways showed considerable variability in area over time, with some individual airways showing changes as great as twofold. The variability showed no obvious relation to the time of the year. To quantify the variability of each airway in each dog, the coefficient of variation for each airway was calculated and plotted as a function of airway size (Figure 3). As can be seen in this figure, the variability was not related to the size of the airway. Larger airways showed a similar range in the coefficients of

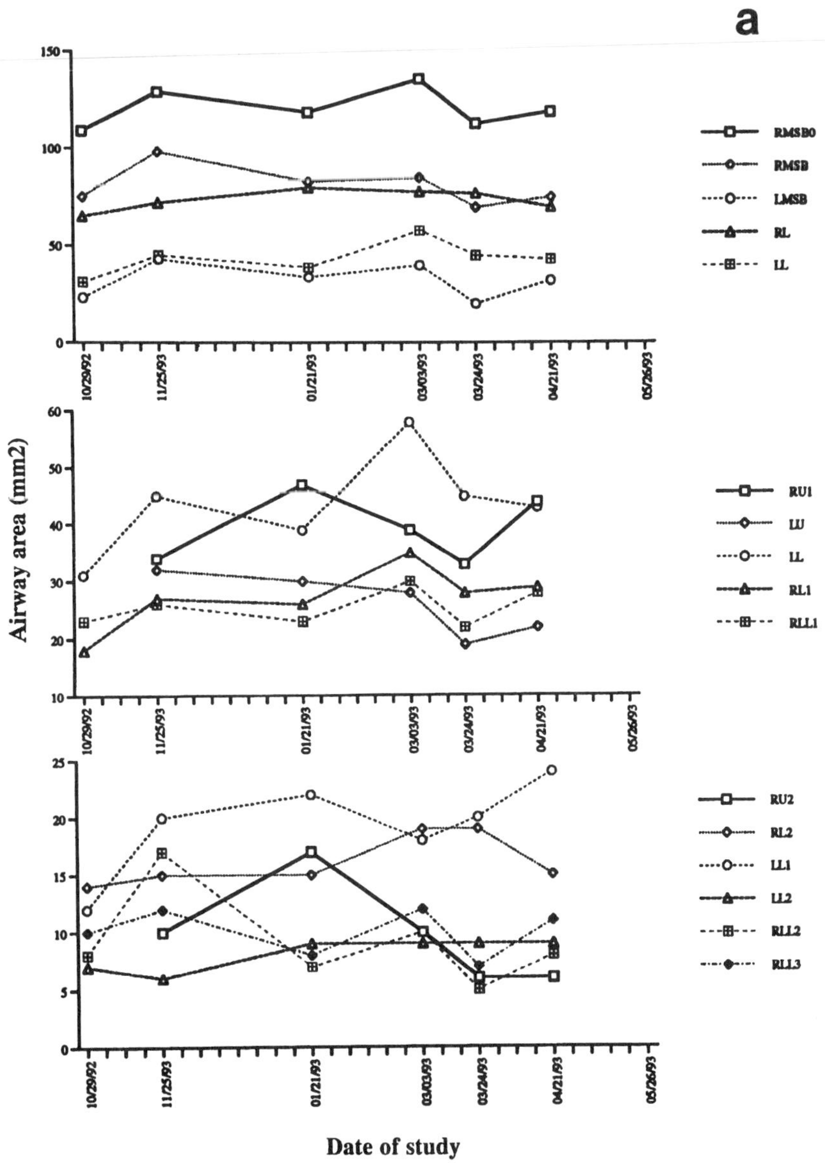

Figure 2 Individual airway areas in each of five dogs (a–e) as a function of time. For clarity, the data for each dog are presented on two or three separate graphs. The upper case letters in the key refer to the location of the airway measurement in different regions of the bronchial tree, and the numbers refer to different airways at the same CT slice. Abbreviations: R and L = right and left; U and L = upper and lower; MSB = main stem bronchus.

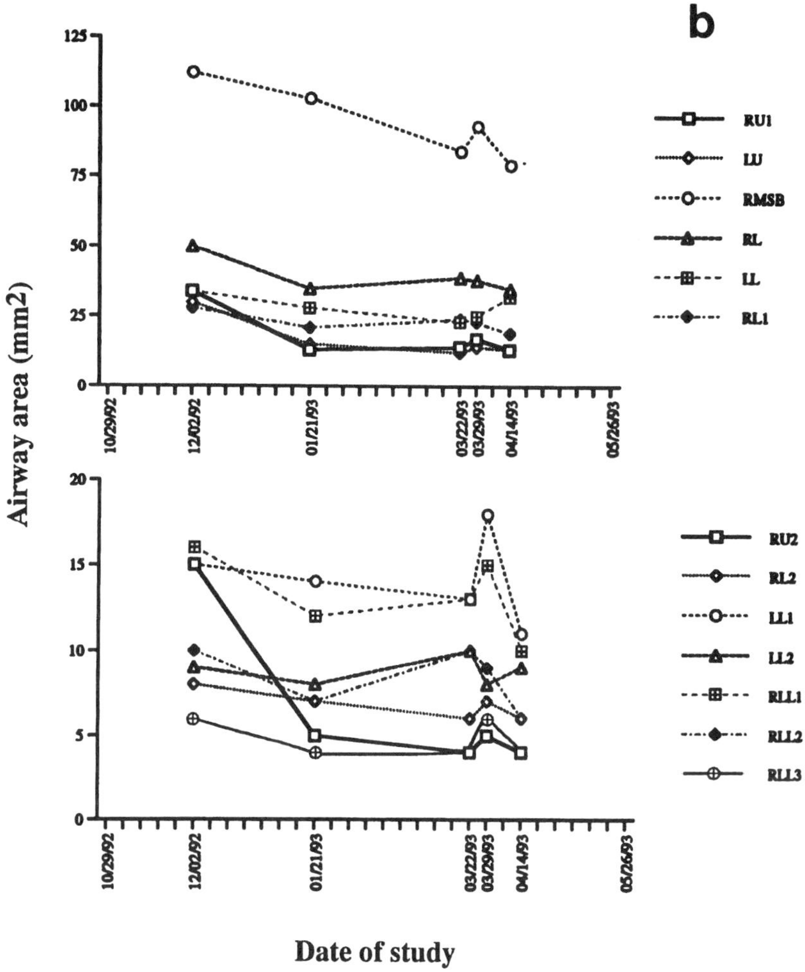

Figure 2 Continued

variation as in smaller airways. There was no statistically significant relationship between the coefficient of variation of an individual airway's diameter and the mean airway diameter ($p = 0.23$). However, the extent of variability in individual airways did vary significantly among dogs. Compared to the high airway variability in dog *e*, dogs *a* and *b* had significantly lower airway variability overall ($p < 0.01$), whereas dogs *c* and *d* had overall airway variability that fell between these extremes (see Figure 3). Additionally, as a crude estimate of overall airway function, similar to what might be measured with conventional

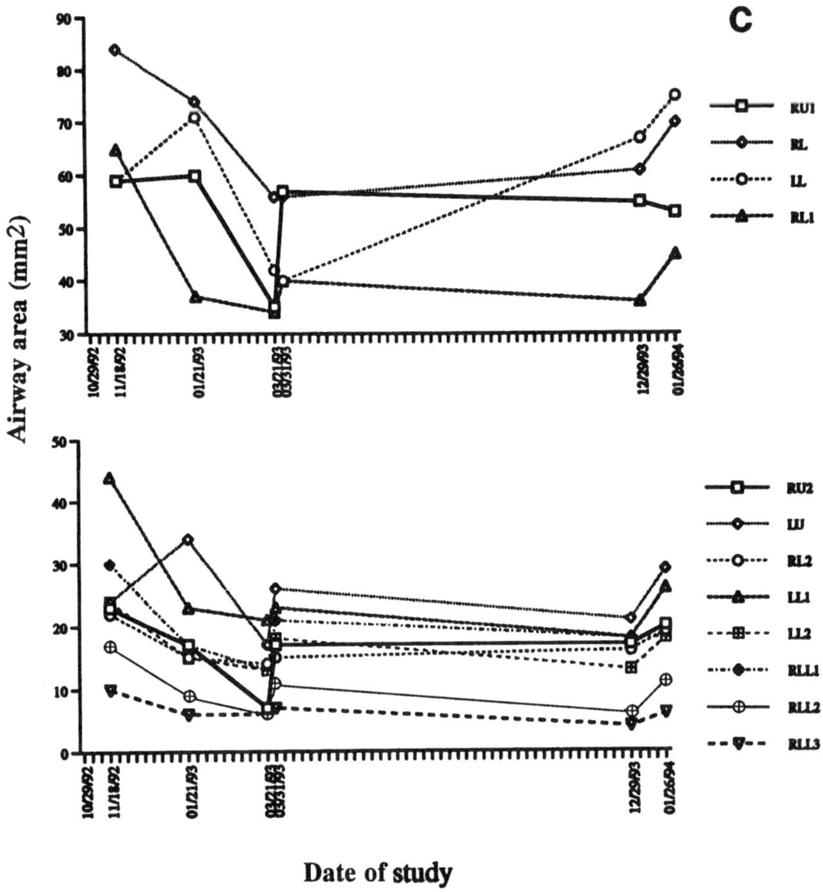

Figure 2 Continued

pulmonary function testing, we calculated the average airway area of all airways measured in each dog for each study. The mean airway areas within each dog for all the study times were not significantly different over time (see reference 3). Moreover, the mean airway areas between all the dogs over time were also not significantly different ($p = 0.23$).

In this study, we found that individual airways within a dog can vary as much as twofold in size over time. These changes occurred over the course of 1 year, but there were no correlations with either repeated measurements or

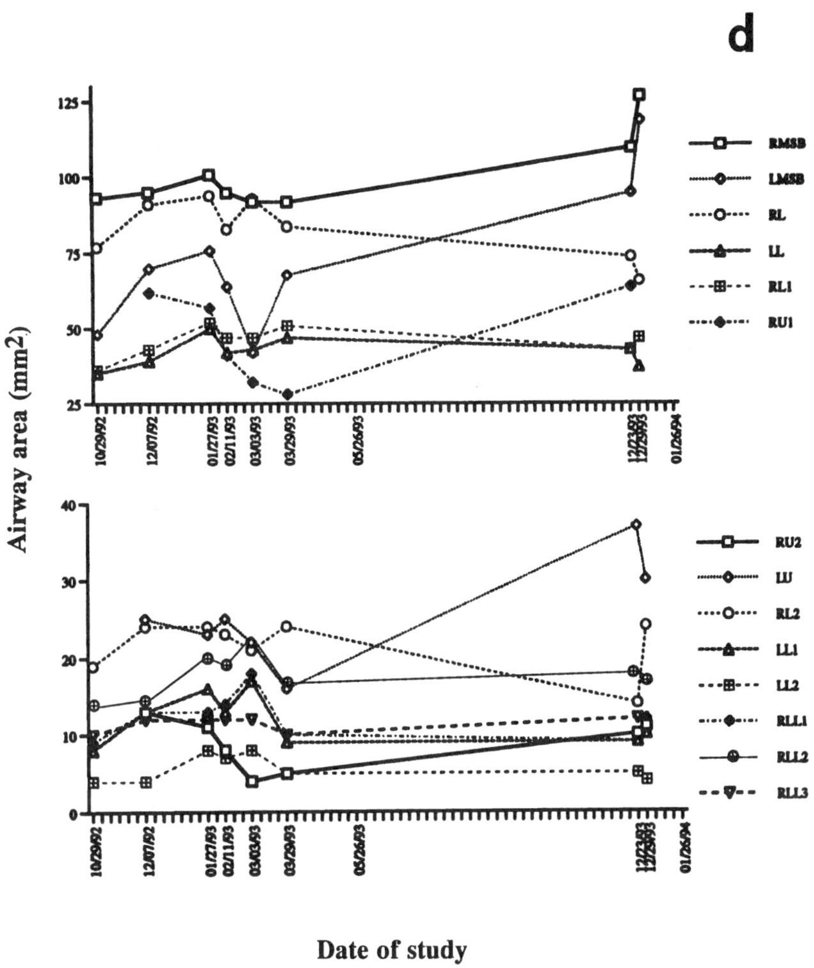

Figure 2 Continued

season. In other words, for individual airways within a dog, the variation seemed to be random. However, there were clear differences in the extent of the airway variability among the individual dogs. At the present time, we do not know the cause of this variability either within or among animals, but there are several possible considerations. First, because computational and technical errors have been shown to lead to variability in conventional pulmonary function test results (4), there is the potential for similar measurement variability in our study. We do not believe that this could account for our present observations, because we

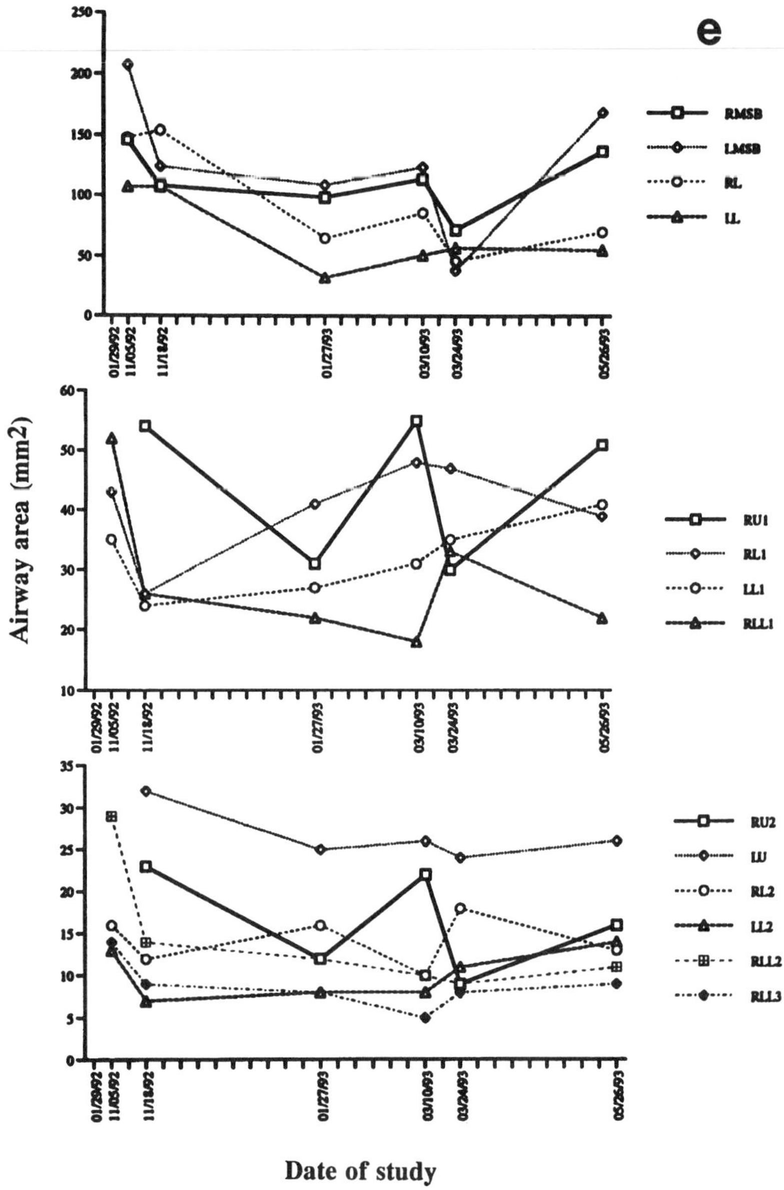

Figure 2 Continued

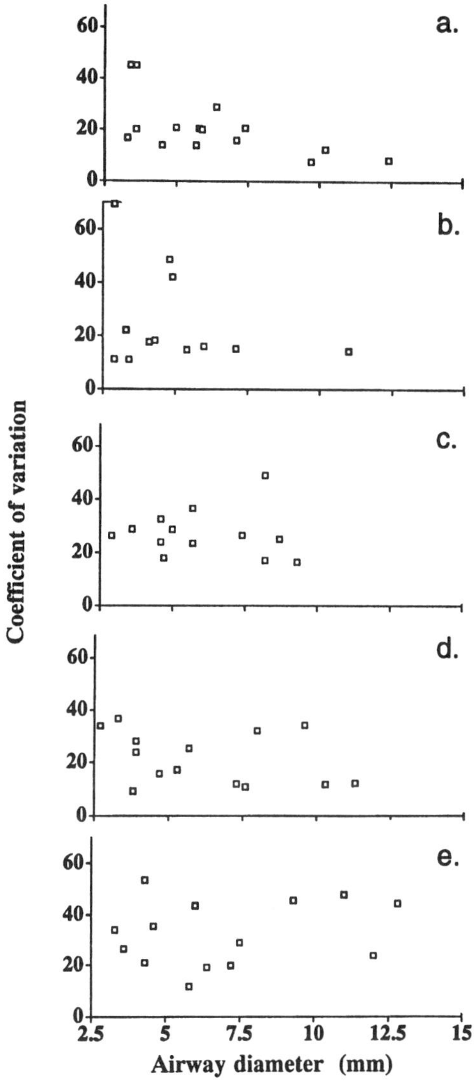

Figure 3 Coefficient of variation as a function of mean airway diameter in each dog. Whereas two dogs showed a significantly lower overall CV of individual airway areas (dogs a and b) ($p < 0.01$), one showed a significantly higher overall CV (dog e).

(5) and others (2) have previously demonstrated the intraobserver and interobserver accuracy and reproducibility of airway area measurements using this HRCT technique in phantoms consisting of rigid tubes (5). Also, because the smallest airways were not more variable than the larger airways, minimum resolution cannot explain the variability we observed even in the smallest airways.

Thus, the variation results from actual changes in airway size. Diurnal variation in pulmonary function has been shown to cause decreases in airway resistance during the morning hours with an increase toward late afternoon and evening (6). Because all of our studies were performed in the evening within the same 3-hour time interval, diurnal variation could not account for our observed airway variability. In human subjects, poor cooperation can lead to increased variability of pulmonary function tests. This potential source of variability clearly does not pertain to our study of anesthetized and ventilated dogs. Scans were acquired during a breath hold at end expiration. Any ventilatory effort during the scanning is easily detected as motion artifact, which leads to image degradation, and such scans were not used for analysis. However, because the animals were all anesthetized during the experiments, it is possible that variability in the level of anesthesia could lead to changes in airway size, perhaps from varying levels of catecholamines in the blood or changes in neural tone (37). In our studies, each dog received the same dose of anesthetic for each series of scans during the study period. Additionally, we used comparable induction doses of a thiobarbiturate in all the dogs, and anesthesia was maintained by a continuous infusion of thiobarbiturate adjusted for weight. Depth of anesthesia was monitored in all dogs by heart rate and eyelash responses, with all dogs exhibiting adequate depth of anesthesia for the duration of the study (approximately 15 minutes per study period). Furthermore, with even substantial changes in the depth of anesthesia in two dogs (data not shown here), there were trivial changes in airway size. Thus, it seems unlikely that variations in the level of anesthesia could account for the large differences in airway size we observed over the course of a year.

Another possible cause of the changes in airway size over time is a variable neural input. If generalized neural effects responsible for the temporal variability, one might expect to see some correlation between the changes in the different airways within an animal at the different time points. We analyzed for this statistically using a binomial model (3). We tested whether the majority of airways increased or decreased in the same direction from one experimental day to another. With this statistical analysis, four of the five dogs had $p < 0.05$ for the number of significant intervals, that is that the majority of airways increased or decreased in the same direction during the majority of time intervals in four of the dogs. This conclusion is not a very strong one, however, because there were still many intervals where the airways behaved randomly. Nevertheless, it does support the likelihood of global effects throughout the lung regulating the complexity at many of the time points studied.

There does not seem to be any correlation between the magnitude of variability in individual airways and its location within the lung. In Figure 2, the letter designations identify airways in similar locations in different dogs. These figures show no differences in airway variability between right and left or upper and lower airways. In addition, there was no consistent variability in any one location. For example, an airway (RU1) that demonstrated large variability from study to study in one dog (number 5) showed little variability in another dog (RU1 in dog number 2). We might have also expected to find some correlation between changes in airway size and the seasons, because seasonal variation in the severity of asthma or allergies is common. However, in the dogs studied, we observed no correlation with seasonal variations.

We know of no comparable in vivo studies that examined the changes in individual airway size over time. There are studies in man and dog that have shown reproducibility of traditional pulmonary function tests over time (8–10). However, these measurements reflect a summation of hundreds or thousands of airways. Indeed, as already noted, if we do a simple average of all the airway areas measured in each dog, we also find no significant changes over time in this mean. Thus, mean values or global pulmonary function measurements provide no insight into the extent of individual airway variability.

These results raise several questions that contribute to the complexity inherent in interpreting global pulmonary function tests. For instance, does the variable size simply reflect some normal variation in smooth muscle contractility, or is it related the local environment of an airway? Could the variability in airway size contribute to the pathogenesis and localization of lung disease? That is, if one airway were consistently smaller, the flow velocity might be higher, leading perhaps to increased particle deposition, epithelial shear, or dehydration. It would be interesting to follow individual airways over time in patients at risk for the development of obstructive lung disease.

More recent studies have begun to address a question that was not considered in the above measurements of baseline size. That is, how much is the airway actually constricted at any point in time? To answer this question, it is necessary have some way to normalize the degree of contraction in different size airways. We were able to do this by first causing a maximal relaxation of airway smooth muscle tone, and then showing that this maximally relaxed size did not change on subsequent experimental days. Figure 4 shows the individual airway baseline tone in five dogs on 2 different experimental days, 2 weeks apart. Airway size is presented as a percent of the fully relaxed size. As can be appreciated, the range of baseline size is enormous, with some airways residing near maximum and others near closure within the same dog. This figure does

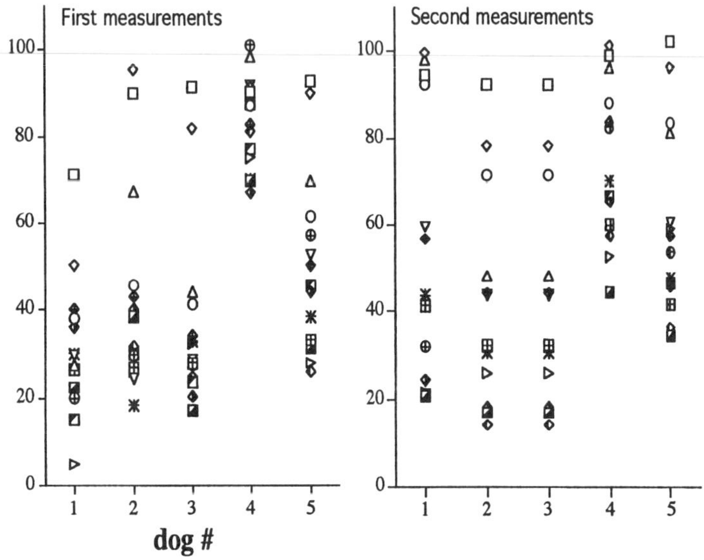

Figure 4 Plot of baseline airway area as a percentage of maximally relaxed size in individual airways in five dogs on two separate occasions 2–3 weeks apart. Symbols for individual airways correspond in each dog. There is some consistency over this time period in some dogs (e.g., dog 4 has relatively dilated airways and dog 2 is moderately constricted). Dog 1 shows the most variability, with most airways being quite constricted (one airway almost closed) on the first day and several airways being fully dilated on the next.

not show any data regarding the degree of baseline constriction and the airway size, but we did find that larger airways on average had slightly less baseline tone compared with medium and smaller airways. The impact that such variability has on measurements of airway responsiveness with subsequent exogenous challenges has not been systematically investigated.

III. Heterogeneity in Individual Airway Responsiveness to Agonist Challenge In Vivo

Given the previously stated variation in baseline size, it might not be unreasonable to suggest that, at specific time points, the airway responsiveness to agonist challenge might vary considerably throughout the lung. Indeed, in an early CT study (11), a striking degree of variability in responsiveness was found. Figure 5 shows the response of individual airways of several dogs to an aerosol histamine challenge. Airway size did not seem to have much effect on this variability. One explanation for this variability was that it was entirely a function of the variability associated with aerosol challenge. Intuitively, one might expect aerosol challenge to have more variability in responsiveness than intravenous challenge. Particle size variation, aerosol delivery rate, gas flow rate during aerosol delivery, and particle deposition would all provide additional sources of variability related to agonist delivery. In a subsequent study, we compared the extent of the airway response variability with intravenous versus aerosol challenge.

Four dogs were studied after both challenges, with the aerosol and intravenous challenges done on separate days at least 2 weeks apart. Figures 6 and 7 show the dose response curves for all individual airways in all dogs for aerosol and intravenous challenges, respectively.

Twenty minutes after induction of anesthesia, stepwise changes in the concentration of the aerosolized histamine were administered. Five breaths at each dose were administered to a peak airway pressure of 15 cm H_2O, held for 1 second, and released to atmospheric pressure. Under test parameter conditions with an operating pressure of 50 psi and an atomization flow rate of 10 L/min, the nebulizer produces particles of mass median diameter of 3.1 μm with a geometric standard deviation of 3.2. Given such a relatively disperse particle size distribution, good central and peripheral distribution should have been achieved (12). The HRCT scans were performed subsequent to the standard 1-minute apneic period. Two sighs, each equal to twice the tidal volume, were given before each challenge, and peak airway pressure was allowed to return to near baseline level (within 10%) before initiating the next challenge.

Twenty minutes after induction of anesthesia, stepwise changes in the infusion rate of the intravenous histamine in doses of 100, 200, and 300 μg/min were administered. Intravenous challenges were administered through a dedicated intravenous catheter by a continuous infusion pump. After increases in airway pressure plateaued, the HRCT scans were performed. Following completion of the HRCT scans, the infusion was stopped, the animals were sighed twice with a volume equal to two times the tidal volume, and airway pressure was allowed to return to approximately baseline levels (within 10%) before infusion at a new dose was started. Doses higher than 300 μg/min were not used because they resulted in delayed recovery of the cardiovascular changes.

We used multiple linear regression models to assess the effect of dose and initial airway size on airway construction. The regression equation used was $y = \beta_0 + \Sigma\beta_i x_i$, where the parameters are defined as follows. Because interpretation and comparison of constriction in different size airways is problematic, we did the model analysis three ways. First, we used the absolute airway size after each challenge as the dependent variable. Second, we analyzed the model with the use of log transformation of the airway size after challenge. Third, we used the change in airway size as the dependent variable to normalize the changes in airways. The independent variables were initial airway size (x_1), which was included only in the first two models, and dose (x_2), both expressed as continuous variables, and dog (modeled categorically, x_3–x_6 for aerosol histamine model and x_3–x_7 for intravenous histamine model to account for the five and six dogs in the models, respectively). The coefficients β_1, and β_2, describe the amounts of change in the outcome variable y for given unit changes in the independent variables x_1, and x_2, respectively. The independent variable of initial airway size was not included in the third model examining the percent change in airway size. All two-way and three-way interaction terms were explored, but they did not add significantly to the model so were not included. The *p*-value associated with the respective β coefficient describes the statistical significance of the associated independent variable. Aerosol and intravenous challenges were modeled separately. A residual mean square value for each model for each route was calculated as a measure of the overall variability in the change in airway size. To compare the overall variability in airway constriction between the two routes of histamine administration, we performed an F-statistic on the ratio of the residual mean square values of the aerosol and intravenous models using their respective residual degrees of freedom.

The net result of all this statistical analysis was negative. The residual mean square values for the multiple linear regression models for the absolute change in airway size for aerosol and intravenous histamine challenges were 17.73 and 15.42, respectively. We compared the residual mean square values from the aerosol and intravenous histamine linear regression models, controlling the independent variables of initial airway size, dose, and dog. Initial airway size was accounted for by either including it as an independent variable in the analysis of absolute airway size after challenge or by converting absolute airway size to change from initial airway size. We found no significant difference between the residual mean squares for aerosol and intravenous administration $F(331,166) = 1.15$, $p = 0.32$ (two-tailed test). We found a similar lack of significant difference when we modeled for the log transformation of the airway size ($F = 1.16$, $p = 0.30$) or for the change in the airway size ($F = 1.14$, $p = 0.32$).

The intravenous route, when allowed to reach steady state should be homogeneous in its systemic and pulmonary distribution. The concentration in the blood and tissues is relatively constant, as long as there is not a local sink of rapid histamine metabolism. The original rationale for this study was that, if uniform drug delivery was the problem with aerosols, then intravenously administered drug should cause less heterogeneity in airway constrictor responses.

Figure 5 Percent changes in airway area after histamine (*solid bars*) and subsequent deep inspiration (*hatched bars*) challenges measured in each airway in each of five dogs. The numbers along the abscissa indicated the area of each airway measured in the control state. The percent changes plotted are calculated from this control area.

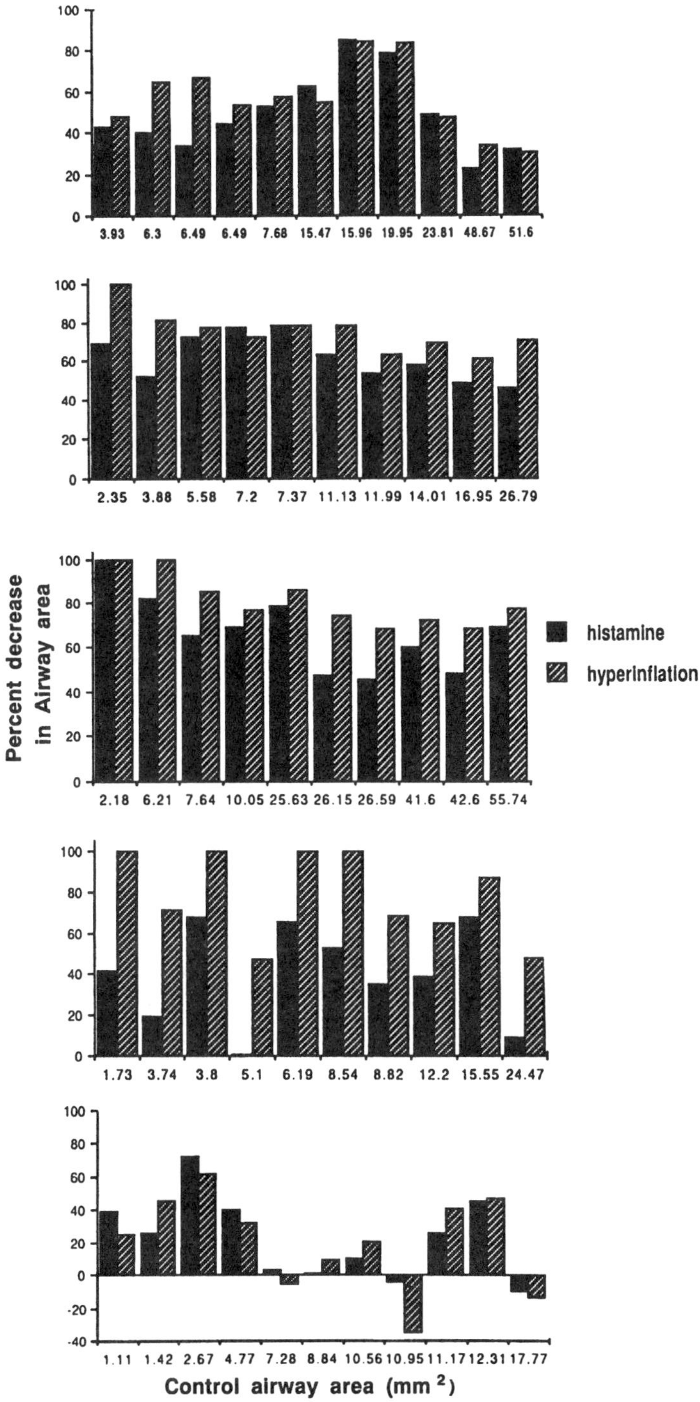

3.93 6.3 6.49 6.49 7.68 15.47 15.96 19.95 23.81 48.67 51.6
2.35 3.88 5.58 7.2 7.37 11.13 11.99 14.01 16.95 26.79
Percent decrease in Airway area
2.18 6.21 7.64 10.05 25.63 26.15 26.59 41.6 42.6 55.74
histamine
hyperinflation
1.73 3.74 3.8 5.1 6.19 8.54 8.82 12.2 15.55 24.47
1.11 1.42 2.67 4.77 7.28 8.84 10.56 10.95 11.17 12.31 17.77
Control airway area (mm²)

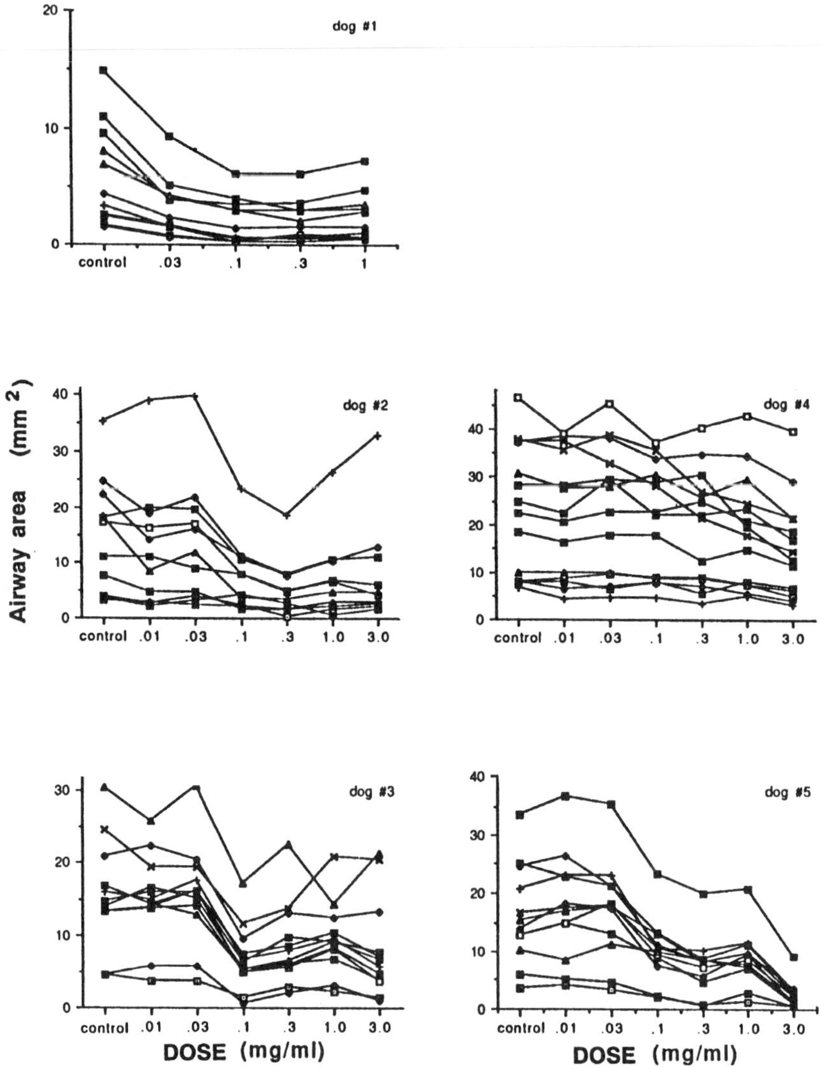

Figure 6 Dose-response curves to aerosol histamine in individual airways in each dog. Ordinate scales are different for different dogs, reflecting different sizes of airways that were visible in slices analyzed.

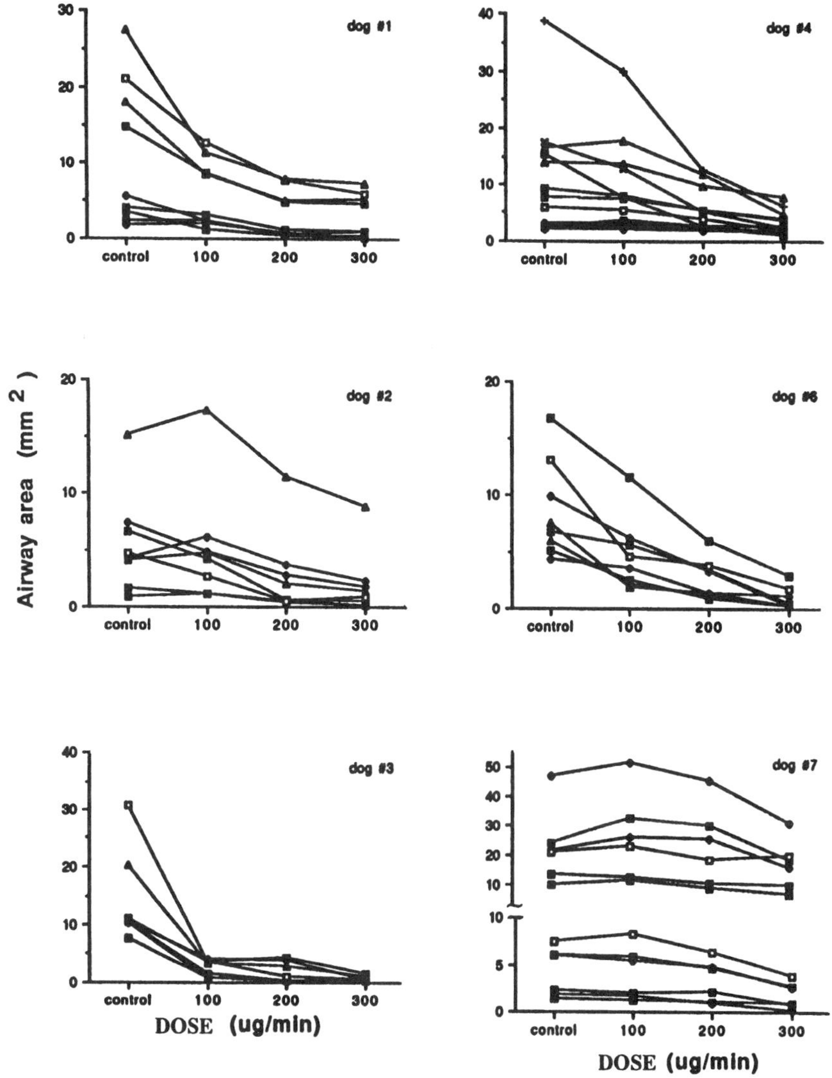

Figure 7 Dose-response curves to intravenous histamine in individual airways in each dog. Ordinate scales are different for different dogs, reflecting different sizes of airways that were visible in slices analyzed. Dogs 1–4 are the same as those in Figure 5, but the airways are not necessarily the same.

However, this rationale is somewhat naive, in that there are several important other differences between aerosol and intravenous histamine challenges. The two routes of histamine administration deliver the drug to different sides of the airway wall. Although we generally think of perfusion as uniform, there might be considerable variability in the local bronchial vascular perfusion of airway smooth muscle. Because it is through the bronchial circulation that intravenous agonists reach the airway muscle (13), such variability would have a direct effect on the magnitude of smooth muscle contraction. The possible release of epithelial derived factors may also contribute additional heterogeneity to the aerosol histamine challenge. With the intravenous administration of histamine, there can be substantial systemic effects affecting all organ systems, such as the marked stable reduction in systemic arterial blood pressure. In contrast, aerosol histamine deposited on the lumenal surface of the airway wall has relatively negligible systemic absorption and thus negligible direct cardiovascular effects. Intravenous histamine can also cause catecholamine release from the adrenal gland (14,15), and such catecholamine release may lead to bronchodilation (16–18). However, this catecholamine release is systemic and therefore should affect all airways equally along with the intravenous histamine. Aerosol histamine may stimulate irritant receptors in addition to histamine receptors on the airway lumenal wall, and multiple receptor activation may account for a portion of the heterogeneity in airway responsiveness. An aerosol irritant effect would be more dominant at lower concentrations of histamine challenge where the irritant receptor response would not be overwhelmed by the histamine receptor activation response.

One-dimensional bronchograms of the lungs have been performed using insufflated tantalum (19). Using such bronchograms, Shioya et al. (20) examined the distribution of airway contractile responses to several intravenously administered bronchoconstrictors. Although they did not directly address the airway response heterogeneity, they noted the distribution of constrictor responses among airways varied substantially with each agonist. More recently, Dandurand et al. (21) studied the heterogeneous response of individual airways in situ. They used a rat lung explant model to measure individual airway responsiveness to methacholine. They found that the responsiveness of individual airways to methacholine in a given animal was far more variable than that between animals.

Other studies examining airway response heterogeneity have measured global responses of the lungs and the factors that influence these responses. Even though these studies cannot corroborate our present findings of individual airways response heterogeneity, similar mechanisms may apply. Fredberg et al. (22) used alveolar capsules in an attempt to assess heterogeneity of lung response to inhaled histamine. They sampled alveolar pressures simultaneously in a number of peripheral regions in canine lungs oscillated at the airway opening.

This method permitted examination of the homogeneity of the pressure field among parallel pathways. The local behavior of airways could also be inferred from the pressure differences across the measured regions. These investigators observed wide variation in the responses to inhaled histamine, from relatively slight constriction in some regions to complete airway closure in others. They suggested that local differences in contractile elements might be more important than differences in deposition pattern. Although these investigators were only able to narrow the field of study to a few hundred or thousand airways, they observed marked regional heterogeneity in airway responses to aerosol histamine. Our direct measurements of individual airways confirm this heterogeneity to histamine on a much smaller scale.

Anderson et al. (23) also examined the association of the heterogeneity in airway responsiveness across human subjects to the variability in deposition of methacholine aerosol challenges. They found that a large proportion of the inhaled methacholine was deposited, and the deposited dose was reasonably uniform among subjects. Consistent with our results, they concluded that the variability in the degree of bronchoconstriction must be a function of inherent properties of airway epithelium, the autonomic nervous system, or smooth muscle, rather than variability in the deposited dose of drug. In our study, we used a polydispersed aerosol, and therefore expected deposition of aerosol particles to occur in both large and small airways (12). Our finding of no difference in the percent change in airways areas related to the initial size of the airway is consistent with a relatively homogeneous distribution of aerosol histamine along the airways throughout the size airways that we measured. The equivalent heterogeneity we observed in airways responses to both aerosol and intravenous histamine suggests an intrinsic etiology independent of the mode of agonist delivery.

Thus, the absence of a difference in the degree of variability by intravenous or aerosol challenge suggests that the variability rests in pathways distal to the receptor stimulation. Local differences in muscle mass, receptor density, or signal transduction pathways may be responsible, but further studies are needed to elucidate these possibilities.

IV. Heterogeneity of Relaxed Airways in Response to Lung Inflation

That airways enlarge as the lung is inflated has been known since the time of Leonardo da Vinci (24). However, the magnitude and variability of this dilation in different airways are unknown. If the lung behaved as a homogeneous isotropic material (as it is often modeled), then one might expect all relaxed airways to dilate in a quite homogeneous manner as the lung inflates.

This question was recently addressed in studies performed on five anesthetized dogs in vivo. A thin-walled latex esophageal balloon inflated with 0.8 mL air was positioned in the lower third of the esophagus to estimate pleural pressure changes (25). Transpulmonary pressure, measured with a differential pressure transducer, was estimated as the difference between the esophageal pressure and the airway pressure measured at the end of the endotracheal tube. To measure lung volume, the total lung area of each standard resolution CT slice (8-mm thickness) was measured. The area of the lung on each standard CT scan was defined as the area within the pleural border excluding the heart and diaphragm. The edge of the lung was defined by the same "full-width-half-maximum" principle used in the airway measurements. All lung standard CT slice areas were multiplied by the slice thickness and summed to calculate the total lung volume for each condition. Airways were studied at fixed airway pressures after deflation from total lung capacity (TLC). Between each experimental condition, the animals were ventilated normally.

In each dog, 13 airways (range 1.8 to 19.1 mm in diameter) were identified and measured under all conditions. Data are expressed as absolute area and as a percent of maximal airway area at 30 cm H_2O after atropine. Data were analyzed by linear regression, and significance of the slope of the regression lines being different from zero were tested.

The graphs in Figure 8 show the relation between transpulmonary pressure and airway area after relaxation with atropine for each individual airway in each of five dogs. Figure 8 clearly demonstrates that relaxed airways reach a maximal area at a very low transpulmonary pressure; there were no significant changes in area in any airway above 7 cm H_2O ($p = 0.71$). Below 7 cm H_2O in each lung, the airways are extremely distensible, with area increasing 7.2% of maximal area for each centimeter of water increase in Ptp. Indeed, below 7 cm H_2O, the airways appear even more distensible than the lung parenchyma; below 7 cm H_2O, parenchymal area $[(V_L)^{2/3}]$ changes only about 5% of maximal volume for each centimeter of water increase in Ptp.

These results clearly demonstrate a level of complexity intrinsic to the interdependence between airways and parenchyma. Not only do airways not expand isotropically with the lung, but this anisotropic behavior also shows substantial variability among individual airways. In a completely relaxed condition, airway area reaches a plateau at very low Ptp, and further increases in Ptp cause negligible changes. Recent histological studies have assumed that the epithelial basement membrane is not distensible, thereby allowing its fixed perimeter to be used to determine the size of the relaxed airways (26). Our results in vivo support this conjecture. Below the plateau, we found the relaxed airways to be extremely compliant, with changes in airway area at least as great as area changes in the lung parenchyma. This is a surprising finding, because one might expect the highly structured airway wall to have greater stiffness than the lung

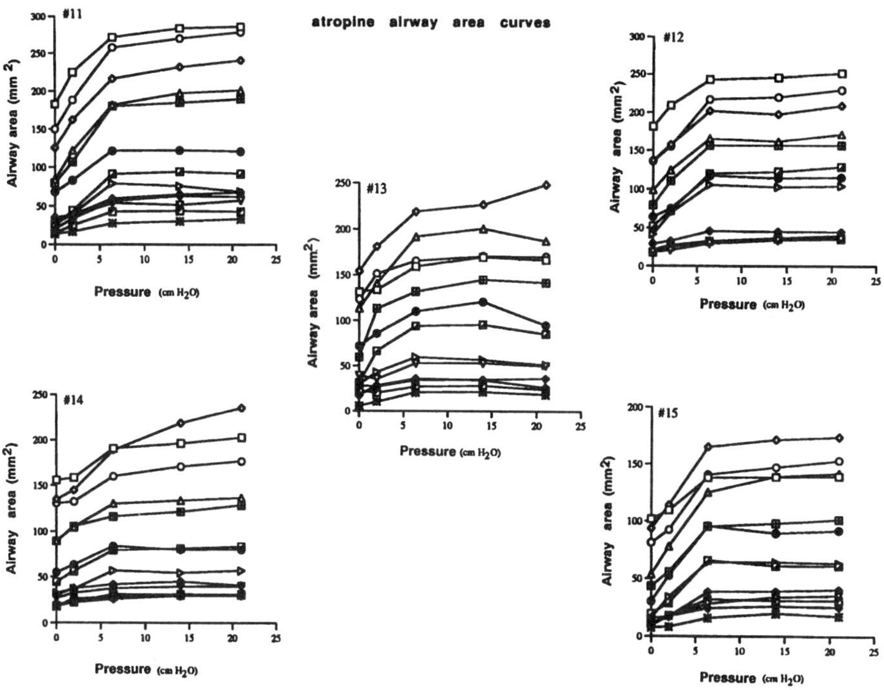

Figure 8 Transpulmonary pressure versus lumenal area curves of atropine-relaxed individual airways in five dogs. (Dog numbers correspond to those in Figure 9.)

parenchyma. However, how the actual airway wall changes with Ptp in relation to how an imaginary circular wall in the lung parenchyma changes with Ptp depends not only on the structure of the wall but also on what exists inside the epithelial border. This situation can be modeled with a continuum mechanics analysis, considering the shear moduli of airway and parenchyma (27). However, one can intuitively envision an imaginary thin circular wall in the lung, where there would be parenchymal tissue inside as well as outside the wall. In such a case, the diameter of that imaginary wall must then increase proportional to the cube root of lung volume. If we add a normal structure to the airway wall, maintaining the imagined parenchyma inside as well as outside the wall, this added wall structure might be expected to make this composite airway tube less distensible than the lung. However, if we next remove this theoretical elastic parenchyma inside the airway wall, this must increase the distensibility of the tubular airway. How much it would increase is not known, but it is conceivable that if the airway wall is not very stiff, the airway could appear more compliant than the lung. Indeed, if the airway gets smaller by buckling its lumen, then it is reasonable to expect the relaxed airway to be very compliant over the pressure range where the compressed lumen is simply being unstressed (unfolded).

Another source of complexity is related to our observation that some individual airways actually decreased in size at the highest transpulmonary pressures. This finding is consistent with several published studies (28,29) that have assessed more global indices of airway size. Every dog in the study showed some airways that decreased in diameter when airway pressure was increased from 20 to 30 cm H_2O. The number of airways that showed a decrease in diameter ranged from one to six airways in each dog (see Figure 8). There did not appear to be a specific effect by size or location of the airway (right versus left lung). This decrease in size may be due to increased axial stresses with continued increases in Ptp. Increasing stress on the spirally oriented airway smooth muscle and elastic fibers could narrow the airway diameter, but why this would occur only in selected airways is not clear.

V. Heterogeneity of Contracted Airways in Response to Lung Inflation

In the same animals as discussed in Section IV, we examined the variability of the interaction between methacholine and lung inflation. Given the complexity that we have already shown in each response, it may not be surprising to find even greater variability in how contracted airways respond to lung inflation.

On separate days, the dogs received a continuous intravenous infusion of methacholine (67 μg/min), a dose previously demonstrated to decrease the size of the airways to about 60% of baseline (30). To standardize lung volume history, prior to each measurement, the airway pressure was increased to 35 cm H_2O, held for 5 seconds, and then decreased and maintained at the designated airway pressure for the duration of each set of scans. At each pressure, HRCT scans were acquired to measure airway areas and standard CT scans were acquired to measure lung volumes. During methacholine infusion, scans were acquired at airway pressures of approximately 0, 10, 20, and 30 cm H_2O. Between each experimental condition, the animals were ventilated normally.

Contraction of the airways with methacholine had a strikingly variable effect among dogs on the airway pressure-area relation (Figure 9). At functional residual capacity (transpulmonary pressure = 2.5 cm H_2O), mean airway area during methacholine infusion was decreased to $22 \pm 2\%$ (mean ± SEM) of atropine at maximum Ptp. Increases in Ptp resulted in linear, convex, or S-shaped mean relations in the different animals. In only one animal (dog number 15) did the individual airway sizes tend to plateau at the highest Ptp. In each animal, some individual airways appear extremely stiff below 15 cm H_2O and become quite compliant at higher pressure. In other airways, even small changes in lung inflation from FRC cause an immediate airway dilation.

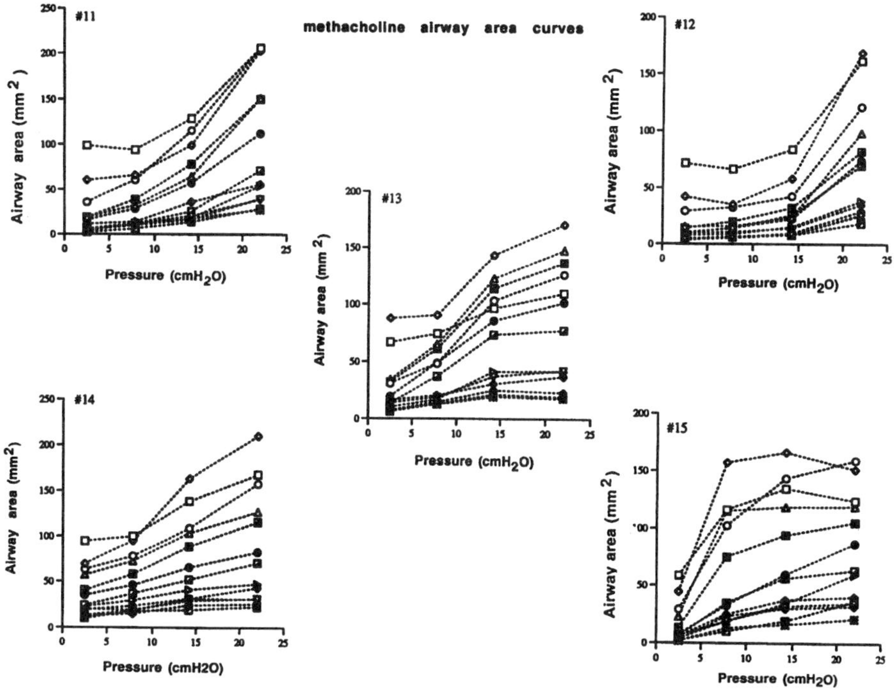

Figure 9 Transpulmonary pressure versus lumenal area curves of methacholine-contracted individual airways in the same five dogs as in Figure 8. The individual airways in each animal are also the same as those in Figure 8 and can be identified from the corresponding symbols.

These results confirm that when the airways have tone, not only is their baseline size reduced, but also their response to increasing pressure is quite variable in different animals. Variations in lung volume cannot account for this variability, because lung volume does not show this extensive variability among animals. At the present time, we have no satisfying explanation for this variability among and within animals. It seems not directly related to the initial response to methacholine, because the initial constrictions at FRC in most dogs were similar. However, it is our expectation that, given enough contractile agonist, the airway pressure area curves in all the animals would show minimal dilation even at the highest pressure. Gunst et al. (31) have suggested that if the smooth muscle contraction is high enough, physiological increases in Ptp might be insufficient to cause any increase in airway size. This latter speculation has obvious and direct clinical implications. In clinical asthma, the intrinsic forces of constriction may be greater than that which lung inflation can overcome. This would be consistent with several observations showing that a deep inspiration does not relieve bronchoconstriction in asthmatic patients (32–38). A model of asthma based on this ineffectiveness of a deep inspiration has recently been described by Skloot et al. (39). If humans showed the same degree of variability that we have seen in our animals, then we might speculate that those subjects with less distensible contracted airways might be more prone to development of asthma.

Several other studies done in isolated lobes and bronchi of dogs using tantalum bronchography are consistent with the above findings. Hahn et al. (28) found that, when airways had low tone, they were very compliant below 10 cm H_2O, but quite stiff above 10 cm H_2O. With high airway tone, airway diameter did not plateau up to a transpulmonary pressure of 25 cm H_2O. Additionally, they found that the airways correlated in a linear fashion with the cube root of lung volume in the high airway tone state but not in the low airway tone state. Marshall (29) found similar results in isolated canine lungs, where maximal airway diameter was quickly reached at pressures less than 10 cm H_2O. In isolated canine bronchi in vitro without tone, Gunst et al. (31) also found that maximal airway diameters were reached below 10 cm H_2O. With high tone, sufficient to contract the airways to less than 10% of maximal size, the airways were not distensible even up to pressures of 25 cm H_2O. The rigidity they observed in the contracted airways likely results from much greater contraction they were able to elicit in vitro. Sasaki et al. (40) also found that the relaxed airways increased in diameter up to 10 cm H_2O and then plateaued above that pressure. However, in constricted airways they found airway diameter plateaued at a decreased maximal size. Such a decrease in maximal diameter was also observed by Murtagh et al. (41) in situ and Gunst and Mitzner (42) in vitro. In the present in vivo experiments, however, we never observed such a decreased plateau. At present, we can only speculate on what might cause such a plateau to occur in excised lungs and in vitro bronchi. The difference may result from variations in methodology, especially those related to dose and volume history. Allowing the contracted airways to reach very low (unphysiological) distending pressures may allow the smooth muscle to approach a latch state, and this could be manifested as a decreased plateau.

VI. Limits of Airway Heterogeneity Along the Axis of an Airway Branch

In considering airway constriction, there is usually an implicit assumption that the constriction between branch points is reasonably uniform. Although this assumption thus allows one to model the airway tree as a group of discrete airway segments separated by branch points, there is no information available that has attempted to validate this assumption. Although it is clear both from the studies discussed and the work of several others, that airways along different branches of the tree can behave differently, no studies address what is the axial limit of an airway contraction in a given branch. Does a daughter branch have to behave similarly to the parent branch? With conventional global challenges to all airways, this question clearly cannot be addressed. We, therefore, sought a method that would allow us the ability to apply a very local stimulus to a restricted region of an airway and measure its size in vivo. To accomplish this, we adapted a method that was used to deliver a local aerosol for clearance studies (43). This method involves localization of a catheter placed through the suction port of a fiberoptic bronchoscope. This catheter (PE 100) has an atomizer nozzle with six equally spaced lateral 0.16-mm holes placed in the end; the distal end is plugged. In use, the catheter is first filled with the solution to be used. Rapid injection of a 20-μL bolus than atomizes solutions, causing lateral deposition in a small region of the airway wall.

We have used this method to study local airway contraction near the initial injection site. Figure 10 shows the contraction at three doses of histamine in a

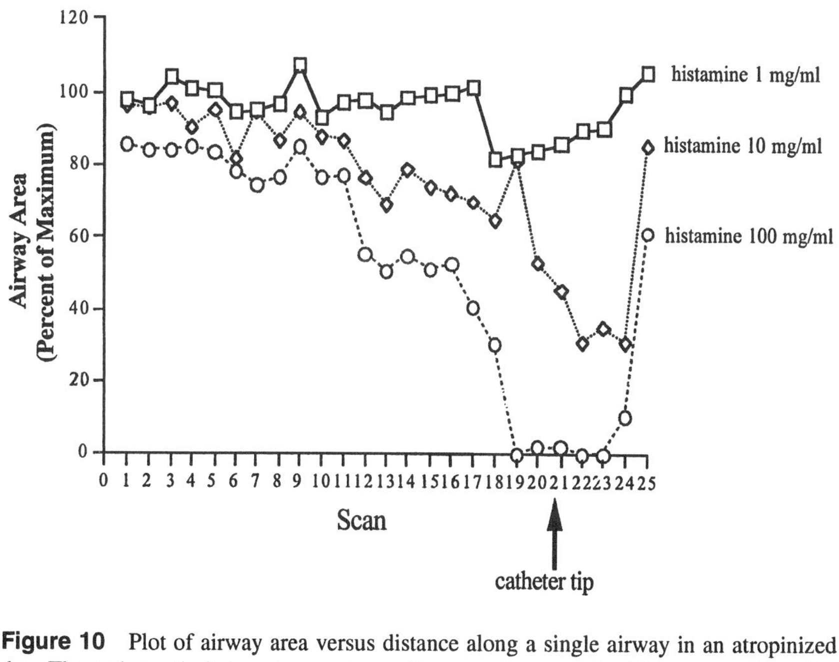

Figure 10 Plot of airway area versus distance along a single airway in an atropinized dog. The catheter tip is in a 4-mm airway. Scan numbers equal millimeters, and smaller scan numbers are more proximal. Shown is the percent of maximal airway area at each position along the airway at three sequential doses of histamine delivered locally (each in 20 μL-sprays) at the catheter tip. At the highest dose, the airway can be seen to close over a very limited 5-mm range.

single 10-mm diameter conducting airway from one dog. For this study, the animal was atropinized to determine the maximal airway size. The 25 CT images were obtained 2 minutes after each sequential (increasing) histamine dose. With the lowest dose, a slight constriction is seen in a few millimeters proximal and distal to the catheter tip. The increasing doses show increasing constriction near the catheter tip. The most striking features of this experiment are, first, that the airway reaches closure, and, second, just how local is this maximal constriction. That is, the airway seems capable of a truly remarkable degree of distortion in the axial direction. Two to 3 mm on either side of an airway segment constricted to closure, the area is about 50% of maximum. This observation is in keeping with the notion supported by the above pressure-area curves, that a fully relaxed airway is very compliant. Apparently this is as true in the axial as it is in the radial direction. That this intense local constriction to closure occurs in a relatively large cartilaginous airway is even more astounding. This result demonstrates an important role for airway smooth muscle tone to provide the airway with structural integrity. Without muscle tone, the airway behaves like a hole in the lung parenchyma. This observation also provides for another level of complexity by allowing almost no limit to the possible extent of axial heterogeneity in the normal lung.

VII. Ramifications of Airway Heterogeneity on Pulmonary Function Tests and Lung Disease

In humans, the airways are ubiquitously studied by spirometry and less often by body plethysmography. In both of these cases, all of the complexity that might exist among the airways is averaged out to arrive at a single variable representing all the airways of the lung in parallel and series. With such an averaging, one might not expect to find much variability in perhaps a forced expiratory volume in 1 second (FEV_1), measured sequentially or on different days. Yet this variability does exist, and it is often substantial. For this reason, the American Thoracic Society has issued a standard on what kind of variability is considered acceptable (44).

In the presence of regional airway disease, normal pulmonary function tests would clearly be of limited value. The importance of this limitation depends on the severity and extent of the local disease. We presently have little information that bears directly on this question. However, preliminary work has indicated that, even in a normal human lung, the FEV_1 is not directly related to conducting airway size. We measured the airway response in four normal subjects to a dose of methacholine aerosol. After baseline spirometry was performed, the subjects were positioned supine in the CT scanner. From RV, they inhaled a measured volume of air to approximately FRC, and CT scans were

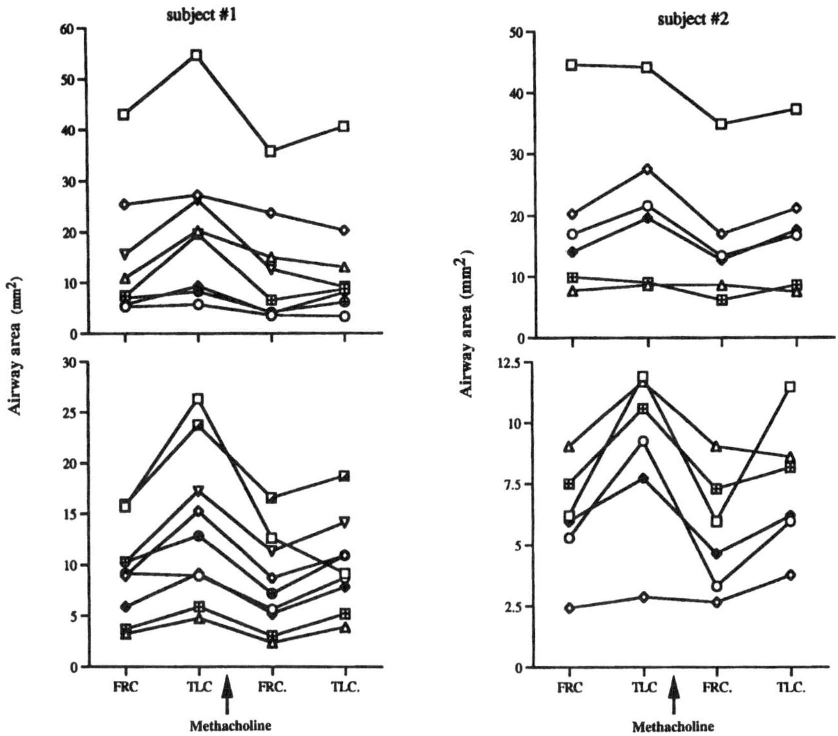

Figure 11 Individual airway responses in four human subjects. For each subject, changes in airway area are shown going from FRC to TLC before and after methacholine challenge. The graphs show absolute airway areas (mm^2), with each line representing an individual airway in each subject. For clarity, the individual airways in each subject are presented on two separate graphs.

obtained while the subjects held their breath. This maneuver was repeated while inhaling a measured volume of air from RV to TLC. While the subjects remained supine, methacholine was administered through a nebulizer during quiet breathing at doses of either 10 mg/mL (subject number 1) or 25 mg/mL (subject numbers 2, 3, and 4) for 2 minutes. Five minutes after completion of the challenges, the inspiratory maneuvers and scans were repeated. After completion of the scans, spirometry was repeated. Figure 11 shows individual airway responses for all four conditions in each subject. The airways are separated into two graphs in each subject for clarity. As can be appreciated from these graphs, there is considerable variability among individual airways in the response to lung inflation before and after methacholine. After methacholine, in all but a few airways, lung inflation failed to dilate airways to the same extent as was

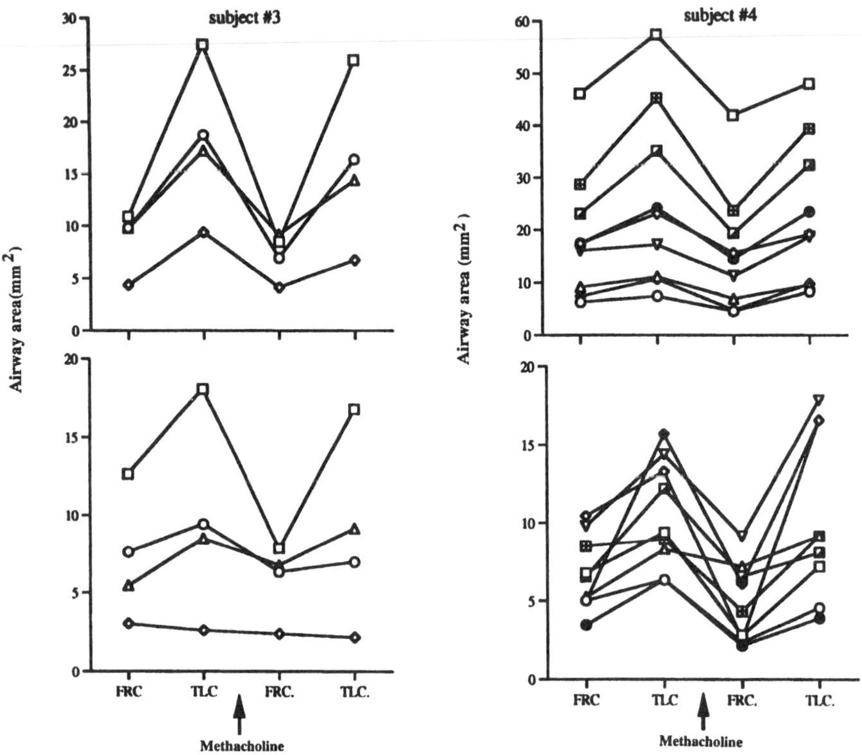

Figure 11 Continued

observed before methacholine. This behavior is consistent with what we observed in the dog. Figure 12 shows the mean responses of all airways in the different subjects present as a percent of their baseline areas at FRC before methacholine. In all subjects, the mean airway area at FRC was decreased by about 10%–15%, a change that should cause conducting airway resistance to increase approximately 24%–38%. All of the subjects showed a decrease in FEV_1 after the methacholine challenge (range 12%–28%).

VIII. Summary

An individual branch of the airway can demonstrate substantial variability in its resting or baseline size, its responsiveness to exogenous challenge, and its response to lung inflation. This variability can occur, not only in parallel airway branches but also along the axis of a single branch. Variation in smooth muscle tone in the longitudinal or axial direction can lead to wide variations in airway

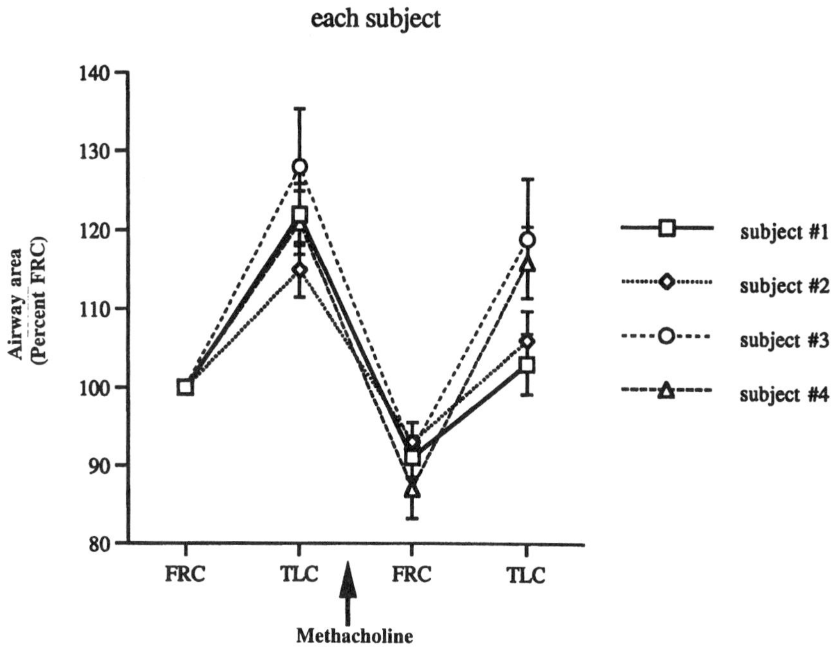

Figure 12 Mean (± SEM) airway responses as a percent of baseline airway area at FRC in the four human subjects. For each subject, changes in airway area are shown going from FRC to TLC before and after a methacholine challenge.

size over the distance of just a few millimeters. This variability in individual airway serial and parallel segments leads to a global complexity in the entire airway tree. Although the specific mechanisms underlying this heterogeneity remain poorly understood, it is clear, that the existence of such widespread heterogeneity in the airway tree produces a complexity in the lung that must have substantive impact on lung function. Local narrowing of airway segments must lead to increased airflow in other regions. This phenomenon could lead to altered regional shear stress on the epithelium, to altered particle deposition, and to altered airway water balance, all processes that may impact on the development of lung disease.

References

1. Wood SA, Zerhouni EA, Hoford JD, Hoffman EA, Mitzner W. Measurement of three-dimensional lung tree structures by using computed tomography. J Appl Physiol 1995; 79:1687–1697.

2. Amirav I, Kramer SS, Grunstein MM, Hoffman EA. Assessment of methacholine-induced airway constriction by ultrafast high-resolution computed tomography. J Appl Physiol 75:2239–2250.
3. Brown RH, Zerhouni EA, Mitzner W. Variability in the size of individual airways over the course of one year. Am J Respir Crit Care Med 1995; 151:1159–1164.
4. Snider GL, Rieger RA, Demas T, Doctor L. Variations in the measurement of spirograms. Am J Med Sci 1967; 254:679–684.
5. Herold CJ, Brown RH, Mitzner W, Links JM, Hirshman CA, Zerhouni EA. High resolution computed tomography: a new method to assess pulmonary airway reactivity. Radiology 1991; 181:396–374.
6. Hruby J, Butler J. Variability of routine pulmonary function tests. Thorax 1975; 30:548–553.
7. Sant'Ambrogio G. Information arising from the tracheobronchial tree of mammals. Physiol Rev 1982; 62:531–569.
8. Dawson A. Reproducibility of spirometric measurements in normal subjects. Am Rev Respir Dis 1966; 93:264–269.
9. Nickerson BG, Lemen RJ, Gerdes CB, Wegmann MJ, Robertson G. Within-subject variability and per cent change for significance of spirometry in normal subjects and in patients with cystic fibrosis. Am Rev Respir Dis 1980; 122:859–866.
10. Rozas CJ, Goldman AL. Daily spirometric variability: normal subjects and subjects with chronic bronchitis with and without airflow obstruction. Arch Intern Med 1982; 142:1287–1291.
11. Brown RH, Herold CJ, Hirshman CA, Zerhouni EA, Mitzner W. In vivo measurements of airway reactivity using high-resolution computed tomography. Am Rev Respir Dis 1991; 144:208–212.
12. Lippmann M. Regional deposition of particles in the human respiratory tract. In: Lee DHK, Falk HL, Murphy SD, Geiger SR, eds. Handbook of Physiology: A Critical, Comprehensive Presentation of Physiological Knowledge and Concepts. Bethesda: American Physiological Society, 1977:213.
13. Wagner EM, Mitzner W. Contribution of pulmonary versus systemic perfusion of airway smooth muscle. J Appl Physiol 1995; 78:403–409.
14. Schellenberg RR, Ohtaka H, Paddon HB, Bramble SE, Rangno RE. Catecholamine responses to histamine infusion in man. J Allergy Clin Immunol 1991; 87:499–504.
15. Staszewska-Barczak J, Vane JR. The release of catecholamine from the adrenal medulla by histamine. Br J Pharmacol 1965; 25:728–742.
16. Berkin KE, Inglis GC, Ball SG, Thomson NC. Effect of low dose adrenaline and noradrenaline infusions on airway calibre in asthmatic patients. Clin Sci 1986; 70: 347–352.
17. Larsson K, Grönneberg R, Hjemdahl P. Bronchodilatation and inhibition of allergen-induced bronchoconstriction by circulating epinephrine in asthmatic subjects. 1985; J Allergy Clin Immunol 75:586–593.
18. Sands MF, Douglas FL, Green J, Banner AS, Robertson GL, Leff AR. Homeostatic regulation on bronchomotor tone by sympathetic activation during bronchoconstriction in normal and asthmatic humans. Am Rev Respir Dis 1985; 132:993–998.

19. Nadel JA, Wolfe WG, Graf PD. Powdered tantalum as a medium for bronchography in canine and human lungs. Invest Radiol 1968; 3:229–238.
20. Shioya T, Solway J, Munoz NM, Mack M, Leff AR. Distribution of airway contractile responses within the major diameter bronchi during exogenous bronchoconstriction. Am Rev Respir Dis 1987; 135:1105–1111.
21. Dandurand RJ, Wang CG, Phillips NC, Eidelman DH. Responsiveness of individual airways to methacholine in adult rat lung explants. J Appl Physiol 1993; 75: 364–372.
22. Fredberg JJ, Ingram RH Jr, Castile G, Glass GM, Drazen JM. Non-homogeneity of lung response to inhaled histamine assessed with alveolar capsules. J Appl Physiol 1985; 58:1914–1922.
23. Anderson PJ, Garshick E, Blanchard JD, Feldman HA, Brain JD. Intersubject variability in particle deposition does not explain variability in responsiveness to methacholine. Am Rev Respir Dis 1991; 144:649–654.
24. Mitzner W. Leonardo and the physiology of respiration. In: Proctor D, ed. The Physiology of Breathing. New York: Marcel Dekker, 1995.
25. Milic-Emili J, Mead J, Turner JM, Glauser EM. Improved technique for estimating pleural pressure from esophageal balloons. J Appl Physiol 1964; 19:207–211.
26. James AL, Hogg JC, Dunn LA, Pare PD. The use of the internal perimeter to compare airway size and to calculate smooth muscle shortening. Am Rev Respir Dis 1988; 138:136–139.
27. Lai-Fook SJ, Kallok MJ. Bronchial-arterial interdependence in isolated dog lung. J Appl Physiol: Respirat Environ Exercise Physiol 1982; 52:1000–1007.
28. Hahn HL, Watson A, Wilson AG, Pride NB. Influence of bronchomotor tone on airway dimensions and resistance in excised dog lungs. J Appl Physiol 1980; 49: 270–278.
29. Marshall R. Effect of lung inflation on bronchial dimensions in the dog. J Appl Physiol 1962; 17:596–600.
30. Brown RH, Zerhouni EA, Hirshman CA. Reversal of bronchoconstriction by inhaled nitric oxide: histamine versus methacholine. Am J Respir Crit Care Med 1994; 150:233–237.
31. Gunst SJ, Stropp JQ, Service J. Mechanical modulation of pressure-volume characteristics of contracted canine airways in vitro. J Appl Physiol 1990; 68:2223–2229.
32. Beaupre A, Badier M, Delpierre S, Orehek J, Grimaud C. Airway responses of asthmatics to carbachol and to deep inspiration. Eur J Respir Dis 1983; 64:108–112.
33. Beaupre A, Orehek J. Factors influencing the bronchodilator effect of a deep inspiration in asthmatic patients with provoked bronchoconstriction. Thorax 1982; 37: 124–128.
34. Fish JE, Ankin MG, Kelly JF, Peterman VI. Regulation of bronchomotor tone by lung inflation in asthmatic and nonasthmatic subjects. J Appl Physiol 1981; 50: 1079–1086.
35. Fish JE, Peterman VI, Cugell D. Effect of deep inspiration on airway conductance in subjects with allergic rhinitis and allergic asthma. J Allergy Clin Immunol 1977; 60:41–46.

36. Gayrard P, Orehek J, Grimaud C, Charpin J. Bronchoconstrictor effects of a deep inspiration in patients with asthma. Am Rev Respir Dis 1975; 111:433–439.
37. Orehek J, Charpin D, Velardocchio JM, Grimaud C. Bronchomotor effect of bronchoconstriction-induced deep inspirations in asthmatics. Am Rev Respir Dis 1980; 121:297–305.
38. Orehek J, Nicoli MM, Delpierre S, Beaupre A. Influence of the previous deep inspiration on the spirometric measurement of provoked bronchoconstriction in asthma. Am Rev Respir Dis 1981; 123:269–272.
39. Skloot G, Permutt S, Togias A. Pathophysiology of asthma: reduced airway-parenchyma interdependence, not smooth muscle hyperresponsiveness (abstr). Am J Respir Crit Care Med 1994; 149:A585.
40. Sasaki H, Hoppin FG, Takishima T. Peribronchial pressure in excised dog lungs. J Appl Physiol 1978; 45:858–869.
41. Murtagh PS, Proctor DF, Permutt S, Kelly B, Evering S. Bronchial closure with mecholyl in excised dog lobes. J Appl Physiol 1971; 31:409–415.
42. Gunst SJ, Mitzner W. Mechanical properties of contracted canine bronchial segments in vitro. J Appl Physiol: Respirat Environ Exercise Physiol 1981; 50(6): 1236–1247.
43. Sweeney TD, Cipolla D, Gonda I. Localized delivery of particles to a small region of the airways (abstr). Am J Respir Crit Care Med 1995; 151:A61.
44. American Thoracic Society, Lung function testing: selection of reference values and interpretative strategies. Am Rev Respir Dis 1991; 144:1202–1218.

2

Alveolar Lining Layer

Functions, Composition, Structures

SAMUEL SCHÜRCH

University of Calgary
Calgary, Alberta, Canada

HANS BACHOFEN

University of Berne
Inselspital
Berne, Switzerland

FRED POSSMAYER

University of Western Ontario
London, Ontario, Canada

I. Introduction

The importance of the lung air–liquid interfacial forces for lung mechanics was first indicated by studies reported in 1929 by von Neergaard. He attributed the differences in the retractive forces between air-filled lungs and lungs filled with an aqueous medium to the action of surface tension (1). However, this new idea was not studied further until a quarter of a century later when Pattle deduced that the lung contained surfactant substances capable of stabilizing small air bubbles in the range of 40 μm in diameter (2). Clements (3) measured the surface tensions of extracts at different surface areas in a Langmuir-Wilhelmy balance. He found that the surface tension declines toward zero on compression of the surface film and increases during film expansion. These investigations pointed to a lack or dysfunction of such surfactants in the lung of newborns with respiratory distress syndrome (4). Direct measurements of surface tension in intact lungs (5,6) and energy analysis based on well-defined structure–function relationships of isolated, air-filled and perfused lungs (7) confirmed that the surface tension within alveoli at lung volumes of normal breathing varies between 25 and 30 mN/m and near zero.

The most prominent component of lung extract surfactants proved to be the phospholipid dipalmitoyl-phosphatidylcholine (DPPC) along with unsaturated phosphatidylcholines, phosphatidyl-glycerol, cholesterol, other trace lipids, and at least three surfactant-specific proteins (SP-A, SP-B, and SP-C) (8,9). It is interesting to note that other animals stabilize their alveolar surfaces in a manner similar to that of mammals (10,11). There is also experimental and theoretical evidence that surfactant stabilizes small airways to avoid airway closure (12), balances lung fluids (13), and modulates alveolar and airway defense reactions of the host against invading pathogens (14).

As outlined by Pattle (15), the lining layer of surfactant should be composed of two parts: a monomolecular film of phospholipids, associated with some proteins, and the lining complex of saline-dispersible lipoprotein serving as a reserve material. This concept of a monomolecular film lining an aqueous subphase, containing surfactant structures, represents the well accepted traditional view of the acellular lining complex, as deduced from physiological experiments and biochemical analysis (16,17).

Weibel and associates demonstrated for the first time by electron microscopy the existence of an extracellular duplex lining layer of lung alveoli (18–20). Weibel and Gil (18) observed that parts of the surface film appeared as a lamellar superficial layer with repeating distances of 3.8 to 5.1 nm adsorbed to the surface film. Grossmann and Robertson (21) also found the surfactant film to be multilamellar and so did Ueda et al. (22) in their ultrastructural studies on the alveolar lining layer, using a variety of fixation methods. However, the postulated continuity of the lining layer, as demonstrated recently by Bastacky and associates (23), could never be proven by chemical fixation.

Recent experiments (24–26) have been more successful in preserving and demonstrating the lining layer. By high-pressure perfusion of excised rabbit lungs with 6% albumin solution, alveolar edema was introduced such that the surface film was lifted off the epithelial cell layer. High-power magnification of the film showed a polymorphous structure. At some sites, triple or even higher order multilayers covered the increased volume of the hypophase whereas other sites of the lining layer appeared amorphous.

These observations are in line with the concept of a surface-associated surfactant reservoir observed in experiments in which the subphase below the surfactant film of a captive bubble was replaced by a salt solution that contained no surfactant. On expansion of this bubble, film material from the interface in excess of a monolayer was incorporated into the surface active film (24,25).

In this chapter, we focus on the formation, the extent, and the complex structure-function relationship of this excess surface-associated surfactant material, the "reserve material" already suggested by Pattle (15) and illustrated by Weibel and Gil (18). We address the question of whether the surface-associated surfactant material acts as reserve material to be incorporated into the monolayer, without essentially modifying the mechanical properties of the monolayer, or whether the associated material is mechanically coupled with the monolayer such that the mechanical properties of the interfacial film between the vapor and the liquid phase are different from those of a monolayer. That is, mechanical properties such as film stability and compressibility below the equilibrium surface tension might be modified by the linkage between the first layer of molecules adjacent to the air phase and multilamellar structures bound to the first layer. We demonstrate the complex interrelationship between structure and function in the lung from studies on intact lungs. Complexities of the pulmonary surfactant film are addressed by structural analysis in situ and in vitro by electron microscopy and by in vitro studies on surfactant films using the captive bubble approach (27,28). Finally, we discuss the surface activity of pulmonary surfactant and the complex role of individual surfactant components and their interplay in the formation and surface activity of the surfactant film.

II. The Surface Film

A. Complexity of Function

1. *Studies on Whole Lungs*

a. Pressure–Volume Relations

The viscoelastic behavior of lungs can be described by the relationship between the recoil pressure (P) and the lung volume (V), that is, by pressure–volume (PV) curves (29,30). Already in normal air-filled lungs, the PV relations are extremely complex, depending on many factors, but in particular, on time, volume history, and degree of lung inflation (29–31). Both the recoil force of air-filled lungs and its PV hysteresis have tissue and surface components (32). Numerous experiments have clearly shown that the complexity of the PV behavior of air-filled lungs is, in part, the result of the complex properties of the alveolar surface lining layer: by eliminating alveolar interfacial forces, that is, by filling the lungs with isosmotic water solutions (32) or with hexadecane (33), the PV behavior of lung parenchyma is rather reproducible and predictable.

This latter observation was the basis of the hypothesis that the size and variability of alveolar surface forces, in situ and in vivo, and, in particular, the physical properties of the surface-active material can be determined by comparisons between PV curves of liquid-filled and air-filled lungs (32). This hypothesis included the assumptions that 1. the geometry of the delicate network of alveolar tissue remains similar during inflation and deflation of air- and liquid-filled lungs, and 2. the tissue forces and the surface forces act mechanically in parallel, that is, the difference between the recoil pressures of air- and liquid-filled lungs in exclusively due to the surface forces in the air-filled lung. Comparative measurements were profitable in so far as they unequivocally demonstrated extremely low surface tensions in the volume-range of normal breathing.

However, important features of lung mechanics could not be explained by this approach, and, in particular, the inconsistent results between in situ and in vitro (Langmuir-Wilhelmy balance) experiments could not be reconciled.

Some problems could be resolved when Schürch developed the microdroplet method to directly determine alveolar surface tensions in intact lungs (5,6). This technique allowed measurements within limited PV ranges under rather static conditions. The experiments confirmed that, within the normal range of breathing, that is, between 40% and 60% of total lung capacity (TLC), surface tensions are close to zero, and they further showed that the maximal γ at TLC is approximately 30 mN/m. In addition a γ–V hysteresis similar to the corresponding PV hysteresis could be observed (Figure 1). And, most importantly, further evidence could be provided that single alveoli are not individual units modeled by bubbles on a tube. At a given lung volume under static conditions, surface tension was found to be the same in all of the alveoli accessible to direct measurement of surface tension, regardless of their size (35). Mechanical stability is provided by both the tissue interdependence and the alveolar lining layer, which form a fluid continuum with a continuous surfactant film of uniform surface tension at the air–fluid interface (23,24,34,35).

Calculations readily revealed that the old and new data were not yet sufficient to create a mechanical model consistent with the real behavior of the lung or to answer questions about the micromechanics of lung parenchyma. In fact, morphological and morphometric studies of lungs fixed under well-controlled physiological conditions showed that the basic hypothesis was incorrect. Tissue forces and surface forces do not act independently. Rather, the surface forces are effective in two ways: directly, they do contribute to the recoil force of the

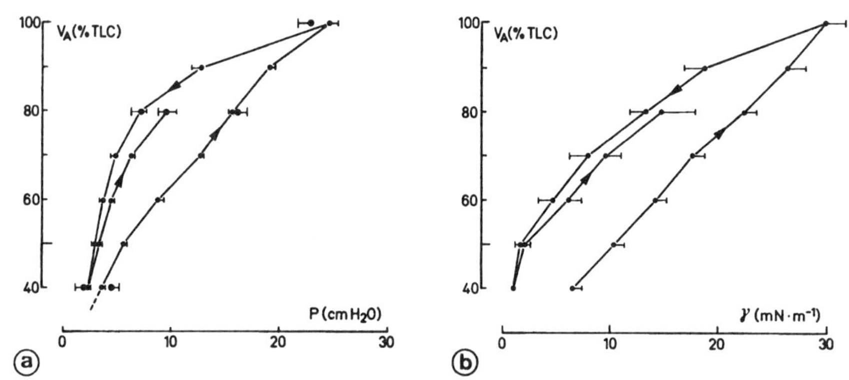

Figure 1 (a) Average pressure–volume relation of 11 rabbit lungs in which alveolar surface tensions were measured by use of the microdroplet method. (b) Surface tension–volume relationship corresponding to pressure–volume relation of *a*.

lung, and, indirectly, they alter the configuration of peripheral air spaces and the alveolar surface area, thus increasing the tissue forces (7). This complex interplay called for a detailed analysis of the structure–function relationships of lung parenchyma.

b. Structure–Function Relations

The delicate structural framework of lung parenchyma is difficult to visualize by microscopy in a state that faithfully reflects the physiological conditions that prevailed at the time of fixation. To study the surface lining layer and the interplay between surface forces and the architecture of alveolar microstructures, particular care is required that the fixation technique does not interfere with the alveolar surface. Fixation of the lung by vascular perfusion comes closest to this requirement, although this method clearly introduces a number of artifactual conditions and adds to the complexity of analysis (36).

In a first attempt, this method was used to reevaluate the basic experiments of lung mechanics, that is, to compare the structure–function relations to liquid-filled and air-filled lungs. In the first case, the surface forces are eliminated, but, in the latter case, they remain active so that one can study the relative importance of tissue mechanics and surface forces on molding the peripheral air spaces and the dimension of the alveolar surface. The influence of surface forces on alveolar architecture can best be visualized on scanning electron micrographs (Figure 2) of air- and fluid-filled lungs fixed at the same lung volume (about 70% TLC). In fluid-filled lungs, the alveolar surface texture is highly irregular because of freely bulging capillaries. Some alveolar septa appear inhomogeneously expanded. The alveolar ducts are relatively narrow and their free edges appear crinkly. In contrast, in air-filled lungs, the alveolar architecture resembles a system of irregular polyhedrons: the walls are mostly flat and form angles with each other. Line elements can be recognized at the alveolar openings of the more expanded duct. Evidently, there is a modeling effect of surface forces on the microstructure, and the rearranged capillaries and septal tissue are accommodated beneath a smooth alveolar surface. This transition is most conspicuous if surface tension is abnormally increased by rinsing the lungs with fluorocarbon or with a detergent (Figure 3): the peripheral air spaces are wider, the fibrous cables forming the alveolar opening rings appear to be stretched, and the arrangement of capillaries indicate numerous pleats of alveolar septa (i.e., a derecruitment of alveolar surface). The qualitative impression that the alveolar surface area is smaller in air-filled than in fluid-filled lungs can be verified by morphometry. In fact, with increasing surface tensions brought about either by physiological pressure-volume maneuvers (37) or artificially by rinsing the alveoli with foreign liquids (fluorocarbons, hexadecane, or detergents [33]), the alveolar surface area progressively decreases (Figure 4). This effect of surface forces on surface area and hence on septal architecture is pronounced at lung volumes

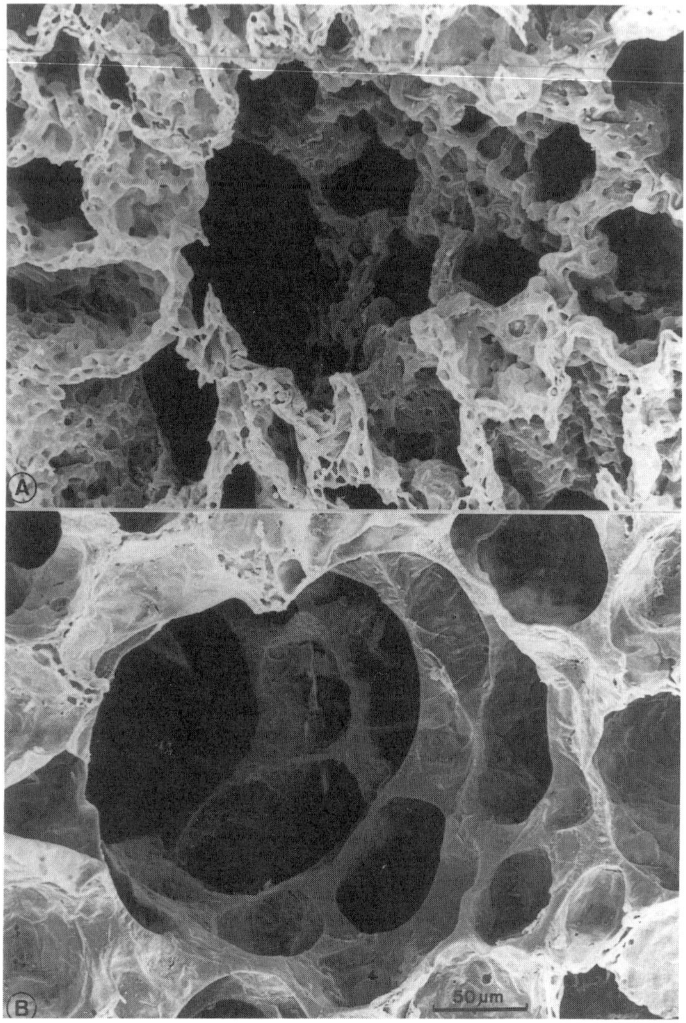

Figure 2 Saline-filled (**A**) and air-filled (**B**) rabbit lungs, fixed at the same volume of about 70% total lung capacity. Note the different alveolar texture and the differences in width of alveolar ducts.

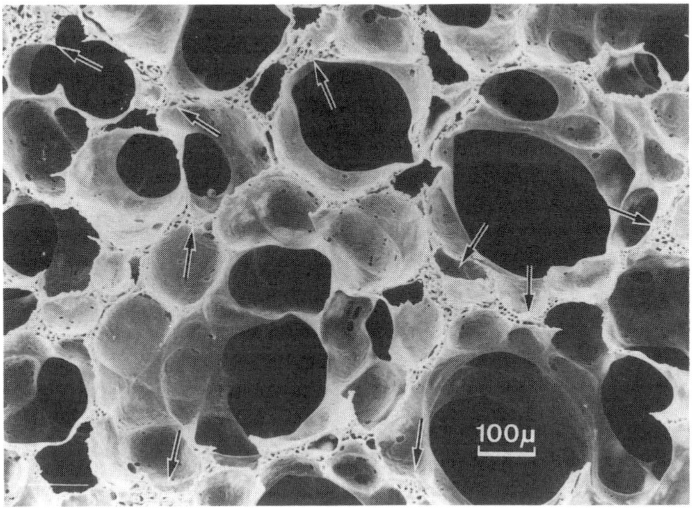

Figure 3 Alveolar morphology of rabbit lung rinsed with fluorocarbon (FC-77; $\gamma \sim 15$ mN/m). Note the smooth alveolar surface, the distended alveolar opening rings, and the clusters of capillaries (*arrows*) indicating numerous pleats of alveolar septa.

of normal breathing (i.e., at 40% TLC). However, at higher lung volumes, the molding effect gradually disappears, suggesting the predominance of tissue forces in determining the dimensions of peripheral air spaces (37). These observations and data have been incorporated in the model by Wilson and Bachofen (7). A first check showed that this model is consistent with data relating surface tension, alveolar surface area, recoil pressure, and lung volume obtained in lungs on the deflation limb of the PV curve between 80% and 40% TLC. Beyond this range, the behavior of the surface lining layer in situ and its complex interplay with pulmonary microstructures still eludes a quantitative description. The problem seems particularly complex if PV cycles are started from below the residual volume (i.e., from volumes below the physiological range).

2. *In Vitro Model Studies*

a. Methods

An examination of the results on surface activity obtained with various methods demonstrates clearly that the criteria for good surface activity depend on the instrument used and, for a particular instrument, on the way a certain test is performed. A test of the surface activity of a surfactant may include measurements on film formation (adsorption), minimum surface tension, film compressibility, and stability (28). Although the therapeutic efficacy of a particular sur-

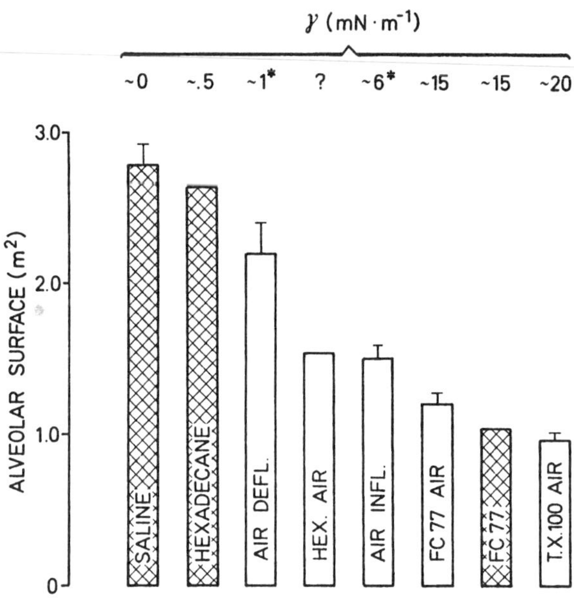

Figure 4 Alveolar surface areas of rabbit lungs fixed by vascular perfusion at lung volume of 40% total lung capacity. From left to right: saline-filled lung, hexadecane-filled lung, normal air-filled lung on deflation, hexadecane-rinsed lung, air-filled lung on inflation (compare Figure 1), fluorocarbon-rinsed lung, fluorocarbon-filled lung, and detergent-rinsed lung. Values were obtained by in situ measurements using the microdroplet method. Abbreviations: γ = alveolar surface tension.

factant preparation has to be tested in animal models of surface deficiency (38), in vitro studies provide valuable guidelines for choosing or preparing a physiologically active surfactant. A standardized approach with a particular instrument may give results on surface activity that correlate well with physiological parameters measured in animals even if the approach does not mimic the situation in the lung.

Unfortunately, the standardization of a particular approach to measure surface activity for a given instrument is difficult. This can be demonstrated for the Langmuir-Wilhelmy balance (39), the pulsating bubble surfactometer (40), and the more recently developed captive bubble surfactometer (27,28). Goerke and Gonzales (41) primed the Teflon walls and barrier of their balance with long-chain saturated phosphatidylcholine and a solution of lanthanum chloride to make the Teflon walls below the water line hydrophilic. Primed surface balances appear to contain the surfactant film better within a well-defined surface area than do untreated balances. In addition, continuous Teflon ribbons or bands standing on edge were used in the 1960s by Clements in rectangular troughs (42) with rhombic frames (43) or a frame in the shape of a rounded triangle (44).

Thus, minimal surface tension and film stability at tension below the equilibrium, typically about 25 mN/m for lung surfactants, depend on the careful preparation of the surface balance because films that produce low and stable minimal surface tensions in a leak-proof system show instability in a balance with untreated walls, regardless of the geometry or arrangement of the moveable barrier.

To overcome the difficulties with the Langmuir-Wilhelmy balance, some investigators have been using small air bubbles formed on subsurface tubes in cuvettes containing as little as 20 μL of fluid. In 1977, Enhorning (40) described his version of an oscillating bubble on a tube. This apparatus, known as the pulsating bubble surfactometer, has been widely used and has yielded a considerable amount of insight into dynamically compressed and expanded films from natural surfactant or compounds related to pulmonary surfactant. The apparatus consists of a bubble drawn from the atmosphere into a disposable plastic chamber at 37°C containing as little as 20 μL of a suspension of the material to be tested. The bubble is oscillated between a maximum radius of 0.55 mm and a minimum radius of 0.40 mm, which produces a surface area reduction of approximately 50%. The cycling frequency is usually about 20 cycles/min, but frequencies of 10 to 80 cycles/min have also been used. The pressure across the bubble is continuously monitored with a pressure transducer. The surface tension is calculated by using the Laplace equation for a spherical interface.

As in the Langmuir-Wilhelmy balance, there are still problems with surface leaks. They occur up the inner surface of the tube at the plastic–air interface as well as at the outer surface of the tube at the plastic–fluid interface by surfactant spreading, similarly to that in the surface balance at the Teflon-water interface. Leakage at the inner surface of the tube can be reduced by keeping the tube dry (45). The method is not suitable to investigate the film stability at minimum surface tension (surface tension versus time) at minimum bubble volume in the nonpulsating mode. The pulsating bubble is convenient for examining the surface activity, commonly named "biophysical activity," of samples under dynamic compression, because leakage is less of a problem if relatively high cycling frequencies are chosen.

The captive bubble surfactometer (CBS) introduced by Schürch and coworkers (27,28) offers a leak-proof system because the surface film is not interrupted by plastic walls, barrier, or outlets. In this apparatus, the air bubble floats against a hydrophilic roof, such as a 1% agarose gel, by buoyancy (Fig. 5). At the air–agarose interface, the water layer is thin but sufficiently thick to prevent adhesion of the bubble to the gel itself. Bubble volume is controlled by varying the pressure in the sample chamber. As bubble volume is reduced, the surface area is reduced and the surface tension of the surfactant film at the bubble

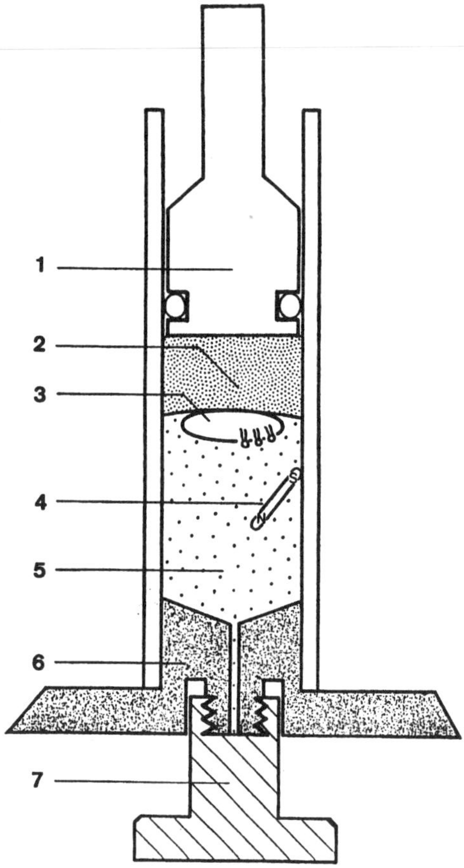

Figure 5 Captive bubble surfactometer. 1 = piston; 2 = 1% agarose gel; 3 = air bubble with surfactant film; 4 = magnetic stir bar; 5 = Surfactant suspension, 6 = stainless steel base with inlet, 7 = pressure-tight plug.

surface decreases. The bubble shape changes depending on the surface tension, from more spherical to an oval shape. For bubbles larger than about 5 mm in initial diameter, the bubble shape assumes that of a thin disk as the surface tension falls toward zero. For surface tensions of less than 1 mN/m to about 30 mN/m, bubbles as small as 4 μL in volume (2 mm diameter) may be used in a sample volume of about 40 μL. However, usually bubbles of about 200 μL in volume (~7 mm diameter) are used in a sample volume of about 0.5 to 1.0 mL. Surfactant concentrations, usually expressed in total phospholipid per volume (mg/mL), can be used from as little as 50 μg/mL to a maximum of 1–2 mg/mL for the large chamber, 10 mm in diameter. In the small chamber, 5 mm in diameter, surfactant concentrations of 2–3 mg/mL may be used. The maximum concentration is given by the optical limitations, because surfactant suspensions become murky at higher concentrations.

Surface tension, area, and volume are calculated from bubble height and diameter, from video images (46). Precision and accuracy of the method are described by Schoel et al. (46).

By comparing the results obtained in the pulsating bubble surfactometer with those in the captive bubble surfactometer, Putz et al. (45) concluded that the captive bubble surfactometer should be used when accurate film area compressions are required to explain mechanisms that determine near zero minimum surface tension, film compressibility, stability, and hysteresis.

A number of novel insights into surface properties have been obtained with the captive bubble. Adsorption from the stirred subphase proceeds rapidly with natural and organic solvent lipid extract surfactants, with equilibrium surface tensions being achieved in seconds with bulk concentrations of less than 1 mg/mL. With this method, more reliable information about the mechanisms related to adsorption, film stability, hysteresis, and compressibility are obtained. For example, the mode of bubble cycling and the extent of film compression and collapse determine various amounts of hysteresis in surface tension–area relations. However, as with all the other methods, it is no trivial task to obtain high-quality surface tension–area relations. For example, in the captive bubble surfactometer, the surface area and the surface tension are interrelated. Hence, volume changes can be predetermined accurately, but area changes cannot (28).

It appears that the surface activity tests conducted with any available method are more complex than hitherto assumed. In the following discussion, we focus on the complexities that determine film formation and the shape of surface tension–area relations.

b. Characteristics of Surface Tension-Area Relations

Surface tension–area relations obtained with lipid extract surfactants, bovine (bLES Biochemicals, London, Ontario, Canada) and porcine (Curosurf, Chiesi Farmaceutici, Parma, Italy), with and without added SP-A, have revealed a number of factors important in film formation, film stability, and the extent of hysteresis in these relations. In addition, detailed knowledge has been obtained from well-defined phospholipid dispersions with and without added surfactant-specific proteins.

i. Adsorptions. Adsorption means the accumulation of material at an interface. An effective pulmonary surfactant adsorbs rapidly to form a film within a few seconds to around 25 mN/m, the plateau or equilibrium surface tension at the air–liquid interface (39). Rapid adsorption toward equilibrium means that adsorption will keep the surface tension in the lung near equilibrium during inspiration to total lung capacity. This keeps the surface component of lung recoil pressure as low as possible, which helps to minimize the work of breathing (39). For lipid extract surfactants and natural lung surfactant extract, the plateau or equilibrium surface tension is between 23 and 25 mN/m at 37°C for concentrations above about 50 µg/mL of total phospholipids (28,47,48). The rate of adsorption is strongly dependent on the concentration of the lipid in the bulk suspension and whether SP-A is added to low-concentration lipid extract surfactant (47). In general, rapid adsorption appears to be followed by low film compressibility and near zero and stable minimum surface tensions on quasi-static or dynamic compressions (48), although longer waiting periods for a slow adsorption process to reach equilibrium surface tension may also be rewarded by low values of minimum surface tension, film compressibility, and a mechanically stable film (48,49). However, these parameters are also dependent on the organization of the surface-associated surfactant material, which can be optimized with regard to the surface activity of the film by a particular mode of adsorption by stepwise area expansion.

Recent work on adsorption (48) demonstrates that fresh lipid extract surfactants that contain SP-B and SP-C have the capacity to adsorb by a cooperative movement of large collective units of molecules into interface during adsorption. The phenomenon of adsorption by the transport of lipid aggregates has been discussed previously (39,50,51) and recently in captive bubble studies (48). In contrast to the clicks that characterize a sudden increase in surface tension accompanied by a decrease in surface area (27,28), the sudden adsorption jumps caused by the movement of lipid aggregates into the interface have been called adsorption clicks (48). Adsorption clicks are characterized by a stepwise decrease in surface tension of 5–10 mN/m corresponding to aggregates of 10^{14} phospholipid molecules. This phenomenon does not depend on the surface-associated protein SP-A, because lipid extract surfactants contain SP-B and SP-C but not SP-A (47). Furthermore, these adsorption clicks cannot be related to tubular myelin, because these structures contain SP-A. Without exception, films formed in this manner appear already highly enriched in DPPC as seen by the extremely low compressibility close to that of DPPC. In contrast, films formed by gradual adsorption during several seconds to minutes may or may not show the same low compressibility as those formed by adsorption clicks. These latter films may then be purified by squeezing-out mechanisms (51). Thus, both mechanisms of selective enrichment in DPPC are not mutually exclusive.

In addition, lipid extract films formed by rapid gradual adsorption within 1 to 2 seconds, or by adsorption ciicks, to the equilibrium surface tension of 23–25 mN/m tend to have film material in the surface-associated surfactant reservoir (see below) in excess of three monolayers, and this excess material appears to be enriched in DPPC.

ii. Dynamic Cycles and Hysteresis. The area enclosed by cyclic, isothermal pressure-volume and surface tension–area plots represents the irreversible heat loss that must be provided by additional work in the cycle. Such added work for pressure-volume or surface tension–area relations of lungs is called "hysteresis" (literally, lagging behind) and is provided by the respiratory muscles.

Since Clements (3) introduced the Langmuir-Wilhelmy surface balance to study pulmonary surfactant, surface tension–area relations obtained in that apparatus have been thought to represent the in situ behavior of the alveolar film. The mechanisms involved in the hysteresis of surface tension–area relations have been discussed (28,47,51). Briefly, with the Langmuir-Wilhelmy method, surfactant films are usually compressed to a fixed residual area of 50% to 10% of the initial area. This manner of film compression has frequently led to large hysteresis areas because films are compressed beyond the point where minimum surface tension is attained (48). Overcompression at near zero minimum surface tensions is characterized by a horizontal plateau at minimum surface tension, indicating film collapse. Furthermore, overcompression leads to the formation of a collapse phase, which, in turn, may reduce the adsorption of fresh material from the bulk phase into the interface, the formation of a shoulder at around 30 mN/m in the expansion part of the hysteresis loop, and the formation of a nearly horizontal plateau of high film compressibility at approximately 20 mN/m in the compression part of the loop (47,48). Recent experiments have demonstrated that overcompression with film collapse may occur at any level of minimum surface tension below the equilibrium film tension of approximately 25 mN/m, if the surfactant quality is compromised by impurities, by peroxidation, or by the presence of inhibitors (e.g., components of blood serum). Thus, overcompression may occur after a very moderate reduction of the film area, far below 30%, which is likely the upper limit of physiological film area changes in the normal lung (37).

We have used the captive bubble surfactometer (Fig. 5) to investigate the interrelated film properties that are involved in quasistatic or dynamic surface tension area relations (28,48). Quasistatic cycling involves a series of small discrete alterations in bubble area where the surface film is allowed to "relax" during the compression-expansion process. These processes are not quasistatic processes as defined in thermodynamics, in which a quasistatic process is an idealized concept defined as a succession of equilibrium states (52). With dynamic cycling, in which the bubble volume is continuously altered at 20–30 cycles per minute (cpm), there is less opportunity for adsorption during the expansion phase and a greater possibility of overcompression (collapse at minimum tension) during the compression phase.

In Figure 6, the initial total film area compressions were approximately 50% of the initial bubble area. Whereas, in Figures 6*B* and 6*C*, the area changes to obtain near zero surface tension for the stationary loops remained 28%–30%. The loops in Figure 6*A* show that more than 80% film area reduction was required to obtain near zero minimum surface tension for the stationary loops centering on cycle 20. The lipid extract surfactant (bLES) concentration in Fig-

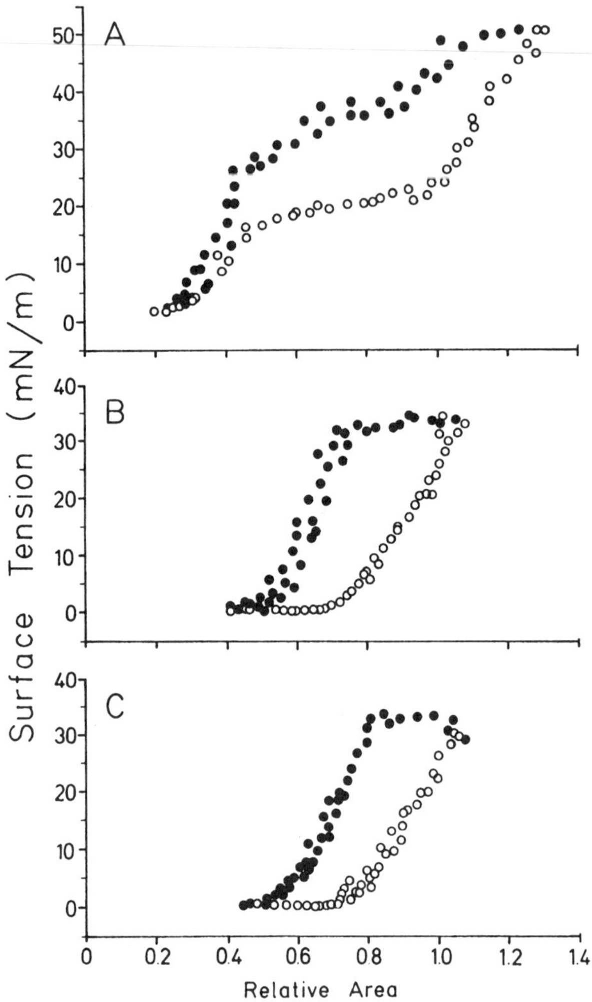

Figure 6 Effect of concentration and SP-A on dynamic hysteresis loops of lipid extract surfactant (bLES). Surface tension is plotted versus relative area. Plots are the summaries of four consecutive dynamic cycles centering on the 20th cycle. Open symbols indicate measurements made during compression; filled symbols indicate measurements made during expansion. Samples were suspended in 0.9% NaCl, 1.5 mM $CaCl_2$. (**A**), bLES at 200 μg/mL. (**B**), bLES at 1000 μg/mL. (**C**), bLES at 200 μg/mL supplemented with 4% SP-A.

ure 6*A* was 0.2 mg/mL in 0.9% NaCl and 1.5 mM $CaCl_2$. In Figure 6*C*, bLES was 0.2 mg/mL supplemented with 4% (w/w) SP-A. In Figure 6*B*, bLES was at 1.0 mg/mL. Thus, stationary loops with moderate film area compressions to near zero surface tensions are obtained with surfactant either at a substantially higher concentration than that for Figure 6*A* or when the low surfactant concentration is supplemented by SP-A (47).

A number of interesting features can be observed at low surfactant concentrations (0.2 mg/mL bLES). During dynamic compressions with low bLES concentrations, a distinct plateau occurs below 25 mN/m where a decrease in surface area of 30% results in only a small reduction in surface tension. Previous studies with the Langmuir-Wilhelmy balance have termed this phenomenon the "purification" or "squeeze-out" plateau, because it appears as though non-DPPC lipids are being removed as opposed to simple packing of monolayer lipids, which would result in the reduction of surface tension below the equilibrium tension of 25 mN/m (39,51,53,54). It has been suggested that squeeze-out corresponds to the exclusion of the lipid-expanded phase and an increase in the percentage of condensed DPPC domains, resulting in a partial enrichment in DPPC (53). However, recent experiments have demonstrated that films from porcine lipid extract surfactant exhibit a very low film compressibility, close to that of pure DPPC films (~0.005 m/mN) after de novo adsorption, and near zero and stable surface tensions after a moderate area compression between 15% and 20% (48). In addition, dynamically overcompressed films from lipid extract surfactant show the distinct plateau (48) previously termed squeeze-out or purification plateau (see above). The conclusion is that there are several mechanisms involved in plateau formation in the compression part, including film collapse at near zero surface tension, which causes a reorganization of film structure, an important feature in the overall film surface activity.

Another feature of the dynamic cycles at low concentration of bLES is a shoulder above 35 mN/m in the expansion portion of the curve (see Figure 6*A*). The conclusion was that this shoulder is caused by adsorption from a distinct pool of lipids referred to as the "surface reservoir" (47) because adsorption from the bulk suspension at low lipid concentration is too slow to explain the relatively rapid adsorption that causes the shoulder. In addition, there is a delay in the increase in surface tension, clearly seen in Figures 6B and 6C at the start of film expansion. This feature is not consistent with the characteristics of monolayer expansion (47).

To clarify the mechanisms involved in the formation of the characteristic features of hysteresis loop, such as those observed in Figure 6A at low lipid concentrations in the bulk phase, we have reduced the bulk lipid concentration to zero by depleting the subphase of surfactant after the initial film formation by adsorption. By this approach, phenomena related to the "reservoir" can clearly be distinguished from those related to the bulk surfactant phase.

c. Subphase Depletion: The Surface-Associated Surfactant Reservoir

Recent experiments have demonstrated the presence of "surplus" material in the air–liquid interface resulting from the presence of surfactant proteins upon de novo adsorption of surfactant derived from natural sources. This material in excess of a monolayer has been termed "the surface-associated surfactant reservoir" (24,25).

In this section, we discuss the surfactant film surface activity including adsorption, compressibility, minimum surface tension, and mechanical stability. These parameters are related to the surfactant reservoir.

i. Quasistatic Expansion Cycles for Lipid Extract Surfactant. Figure 7 represents a typical series of consecutive quasistatic compression-expansion cycles, with each compression being conducted with a slightly larger bubble area than that of the preceding bubble. After film formation by adsorption, the surfactant was depleted and the subphase replaced by 0.9% NaCl, 1.5 mM $CaCl_2$. The surfactant was bovine lipid extract surfactant, the suspension contained 1 mg/mL of phospholipid in 0.9% NaCl, 1.5 mM $CaCl_2$ at pH 5.5. A small atmospheric bubble was introduced into the bubble chamber and the surface tension was allowed to reach the equilibrium value of 23 mN/m. The bubble was then compressed until a low surface tension of less than 2 mN/m was achieved. The reduction of the film surface area was 22% of the original bubble area. With succeeding cycles, compressions of 20%, 25%, and 38% were required to reach minimum surface tensions near zero (about 2 mN/m). The maximum surface tensions observed after 2-minute adsorption times were 23, 24, 29, and 40 mN/m, respectively. The bubble areas at minimum surface tension increased from 0.33 to 0.65, to 0.85, and to 0.87 cm^2, respectively.

In this manner, the successive area expansions to surface tensions slightly above equilibrium were used to incorporate or adsorb "excess" surfactant material from the bubble lining layer into the surface active film. This resulting surfactant film could then be compressed to near zero surface tension at a larger surface area. Thus, by compressing repeatedly to near zero minimum surface tension, it was possible to estimate the amount of film material in the surface-associated reservoir in terms of densely packed "monolayers" of near zero surface tension. The film area at minimum tension on the last compression, before the surface tension begins to increase substantially to values above 25 mN/m on expansion, was about 0.87 cm^2, or 2.6 times the area at the first minimum (0.33 cm^2). There was an excess of at least two monolayers present in the "surface-associated reservoir" or material, for a total of at least three monolayers after adsorption to 23–25 mN/m. Upon the fifth expansion, adsorption was minimal, indicating that nearly all the excess material had moved from the reservoir to the surface active film.

Figure 8 shows the effect of SP-A on the incorporation of material from the surface-associated reservoir into the surface active film. The experiment

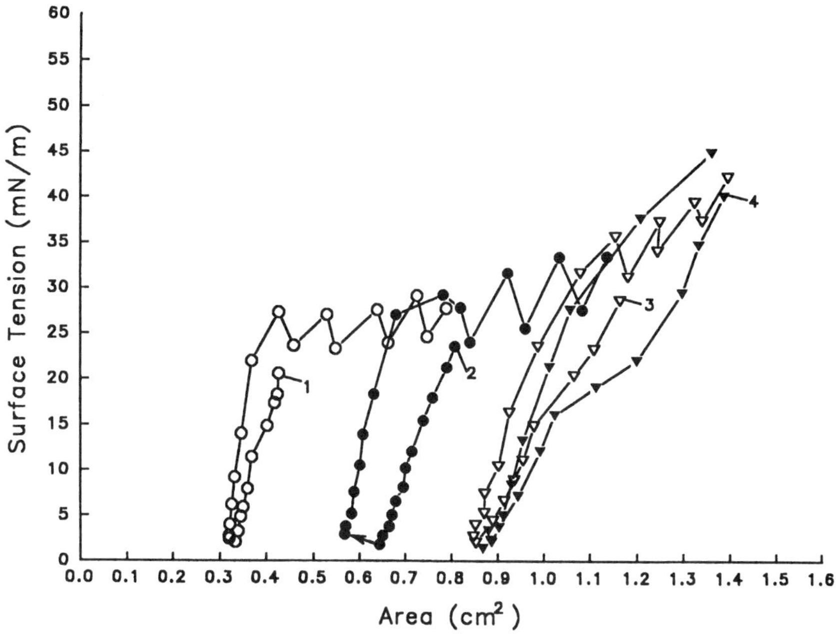

Figure 7 Bovine lipid extract surfactant (bLES). Typical series of consecutive quasi-static compression-expansion cycles conducted at increasing bubble areas in the captive bubble surfactometer, after surfactant depletion and replacement of the subphase with 0.9% NaCl, 1.5 mM $CaCl_2$. Initial bubble formation is 1.0 mg/mL bLES. Numbers (1–4) indicate start of film compression. Peaks represent relatively high surface tensions generated by stepwise, rapid area expansions. Each peak is followed by a decrease in surface tension by adsorption of material from the "surface-associated reservoir." The film area compression to reach near zero tension for the first cycle was 22 and, for the following cycles, 20%, 25%, and 38%. Bubble area at minimum tension for cycles 1 to 4 was approximately three times that of cycle 1. This indicates existence of excess material at the bubble surface after first adsorption.

represents a typical series of consecutive compression-expansion cycles after surfactant depletion for increasing bubble sizes, as described above. However, before the formation of an atmospheric small bubble, 1% SP-A, percent weight relative to the amount of total phospholipid, was added to the suspension, which was incubated while stirring for 5 minutes at 37°C.

The surface tension values after adsorption (2 minutes) for the consecutive isotherms (1–4) were all approximately 25 mN/m. The film area reductions required to achieve near zero (about 1 mN/m) surface tensions were 22%–23% for all four curves. The resulting total amount of material at the interface was equivalent to approximately five monolayers. Whether this additional excess is

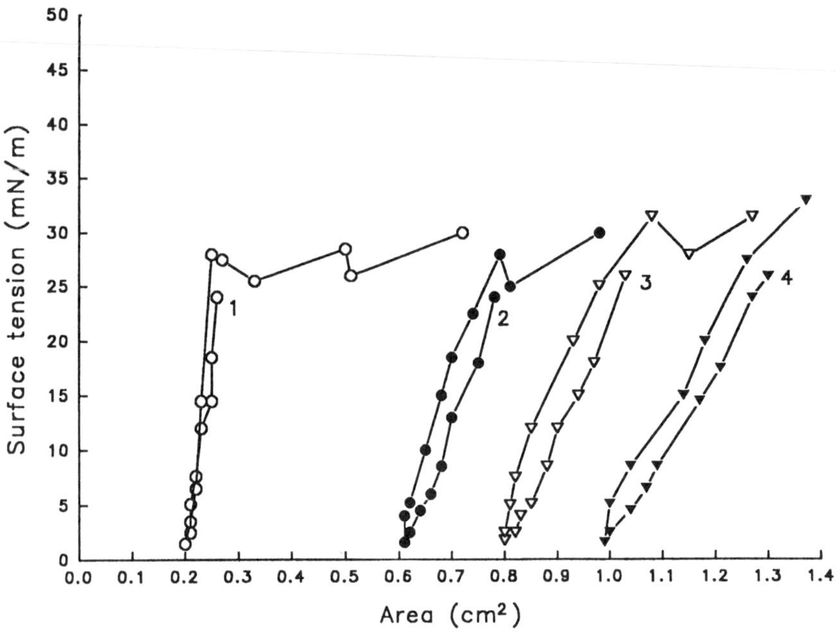

Figure 8 bLES with SP-A. Series of four consecutive quasistatic cycles after adsorption from 1.0 mg/mL bLES with 1% SP-A, followed by surfactant depletion and replacement with a saline-$CaCl_2$ solution. Peaks in surface tension indicated stepwise bubble area expansion followed by adsorption from the "surface-associated reservoir." Film area changes required to achieve near zero tensions were 22%–23% for all four curves. The total amount of surfactant material after initial adsorption was equivalent to five monolayers.

due to the formation of a larger surface-associated reservoir or a more effective incorporation of the material into the surface active film could not be distinguished from these results. The addition of SP-A could lead to the formation of tubular myelin structures (55,56), which remained associated with the interface. Electron microscopic studies are necessary to further investigate this possibility.

ii. Effect of Serum Protein. A number of workers have reported that serum proteins adversely affect surfactant function. Figure 9 represents a typical series of quasistatic cycles of a film formed in the presence of 2.5 mg/mL calf serum protein in a suspension of 1.0 mg/mL bLES in 0.9% NaCl, 1.5 mM $CaCl_2$. The presence of the serum protein resulted in a slower decrease in surface tension, to a final plateau of 28 mN/m, after 5 minutes of adsorption at 37°C. The ability to achieve near zero surface tension was reduced by calf serum protein at the above concentration; the minimum was approximately 10 mN/m. In addition, there was a dramatic effect on the film area reduction required to

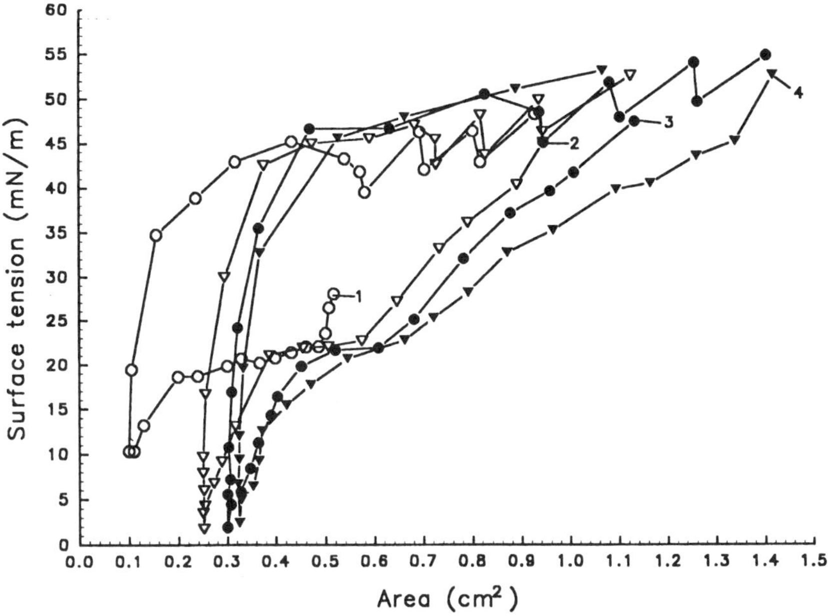

Figure 9 Depletion experiment with bLES and calf serum protein. Effect of calf serum protein on the surface activity of the surface-associated surfactant material, after film formation by adsorption from bLES at 1 mg/mL and calf serum protein at 2.5 mg/mL, both in 0.9% NaCl and 1.5 mM $CaCl_2$, pH 5.5. The surfactant was replaced by the salt solution without surfactant. The film area compression to reach the minimum tension of 10 mN/m from about 28 mN/m was more than 80%. After several expansion-adsorption steps, the area compression needed for the second cycle to compress the film from 28 to near zero minimum tension was about 66%, and, for cycles 3 and 4, about 60%. There was only little increase in the bubble area at near zero minimum surface tension, indicating that little surfactant material adsorbed remained in the film. This is consistent with the "squeeze-out plateau" at approximately 20 mN/m.

compress the film from the equilibrium value of about 30 mN/m (5 minutes of adsorption of 37°C) to the surface tension of approximately 10 mN/m. This area change was about 80%. After stepwise expansion, there was no obvious adsorption initially until the bubble area reached approximately the original bubble size at the start of compression. At that point, the incorporation of material from the reservoir into the interface started, as is seen by the adsorption steps (sawtooth ridge). Upon the second compression, near zero surface tension was achieved after a film area compression of about 74% from the starting point and about 64% from 30 mN/m. Further bubble expansion, as seen from cycles 3 and 4, had only a minimal effect on the surface area at near zero surface tension.

For lower concentrations of calf serum protein added to the bLES suspensions, near zero minimum surface tension was obtained upon the first quasistatic compression but only after relatively large film area compressions. The film area reductions necessary to achieve near zero minimum surface tension increased with increasing concentration of serum protein. These film area reductions were 60% and 73% of the initial bubble area (after adsorption to equilibrium) for calf serum protein concentrations of 0.5 and 1.5 mg/mL, in that order. For higher concentrations of serum protein, near zero minimum surface tension was no longer achieved on the first compression, as seen in Figure 9. However, the mode of bubble expansion appears to determine minimum surface tension, compressibility, and the mechanical stability of films formed from surfactant suspensions with inhibitory proteins added. For these films, the surface activity can be improved by stepwise increases of the film area to values just above the level at which adsorption becomes obvious. The new near-equilibrium position, is illustrated by the low points in the sawtooth ridge on the top of the curves. A continuous slow or fast expansion to the maximum area corresponding to the start position of compression 4 was followed by a much higher minimum surface tension of approximately 20 mN/m (not shown).

Thus, in the presence of serum protein, either very little surface active material entered the surface active film from the reservoir, or the presence of the serum protein prevented the film from attaining a structural arrangement that allows compression through a series of stable mechanical configurations. At present, we do not know whether the process that causes the high compressibility region (plateau at about 20 mN/m) upon compression can be explained by terms such as preferential squeeze-out, film refinement, or other structural modifications. However, depletion experiments demonstrate that the film surface activity is determined to a large degree by the organization of the surface-associated reservoir and that this organization can be optimized to achieve optimal values for film stability, low minimum surface tension, and low film compressibility by choosing a particular mode of film expansion.

When SP-A at 1% (w/w) was added to the bLES suspension of 1 mg/mL in 0.9% NaCl and 1.5 mM $CaCl_2$ with added calf serum protein at 2.5 mg/mL, a completely different series of expansion-compression relations resulted (Figure 10). The characteristics of these films containing SP-A were nearly identical to those without added calf serum protein (see Figure 8).

These depletion experiments and the experiments with low-concentration lipid extract surfactant (see Figure 6C) clearly demonstrate the ability of SP-A to restore the film surface activity when 1. the concentrations are limiting, 2. when the surfactant components are damaged because of peroxidation (47), or 3. when inhibitors from blood protein are present (25,47).

The ability of serum proteins to adversely affect pulmonary surfactant and the physiological consequences of such inactivation is well documented (38,57).

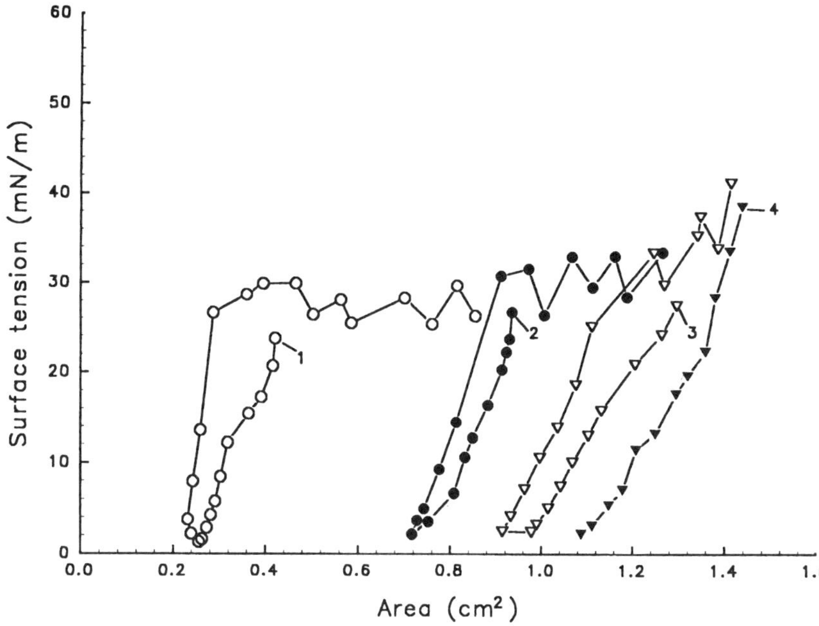

Figure 10 Depletion experiment with bLES, calf serum protein, and SP-A. The inhibitory effect of 2.5 mg calf serum protein on the surface-associated material from 1 mg/mL bLES in 0.9% NaCl and 1.5 mM $CaCl_2$, pH 5.5, was nearly eliminated by the addition of 1% SP-A to the suspension before the washout procedure. The area at near zero minimum surface tension for cycle 4 is approximately four times that of cycle 1, indicating an excess of three monolayers after compression 4.

Holm (57) suggested that, by adsorbing rapidly, serum proteins can monopolize the surface, thereby interfering with phospholipid adsorption. It appears that some serum proteins, like fibrinogen, interact with surfactant components, although the inhibitory mechanism is not clear. Addition of SP-A to lipid extract surfactants counteracts the inhibitory effects of serum proteins, presumably, in part, because of the ability of SP-A to enhance adsorption (58,59). The present studies suggest a mechanism by which serum proteins can limit surfactant function. The depletion experiment illustrated in Figure 9 reveals that, in the presence of serum proteins, the area of the compressed bubble at minimum surface tension remains essentially unaltered with repeated cycling. This demonstrates that, under these conditions, additional surface active material cannot be recruited into the surface active film as discussed above.

It remains to be demonstrated by morphological analysis whether this inactivation has structural consequences, that is, whether the film shows increased polymorphism compared with normal surfactant layers. Figure 9 shows an additional interesting characteristic, namely the appearance of an area of relatively high film compressibility at about 20 mN/m on the compression part of the curves. Such regions have been termed "squeeze-out" plateaus, as previously discussed. The present plateaus cannot be related to the formation of a collapse phase formed by overcompressing films at near zero tension as discussed recently, because the present films were only compressed to minimum surface tension and collapse at that tension was avoided. Figure 9 shows that large film area compressions are required to obtain near zero surface tension, about 70% compared with 20%–25% for normal bLES, indicating interference with a possible surface-associated reservoir resulting from the presence of serum protein.

d. Effect of Calcium on Surfactant Inhibition

Studies with lipid extract surfactant (48) have shown that films compressed in quasistatic or dynamic fashion beyond the point of collapse at minimum surface tension form a collapse phase of unknown structure, which remains associated with the surface film. This collapse phase represents a reservoir that is not identical to that formed de novo. Its presence reduces adsorption of surfactant from the bulk phase and increases film compressibility during film compression, and it may prevent the ability to the film to achieve near zero minimum surface tension by reducing the mechanical stability of the film, as seen by increased bubble clicking. Reducing overcompression promotes recovery of film material from the collapse phase into the surface active film. This recovery is greatly enhanced by calcium (48).

In the presence of inhibitory agents, films can be overcompressed easily because they may collapse at surface tensions well above near zero minimum values, after only 10%–20% reduction in area. To study the effect of added calcium on surface tension–area relations of lipid extract surfactant films, we conducted a series of dynamic compression-expansion cycles with bLES at 1 mg/mL in 0.9% NaCl in the presence of calf serum protein with or without added calcium at a concentration of 1.5 mM $CaCl_2$. Figures 11 and 12 depict cycles 10, 11, and 12 of 30 consecutive dynamic cycles at 20–30 cpm conducted with total film area compressions of 50%–60%. In Figure 11, the surfactant suspensions contained 20 mg/mL calf serum protein and no additional calcium. With progressive cycling, the area compressions had to be increased to more than 80% to achieve minimum surface tensions, which remained between 18 and 20 mN/m. In contrast, in Figure 12, when calcium was added at 1.5 mM to the surfactant with serum, very different surface tension–area characteristics resulted. Near zero minimum surface tensions were obtained upon a film area compression of about 25% from 25 mN/m to the minimum. The stationary loops demonstrate the beneficial effect of added calcium, probably by enhancing recovery of the collapse material into the surface active film.

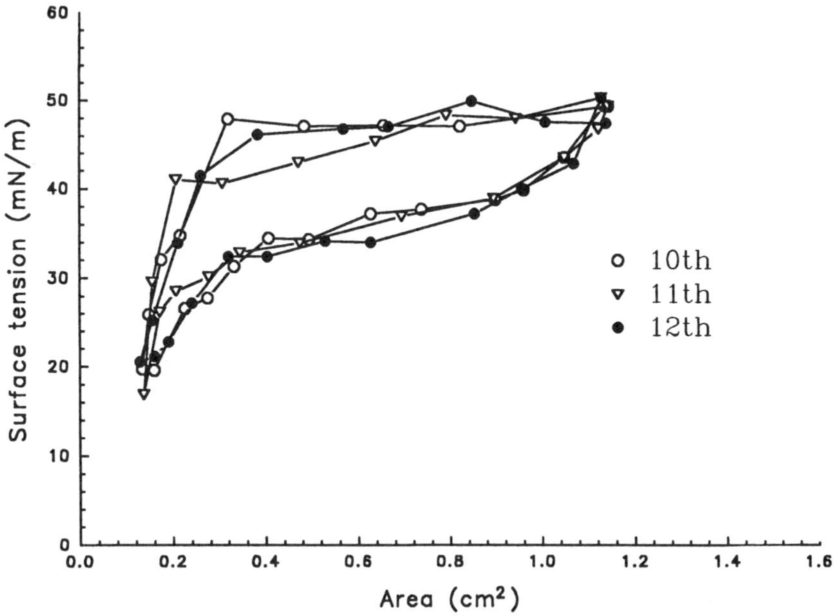

Figure 11 Dynamic cycles at 20–30 cpm, centering on number 11, at bLES at 1 mg/mL and 20 mg/mL calf serum protein, in 0.9% NaCl, pH 5.5. Note the large area compression (more than 80%) required to reach minimum surface tension of 17 mN/m. No extra calcium was added.

In the present work, we have drawn attention to the formation of an active surface-associated reservoir; however, the significance of this reservoir in lung function has not yet been determined. Additional work that combines biophysical, biochemical approaches with structural analysis is required.

B. Complexity of Film Formation: The Role of SP-B and SP-C

Both SP-B and SP-C enhance lipid adsorption to equilibrium, but the mechanisms by which adsorption is promoted by SP-B or SP-C have not been clarified (60,61). SP-B but not SP-C induces fusion of lipid vesicles (62). SP-B appears to interact specifically with acidic phospholipids like phosphatadylglycerol (63–66). The positively charged head groups near the N-terminal of SP-C could interact with negatively charged lipids, but this is less certain (62,67). Studies conducted with the pulsating bubble surfactometer suggested that SP-C enhances adsorption of surfactant phospholipids into the surface active film (63–65). In contrast, recent studies in which spread monolayers of DPPC : PG containing SP-B or SP-C were compressed in a Langmuir-Wilhelmy surface balance sug-

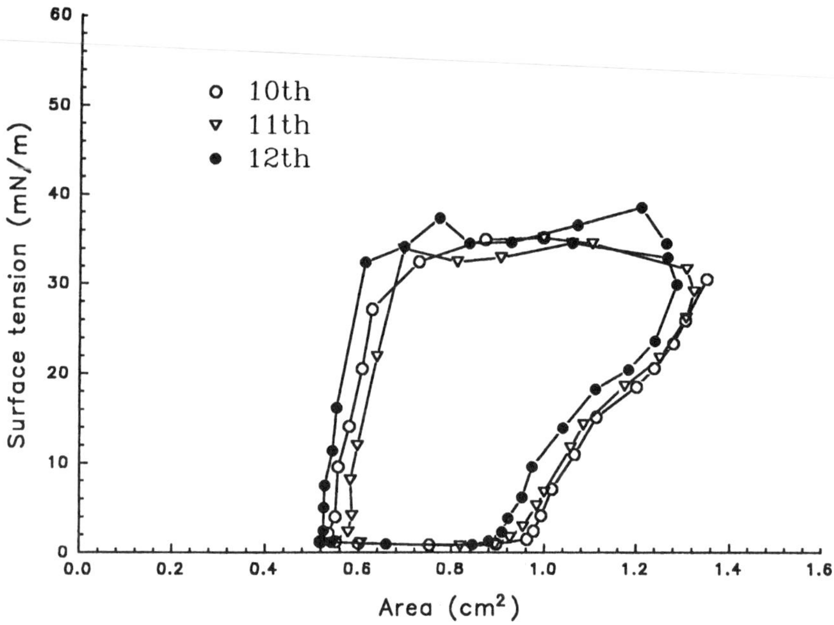

Figure 12 Dynamic cycles at 20–30 cpm, centering on number 11, of bLES at 1 mg/mL and 20 mg/mL calf serum protein, in 0.9% NaCl and 1.5 mM $CaCl_2$, pH 5.5. Hysteresis cycles were performed with a total area compression of approximately 55%. The area compression required to compress the film from 32 to 1 mN/m was 27%. Note the low minimum surface tension and small area compression needed to reach near zero surface tension.

gested that SP-C does not enhance lipid adsorption but was effective in purifying the film by removing non-DPPC phospholipid from the surface film at high surface pressures (68). These apparently conflicting conclusions can be readily resolved by considering the possibility of selected adsorption of DPPC into the surface active film in the pulsating bubble studies.

Oosterlaken-Dijksterhuis et al. (69) have reported that SP-B and SP-C promoted incorporation of lipid vesicles associated with the surface into preformed phospholipid monolayers at surface tensions below equilibrium, demonstrating that these hydrophobic proteins are involved in film formation. These workers observed that phospholipid vesicles associated with monolayers are tightly bound and are highly resistant to flushing even in the absence of calcium. These observations are in excellent agreement with the present concept of a surface-associated reservoir that supplies highly surface active material to the surface active film during film expansion.

To obtain further insight into potential mechanisms involved in the formation of the surface-associated reservoir and the incorporation (adsorption) of material from this reservoir into the surface active film, studies were conducted with a lipid mixture containing the major surfactant phospholipids, DPPC and PG 7:3 by weight, dispersed in 0.9% NaCl, 1.5 mM $CaCl_2$, pH 6.0 (Figure 13). Several differences were noted between the properties of the DPPC:PG 7:3 and the lipid extract surfactants bLES and Curosurf. First, whereas the lipid extract surfactants achieved equilibrium surface tensions in seconds, the lipid mixtures reached a plateau at a surface tension of 34 mN/m in 5 minutes by adsorption. This difference can be attributed to the ability of the low-molecular-weight hydrophobic proteins SP-B and SP-C to enhance surface film formation. Furthermore, to attain surface tensions near zero, the area of the surface film derived from the lipid mixture had to be reduced by 70%–80% during the first compression from 34 mN/m and by greater amounts during subsequent com-

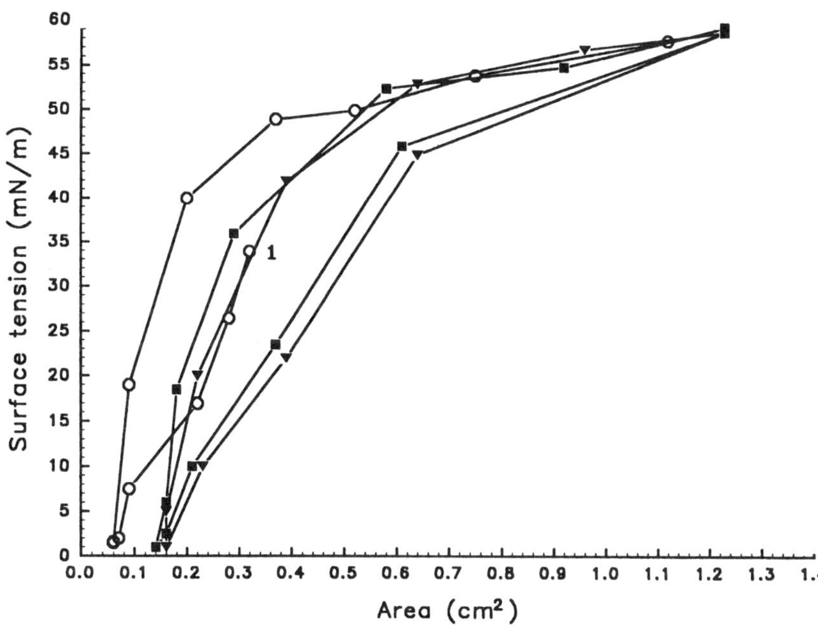

Figure 13 DPPC:PG, 7:3 by weight. Series of five consecutive quasistatic cycles after 5 minutes of adsorption to 34 mN/m (start of cycle 1). Cycles 1, 2, and 3 are shown; cycles 4 and 5 were equivalent to cycles 2 and 3. There was negligible adsorption on stepwise area expansion. Film area compressions required to achieve near zero surface tension remained between 80% and 90%. The total amount of surfactant material, after initial adsorption, was equivalent to approximately 1.5 monolayers.

pressions. In contrast, films formed from lipid extract surfactants at equilibrium require only a 20% reduction in surface area to achieve surface tensions of 1–2 mN/m. Hence, these films behave as if they were highly enriched in DPPC. The fact that similar film area compressions for lipid extract surfactant are sufficient to reduce the surface tension to low values in subsequent compressions from larger surface areas indicates that the material incorporated from the surface-associated reservoir does not modify the initial film structure or composition (see Figure 7). Finally, in contrast to the lipid extract surfactants in which surface active material corresponding to several monolayers could be incorporated into the surface film, only material equivalent to approximately half a monolayer could be incorporated from the surface-associated reservoir of the mixed films without the surfactant proteins.

The suggestion that the low-molecular-weight hydrophobic surfactant apoproteins could be involved in the formation of the surface reservoir led to reconstitution studies involving SP-B and SP-C. Preliminary results from depletion experiments revealed that when SP-B (1%, w/w) was added to DPPC : PG 7 : 3, an area reduction of only 28% was sufficient to lower the surface tension from equilibrium (25 mN/m) to less than 1.0 mN/m during the first compression. Furthermore, similar area reductions resulted in surface tensions near zero as the bubble was systematically expanded. Excess material equivalent to approximately two additional monolayers could be incorporated into the surface active film. Reconstitution studies with the captive bubble surfactometer involving DPPC : PG samples containing SP-C (1%, w/w) showed that an area reduction of 40% was required to achieve surface tensions near zero mN/m with the first and subsequent compressions. This value was intermediate between the value of 80% observed with DPPC : PG 7 : 3 alone and the 28% observed with DPPC : PG 7 : 3, containing 1% SP-B. Depletion experiments showed that when SP-C (1%, w/w) was added to DPPC : PG 7 : 3, excess material equivalent to approximately four additional monolayers could be incorporated into the surface active film.

These studies are consistent with the concept that both SP-B and SP-C contribute to alveolar stability, but that these hydrophobic proteins contribute distinct properties to the alveolar lining layer. SP-B appears to be more effective than SP-C in enhancing selective adsorption of DPPC, whereas SP-C appears to be more effective in promoting incorporation of additional material from the surface-associated reservoir into the surface active film. In addition, SP-C likely enhances the mechanical stability of pulmonary surfactant films at near zero minimum surface tension. This is supported by the recent results of Qanbar and coworkers (70), which demonstrated that mixed films of DPPC and PG possessed greater mechanical stability in the presence of SP-C than when formed in the presence of SP-B or in the absence of the two hydrophobic proteins.

In summary, the surfactant-associated proteins SP-B and SP-C enhance the surfactant film formation by promoting selective adsorption of DPPC and/

or squeeze-out of components other than DPPC upon film compression. SP-B appears more effective than SP-C for selective adsorption, whereas SP-C is more effective than SP-B in stabilizing mechanically the surfactant film at near zero minimum surface tension.

C. Complexity of Film Structure

1. *Alveolar Surface Film In Situ*

Illustrations in textbooks of physiology attribute to the alveolar lining layer the following structural properties: 1. It is a continuous duplex layer consisting of an aqueous hypophase covered by a thin surfactant film. 2. The surfactant film is a monolayer with dipalmitoyl-phosphatidylcholine as the most important component. 3. The surface film is stable in the lung volume range of normal breathing.

There are numerous studies of the structure of the lining layer, all of which are fragmentary. Indeed, the preservation and sample preparation of this delicate structure for microscopy is extremely difficult; there is no standard to distinguish between facts and artifacts, and it is not readily conceivable how monolayers of saturated phospholipids can be preserved and visualized by the usual fixatives (71). As to the first postulate, that is, the existence and continuity of a duplex layer, Weibel and Gil were the first to convincingly demonstrate a two-phase lining layer by transmission electromicroscopy (18–20). They found a hypophase of variable thickness and composition that could best be recognized in the numerous depressions of the epithelial surface and in alveolar corners. The surface film appeared as osmiophilic layer at sites where the hypophase was clearly visible. However, the film was often fragmented and disposed in patches, and could not be detected on flat parts of the alveolar walls. Although studies of freeze-fractured preparations suggested its continuity (72), the exact structure of the lining layer in situ remained a matter of debate. Quite recently, however, Bastacky et al. (23), clearly demonstrated the continuity of the lining layer by low-temperature electron microscopy: it varies from a few nanometers to several micrometers in thickness such that surfactant can be absorbed and spread over the entire surface. Improved tissue preparations resulted also in a better visualization of the surfactant film (Figure 14) such that all evidence available suggests a continuum of the duplex layer.

As to the second postulate, that is, a monolayer as surface film, the structural evidence is scanty. Already the micrographs of Weibel as well as more recent high-power magnifications of the film revealed a polymorphous structure. At some sites, the surface film appears to be an amorphous material; at other sites, triple layers or even multilayers can be recognized, and, generally, it appears to be thicker than a monolayer of phospholipids. Certainly, the latter finding might be an artifact caused by the heavy metals used as staining material.

As to the third postulate, that is, film stability at lower lung volumes, the

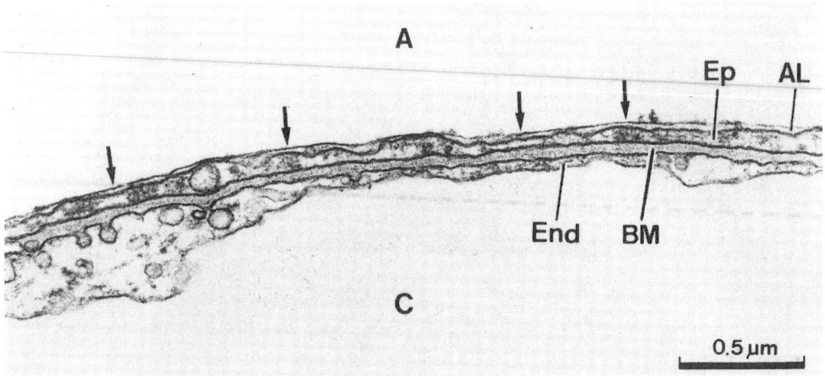

Figure 14 Continuous surface film (*arrows*) covering the thin and flat parts of alveolar septa. In this hexadecane-filled lung, a slight high-pressure edema was induced to augment the hypophase. Abbreviations: A = alveolar space; C = capillary lumen; AL = alveolar liquid (hypophase); Ep = epithelial cell layer; BM = basement membrane; End = endothelial cell layer.

structural findings are not revealing so far. However, microscopic observations of alveolar microdroplets show extremely slow increases in the surface tension and minimal γ-V hysteresis within the volume-range of normal breathing (6,37, 73), thus giving indirect evidence of a rather stable surface film.

2. *Disturbance of the Alveolar Film In Situ*

Normal surfactant can easily be destroyed and washed by rinsing the lung with a detergent solution. The ensuing increase in interfacial tension results in a substantial decrease of alveolar surface area, and conspicuous alterations of alveolar microstructures and micromechanics (74). However, this radical treatment of lung parenchyma is not the objective of this discussion. Of more interest are the effects of hydrophobic liquid films with well-defined surface tensions on lung mechanics, and microstructure, and their interplay with the lining layer. To this aim, normal rabbit lungs were rinsed with the fluorocarbon FC-77 (in vitro surface tension ~15 mN/m) or hexadecane (~25 mN/m) (33). The mechanical behavior and the alveolar microstructure of FC-77 rinsed lungs indicate that the surface forces of surfactant are replaced by FC-77. Electron micrographs showed that osmiophilic lining layers and specks of tubular myelin still were present. However, the surfactant film is not preserved continuously, but frequent fragmentations can be observed, suggesting a "sequestration" of the natural surfactant within the fluorocarbon layer.

In contrast, rinsing lungs with hexadecane results in complex structural and functional alterations. Such lungs exhibit an unusual PV curve: at low lung volumes, the width of the hysteresis is large but decreases with increasing lung volume. The high inflation pressures, which exceed those of fluorocarbon-rinsed lungs, reflect the high surface forces of hexadecane. On deflation, however, the recoil pressures rapidly decrease and approach to values observed in normal air-filled lungs. This remarkable finding can be explained by in vitro experiments and by observations of alveolar microstructures. On deflation of the lung, the alveolar surfactant film still appears to be compressible and hence able to reduce the surface tension. The hexadecane film, overlying the surfactant film on inflation and at high lung volumes, becomes sequestered into small droplets, which are molded into the highly plastic lung tissue at low lung volumes (Figure 15). Certainly, the surfactant film interposed between air and hexadecane is no longer a monolayer but a multilayer. On reinflation of the lung, the surface

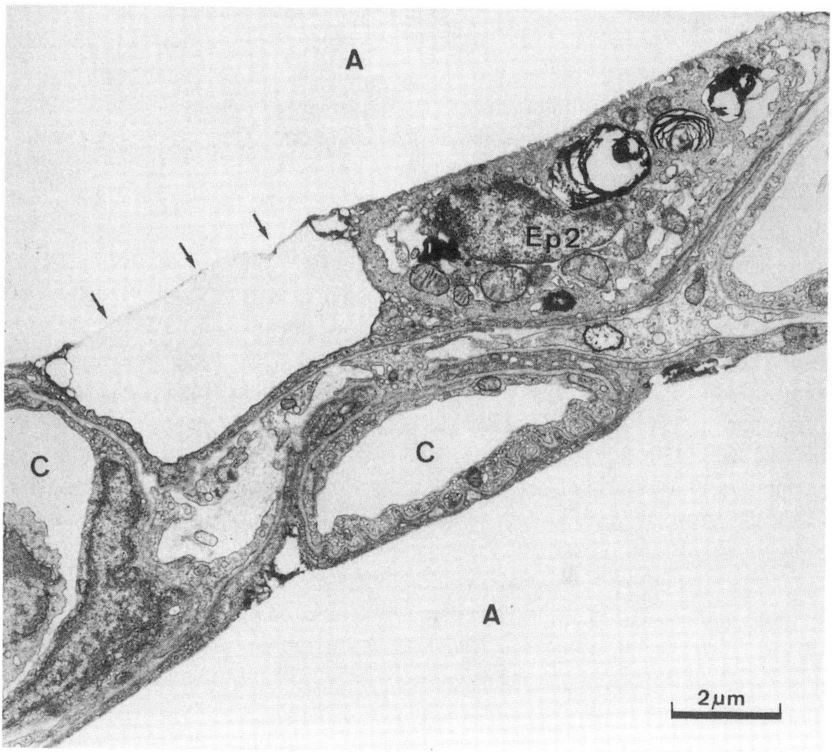

Figure 15 Alveolar septum of air-filled rabbit lung rinsed with hexadecane. Note indentation between epithelial type II cell (Ep 2) and capillary (C, left) covered by a continuous surfactant film. The empty space presumably was filled with (nonfixable) hexadecane. Abbreviations: A = alveolar spaces.

tension rapidly increases and the hexadecane again spreads at the surface and forms the top part of the surface lining layer with a relatively high interfacial tension (>20 mN/m).

These observations demonstrate that the effects of foreign liquids introduced into the lung cannot be predicted exclusively from their surface tension. Other factors, such as molecular size, configuration, and polarity (which also determine the interfacial phenomena with the preexisting surface and also the amount and condition of alveolar surfactant) play a role. All these interactions must be taken into account in the design of therapeutic surfactants (24,33).

3. Surface Film In Vitro: Electron Microscopy

By far, most current knowledge about the biophysical properties of lung surfactant and its biophysical-biochemical relation have been obtained in vitro, that is, by using Langmuir-Wilhelmy balances, pulsating surfactometers, captive bubble techniques, and so on. In addition, the lipid structures of surfactant in solution have been extensively studied (56,75). Few attempts have been made to study the structure–function relationship of surface films in vitro and, in particular, at different points of compression-expansion isotherms. The reason for this lack of experimental data is that the fixation of an extremely fragile surface film together with an undisturbed layer of aqueous hypophase to preserve the molecular arrangement is a seemingly impossible task.

Reiss and collaborators (76) succeeded in transferring pieces of surfactant film from the surface balance to coated copper grids for shadow casting and analysis with the electron microscope. At low degrees of film compression, they found an irregular pattern of islands separated by open spaces. At high compression, that is, at low surface tensions, only inhomogeneous collapsed films with highly irregular surfaces could be observed. These results suggest that the very low surface tensions, which are postulated to exist at low lung volumes, are not compatible with the theory of a smooth, uniform monolayer lining the alveolar surface, but envisage the possibility of metastable films at high degrees of compression (77).

More recently, a new attempt has been made to analyze the structure–function relationship of the surface film of bubbles in a "captive bubble surfactometer." The usual aqueous surfactant suspension (from which surfactant is adsorbed to the surface of the bubble) is replaced by an alginate surfactant suspension. Preliminary experiments have shown that the alginate solution does not interfere with the function of surfactant. By addition of calcium, the alginate solution is solidified together with the bubble and its surface without a detectable change of shape and size. The block is then fixed, cut, and processed for electron microscopy. Some preliminary findings are noteworthy: 1. With a surfactant suspension of low concentration (0.3 mg lipid extract surfactant in 1 mL of alginate solution), only a faint, amorphous, and seemingly fragmented film can be visualized at the bubble surface (Figure 16*A*), although the behavior

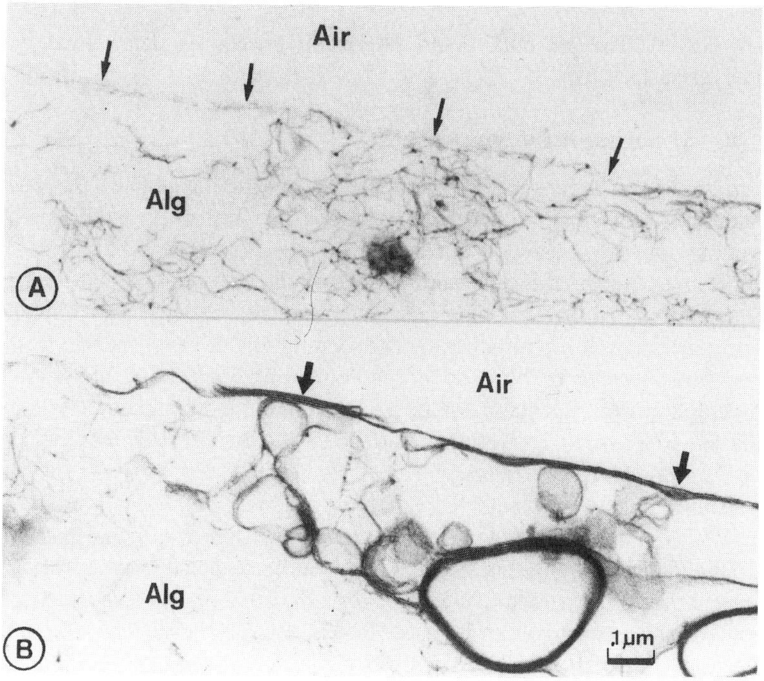

Figure 16 Surfactant films of captive bubbles showing perfect surface activity. **A**, Faint and fragmented surfactant film (*arrows*) if the alginate solution contained 0.3 mg/mL lipid extract surfactant (Curosurf) only. **B**, Conspicuous film formation on suspensions of high concentration (1 mg/mL) with frequent multilayers (*arrows*). Abbreviations: Air = air of captive bubble; Alg = solidified alginate solution.

of the bubble before solidification of its hypophase demonstrated clear-cut surface activity. 2. With suspensions of high concentration (1 mg/mL), a more distinct and continuous film is formed at the bubble surface. Remarkably, this film is of variable thickness, and multilayer formations are frequent (see Figure 16*B*). So far, one can only speculate about these findings, and more research is needed. However, all structural observations indicate that the properties of the alveolar surface film are more complex than those of a simple monolayer.

D. Monolayer and Nonmonolayer Properties of the Surfactant Film

1. *Monolayer Hypothesis*

In the traditional, widely accepted view, the lining layer of surfactant should be composed of two parts, a monomolecular film of phospholipids with partially integrated (SP-B, SP-C) and partially associated specific surfactant proteins

(SP-A, SP-D). The air–bulk liquid interfacial tension is determined by the monolayer surface tension.

2. Monolayer Approximation

According to our recent work (24,26,33) by in situ imaging of the alveolar surfactant with electron microscopy, we found the film to be multilamellar or amorphous, but it was always thicker than the cell membrane of a type I cell. Electron micrographs of the surfaces of air bubbles within a lipid extract surfactant suspension (captive bubbles) disclosed complex structures of the surface film. In particular, at high lipid extract concentrations of the suspensions, multilayered films became visible. The morphological findings are in line with the in vitro depletion experiments using the captive bubble method, showing that surfactant material associated with the interface can be incorporated into the surface active film upon bubble expansion.

Although the surfactant film is partially made up of three or more molecular layers, these layers may be free to slide relative to one another, that is, they are uncoupled, and would not develop mechanical moments because of change of curvature (see Evans and Skalak [78] for a discussion). For this situation, the monolayer approximation can be used, that is, the interfacial area is consistent with a Laplacian shape, as discussed below.

3. Surface Tension: Mechanical Equilibrium

The tension between the vapor phase and the bulk liquid phase in the lung is lowered by the presence of a film at the vapor–liquid interface. The most general interface separating a liquid and a gas or two immiscible liquids will have, at any point, a maximum and a minimum radius of curvature R_1 and R_2, respectively. These are the principal radii of curvature and occur in planes that are perpendicular to each other, and are both perpendicular to the tangent plane to the surface. The Laplace equation of capillarity relates the pressure difference P across the interface at any point to the radii of curvature at the point by

$$P = \gamma(1/R_1 + 1/R_2)$$

where γ is the surface tension for the liquid–gas interface, or the interfacial tension for a fluid–fluid interface (79). The shape of such an interface, even if it is modified by a monolayer or a thin film, is denoted "Laplacian" if the equation above applies to any point of the interface. The Laplace equation describes the equilibrium of the mechanical forces within the interface, even though the system as a whole is often in a termodynamically nonequilibrium state.

Our use of the term "surface tension" follows the theory of Ono and Kondo (80) and of Defay and Prigogin (81). Thus, we use "surface tension" for the vapor–water interfacial tension for any surfactant film whose shape is "Laplacian."

To test whether the shape, for example, of a captive bubble is "Laplacian" we have used the approach by Neumann and associates as originally published by Rotenberg et al. (82). This axisymmetric drop shape analysis (ADSA) has been adapted to many experimental situations (83).

4. Nonmonolayer Properties

The time-dependent response of film or membrane deformation to applied forces is determined by the rate of viscous dissipation in the material. This viscoelastic behavior does not involve irrecoverable (plastic) material deformation (78). The following observations on surfactant films are not consistent with the concept of a monolayer or of a multilayered film in mechanical equilibrium, although the films might be characterized by a "local mechanical equilibrium" (78).

1. There is a small delay in surface tension upon area expansion in dynamically cycled films of lipid extract surfactant, compressed beyond the area at which near zero minimum surface tension is obtained (overcompression) (see Figure 6).
2. Surfactant-associated proteins substantially decreased film compressibility of mixed phospholipid films and modify their structure such that the bubble shape at surface tensions below 1 mN/m clearly starts to deviate from a Laplacian shape.
3. Lipid extract films and phospholipid mixtures with added SP-B and/or SP-C compressed to low surface tension are mechanically far more stable than phospholipid monolayers, DPPC, or mixtures of DPPC and PG in the absence of SP-B or SP-C. Whereas the films with added SP-B and/or SP-C can tolerate mechanical disturbances and revert to the undisturbed original bubble shape in a time-dependent manner at low minimum surface tensions. The bubbles with spread phospholipid monolayers always revert spontaneously and rapidly to higher surface tensions (bubble clicks) upon mechanical deformation by stir bar action in the captive bubble chamber.

III. Summary

There is " surplus" surfactant material at the air–liquid interface upon de novo adsorption of surfactants derived from natural sources. The mode of cycling in vitro and possibly the mode of ventilation of lungs can be chosen such that the excess material can be incorporated into the surface active film. The mechanisms governing this incorporation appear to be influenced by the presence of inhibitory proteins.

The deviation of the bubbles from a Laplacian shape at very low surface tension in combination with the depletion experiments and the morphological observations in situ and in vitro strongly suggest that the surfactant film is not a monomolecular layer. Its mechanical behavior can be estimated by shape analysis of the captive bubble, a method that measures the whole film tension across the interface from the bulk (air) to bulk (fluid) phases.

There is no doubt that future experiments will be directed toward the structural analysis of the surfactant film and toward the role of the surfactant-associated proteins in the three-dimensional organization of the surfactant lipids. The knowledge with regard to the film architecture is most relevant for the understanding of the inhibitory action of blood proteins. We believe that the film structure, its surface activity and resistance to mechanical disturbances, and inhibitory action of blood proteins are determined not only by the biochemical composition of the film but also by its structural modification resulting from the mode of cycling.

Acknowledgments

This work was supported by the Medical Research Council of Canada, the Alberta Heritage Foundation for Medical Research, the Swiss National Science Foundation, and the Stanley Thomas Johnson Foundation. We thank bLES Biochemicals Inc., London, Ontario, and Dr. T. Curstedt, Karolinska Institute, Stockholm, for the lipid extract surfactants bLES and Curosurf, respectively, used in this study.

References

1. von Neergaard K. Neue Auffassungen über einen Grundbegriff der Atemmechanik. Die Retraktionskraft der Lunge, Abhängig von der Oberflächenspannung in den Alveolen. Z Gesamte Exp Med 1929; 66:373–394.
2. Pattle RE. Properties, function and origin of the alveolar lining layer. Nature 1955; 175:1125–1127.
3. Clements JA. Surface tension of lung extracts. Proc Soc Exp Biol Med 1957; 95: 170–172.
4. Avery ME, Mead J. Surface properties in relation to atelectasis and hyaline membrane disease. Am J Dis Child 1959; 97:517–523.
5. Schürch S, Goerke J, Clements JA. Direct determination of surface tension in the lung. Proc Natl Acad Sci U S A 1976; 73:4698–4702.
6. Schürch S, Goerke J, Clements JA. Direct determination of volume- and time-dependence of alveolar surface tension in excised lungs. Proc Natl Acad Sci U S A 1978; 75:3417–3421.
7. Wilson TA, Bachofen H. A model for mechanical structure of the alveolar duct. J Appl Physiol 1982; 52:1064–1070.

8. Van Golde LM, Batenburg JJ, Robertson B. The pulmonary surfactant system: biochemical aspects and functional significance. Physiol Rev 1988; 68:374–455.
9. Johansson J, Curstedt T, Robertson B. The proteins of the surfactant system. Eur Respir J 1994; 7:372–391.
10. Lum H, Mitzner W. A species comparison of alveolar size and surface forces. J Appl Physiol 1987; 62:1865–1871.
11. Keyhani E. The surfactant system of the lung in the Mexican axoloth *Ambystoma mexicanum*. Cell Biol Int Rep 1987; 11:197–204.
12. Kamm RD, Schroter RC. Is airway closure caused by a liquid film instability? Respir Physiol 1989; 75:141–156.
13. Bredenberg CE, Nieman GF, Paskanik AM, Hart KE. Microvascular membrane permeability in high surface tension pulmonary edema. J Appl Physiol 1986; 60: 253–259.
14. Pison U, Max M, Neuendank A, Weissbach S, Pietschmann S. Host defence capacities of pulmonary surfactant: evidence for "non-surfactant" functions of the surfactant system. Eur J Clin Invest 1994; 24:586–599.
15. Pattle RE. Surface tension and the lining of the lung alveoli. In: Caro CG, ed. Advances in Respiratory Physiology. London: Edward Arnold Ltd., 1966.
16. Pattle RE, Thomas LC. Lipoprotein composition of the film lining of the lung. Nature 1961; 189:844–846.
17. Klaus MH, Clements JA, Havel RJ. Composition of surface-active material isolated from beef lung. Proc Natl Acad Sci U S A 1961; 47:1858–1859.
18. Weibel ER, Gil J. Electron microscopic demonstration of an extracellular lining layer of alveoli. Respir Physiol 1968; 4:42–57.
19. Gil J, Weibel ER. Improvements in demonstration of lining layer of lung alveoli by electron microscopy. Respir Physiol 1969/70; 8:13–36.
20. Gil J, Weibel ER. Extracellular lining of bronchioles after perfusion-fixation of rat lungs for electron microscopy. The Anatomical Record 1971; 169(2):185–200.
21. Grossmann G, Robertson B. Lung expansion and the formation of the alveolar lining layer in the full-term newborn rabbit. Acta Paediatr Scand 1975; 64:7–16.
22. Ueda S, Ishii N, Masumoto S, Hayashi K, Okayasu M. Ultrastructural studies on surface lining layer of the lungs: part II. J Jpn Med Soc Biol Interface 1983; 14: 30–35.
23. Bastacky J, Lee CYC, Goerke J, Koushafar H, Yager D, Kenaga L, Speed TP, Chen Y, Clements JA. Alveolar lining layer is thin and continuous: low-temperature scanning electron microscopy of rat lung. J Appl Physiol 1995; 79(5):1615–1628.
24. Schürch S, Bachofen H. Biophysical aspects in the design of therapeutic surfactant. In: Robertson B, Taeusch HW, eds. Surfactant therapy for lung disease. In: Lenfant C, ed. Lung Biology in Health and Disease. New York: Marcel Dekker, 1995: 3–32.
25. Schürch S, Qanbar R, Bachofen H, Possmayer F. The surface associated surfactant reservoir in the alveolar lining. Biol Neonate 1995; 67(suppl 1):61–76.
26. Bachofen H, Schürch S, Michel RP, Weibel ER. Experimental hydrostatic pulmonary edema in rabbit lungs. Morphology. Am Rev Respir Dis 1993; 147:989–996.

27. Schürch S, Bachofen H, Goerke J, Possmayer F. A captive bubble method reproduces the in situ behavior of lung surfactant monolayers. J Appl Physiol 1992; 67: 2389–2396.
28. Schürch S, Bachofen H, Goerke J, Green F. Surface properties of rat pulmonary surfactant studied with the captive bubble method: adsorption, hysteresis, stability. Biochim Biophys Acta 1992; 1103:127–136.
29. Hoppin FG Jr, Hilderbrandt J. Mechanical properties of the lung. In: West J, ed. Bioengineering Aspects of the Lung. New York: Marcel Dekker, 1977:83–162.
30. Hoppin FG Jr, Stothert JC Jr, Greaves IA, Lai YL, Hildebrandt J. Lung recoil: elastic and rheological properties. In: Handbook of Physiology. The Respiratory System. Mechanics of Breathing. Vol. III. Part 1. Bethesda, MD: American Physiological Society, 1986: 195–215.
31. Horie T, Hildbrandt J. Dynamic compliance, limit cycles, and static equilibria of excised cat lung. J Appl Physiol 1971; 31:423–430.
32. Bachofen H, Hildebrandt J, Bachofen M. Pressure-volume curves of air- and liquid-filled excised lungs—surface tension in situ. J Appl Physiol 1970; 29:422–431.
33. Bachofen H, Schürch S, Possmayer F. Disturbance of alveolar lining layer: effects on alveolar microstructures. J Appl Physiol 1994; 76:1983–1992.
34. Weibel ER. Functional morphology of lung parenchyma. In: Handbook of Physiology. The Respiratory System. Mechanics of Breathing. Vol. III. Part 1. Bethesda, MD: American Physiological Society, 1986:89–111.
35. Schürch S. Surface tension at low lung volumes: dependence on time and alveolar size. Respir Physiol 1982; 48:339–355.
36. Bachofen H, Ammann A, Wangensteen D, Weibel ER. Perfusion fixation of lungs for structure-function analysis: credits and limitations. J Appl Physiol 1982; 53: 528–533.
37. Bachofen H, Schürch S, Urbinelli M, Weibel ER. Relations among alveolar surface tension, surface area, volume and recoil pressure. J Appl Physiol 1987; 62:1878–1887.
38. Robertson B. Animal models in neonatal surfactant dysfunction. In: Robertson B, Van Golde LMG, Batenburg JJ, eds. Pulmonary Surfactant: From Molecular Biology to Clinical Practice. Amsterdam: Elsevier, 1992:459–484.
39. Goerke J, Clements JA. Alevolar surface tension and lung surfactant. In: Handbook of Physiology. The Respiratory System. Mechanics of Breathing. Vol. III. Part 1. Bethesda, MD: American Physiological Society 1986:247–261.
40. Enhorning GA. A pulsating bubble technique for evaluating pulmonary surfactant. J Appl Physiol 1977; 43:198–201.
41. Goerke J, Gonzales J. Temperature dependence of dipalmitoyl phosphatidylcholine monolayer stability. J Appl Physiol 1971; 51:1108–1114.
42. Clements JA, Hustead RF, Johnson RP, Gribetz I. Pulmonary surface tension and alveolar stability. J Appl Physiol 1961; 16:444–450.
43. Schoedel W, Slama H, Hansen E. Zeitabhängiges Verhalten von Filmen von oberflächenaktivem Material aus Lungenalveolen. Pflügers Arch 1971; 322:336–346.
44. Qiu R, MacDonald RC. A nonleak trough for monolayers at the air/water interface. Rev Sci Instrum 1994; 65:500–502.
45. Putz G, Goerke J, Taeusch HW, Clements JA. Comparison of captive- and pulsat-

ing-bubble surfactometers using lung surfactant. J Appl Physiol 1994; 76:1425–1431.
46. Schoel WM, Schürch S, Goerke J. The captive bubble method for the evaluation of pulmonary surfactant: surface tension, area and volume calculations. Biochim Biophys Acta 1994; 1200:281–290.
47. Schürch S, Possmayer F, Cheng S, Cockshutt AM. Pulmonary SP-A enhances adsorption and appears to induce surface sorting of lipid extract surfactant. Am J Physiol 1992; 263:L210–L218.
48. Schürch S, Schürch D, Curstedt T, Robertson B. Surface activity of lipid extract surfactant in relation to film area compression and collapse. J Appl Physiol 1994; 77:974–986.
49. Putz G, Goerke J, Clements JA. Surface activity of rabbit pulmonary surfactant subfractions to different concentrations in a captive bubble. J Appl Physiol 1994; 77(2):597–605.
50. Keough KMW, Farrell E, Cox M, Harrell G, Tauesch HW. Physical, chemical and physiological characteristics of isolates of pulmonary surfactant from adult rabbits. Can J Physiol Pharmacol 1985; 63:1043–1051.
51. Keough KMW. Physical chemistry of pulmonary surfactant in the terminal air spaces. In: Robertson B, Van Golde LMG, Batenburg JJ, eds. Pulmonary Surfactant: From Molecular Biology to Clinical Practice. Amsterdam: Elsevier, 1992:109–164.
52. Callen HB. Thermodynamics. New York: John Wiley, 1960:1–376.
53. Boonman A, Machiels FHJ, Snik AFM, Egberts J. Squeeze-out from mixed monolayers of dipalmitoyl phosphatidylcholine and egg phosphatidylglycerol. J Colloid Interface Sci 1987; 120:456–468.
54. Egberts J, Sloot H, Mazure A. Minimal surface tension, squeeze-out and transition temperatures of binary mixtures of dipalmitoyl phosphatidylcholine and unsaturated phospholipids. Biochim Biophys Acta 1989; 1002:109–113.
55. Suzuki Y, Fujita Y, Kogishi K. Reconstitution of tubular myelin from synthetic lipids and proteins associated with pig pulmonary surfactant. Am Rev Respir Dis 1989; 140:75–81.
56. Williams MC, Hawgood S, Hamilton RL. Changes in lipid structure produced by surfactant proteins SP-A, SP-B, and SP-C. Am J Respir Cell Mol Biol 1991; 5: 41–50.
57. Holm BA. Surfactant inactivation in adult respiratory distress syndrome. In: Robertson B, Van Golde LMG, Batenburg JJ, eds. Pulmonary Surfactant: From Molecular Biology to Clinical Practice. Amsterdam: Elsevier, 1992:665–684.
58. Cockshutt AM, Weitz JL, Possmayer F. Pulmonary surfactant-associated protein A enhances the surface activity of lipid extract surfactant and reverses inhibition by blood proteins in vitro. Biochemistry 1990; 29:8424–8429.
59. Venkitaraman AR, Hall SB, Whitsett JA, Notter RH. Enhancement of biophysical activity of lung surfactant extracts and phospholipid-apoprotein mixtures by surfactant protein A. Chem Phys Lipids 1990; 56:185–194.
60. Possmayer F. The role of surfactant-associated proteins. Am Rev Respir Dis 1990; 142:749–752.
61. Haagsman HP. Structure-function relationships in lung surfactant: protein-lipid interactions. Progr Respir Res 1994; 27:15–24.

62. Shiffer K, Hawgood S, Haagsman HP, Benson B, Clements JA, Goerke J. Lung surfactant proteins SP-B and SP-C altered the thermodynamic properties of phospholipid membranes: a differential colorimetry study. Biochemistry 1993; 32:590–597.
63. Yu S-H, Possmayer F. Comparative studies on the biophysical activities the low-molecular-weight hydrophobic proteins purified from bovine pulmonary surfactant. Biochim Biophys Acta 1988; 961:337–350.
64. Yu S-H, Possmayer F. Role of bovine pulmonary surfactant-associated proteins in the surface active property of phospholipid mixtures. Biochim Biophys Acta 1990; 1046:233–241.
65. Yu S-H, Possmayer F. Effect of pulmonary surfactant protein B (SP-B) and calcium on phospholipid adsorption and squeeze-out of phosphatidylglycerol from binary phospholipid monolayers containing dipalmitoylphosphatidylcholine. Biochim Biophys Acta 1992; 1126:26–34.
66. Baatz JE, Elledge B, Whitsett JA. Surfactant protein SP-B induces ordering at the surface of model membrane bilayers. Biochemistry 1990; 29:6714–6720.
67. Simatos GA, Forward KB, Morrow MR, Keough KMW. Interactions between perduterated dimeristol phosphatidylcholine and low molecular weight pulmonary surfactant protein SP-C. Biochemistry 1990; 29:5807–5814.
68. Taneva S, Keough KMV. Pulmonary surfactant proteins SP-B and SP-C in spread monolayers at the air-water interface. I. Monolayers of pulmonary surfactant protein SP-B and phospholipids. Biophys J 1994; 66:1137–1148.
69. Oosterlaken-Dijksterhuis MA, Haagsman HP, Van Golde LMG, Demel RA. Characterization of lipid insertion into monomolecular layers mediated by lung surfactant proteins SP-B and SP-C. Biochemistry 1991; 30:10965–10971.
70. Qanbar R, Cheng S, Possmayer F, Schürch S. The role of the palmitoylation of surfactant-associated protein C in surfactant film formation and stability. Am J Physiol (Lung Cell Mol Physiol 15) 1996; 271:L572–L580.
71. Dermer GB. The fixation of pulmonary surfactant for electron microscopy. J Ultrastruct Res 1969; 27:88–104.
72. Untersee P, Gil J, Weibel ER. Visualization of extracellular lining layer of lung alveoli by freeze etching. Respir Physiol 1971; 13:171–185.
73. Schürch S, Bachofen H, Weibel ER. Alveolar surface tensions in excised rabbit lungs: effect of tmeperature. Respir Physiol 1985; 62:31–45.
74. Bachofen H, Gehr P, Weibel ER. Alterations of mechanical properties and morphology in excised rabbit lungs rinsed with a detergent. J Appl Physiol 1979; 47: 1002–1010.
75. Chapman D, Fluck DJ. Physical studies of phospholipids. III. Electron microscope studies of some pure fully saturated 2,3-diacyl-dl-phosphatidyl-ethanolamines and phosphatidylcholines. J Cell Biol 1966; 30:1–11.
76. Reiss OK, Paul GW, Gil J. An electron microscopic study of thin films of alveolar surfactants and dipalmitoyl phosphatidylcholine: film collapse at high surface pressures. Prog Respir Res 1984; 18:29–35.
77. Wolfe DH, Brockman HL. Regulation of the surface pressure of lipid monolayers and bilayers by the activity of water: derivation and application of an equation of state. Proc Natl Acad Sci U S A 1988; 85:4285–4289.

78. Evans EA, Skalak R. Mechanics and Thermodynamics of Biomembranes. Boca Raton, FL: CRC Press, 1980:1–254.
79. Adamson AW. Physical Chemistry of Surfaces. 4th ed. New York: John Wiley, 1982:1–664.
80. Ono S, Kondo S. Molecular theory of surface tension in liquids. In: Flügge S, ed. Encyclopedia of Physics. Berlin: Springer Verlag 1960:134–280.
81. Defay R, Prigogine I. Surface Tension and Adsorption. New York: John Wiley & Sons, 1966.
82. Rotenberg YL, Boruvka L, Neumann AW. Determination of surface tension and contact angle from the shapes of axisymmetric fluid interfaces. J Colloid Interface Sci 1983; 93:169–183.
83. Skinner FK, Rotenberg Y, Neumann AW. Contact angle measurement from the contact diameter of sessile drops by means of a modified axisymmetric drop shape analysis. J Colloid Interface Sci 1989; 130:25–34.

3

Parenchymal Macromechanics

THEODORE A. WILSON

University of Minnesota
Minneapolis, Minnesota

I. Introduction

The study of the mechanical properties of the lung began with the measurement of the pressure-volume (PV) curve (1). The PV curve provides fundamental, but limited, information about the mechanics of lung parenchyma. It provides the data that are required for the simplest model of parenchymal mechanics, the model in which the parenchyma is described as a uniform isotropic material that is uniformly inflated.

The realization that the lung does not expand uniformly stemmed from Fowler's observation that the concentration of nitrogen in the gas expired after a breath of oxygen is not constant; it continues to increase during the course of expiration (2). From this, Fowler deduced that the residual nitrogen in the lung must be diluted by the delivery of different amounts of oxygen to different regions and that different regions must empty asynchronously, with regions with lower nitrogen concentrations contributing a bigger fraction of expired gas at the beginning of expiration than at the end. Nonuniform lung expansion was first explained by a model that stayed within the bounds of the PV description of lung mechanics (3). It was argued that the weight of the lungs must be supported and, therefore, that pleural pressure must be higher at the bottom of the lung than at the top. The vertical gradient in pleural pressure, and hence in transpulmonary pressure (Ptp), placed different regions at different points on the PV curve. Because lung compliance increases as transpulmonary pressure decreases, the base of the lung, where pleural pressure is larger and transpulmonary pressure is smaller, is more compliant at the beginning of expiration than the apex and reaches residual volume earlier in expiration than the apex. Thus, the base contributes more at the beginning, and the apex contributes more toward the end of expiration. Studies using radioactive xenon showed differences in regional expansion that were consistent with the predictions of this model, and the predicted vertical gradient of pleural pressure was observed. The model was never tested quantitatively by comparing gas mixing predicted from the model against nitrogen washout data, and for many years, it remained the accepted model for nonuniform lung expansion despite observations that did not fit the model; in particular, the observation that expired gas collected from airways that fed regions too small to be affected by the gravitational gradient also showed an increasing nitrogen concentration (4).

Interest in the gravitational distortion of the lung led to questions about the mechanics of lung distortion. Methods that had been developed to analyze the deformation of engineering materials were applied to the lung. Lung parenchyma was modeled as a linear isotropic elastic material (5,6). In this model, the mechanical properties of the lung are described by two elastic moduli: the bulk modulus and shear modulus. The bulk modulus was obtained from the PV curve, and the shear modulus was obtained by measuring the force required to indent the surface of the lung. This model entails some simplifications. For example, nonlinearities associated with the large strains that occur in the lung are only partially included in the model by allowing the elastic moduli to depend on lung volume, and hysteresis is usually ignored. Nonetheless, with this model, the techniques of engineering analysis of deformable materials could be brought to bear, and this has been helpful in analyzing the deformations and stress distributions around inclusions such as vessels and bronchi as well as in analyzing the gravitational deformation of the lung.

The PV curve and the linear elasticity model provide empirical descriptions of the average macroscopic properties of lung parenchyma. Studies of the micromechanical source of these macromechanical properties have been constant companions to the empirical studies. These studies have included the measurement of PV curves of lungs that were filled or rinsed with fluids of different surface tension (7,8), measurement of surface tension in situ (9–11), measurements of alveolar surface area as a function of lung volume (12–14) and in distorted lungs (15) and lungs with altered surface tension (7,16), measurements of the geometry of the acinus (17) and the alveolar septal junctions (18,19), and measurements of the mechanical properties of the pleural membrane (20,21) and of the distribution of elastin and collagen (22–24). Efforts to incorporate these data into models of parenchymal mechanics and to deduce the contributions of tissue and surface forces to lung recoil have a long history. In fact, the first modeling of the micromechanics of shear deformations (25) preceded the measurement of the shear modulus (6).

In the work described above, lung properties were assumed to be uniform. To be sure, structural heterogeneities such as the pleural membrane and the bronchial and vascular trees were recognized, but parenchymal properties, averaged over a sample larger than several alveoli, were assumed to be uniform. The first direct evidence that the lung expands nonuniformly, independent of nonuniformities of transpulmony pressure, was obtained by the parenchymal marker technique in 1983 (26). In this technique, radiopaque markers are implanted in the parenchyma, and the markers are tracked by biplane video fluoroscopy. During deflation from total lung capacity (TLC), regional rates of emptying were found to vary by ±10% from the mean. In the supine dog, a vertical gradient of regional emptying was observed, but this accounted for only 30% of the total variability. Because these results were unexpected, the authors searched for a spatial organization for the nongravitational component of the variability of regional expansion, but with no success. It appears that this variability has a scale as small as an acinus and no large-scale spatial organization. Using these new techniques, the earlier work on the gravitational gradient of ventilation was confirmed, but the gravitational gradient was shown to be the smaller component of the total variability. Recent reports of gas mixing experiments in humans under zero gravity conditions aboard Spacelab SLS-1 are consistent with this conclusion (27). Presumably, nonuniform parenchymal expansion is caused by nonuniformities in the volume densities of connective tissue and surface area, but, at this point, no data on the nonuniformity of lung morphology are available.

Recently, attention has returned to an aspect of parenchymal macromechanics that is poorly understood, that is, active changes in parenchymal properties. It has been known for some time that lung compliance changes during bronchoconstriction. Severinghaus et al. (28), in their seminal paper on hypocapnic bronchoconstriction, pointed out that, at resting breathing frequencies, resistance is a small part of lung impedance, and ventilation is determined by lung elastance. They concluded that changes in lung elasticity, not changes in airway resistance, caused the shifts in ventilation that followed shifts in perfusion. A much stronger state of bronchoconstriction can be produced by exposing the lung to bronchoconstricting drugs. It has been difficult to sort out the contributions of airway resistance and parenchymal elasticity to the large changes in lung impedance that occur during severe bronchoconstriction, but it appears that bronchoconstriction can cause lung recoil and elastance to increase by up to 50% (29,30), about the same magnitude as the changes associated with hypocapnic bronchoconstriction. A variety of micromechanical mechanisms for the active component of parenchymal elastance have been suggested, but these suggestions are speculative.

This chapter addresses each of the topics mentioned in this introduction. First, current knowledge about average parenchymal mechanical properties and current understanding of the micromechanical source of these properties are reviewed. Then, lung deformations, including gravitational deformations and local deformations around airways and vessels, are described. Finally, in a more speculative section, the source of the active component of parenchymal elastance is discussed. Some important topics in parenchymal mechanics, such as dissipative mechanisms (31) and parenchymal stability (32), are not discussed.

II. The Pressure–Volume Curve

A. Macroscopic Properties

A typical PV curve is shown in Figure 1. The curve shows an inflation limb initiated from functional residual capacity (FRC) and the deflation limb returning from TLC to FRC. Smaller tidal volume loops initiated from 40% and 60% TLC on the deflation limb are also shown. At a given volume, the pressure is higher on the inflation than the deflation limb of any PV loop. The area of the

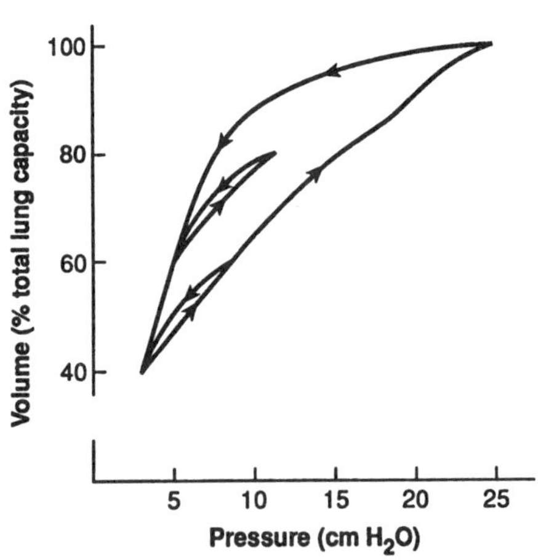

Figure 1 Pressure-volume (PV) curve of the lung. Pressure depends on volume, volume history, and direction of volume change. Pressure is higher on the inflation limb of a PV loop than on the deflation limb. The area within a PV loop, as a fraction of the area of the rectangle enclosing the loop, is smaller for smaller volume excursions than for larger volume excursions.

loops, as a fraction of the rectangle enclosing the loops, is smaller for smaller tidal volumes than for the large volume excursion to TLC.

Figure 1 shows that the volume elasticity of the lung cannot be described simply; it depends on volume, volume history, and the direction of volume change. Two methods have been used to describe volume elasticity. In the first, approximations are made to obtain a description that is consistent with classical elasticity (5). A bulk modulus K is defined as the increase in pressure per fractional increase in volume, V(dP/dV). K is allowed to be a function of lung volume, and K(V) is determined from the mean slope of small tidal volume loops at each volume (6). In the second, quasielastic model, different PV trajectories are allowed for inflation and deflation (33). The second is more accurate, but it is more difficult to apply.

The bulk modulus K increases with increasing lung volume because the stiffnesses of the tissue and surface forces increase with increasing volume and because stiff collagen fibers are slack at lower lung volume and become taught at higher lung volume. The elastic moduli have units of pressure, and it is convenient to relate the values of K to the value of Ptp. K increases more rapidly than linearly with Ptp, but in the mid range of lung volumes, the value of K is approximately 4 Ptp.

B. Structural Morphology

Weibel (34) states that "the mechanical properties of lung parenchyma are determined to a large extent—though not exclusively—by a tension skeleton made of connective tissue fibers that pervade the lung according to a strictly hierarchical design pattern." He identifies three components of the tissue structure: 1. an axial fiber system that runs along the airways and extends from the terminal bronchioles to form cables at the free edges of the alveolar openings, 2. a peripheral system that consists of the pleural membrane and extensions that penetrate the lung to form intersegmental septa and sheaths around the airways, and 3. a network of fine septal fibers that interweave with the capillary network in the alveolar walls. A schematic diagram of these components is shown in Figure 2. Tension in these tissue components provides part of the recoil pressure of the lung.

Surface tension at the air–liquid interface that covers the alveolar walls provides a second contribution to lung recoil. Although surface tension in the lung is low, of the order of a few dynes per centimeter, surface area density is high, of the order of hundreds of square centimeters per milliliters, and surface energies are comparable to recoil pressure. Data on surface area and surface tension versus lung volume are shown in Figure 3. These data show that surface area depends on both lung volume and surface tension. Because surface

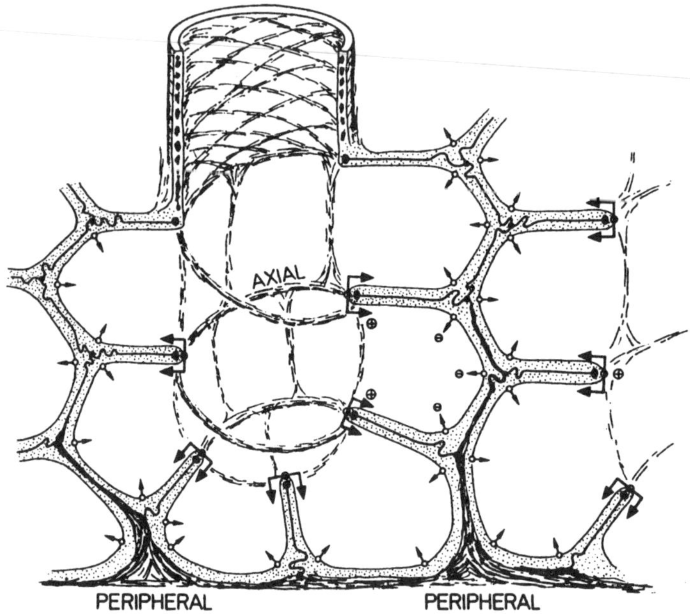

Figure 2 Schematic diagram of the tissue structure of the lung. The peripheral tissue system includes the pleural membrane and extensions of the membrane that penetrate the lung and connect to the outer sheaths of the airways. The axial fiber system extends from the airways to form cables that define the alveolar openings. The action of surface forces on the tissue cables at the free ends of alveolar walls is shown by arrows. (From Ref. 34. Reprinted with permission. Copyright 1984 by the President and Fellows of Harvard College.)

tension depends on surface area and surface area changes with lung volume, surface tension changes with volume.

C. Contributions of Tissue Forces and Surface Tension to Recoil

Weibel's description of the tissue structure of parenchyma and data on surface area and surface tension have been incorporated into a model that describes the mechanics of the pressure-volume curve (35). This model is reviewed by setting the objective of answering a specific question: What are the contributions of tissue forces and surface tension to recoil pressure at a lung volume of 60% TLC? Recoil pressure at 60% TLC is ~5 cm H_2O. Part of this pressure is balanced by tension in the curved pleural membrane and tension in the extensions of the peripheral fiber system that connect to the outer surface of the

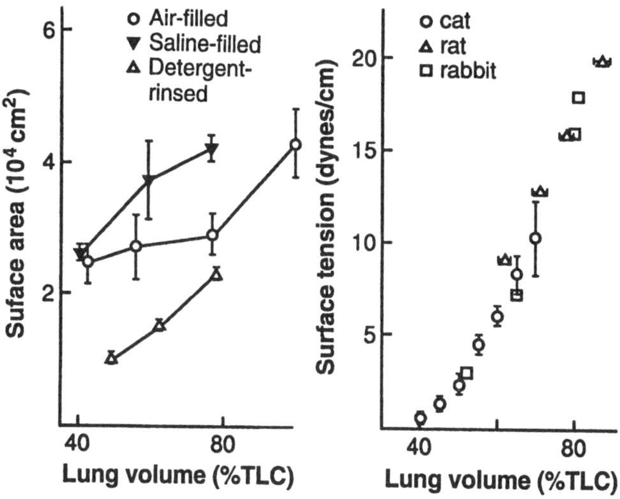

Figure 3 Data on surface area and surface tension versus lung volume. **Left panel**, surface area versus lung volume in saline-filled and air-filled (14) and detergent-rinsed (9) rabbit lungs. Surface area depends on both lung volume and surface tension. **Right panel**, surface tension versus lung volume, as percent total lung capacity (TLC), during deflation from TLC in cat lungs (10), rat lungs (11), and rabbit lungs (8).

bronchial tree, and part is balanced by the stress in the fine tissue structure of the acinus and surface tension on the alveolar walls. First, the contributions of the peripheral fiber system and the bronchial tree to recoil are discussed, and then the contributions of parenchymal tissue and surface forces are described.

The pleural membrane contains ~20% of the elastin and collagen content of the lung (24). Tension in the pleural membrane depends on animal size. In dogs, tension is $\sim 2 \times 10^3$ dynes/cm at a lung volume of 60% TLC (20). From the tension in the pleural membrane and its area, the work of expanding the membrane can be calculated, and, from this, the contribution of the pleural membrane to recoil can be estimated. This calculation yields the result that the pleural membrane contributes ~20% of recoil on the deflation limb. Thus, 1.0 cm H_2O of the total recoil of 5 cm H_2O is assigned to the pleural membrane. The energy required to expand the intraparenchymal extensions of the peripheral tissue system and to extend the bronchial tree is unknown. If tension in these tissues also contributes 1.0 cm H_2O, the peripheral tissue system and the axial tissue system within the conducting airways provide the recoil of the saline-filled lung, 2.0 cm H_2O. This assumption is discussed further at the end of this section.

In the air-filled lung, an additional inward stress of 3 cm H_2O is required to balance transpulmonary pressure. This inward stress is provided by parenchymal attachments. Stress is the force per unit area transmitted across a plane. It can be shown that the force per unit area transmitted across a plane passing through an array of randomly oriented surfaces carrying surface tension γ is ⅔ $\gamma(S/V)$, where S/V is the surface area per unit volume (36). A plane passing through parenchyma also cuts connective tissue cables, and it can be shown that the force per unit area transmitted across a plane by randomly oriented line elements carrying tension T is ⅓ T(L/V), where L/V is the length of the line elements per unit volume (35). Therefore, the total tensile stress in the parenchyma, or equivalently, the total contribution of parenchyma to recoil pressure P_{par}, is given by the following equation:

$$P_{par} = \tfrac{2}{3}\,\gamma(S/V) + \tfrac{1}{3}\,T(L/V) \tag{1}$$

Surface tension γ and the surface area and cable length densities, S/V and L/V, have been measured, and cable tension T can be estimated. Thus, data on the numerical values of the variables that appear in Equation 1 can be substituted into Equation 1 to test this equation as a model for parenchymal recoil and to determine the relative contributions of surface forces, described by the first term in Equation 1, and tissue forces, described by the second term. At 60% TLC, γ is ~6 dynes/cm and S/V is ~300–400 cm^2/cm^3. Thus, the value of the first term in Equation 1 is about 1.5×10^3 $dynes/cm^2$ or 1.5 cm H_2O. The length density of the cables in the acinus, including cables that form the edges of single alveolar walls and cables that form the edge of two intersecting walls, is ~3×10^4 cm/cm^3 (23). The tension in these cables has not been measured. However, the cables are mechanically coupled to the alveolar walls, and the equation that describes this coupling can be used to estimate T. The hoop stress in the cable, T/r, where r is the radius of curvature of the cable, must balance the outward pull of surface tension on the two surfaces of an alveolar wall extending outward from a cable.

$$T/r = 2\gamma \tag{2}$$

The radius of curvature of the cables has not been measured directly either. Because the cables do not run circumferentially around the duct, but have an axial slant, the radius of curvature of the cable must be somewhat larger than the radius of the lumen of an alveolar duct. An estimate, $r \sim 1.5 \times 10^{-2}$, cm seems reasonable. Then, from Equation 2, $T \sim 0.15$ dynes. The cross-sectional area of the cables is ~2×10^{-8} cm^2 (23). For $T \sim 0.15$ dynes, the stress in the cables is ~7×10^6 $dynes/cm^2$, a value that is in the range of stress that can be carried by elastin. This estimate for T, substituted into Equation 1, yields the value, 1.5×10^3 dynes/cm or 1.5 cm H_2O for the second term in Equation 1. Thus, surface forces and tissue forces contribute about equally to P_{par}, and the sum of the two is ~3 cm H_2O.

In the model that is described above, the tissue component of parenchymal recoil was ascribed to the cables that form the free edges of alveolar walls and define the lumen of the alveolar duct. Cable tension was estimated by invoking the equation that describes the balance between hoop stress and the outward pull of surface tension in the curved cable. This implies that the cables are extended and tensed by the outward pull of surface tension and that their extension and tension change as surface tension changes. This inference is supported by a number of observations. In scanning electron micrographs of saline-filled lungs, in which surface tension is abolished, the free edges of alveolar walls appear to be wavy and flaccid. In contrast, in air-filled lungs, the alveolar openings appear to be supported by smoothly curved line elements, and in detergent-rinsed lungs, in which surface tension is higher than normal, the lumen of the duct is enlarged. It appears that material in the alveolar walls folds into the interior corners of the alveolus as surface tension increases and the cables expand. As a result, surface area at a given lung volume is greatest in saline-filled lungs, less in normal lungs, and least in detergent-rinsed lungs. The same interplay between surface tension and duct expansion occurs in normal air-filled lungs. Surface tension increases rapidly with increasing lung volume (9), and surface tension is higher on an inflation limb that passes through a given volume than on the deflation limb. The duct expands in response to increasing surface tension, and alveolar surface area is smaller on the inflation limb (9,12). Thus, cables and alveolar surface area act like two springs in series. If the force increases in one, the other expands. If the rate of increase of surface tension with surface area were infinite and surface area were fixed, the elastance of the lung would be finite because lung volume could increase via expansion of the cables alone. A more complete version of this model that includes quantitative descriptions of the relations among surface tension, surface area, and lung volume is presented in reference 37.

Although the model described above seems to be consistent with a significant amount of data on lung PV and morphological properties, some questions remain. For example, fine elastic fibers interweave with the capillaries in the alveolar walls, and some authors believe that these fibers carry tension that contributes to the outward pull on the cables at the alveolar openings and contributes directly to recoil (23). It appears that the alveolar walls are stretched at higher lung volumes and that the connective tissue in the alveolar walls limits alveolar wall expansion at high volume.

The properties of the pleural membrane and the geometry and mechanical properties of the bronchial tree have been studied. The geometry and structure of the acinus have been described in detail. However, information about the structure of the lung at the scale between the scale of the lobe and the scale of the acinus is missing. Presumably, extensions of the peripheral tissue system penetrate the parenchyma and connect to the outer surface of the bronchial tree, but intersegmental septa are not apparent in sections of canine parenchyma, and little is known about the extent and connectedness of this system. This mesostructure has been assigned a number of putative functions.

1. It completes the tissue skeleton that supports the finer scale parenchymal structure.
2. It provides the forces that extend the bronchial tree as the lung inflates.
3. It maintains lobe shape.
4. It provides a shear stiffness for the lobe as a whole that is greater than the shear stiffness of parenchyma at smaller scale (38).

More information about the mesostructure is needed in order to test these hypotheses and to fill this gap in current understanding of parenchymal mechanics.

III. Shear

A. Macroscopic Description

Shear is shown in Figure 4. Tangential forces applied to the faces of a cube of elastic material cause a distortion with no change in volume. Shear strain ε_{sh} is defined as the ratio of horizontal displacement *d* to vertical side length *l*. Shear strain in an elastic material is proportional to shear stress σ_{sh}, the force per unit area applied to the surfaces. The relation between stress and strain is written as $\sigma_{sh} = \mu\ \varepsilon_{sh}$, where μ is the shear modulus of the material. The diagonal CB in Figure 4 lengthens under shear, and the diagonal AD shortens. Thus, in the

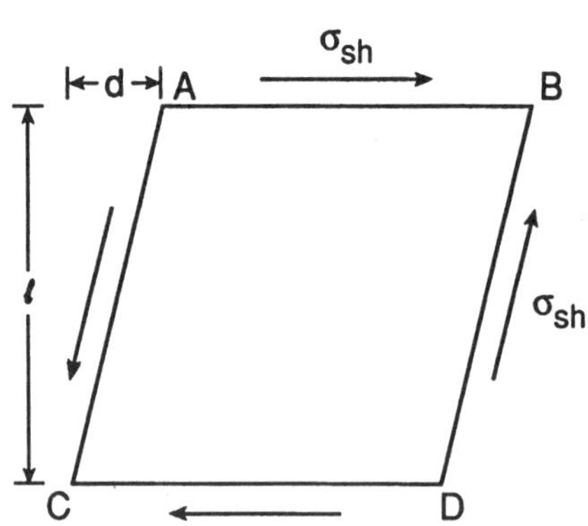

Figure 4 Deformation produced by tangential shear stresses σ_{sh} applied to the surface of a cube. Volume is conserved in the deformation, and shear strain ε_{sh} is defined as the ratio d/l.

coordinate system inclined at 45° from the horizontal, the deformation looks like a combination of extension along the direction CB and compression in the orthogonal direction. The stresses in this coordinate system are a tensile stress in the direction of extension and a compressive stress in the orthogonal direction. The view in the original coordinate system and the view in the rotated coordinated system are alternative descriptions of a shear deformation in which the material deforms by changing shape without changing volume. Any small deformation can be described as a combination of a volume expansion and shear deformations in three orthogonal directions, and, as a result, only two elastic moduli are required to describe the relation between deformation and stress in an elastic material.

The shear modulus of the lung has been measured by measuring the force and displacement when the lung is indented (6,20). This measurement has been made at different lung volumes and at points on the inflation limb as well as the deflation limb of the PV curve. The results are described well by a simple relation, $\mu = 0.7$ Ptp. The value of the shear modulus is considerably smaller than the value of the bulk modulus.

B. Micromechanics of Shear Deformations

Except for the presence of alveolar ducts that provide open pathways to all alveoli, the architecture of the parenchyma is like the architecture of foams. Three alveolar walls intersect along lines with angles of 120° between intersecting walls, and four lines of intersection intersect at equal angles at nodes (18,39). When a shear deformation is imposed, the material deforms as shown in Figure 4, on average, but individual elements of the structure may be displaced by more or less than the average. The microstructure deforms to a configuration that has the lowest energy for the given average shear strain. In a foam, the walls are loosely connected, and the internal geometry has considerable freedom to adjust to the lowest surface energy configuration compatible with the average strain. In fact, it has been argued that, under shear, the walls of foam cells move without rotation (40), with the distance between walls increasing in the direction of stretch, the direction CB in Figure 4, and decreasing in the direction AD. The change in spacing provides the stress that accompanies shear, and the value of the shear modulus depends on surface tension and cell size.

In the paper that stimulated the investigation of the properties of lungs under shear, Mead et al. (25) used models to investigate the relation between stress and strain. One of these was a two-dimensional analogue of a foam; namely, a network of springs that formed hexagonal cells. Kimmel et al. (39) extended the model to three dimensions. The shear modulus of this model, computed by computing the minimum energy configuration of the springs, agrees well with the measured value of the shear modulus of parenchyma. Therefore, this model provides some understanding of the macromechanics of shear distortion of parenchyma. Like foam, the displacements of the microstructure depart from the average displacements. Although the microstructure of parenchyma is more restricted than the microstructure of foam because alveolar walls have material connections at their intersections, the structure responds primarily by translation and rotation of the walls, with little extension. As a result, the value of the shear modulus depends on the forces in the walls, not their stiffness. This explains why the shear modulus is small compared to the bulk modulus and why its value is proportional to Ptp and independent of the extensional stiffness of the tissue.

IV. Lung Deformations

A. Background

First, one general statement can be made about parenchymal deformations. This general statement is a consequence of the fact that the shear modulus of parenchyma is considerably smaller than the bulk modulus. Rubber is a material for which the ratio of shear modulus to bulk modulus is extremely low, and, as a result, rubber is often described as an incompressible material. Rubber is not incompressible; if rubber is subjected to a uniform pressure, its volume decreases. However, if a force is applied locally, the deformation that is produced is essentially a shear deformation and the magnitudes of the displacements that occur are inversely proportional to the shear modulus and independent of the bulk modulus. Therefore, compressibility and the value of the bulk modulus can be ignored. The ratio of the values of the shear and bulk moduli of parenchyma is not as low as that of rubber, and the volume expansion of parenchyma is usually of primary interest. However, deformations that are produced by local forces, such as the forces that indent the surface under a rib, are primarily shear deformations, and the volume changes produced by local forces are relatively small.

Lung parenchyma has been modeled as a linear elastic material to take advantage of the techniques that have been developed to analyze the deformations of these materials. The stresses and displacements of linear elastic materials for some simple deformations are known in closed mathematical form. A computational technique, the finite-element technique, has been developed to generate numerical solutions to more complicated problems. A primary difficulty in using this technique is the problem of obtaining the data that define the problem; namely, the data that describe the shape of the lung and the forces or displacements that are imposed on it. Two simple mathematical solutions that are useful in describing deformations around bronchi and vessels are described first. Then, finite-element solutions that describe the gravitational deformation of the lung are reviewed.

If it is assumed that displacements depend on only the radical coordinant, either in cylindrical or spherical coordinants, the requirements of static equilibrium are satisfied by a radial displacement *u* and radial component of stress σ_r that are simple functions of the radial coordinate *r*. In cylindrical coordinates:

$$u = A/r \qquad \sigma_r = -A(2\ \mu)/r^2 \tag{3}$$

In spherical coordinates:

$$u = B/r^2 \qquad \sigma_r = -\ B(4\ \mu)/r^3 \tag{4}$$

Some general features of these solutions should be noted. First, A and B are constants with arbitrary values. That is, the solutions have the characteristic property of solutions for linear models; they are valid for arbitrary amplitudes. Second, displacement decreases as $1/r$ in cylindrical coordinates and $1/r^2$ in spherical coordinates. Because the surface area of a cylinder and sphere increase in proportion to r and r^2, respectively, the amount of material that crosses a cylindrical or spherical surface, respectively, is independent of r. This means that any volume expansion at an inner boundary of the material is carried out to the outer boundary with no volume change within the material. Each element of the body is compressed in the radial direction, if A or B is positive, and stretched in orthogonal directions so that its volume remains unchanged. The deformations are shear deformations, and the stresses are proportional to strain and to the value of the shear modulus.

B. Deformations Around Bronchi and Vessels

If bronchi expanded similarly to the lung and their diameters increased proportionally with the cube root of lung volume, the parenchyma surrounding the bronchi would expand uniformly. Because the stress carried by the parenchyma is approximately equal to Ptp, parenchymal attachments would exert a tensile stress of approximately Ptp on the outer surface of the bronchus, and the sum of this tensile stress and the stress exerted by alveolar gas pressure would equal pleural pressure. In that case, peribronchial pressure would equal pleural pressure and the transmural pressure that expands the bronchus would equal Ptp. In the normal lung, bronchial diameter increases nearly proportionally with lung volume, and peribronchial pressure is nearly equal to pleural pressure (41).

If the bronchus contracts becasue of smooth muscle activation, the surrounding parenchyma must deform to remain attached to the bronchus. The local deformation is described by Equation 3. The displacement *u* is negative with a magnitude equal to the difference between the diameter for similar expansion and the true diameter. The accompanying stress is a tensile stress that is proportional to the displacement u and the shear modulus μ. As a result, the total tensile stress exerted by the parenchyma is greater than Ptp, and peribronchial pressure is less than pleural pressure. Because the magnitude of u increases with increasing lung volume, and more importantly, μ increases with lung volume, the difference between peribronchial pressure and Ptp increases with increasing lung volume. To obtain a rough estimate of the maximum effect of parenchymal interdependence, the magnitude of u is taken to equal the unconstricted radius. The corresponding stress, from Equation 3, is 2 μ. Because μ = 0.7 Ptp, the added stress is 1.4 Ptp, and the total transmural pressure is 2.4 Ptp. A transmural pressure of 30–40 cm H_2O is required to open airways that are maximally constricted (42). Therefore, at values of Ptp < 15 cm H_2O, airways can close, but at values of Ptp > 15 cm H_2O, the forces of parenchymal interdependence can overcome maximal tension in smooth muscle and open the airway. This estimate has been confirmed experimentally (43). In normal subjects, bronchoconstriction is significantly reduced after a single deep inspiration, presumably by the parenchymal interdependence mechanism (44). Infants are more responsive to bronchoconstricting drugs than adults, perhaps because the parenchymal structure of infants is less developed (45). Also, asthmatics do not respond to a deep inspiration (46). The reason is uncertain. Perhaps it is a result of smooth muscle hypertrophy, or perhaps it is a result of greater airway wall volume so that closure can occur with a smaller displacement of the outer surface of the airway.

The same analysis of parenchymal forces can be applied to the vessels. Their diameter depends on both Ptp and vascular pressure, and Lai-Fook (47,48) has used this analysis to sort out the effects of lung volume and vascular pressure on vascular diameter. The diameter of vessels does not increase proportionally with the cube root of lung volume and perivascular pressure is less than pleural pressure. Because the peribronchial and perivascular spaces are accessible to interstitial fluid, peribronchial and perivascular pressures are important determinants of interstitial fluid flow.

It should be kept in mind that the local parenchymal deformations around bronchi and vessels are shear deformations. These deformations do not affect volume, and they do not contribute to nonuniform ventilation.

C. Gravitational Distortions

Measurements of regional volume in supine dogs, obtained by the parenchymal marker technique, showed a vertical gradient in regional emptying as lung volume decreased from TLC (26,30). Surprisingly, the gradient was not anatomically reversed when the animal was rotated to the prone posture. In the prone posture, regional emptying was uniform. Hoffman confirmed these results using a different technique (49). From multiple slice computed tomography (CT) scans, he obtained mean tissue density in horizontal slices at different vertical heights in the lungs of dogs and supine postures. He found that, at TLC, tissue density is uniform in both postures; at TLC, the lung is uniformly expanded. As lung volume decreases, tissue density increases, but in the supine posture, density increases more rapidly in more dorsal planes that are lower in the gravitational field than in more ventral planes. This implies that the lower "dependent" regions empty more rapidly than the upper "independent" regions. In the prone position, tissue density decreases at the same rate at all vertical levels.

The fact that the vertical gradient of regional volume is different in the prone and supine postures implies that lung deformation cannot simply be a gravitational deformation of the lung within a rigid chest wall. The deformation must be the result of both the direct effect of gravity on the lung and a deformation in response to a change of chest wall shape. Liu et al. (50) included both effects in an analysis of lung deformations. They used experimental data on chest wall shape, obtained from three-dimensional CT scans, as the boundary conditions in a finite-element analysis of lung deformations. The data on the shapes of the chest wall of dogs at TLC and FRC in the prone and supine postures were obtained by Margulies and Rodarte (51). They found that the shape of the rib cage remains similar as lung volume decreases, but, because the volumes of the heart and abdomen do not decrease, the shape of the lung at FRC is not similar to its shape at TLC. Liu et al. (50) assumed that the lung was uniformly expanded at TLC. They constructed a hypothetical chest wall shape that was similar to the shape at TLC, but with a volume reduced to volume at FRC. Boundary displacements were defined as the difference between the hypothetical and measured chest wall shapes at FRC, and the deformation of the lung caused by both the gravitational force on the lung and the boundary displacements were computed.

The results are shown in Figure 5. Transverse sections at two thoracic levels, one that traverses the heart and one that traverses the abdomen, are shown. Regional lung volume, as a fraction of volume at TLC, is described by the isovolume lines in these figures. It can be seen that the fractional volume is much more uniform in the prone posture than in the supine posture. The difference between the two postures is due to the difference in chest wall shapes. In the supine posture, the heart and abdomen extend further dorsally. Computed values of pleural pressure at the dorsal boundaries of the heart and abdomen are higher in the supine than in the prone posture. In the supine posture, the lung bears the weight of the heart and abdomen, and the parts of the lung that lie beneath the heart and lung are compressed. In the prone posture, the heart and abdomen rest on the sternum and abdominal wall, and the lung is more uniformly expanded.

V. Small-Scale Variability in Parenchymal Expansion

The parenchymal marker data showed a gravitational gradient of ventilation, as expected, in the supine dog, but it also revealed small-scale variations in ventilation that were independent of gravity. It has become apparent that the small-

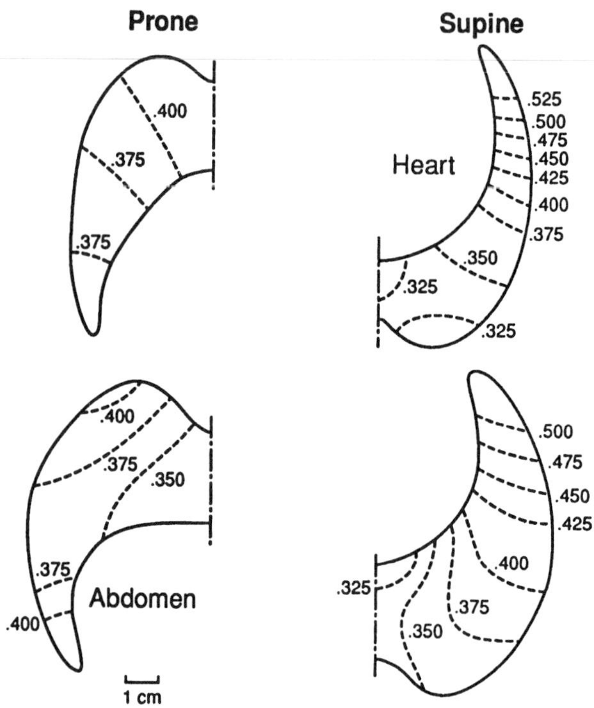

Figure 5 Isovolume lines that describe regional volume as a fraction of volume at TLC in transverse sections of prone and supine dogs. In the supine posture, the vertical gradient of regional volume is greater than in the prone posture because dependent regions are compressed by the weight of the heart and abdomen. (From Ref. 50. Reprinted with permission.)

scale variations are the major component of nonuniform ventilation (52). Recent data show that regional tidal volumes vary by ±20% from the mean during oscillations at frequencies and tidal volumes that correspond to resting breathing. There is evidence that the scale of the variability is smaller than the resolution of the parenchymal marker technique and that at the scale of the acinus, the variability of ventilation is larger than the variability detected by the parenchymal markers (53,54).

The cause of nonuniform volume expansion at small scale is unknown. Presumably, the compliance of the lung is nonuniform because the density of connective tissue and surface area is nonuniform.

The efficiency of gas exchange depends on the variability of the ratio of ventilation to perfusion. Thus, the variability of perfusion and the correlation between ventilation and perfusion must be known to determine the effects of nonuniform lung properties on gas exchange (55). These questions are addressed in Chapters 16, 17, and 18.

VI. Active Component of Lung Recoil

The existence and approximate magnitude of an active component of recoil have been established by a few basic observations. First, De Troyer et al. (56) found that, in awake humans, vagal blockade caused a decrease in lung recoil and an increase in compliance. This shows that normal lung recoil includes an active component with a magnitude of ~25% of total recoil. Second, recoil increases by ~1–2 cm H_2 O during hypocapnic bronchoconstriction (28). Finally, bronchoconstricting drugs cause an increase in recoil and a decrease in compliance (29). Some authors have concluded from alveolar capsule data that dynamic lung elastance increases by factors of 5–10 during severe bronchoconstriction. However, regional expansion becomes nonuniform during bronchoconstriction, and it may be that most of the increase in dynamic lung elastance is caused by maldistribution of lung expansion (29,30). A safer estimate of the increase in recoil during bronchoconstriction is given by the data on recoil at constant volume reported by Bates et al. (29). They found that airway opening pressure increased by 1–3 cm H_2O when the lung was held at constant volume and the bronchoconstricting drug was delivered via the pulmonary circulation.

A number of possibilities have been suggested for the identity and the location of the elements that provide the active component of recoil, but these are speculative, and the micromechanics of active recoil is not understood. However, the magnitude of the effect is known, and the quantitative relations that have been described above can be used to test the plausibility of different hypotheses. In the remainder of this chapter, I describe estimates of the potential effect on recoil of some of the elements that have been suggested as the source of the active component of lung recoil.

The natural place to search for elements that contribute to recoil is in the parenchyma. Strands of smooth muscle are found sporadically running parallel to the elastin and collagin cables that form the free edges of alveolar walls, and it has been suggested that contraction of these strands of smooth muscle provides the active component of recoil. If the smooth muscle contracts, the parallel connective tissue presumably would shorten, and the increase in muscle tension should be partially offset by a decrease in tension in the connective tissue. Conversely, tension would increase in connective tissue that is in series with smooth muscle. Thus, the effect of smooth muscle tension on other tissue is uncertain. Nonetheless, Equation 1 can be used to obtain a rough estimate of the contribution of smooth muscle in the parenchyma to lung recoil. In Equation 1, the contribution of line elements to recoil is given by the term ⅓ T L/V. By multiplying and dividing by the cross-sectional area A of the cables and identifying L A as the volume of the cables and T/A as the stress in the cables, the potential contribution of smooth muscle to recoil P_{sm} can be written as follows:

$$P_{sm} = \tfrac{1}{3}\,\sigma_{sm}\,(V_{sm}/V) \tag{5}$$

where σ_{sm} is the stress in the muscle and V_{sm}/V is the volume density of muscle. It was shown above that a stress in the elastic cable of 7×10^6 dynes/cm^2 provides a recoil of 1.5 cm H_2O. The stress in maximally activated smooth muscle is smaller, $\sim 2 \times 10^6$ dynes/cm^2. Therefore, a volume density of smooth muscle in the parenchyma that is 3.5 times the volume density of the elastin cables would be required for smooth muscle to contribute a recoil of 1.5 cm H_2O. I do not know of any data on the volume density of smooth muscle in parenchyma, but smooth muscle is not a prominent feature in the electron micrographs that I have seen, and I have the impression that the volume density of smooth muscle is too small to provide an active recoil of 1–3 cm H_2O.

It has been suggested that contraction of the lumen of the alveolar duct by contraction of smooth muscle would expand alveolar surface area, thereby increasing surface tension and inducing an increase of surface forces and their contribution to recoil. However, bronchoconstriction of saline-filled lungs also causes an increase in recoil of 1–3 cm H_2O, about the same as the increase in air-filled lungs, and unless the tissue component of alveolar wall tension has been badly underestimated, active recoil is not the result of increased surface or tissue forces in the alveolar walls.

Finally, a contractile apparatus is found in cells other than smooth muscle cells, and it has been suggested that a much more general cell contraction may provide the active component of recoil. The stress that can be generated in other cells must be orders of magnitude smaller than the active stress in smooth muscle cells, and this hypothesis seems questionable.

The second general source of active recoil that has been proposed is smooth muscle in the airways. The total volume of smooth muscle in the airways can be estimated. Gunst et al. (42) report that smooth muscle constitutes ~7% of the volume of the walls of 5-mm airways and that the volume of the airway walls is ~50% of the volume of the airway lumen at a transpulmonary pressure of 5 cm H_2O. The volume of the intraparenchymal conducting airways of dogs is ~50 cm^3, or ~7% of lung volume at 50% TLC. Combining these values yields an estimate for the volume density of airway smooth muscle V_{sm}/V of 2×10^{-3}. Simply substituting this value of V_{sm}/V and the value of $\sigma = 2 \times 10^6$ dynes/cm^2 into Equation 5 yields the estimate $P_{sm} = 1.3$ cm H_2O. Thus, the amount of smooth muscle in the airway walls seems sufficient, if only barely, to provide the active component of recoil. Increased tension in elastic elements that are in series with the muscle may add to the effect.

Mitzner et al. (57) devised an experiment to measure the effect of airway smooth muscle contraction on recoil. They delivered the bronchoconstricting drug via the bronchial circulation and thereby constricted the airways without exposing the parenchyma to the drug. They found that lung elastance doubled during bronchoconstriction. This observation provides strong support for the hypothesis that airway smooth muscle is the primary source of active recoil.

Although constriction of the airways causes a significant increase in recoil and the amount of smooth muscle in the airways seem sufficient to account for the active component of recoil, the mechanism by which airway constriction is converted to lung recoil is not clear. In the following paragraphs, the effects of the circumferential and axial components of smooth muscle force are discussed.

The circumferential component of smooth muscle force causes a radial contraction, and as the airway contracts, the parenchyma must deform to remain attached to the outer surface of the airway. Smith et al. analyzed the effect of radial airway contraction on recoil (58). Near the airway, the deformation has cylindrical symmetry, and, in this near field, Equation 3 describes the stress that accompanies airway constriction. At a distance from the airway greater than the length of the constricted segment, the parenchymal deformation becomes three-dimensional, and Equation 4 can be used to describe the effect far from a constricted airway. The displacement in the far field must accommodate the volume change of the segment. Therefore, $u = -\delta V/4\pi r^2$, where δV is the decrease in the volume of the segment. That is, the parameter B in Equation 4 is assigned the value $\delta V/4\pi$. The corresponding stress is given by $\mu\delta V/\pi r^3$. The value of r at the surface of the lung will be denoted R. An approximate value of R is obtained by setting $\frac{4}{3}\pi R^3 = VL$. Therefore, at the surface, $\sigma_r = \frac{4}{3}\mu\,\delta V/V$, and recoil pressure increases by this amount. Because $\mu = 0.7$ Ptp and the sum of $\delta V/V$ for all airways is ~5%, the increase in recoil caused by parenchymal distortion is ~5% of Ptp. A second contribution to recoil occurs because of the shift of volume between the airways and the parenchyma. The parenchyma must expand to absorb the volume expelled from the airway lumen. The volume of the airways is ~5% TLC. The compliance of the lung on its deflation limb is ~10% TLC/cm H_2O. If the airways were maximally constricted and the expelled volume were uniformly distributed to the parenchyma, recoil would increase by ~0.5 cm H_2O. The total of the two effects of radial contraction is ~1 cm H_2O. The magnitudes of both of these effects are proportional to lung elastance. Lung elastance increases with lung volume, and Bates et al. (29) found that bronchoconstriction causes a bigger increase in recoil at higher volume. However, saline-filled lungs are more compliant that air-filled lungs, and bronchoconstriction causes recoil in saline-filled lungs to increase by about the same amount as in air-filled lungs (59). Therefore, it appears that radial contraction of the airways is not the only cause of increased recoil.

It has also been suggested that the axial component of smooth muscle tension contributes to recoil. Little is known about the axial forces in the airways and how they affect recoil. However, two observations, one empirical and one conceptual, are pertinent. Hoppin et al. (60) report that, when the terminal airways of an excised bronchial tree are sealed and the tree is inflated, the length of the tree is smaller than the length of the intact tree at the same lung inflation pressure. Therefore, tissue connections to the intact bronchial tree must exert an axial force on each airway segment that is greater than the product of Ptp and airway area. Second, it is clear that axial contraction of the airway that occurs during bronchoconstriction (61) cannot be accommodated in the same way that radial contraction is accommodated by the surrounding parenchyma. Radial contraction causes a local distortion at every point along the airway. Airway diameter and surrounding parenchyma form a pair of springs in series, and radial contraction of the airway is accommodated by radial extension of the parenchyma. The parenchymal spring is relatively weak, and the stress that is generated in the parenchyma is small. On the other hand, axial contraction of the airways would accumulate along the length of the airway. A 10% contraction over an axial distance of 10 cm would produce a displacement of 1 cm. Thus, a modest fractional length contraction would produce large displacements, severe parenchymal distortions, and large forces at the end of the 10-cm tree that would, in fact, prevent the contraction. In general, it can be shown that a line element embedded in an elastic body must follow the strain imposed by the surrounding body except at local points near the ends of the line or at a free surface of the body. Therefore, if active smooth muscle exerts an axial force, parenchymal elements provide an opposing force that prevents the airway from shortening. The identity of the parenchymal elements that provide the opposing force is unknown. Perhaps shear forces on the surface of the airways play a role. However, it seems more likely that the connective tissue skeleton of the lung is a complete structure, that the intersegmental septa that connect the pleural membrane and the airways provide the forces that extend the intact bronchial tree, and that axial contraction of the airways increases tension in the connective tissue and increases lung recoil.

VII. Conclusion

The lung is a complex mechanical structure that is difficult to study because its configuration and its mechanical properties are conferred, in part, by transpulmonary pressure. That is, the collapsed lung is a different mechanical structure from the inflated lung. New techniques have been developed to overcome this difficulty in study. The technique of fixing the lung via the pulmonary circulation that was introduced by Weibel and colleagues has been combined with new morphological techniques to produce data on the interplay between surface tension and surface area. Surface tension has been measured in situ. These data have been integrated into quantitative models that describe the balance of forces in the parenchyma. Much of the work has focused on the alveolar and acinar scale, and comparable information about the mesostructure of the lung is not available.

In most of the work on parenchymal mechanics, the lung has been pictured as a passive structure. However, active elements provide the function of control of ventilation during hypocapnia and are responsible for the dysfunction of asthma. At this point, the source of the active component of recoil is unknown, and the mechanisms by which the active elements affect ventilation are unknown. An apparent paradox must be resolved. A local mechanism is required to control ventilation locally, but, in the normal lung, bronchioles, unlike arterioles in the pulmonary circulation, contribute a small part of flow resistance, and, in the normal lung, resistance is a small part of lung impedance. Thus, bronchioles are not on the verge of controlling ventilation, and bronchoconstriction seems to be an unsuitable mechanism for controlling ventilation through resistance. Certainly, small airways can close. Perhaps the small airways operate like switches, offering little resistance when they are open, but closing easily when smooth muscle is activated. Alternatively, bronchoconstriction may be coupled to lung recoil and elastance and local ventilation may be controlled by local elastance. Some of the mechanisms that have been proposed to explain the effect of bronchoconstriction on recoil are well-enough understood so that their magnitude can be estimated, and these mechanisms seem too weak to generate 1–3 cm H_2O of recoil pressure. Too little is known about other mechanisms to decide whether they are plausible. Nonetheless, it may be worthwhile to point out that the anatomy of the intersegmental septa and the connections between the pleural membrane and the bronchial tree have not been thoroughly investigated and that these components of the connective tissue skeleton of the lung, which presumably play a role in the expansion of the passive bronchial tree, may provide a coupling between bronchoconstriction and lung recoil.

Acknowledgment

The writing of this chapter was supported in part by grant HL 49788.

References

1. Otis AB. History of respiratory mechanics. In: Macklem PT, Mead J, eds. Handbook of Physiology. The Respiratory System. Mechanics of Breathing. Vol. III. Bethesda, MD: American Physiological Society 1986:1–12.
2. Fowler WA. Lung function studies. III. Uneven pulmonary ventilation in normal subjects and in patients with pulmonary disease. J Appl Physiol 1949; 2:283–299.

3. Milic-Emili J. Static distribution of lung volume. In: Macklem PT, Mead J, eds. Handbook of Physiology. The Respiratory System. Mechanics of Breathing. Vol. III. Bethesda, MD: American Physiological Society 1986:561–574.
4. Engel LA, Utz G, Wood LDH, Macklem P. Ventilation distribution in anatomical lung unit. J Appl Physiol 1974; 37:194–200.
5. West JB, Matthews FL. Stresses, strain, and surface pressure in the lung caused by its weight. J Appl Physiol 1972; 32:332–345.
6. Lai-Fook SJ, Hyatt, RE, Rodarte JR, Wilson TA. Elastic constants of inflated dog lungs. J Appl Physiol 1976; 40:508–513.
7. Bachofen H, Gehr P, Weibel ER. Alterations of mechanical properties and morphology in excised rabbit lungs rinsed with a detergent. J Appl Physiol 1979; 47: 1002–1010.
8. Smith JC, Stamenovic D. Surface forces in lungs. Alveolar surface tension-lung volume relationships. J Appl Physiol 1986; 60:1341–1350.
9. Bachofen H, Schürch S, Urbinelli M, Weibel ER. Relations among alveolar surface tension, surface area, volume and recoil pressure. J Appl Physiol 1987; 62:1878–1887.
10. Schürch S. Surface tension at low lung volumes: dependences on time and alveolar size. Respir Physiol 1982; 48:339–355.
11. Schürch S, Goerke J, Clements J. Direct determination of volume- and time-dependence of alveolar surface tension in excised lungs. Poc Natl Acad Sci U S A 1978; 4698–4702.
12. Akahori TS, Suzuki S, Suzuki M, Okubo T. Dynamic behavior of alveolar surface-to-volume ratio in live dogs by light-scattering stereology. J Appl Physiol 1993; 75:1624–1629.
13. Butler JP, Miki H, Suzuki S, Takishima T. Step response of lung surface-to-volume ratio by light-scattering stereology. J Appl Physiol 1989; 67:1873–1880.
14. Gil J, Bachofen H, Gehr P, Weibel ER. The alveolar volume to surface area relationship in air- and saline-filled lungs fixed by vascular perfusion. J Appl Physiol 1979; 47:990–1001.
15. Butler JP, Miki H, Squarcia S, Rogers Ra, Lehr JL. Effect of macroscopic deformation on lung microstructure. J Appl Physiol 1996; 81:1792–1799.
16. Suzuki S, Akahori T, Miyazawa N, Numata M, Okubo T, Butler JP. Alveolar surface area-to-lung volume ratio in oleic acid-induced pulmonary edema. J Appl Physiol 1996; 80:742–746.
17. Mercer RR, Crapo JD. Three-dimensional reconstruction of the acinus of the rat. J Appl Physiol 1987; 63:785–794.
18. Butler JP, Oldmixon EH, Hoppin FG Jr. Dihedral angles of septal "bend" structures in lung parenchyma. J Appl Physiol 1996; 81:1800–1806.
19. Oldmixon EH, Butler JP, Hoppin FG Jr. Dihedral angles between alveolar septa. J Appl Physiol 1988; 64:299–307.
20. Hajji MA, Wilson TA, Lai-Fook SJ. Improved measurements of shear modulus and pleural membrane tension of the lungs. J Appl Physiol 1979; 47:175–181.
21. Stamenovic D. Mechanical properties of pleural membrane. J Appl Physiol 1984; 57:1189–1194.

22. Mercer RR, Crapo JD. Spatial distribution of collagen and elastin fibers in the lungs. J Appl Physiol 1990; 69:756–765.
23. Oldmixon EH, Hoppin FG Jr. Distribution of elastin and collagen in canine lung alveolar parenchyma. J Appl Physiol 1989; 67:1941–1949.
24. Oldmixon EH, Hoppin FG Jr. Comparison of amounts of collagen and elastin in pleura and parenchyma of dog lung. J Appl Physiol 1984; 56:1383–1388.
25. Mead J, Takishima T, Leith DE. Stress distribution in the lungs: a model of pulmonary elasticity. J Appl Physiol 1970; 28:596–608.
26. Hubmayer RD, Walters BJ, Chevalier RA, Rodarte JR, Olson LE. Topographical distribution of regional lung volume in anesthetized dogs. J Appl Physiol 1983; 54: 1048–1056.
27. Prisk GK, Guy HJB, Elliott AR, Paiva M, West JB. Ventilatory inhomogeneity determined from multiple-breath washouts during sustained microgravity on Spacelab SLS-1. J Appl Physiol 1995; 78:597–607.
28. Severinghaus JW, Swenson EW, Finley TN, Lategola MT, Williams J. Unilateral hypoventilation produced in dogs by occluding one pulmonary artery. J Appl Physiol 1961; 16:53–60.
29. Bates JHT, Lauzon AM, Dechman GS, Maksym GN, Schuessler TF. Temporal dymanics of pulmonary response to intravenous histamine in dogs: effects of dose and lung volume. J Appl Physiol 1994; 76:616–626.
30. Hubmayr RD, Hill MJ, Wilson TA. Nonuniform expansion of constricted dog lungs. J Appl Physiol 1996; 80:522–530.
31. Fredberg JJ, Stamenovic D. On the imperfect elasticity of lung tissue. J Appl Physiol 1989; 67:2408–2419.
32. Stamenovic D, Wilson TA. Parenchymal stabiiity. J Appl Physiol 1992; 73:596–602.
33. Fung YCB. Biomechanics. Mechanical Properties of Living Tissues. New York: Springer-Verlag, 1981.
34. Weibel ER. The Pathway for Oxygen. Cambridge, MA: Harvard University Press, 1984.
35. Wilson TA, Bachofen H. A model for mechanical structure of the alveolar duct. J Appl Physiol 1982; 52:1064–1070.
36. Hoppin FG Jr, Hildebrandt J. Mechanical properties of the lung. In: West JB, ed. Bioengineering Aspects of the Lung. New York: Marcel Dekker, 1977:83–162.
37. Wilson TA. The mechanics of lung parenchyma. In: Chang HK, Paiva M, eds. Respiratory Physiology: An Analytical Approach. New York: Marcel Dekker, 1989:317–342.
38. Olson LE, Wilson TA, Rodarte JR. Distortion of submerged dog lung lobes. J Appl Physiol 1985; 59:521–527.
39. Kimmel E, Budiansky B. Surface tension and the dodecohedron model for lung elasticity. ASME J Biomech Eng 1990; 112:160–167.
40. Stamenovic D. A model of foam elasticity based upon the laws of Plateu. J Colloid Interface Sci 1991; 145:255–259.
41. Lai-Fook SJ, Hyatt RE, Rodarte JR. Effect of parenchymal shear modulus and lung volume on bronchial pressure-diameter behavior. J Appl Physiol 1978; 44:859–856.

42. Gunst SJ, Stropp JQ. Pressure-volume and length-stress relationships in canine bronchi in vitro. J Appl Physiol 1988; 64:2522–2531.
43. Gunst SJ, Warner DO, Wilson TA, Hyatt RE. Parenchymal interdependence and airway response to methacholine in excised dog lobes. J Appl Physiol 1988; 65: 2490–2497.
44. Nadel JA, Ticrney DF. Effect of a previous deep inspiration on airway resistance in man. J Appl Physiol 1961; 16:717–719.
45. Tepper RS, Stevens J, Eigen H. Heightened airway responsiveness in normal female children compared with adults. Am J Respir Crit Care Med 1994; 149:678–681.
46. Fish JE, Ankin MG, Kelley JF, Peterman VI. Regulation of bronchomotor tome by lung inflation in asthmatic and nonasthmatic subjects. J Appl Physiol 1981; 50: 1079–1086.
47. Lai-Fook SJ. A continuum mechanics analysis of pulmonary vascular interdependence in isolated dog lobes. J Appl Physiol 1979; 46:419–429.
48. Lai-Fook SJ, Kallok MJ. Bronchial-arterial interdependence in isolated dog lung. J Appl Phsyiol 1982; 52:1000–1007.
49. Hoffman EA. Effect of body orientation on regional lung expansion: a computed tomographic approach. J Appl Physiol 1985; 59:468–480.
50. Liu S, Margulies SS, Wilson TA. Deformation of the dog lung in the chest wall. J Appl Physiol 1990; 68:1979–1987.
51. Marguiles SS, Rodarte JR. Shape of the chest wall in prone and supine dogs. J Appl Physiol 1990; 68:1970–1978.
52. Wilson TA, Hill MJ, Hubmayr RD. Regional volume trajectories during expiratory flow in dogs. J Appl Physiol 1996; 80:1144–1148.
53. Rodarte JR, Chaniotakis M, Wilson TA. Variability of parenchymal expansion measured by computed tomography. J Appl Physiol 1989; 67:226–231.
54. Wilson TA, Olson LE, Rodarte JR. Effect of variable parenchymal expansion on gas mixing. J Appl Physiol 1987; 62:634–639.
55. Wilson TA, Beck KC. Contributions of ventilation and perfusion inhomogeneities to the VA/Q distribution. J Appl Physiol 1992; 72:2298–2304.
56. De Troyer A, Yernault JC, Rodenstein D. Effects of vagal blockade on lung mechanics in normal man. J Appl Physiol 1979; 46:217–226.
57. Mitzner W, Blosser S, Yager D, Wagner E. Effect of bronchial smooth muscle contraction on lung compliance. J Appl Physiol 1992; 72:158–167.
58. Smith JC, Butler JP, Hoppin FG Jr. Contribution of tree structures to lung elastic recoil. J Appl Physiol 1984; 57:1422–1429.
59. Colebatch HJH, Mitchell CA. Constriction of isolated living liquid-filled dog and cat lungs with histamine. J Appl Physiol 1971; 30:691–702.
60. Hoppin FG Jr, Hughes JMB, Mead J. Axial forces in the bronchial tree. J Appl Physiol 1977; 42:773–781.
61. Murtagh PS, Proctor DF, Permutt S, Kelly B, Evering S. Bronchial closure with Mecholyl in excised dog lobes. J Appl Physiol 1971; 31:409–415.

4

Micromechanics of the Lung

From the Parenchyma to the Cytoskeleton

JEFFREY J. FREDBERG and NING WANG

Harvard School of Public Health
Boston, Massachusetts

DIMITRIJE STAMENOVIĆ

Boston University
Boston, Massachusetts

DONALD E. INGBER

Harvard Medical School
Boston, Massachusetts

I. Introduction

This chapter discusses pulmonary mechanics and its extension to the levels of tissue, cell, and molecule. It traces a thread of a common biophysical mechanism that may form the basis of function at each of these levels, the connections between levels, and their alterability in selective but biologically important departures from the normal state. This is not meant to imply that mechanical behavior at the level of molecules can necessarily be used to predict mechanical behavior of the lung as a whole, but only that a common mechanism may be reiterated at several levels of organization.

At the level of parenchymal microstructure, the lung is a tensed pressure-supported structure (1). The key distending stress, transpulmonary pressure, is transmitted throughout parenchymal tissues. It distends all intrapulmonary structures. This distending stress confers, in nearly direct proportion to its magnitude, the parenchymal shear modulus and the associated forces of elastic interdependence that are critical in maintaining the shape of organ, region, vessel, airway, and alveolus. At each of these levels, this distending stress is essential to lung function, influencing lung stability, the distribution of perfusion, the distribution of ventilation, ventilation-perfusion matching, airway obstruction, fluid balance in lungs, and expiratory flow limitation. Whereas the central importance of the distending stress in these processes is not in dispute, the specific mechanism of action of the distending stress in health, and its disruption in disease, remains incompletely understood.

At the level of the cell, some of the best evidence for the importance of mechanical events comes from the effects of shear flow on the endothelium. To cite only one example, endothelial cells subjected to shear flow alter synthesis and release of endothelin with increasing shear stress. The mechanism by which these cells transduce shear stress is not understood. A long-standing interpretation of this and related shear-dependent phenomena has been that shear flow influences mass transport of exogenous or endogenous species across the boundary layer above the cell membrane. A more recent interpretation, however, is that the adherent endothelial cell is spread and its cytoskeleton is tensed (2). A change in fluid shear stress alters the preexisting mechanical equilibrium within the cytoskeleton, requiring it to deform until a new equilibrium is attained. Through unknown mechanisms, these mechanical forces are transduced into biochemical signals that lead to genetic expression and protein synthesis.

Even though it is perhaps not surprising that the endothelium functions as a transducing mechanosensitive interface between blood and arterial wall, increasing evidence points to the fact that mechanical regulation of cellular functions may be a general property of adherent cells. For example, recent investigations have addressed dependence of DNA synthesis upon the degree of cellular distention in a hepatocyte system with defined medium, saturating amounts of growth factors and defined composition of extracellular matrix molecules. All other factors being equal, DNA synthesis increases in a dose-dependent fashion with increasing cellular distention (3). Thus, even at the level of the nuclear lattice, a key role for mechanical distention is suggested (4,5). In this connection, the current paradigm holds that adhesion and spreading are preconditions for DNA synthesis but, once the cell is anchored to the substratum and is well spread, key processes regulating DNA synthesis center around chemotactic and soluble growth factors. However, this recent evidence could plausibly be taken to demonstrate just the converse, that whereas chemotactic and growth factors are preconditions, key processes regulating DNA synthesis center around adhesion and spreading. In fact, regulation is unlikely to be a simple linear process. Rather, in a system as complex as the cell, there is probably a multifactorial network of causation, one in which the role of physical forces on cellular functions seems to have been underappreciated and has begun to come to light.

This leads to two interlocking questions of substance. First, by what mechanisms does the cell generate mechanical stresses that resist distortion of shape?

Second, how are such mechanical stresses transduced into biochemical signals? The latter question defines an emerging branch of biological research—cellular mechanotransduction. The first question, however, and its implications at levels spanning cytoskeleton to tissue, is a major focus of this chapter. Indeed, in the lung at each level—the surface film, the extracellular lattice, the focal adhesion complex, and the cytoskeleton (CSK)—the distending stress emerges as a recurring and unifying theme. This is where the trail seems to lead.

A. The Cascade of Force Transmission

In the lung parenchymal network, distending stresses are transmitted by a tensed lattice. This lattice is composed of the extracellular matrix (i.e., parenchymal connective tissue), the interfacial film, and the contractile apparatus. In the normal lung, the tensed extracellular matrix is the scaffolding upon which pulmonary cells of all types adhere, spread, differentiate, proliferate, remodel, contract, and locomote. Like the lung as a whole, in the absence of an external distending stress, the extracellular matrix would collapse under the influence of interfacial surface forces. The interfacial force is central because it sets the state of distention and stress of tissues and cells comprising the alveolar entrance ring, the alveolar septum, and, to a lesser degree, the small airway (Figure 1). Inflammation-induced disruption of surfactant function during adult respiratory distress syndrome leads to elevation of interfacial forces and a tendency for diminished septal area being available for gas exchange and distortion of the capillary bed (see Figure 1*C*), focal parenchymal collapse, or airway closure (6).

In the cytoskeletal network also, distending stresses are transmitted by a tensed lattice. Stress in the lattice is transmitted across the cell membrane at focal adhesions (Figure 2). The focal adhesion complex is composed of integrins (a transmembrane adhesion molecule) attached in the extracellular domain to the extracellular matrix and in the cytoplasmic domain to vinculin, talin, α-actinin, paxillin, tensin, and the microfilament terminus. The role of the focal adhesion complex is in some ways analogous to that of the peg of a pup-tent. The tent requires external distending stress to maintain its shape and stability. Like the lung, the pulmonary extracellular matrix, the pup-tent, or the spider's web, the adherent cell may be dependent upon the external distending stress to maintain its shape and stability. When adherent to the extracellular matrix, cells spread and flatten. As the cell spreads and flattens, the nucleus does so as well (3). In contrast, in the absence of anchorage, cells round up, because the sphere is the shape with minimum surface energy for a given volume.

Taken together, the lung, the pulmonary extracellular matrix, the cytoskeleton, as well as the pup-tent and the spider's web, all seem to belong to the special class of mechanical structures in which a distending stress may be the essential root by which shape stability is conferred (1,7).

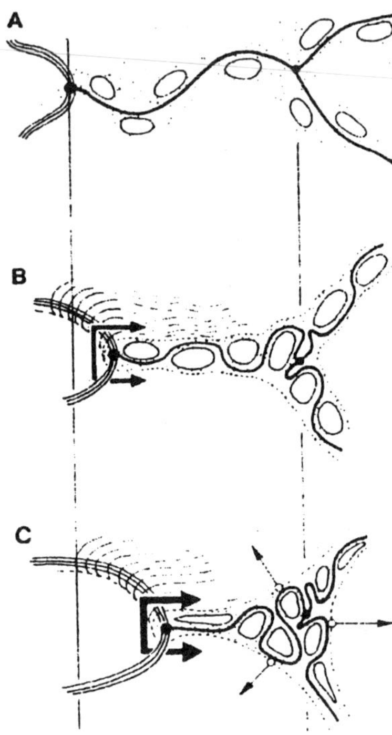

Figure 1 The state of distention of the alveolar entrance ring (*left*) and alveolar septa and capillaries (*right*) with graded surface tension. **A**, Zero. **B**, Moderate. **C**, High. (Adapted from Weibel ER, Bachofen H. How to stabilize pulmonary alveoli: surfactant or fibers? NIPS 1987; 2:72–75.)

B. From Lung Parenchyma to Cytoskeleton

Over the past decade, one of the outstanding conceptual problems in respiratory mechanics was to understand parenchymal resistance to shape distortion. Resistance to shape distortion is the basis of elastic interdependence and the recruitment, distention, patency and stability of all intraparenchymal structures including alveoli, airways, and vessels. Arguably, elastic interdependence, its origins, its physiological implications, and its disruption in disease stand at the epicenter of lung parenchymal pathophysiology. A measure of resistance to shape distortion in the lung is the parenchymal shear modulus. However, structurally based mechanistic predictions of the shear modulus from all existing theories far exceeded observed values. Also, no theory could explain the biologically and clinically crucial observation that the shear modulus of lung parenchyma increases in nearly direct proportion to the distending stress, that is, the transpulmonary pressure. Wilson (8) developed an alternative microstructural analysis that ex-

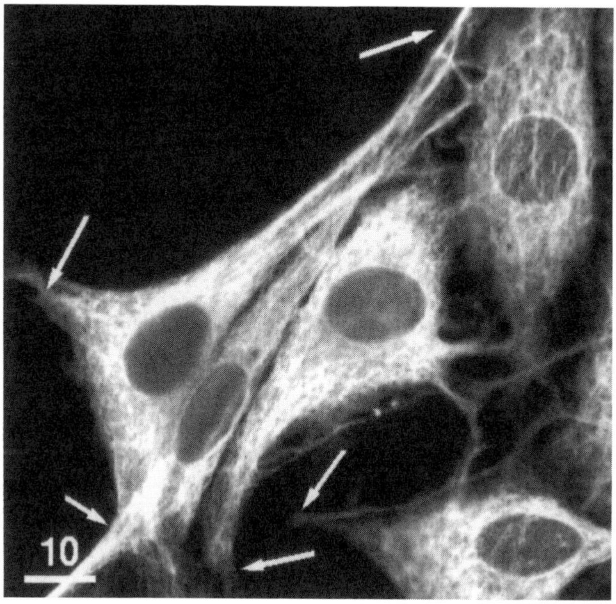

Figure 2 A fluorescent confocal section of C6D10 cells immunostained for vimetin. Because they fall beneath the plane of the section, focal adhesions are not visible but their location is indicated by arrows. Scale-bar is 10 μm. (Courtesy of Dr. Rick A. Rogers, BioMedical Imaging Laboratory, Harvard School of Public Health, Boston, MA.)

hibited that essential feature, but it was not until much later that the importance of his work was appreciated and that the essential origin of that behavior was identified (1).

Previous mechanistic understanding of pulmonary elasticity derived mostly from the theory of continuum mechanics.* Continuum theory holds that, as one proceeds to smaller and smaller scales, the microscale strain of structural members must faithfully follow the macroscale strain of the matrix or network. The approach developed by Budiansky and Kimmel (7) bypassed that assumption as well as others implicit in continuum theory. Instead, it considered the *discrete* (as opposed to continuum) nature of stress-bearing members at the microscale and the nature of their *connectedness*. It is this interconnectedness that turned out to be the radical feature. They showed that, depending on that connectedness, the structural matrix composed of discrete stress-bearing members

*Continuum refers to a concept that disregards the structure of matter, depicting it as being without gaps or empty spaces.

resists shape distortion, not so much by elongation of those microstructural members as in a continuum but, more so, by *reorientation* of those members, that is, reorientation of discrete septal faces and connective tissue cables. Indeed, in such structures, the macroscopic shear modulus can remain finite and small, even as the stiffness of microstructural members becomes infinitely large. This approach not only explained why the shear modulus of lung parenchyma is as small as it is in the face of relatively stiff connective tissue elements but also revealed why the shear modulus *must* be nearly a constant fraction of the *external* distending stress.

The common underlying principle is illustrated in other structures in nature, such as foams, plant leaves, and spider's webs, that share this behavior. In the cases of foams, plant leaves, and lungs, the initial distending stress is provided by the inflating pressure. In the case of the spider's web, the initial distending stress is provided by discrete attachments to surrounding objects, focal adhesions as it were. The pup-tent is a familiar manmade structure that secures resistance to shape distortion from distending stress provided by attachments to surrounding structures. In classic continuum theory, all solids possess *intrinsic* resistance to distortion of shape, but, in the structures cited here, intrinsic resistance to distortion of shape is lacking entirely.

The distinguishing feature accounting for this behavior is that the internal degrees of freedom of the lattice are not fully constrained as in an elastic continuum.* In the absence of an initial distending stress, the structural collapses under shear loading. In the presence of a distending stress, however, the structural elements that carry initial load move relative to one another, changing orientation and spacing until a new equilibrium configuration is attained. The bigger the initial load carried by those elements (i.e., the bigger the distending stress of the structure), the smaller the deformation that the structure must undergo before attaining a new equilibrium configuration. As the prestress increases, the resistance to change of shape increases in proportion.

It seems that the physics elucidated by Budiansky and Kimmel (7) may apply not only to lung parenchymal microstructural elements but also, at a smaller scale still, to the cytoskeletal lattice of the adherent and spread cell (Figure 3). This comes back to the fundamental question of how individual cells, their cytoskeleton, and their nuclear lattice resist distortion of shape. A closely related hypothesis holds that these structures are not adequately described by continuum mechanics (9). Instead, cells and subcellular structures may secure

*The nature of the connectedness defines whether the microstructure has its internal degrees of freedom fully constrained, like a triangular truss, or whether its internal degrees of freedom are not fully constrained, like a swinging gate or a four-bar linkage. To secure mechanical stability, the latter class requires an external distending stress whereas the former does not.

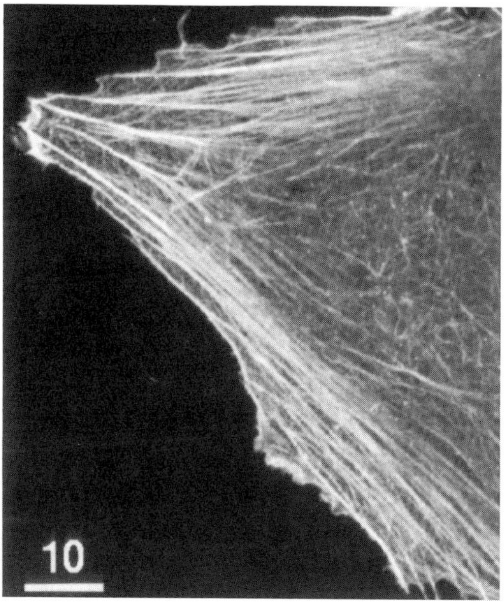

Figure 3 A fluorescent image of the tensed microfilament lattice seen in confocal section of a rat fibroblast immunostained by antiactin antibody. Scale-bar is 10 μm. (Courtesy of Dr. Rick A. Rogers, BioMedical Imaging Laboratory, Harvard School of Public Health, Boston, MA.)

resistance to shape distortion by virtue of an architectural system of tensional prestress that is known as tensional integrity or *tensegrity* (9–13). This concept is related intimately to the theory of Budiansky and Kimmel (7) but explicitly emphasizes the presence of internally generated distending stress that is generated within the cell by discrete contractile proteins using processes that may be ATP-dependent.

II. Magnetic Twisting Cytometry—A Novel Probe of Cytoskeletal Mechanics

To test these ideas, we have recently developed a new technique—the magnetic twisting cytometry (MTC)—that applies controlled mechanical stresses to specific cell surface receptors and measures mechanical responses of adherent cells (Figure 4) (12–15). In this technique, ferromagnetic beads are first coated with a synthetic peptide containing the Arg-Gly-Asp (RGD) sequence that is a known ligand that binds specifically to cell surface integrin receptors (16–18). After

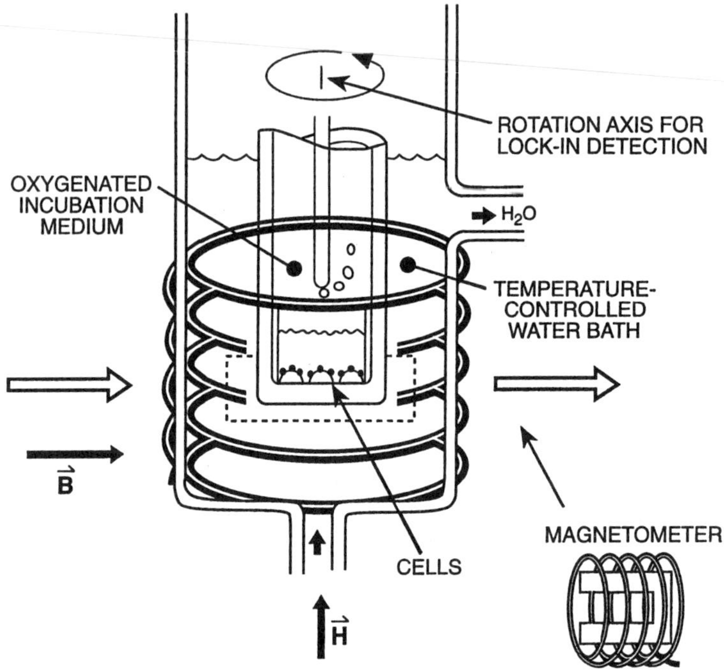

Figure 4 Schematic of the magnetic twisting cytometry system. Individual wells of 96 Removawell plates are placed into the magnetic twisting chamber. The cells are maintained in defined medium that is continuously gassed with 95% O_2/5% CO_2 and held at 37°C using a circulating water bath that is built into the system. The beads are magnetized in the horizontal direction by applying a strong (1000 G) but brief (10 μs) homogeneous magnetic field (*open arrows*). The magnetic signal generated by the beads is measured by a magnetometer in the same direction. A weaker twisting field (0–25 G) is then applied perpendicularly to the original field. Noise from ambient magnetic fields is minimized by appropriately orienting the four probes of the magnetometer, shielding the system with an external supermalloy cylinder and rotating the entire chamber around its vertical axis at 10 Hz. Neither the cells nor culture chamber are drawn to scale. (From Ref. 48.)

the beads are magnetized by a strong pulse in the horizontal direction, a twisting torque is applied to these beads by subsequent application of a weak vertical homogeneous magnetic field, causing the bead to rotate as would a compass needle. In this method, it is possible to quantify the applied stress, the resulting angular rotation of the magnetic beads, and the ratio of the two, that is, stiffness. Therefore, using MTC we are able to probe mechanical properties of cells.

A. Mechanical Coupling Between Integrins and the Cytoskeleton

The magnetic twisting cytometer applies mechanical stresses to specific receptors. Accordingly, one of the first applications of MTC was to address the question of whether the transmembrane integrin receptors are mechanically coupled to the cytoskeleton. We applied mechanical stresses specifically to integrin receptors of endothelial and smooth muscle cells and measured cellular responses. When beads were coated with nonspecific cell attachment ligands, such as acetylated low-density lipoprotein (AcLDL) or bovine serum albumin (BSA), they were not restricted in their rotation as was evident by very small stiffness when compared with RGD-coated beads (Figure 5) (12). To confirm that applied stresses were transmitted to the CSK, we disrupted microfilaments by adding cytochalasin D (CytD). Indeed, the measured stiffness via integrins was decreased by about 50%. Disrupting all major CSK filament systems (microfilaments, microtubules, and intermediate filaments) almost reduced the stiffness to

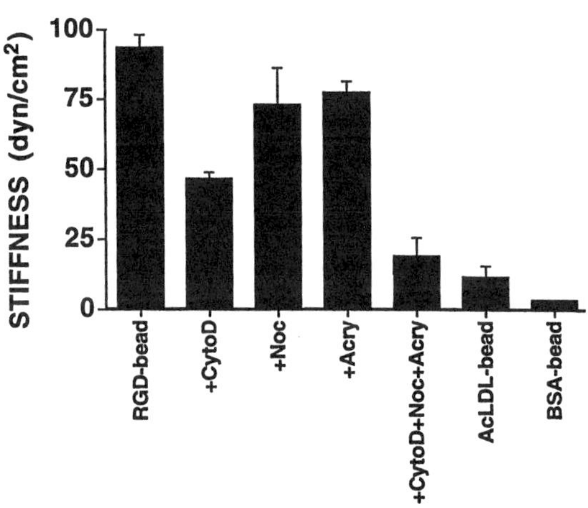

Figure 5 Stiffness measurements in endothelial cells plated on high fibronectin for 8–10 hours in defined medium. Initial applied stress was 40.8 dyne/cm^2. Abbreviations: RGD-bead = RGD-coated beads; +CytoD = 15 minutes after addition of 0.1 μg/mL cytochalasin D to disrupt microfilaments; +Noc = 15 minutes after addition of 10 μg/mL nocodazole to disrupt microtubules; +Acry = 60 minutes after addition of 4 mM acrylamide to disrupt intermediate filaments; +CytoD + Noc + Acry = 60 minutes after addition of all the aforementioned drugs together: CytoD = 0.1 μg/mL, Noc = 10 μg/mL, Acry = 4 mM. AcLDL = acetylated low-density lipoprotein coated beads; BSA = bovine serum albumin coated beads. For RGD-coated beads, stiffness increases to 346 ± 57 dyne/cm^2 after 10 minutes of treatment with 2.5% glutaraldehyde to crosslink all proteins.

the value of that measured via AcLDL-coated beads (see Figure 5). Thus, integrin receptors are mechanically coupled to the CSK. Our results demonstrate that most resistance to bead rotation (that is, most resistance to cell shape distortion) is located at the CSK. Furthermore, our data show that the CSK behaves like an interconnected network and that it is the structural interactions among all three filament systems that are responsible for the cellular mechanical behavior.

B. Coupling Between Changes in Cell Shape and Cytoskeletal Mechanics

If distending stress in the CSK is an important determinant of cell shape stability, then, based on the reasoning offered above, we would predict that increasing cell spreading should result in increases in distending stress and, thus, cell shear stiffness. We have previously shown that CSK stiffness was indeed higher in cells that exhibited more highly extended forms after 6 hours of culture on dishes coated with high fibronectin (FN) densities compared with round cells cultured on low FN (13). To further explore the relation between alterations in CSK mechanics and cell shape changes, we used magnetic twisting cytometry to analyze cells that were undergoing active cell spreading. When suspended endothelial cells were allowed to attach to FN-coated dishes, cell spreading and CSK stiffness were found to both increase in parallel (Figures 6 and 7). Similarly, when spread cells were induced to retract and round by addition of a soluble FN peptide (GRGDSP; 1.5 mg/mL) that competes with immobilized FN for integrin binding, projected cell area and CSK stiffness also decreases coordinately (Figures 8 and 9). The initial stiffness, that is, the stiffness extrapolated to zero applied stress (approximately 10 dyne/cm^2) also was much less than that of the untreated spread cells (about 20 dyne/cm^2), suggesting that cell rounding induced by dislodging integrins resulted in a decrease in the initial distending stress in the CSK that existed before stress application. Recently, we found in human airway smooth muscle cells that treating spread cells with isoproterenol that resulted in muscle relaxation reduced CSK stiffness to the level observed in the round cells (15). This suggests that greater stiffness in spread cells (at least in airway smooth muscle cells) is primarily due to elevated prestress in the CSK.

C. Cytoskeleton Response to Mechanical Stress: Stiffening Effect

We have previously shown that, in cultured endothelial cells, the CSK stiffness increases as the level of mechanical stress applied to integrins is raised (Figure 10) (12). This stiffening response shows that the mechanics of the CSK of endothelial cells is nonlinear. We recently carried out studies to determine whether this stiffening response is a feature shared by other cell types. When pulmonary

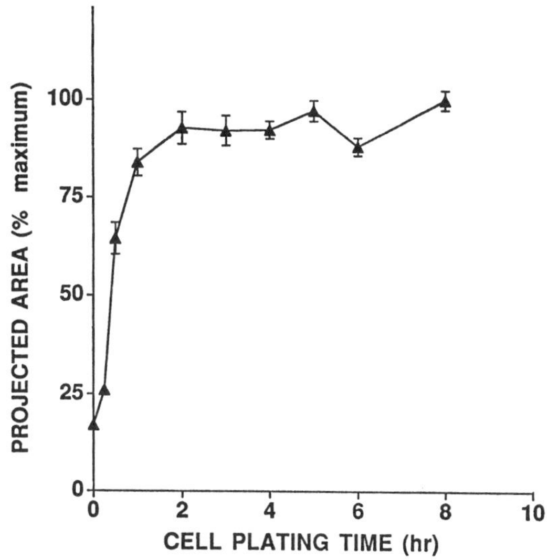

Figure 6 Time course of spreading following cell plating on FN-coated dishes. Capillary endothelial cells were plated on FN-coated dishes and projected areas were determined at different times using a computerized image analysis. Projected cell area was 1815 ± 46 mm^2 at 8 hours (From Ref. 48.)

arterial smooth muscle cells were analyzed using the MTC, CSK stiffness was found to increase from 60 to 175 dyne/cm^2 as the applied stresses were increased from 13 to 68 dyne/cm^2 (Figure 10). The form of this stiffening response is very similar to that exhibited by endothelial cells cultured under similar conditions (see Figure 10). Similar CSK stiffening responses also were observed in adherent hepatocytes and human airway smooth muscle cells (not shown). However, at a given applied stress, smooth muscle cells were found to be stiffer than endothelial cells. Similarly, the initial stiffness (i.e., the stiffness corresponding to zero applied stress) was greater than that found in endothelial cells (27 versus 19 dyne/cm^2) (Figure 10). Therefore, using MTC, we have shown that this stiffening behavior is shared by many cell types, although the degree of stiffening varies between different cells. Importantly, this peculiar stiffening response appears to be a fundamental property of many biological tissues (19). Although the stiffening response can be predicted by empirical relationships (20) or phenomenological models (21) these approaches have not been able to explain the observed phenomena based on first principles (22). We have proposed that the stiffening behavior exhibited by living cells may be due to global rearrangements within the CSK (12). In the following sections, we show that this behavior can be explained starting from first principles, if three-dimensional tensegrity

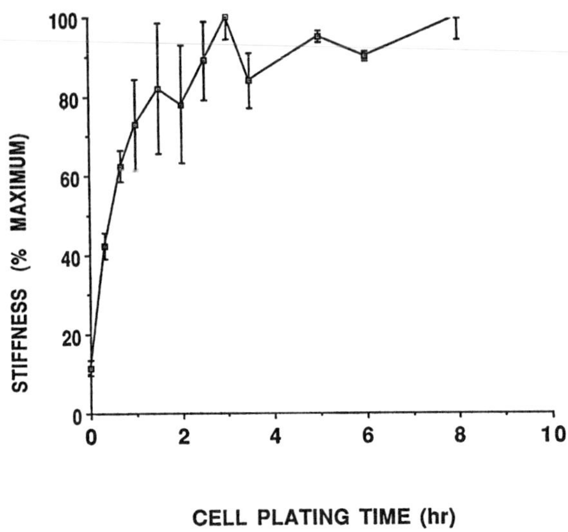

Figure 7 Changes in CSK stiffness measured during the time course of cell spreading on FN-coated dishes. Values are given as a percentage of maximal stiffness measured at 8 hours. Applied stress was 15.2 dyne/cm^2 (30 G twisting field, 4.5 μm-diameter Spherotech beads). Cells were plated exactly as those in Figure 6. Other experiments with different sized beads yielded similar results. (From Ref. 48).

structures are used as a starting point for modeling of mechanics of the CSK. If the CSK behaves like a tensegrity structure, its stiffening response would result from the increased resistance caused by rearranging structural elements within the integrated CSK lattice, rather than solely from deformation of individual filaments. Moreover, CSK stiffness would primarily depend on the distending stress carried by the CSK lattice.

III. Microstructural Analysis of Cytoskeletal Mechanics

Microstructural approaches have been used in the past to study lung deformability (7,8,23–30). Based on these approaches, distending stress (i.e., transpulmonary pressure) and architectural features of lung parenchyma have been identified as unifying principles that underlie lung shape stability. We have extended this idea to cells by focusing on the discrete nature of stress-bearing elements and known properties of the CSK. To illustrate our approach, we present in the following section a conceptual microstructural analysis and show explicitly how distending stresses and interconnectedness of the CSK lattice may come into play in the cell exposed to shear stresses. We then consider a specific class of

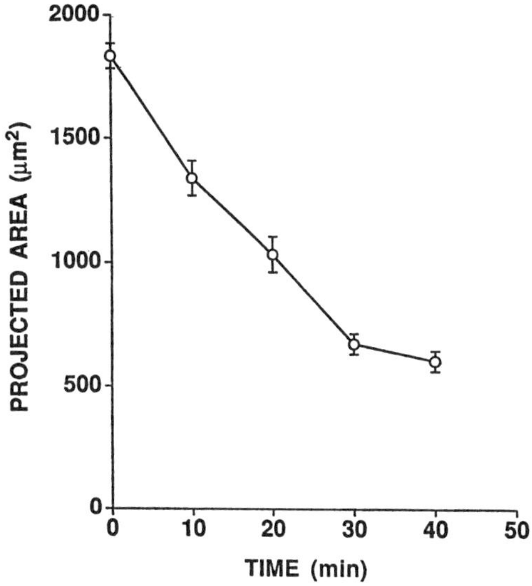

Figure 8 Time course of cell retraction (decrease in projected cell area) induced by addition of soluble GRGDSP (15 mg/mL) to cells adherent to FN-coated dishes. Cells were adherent to FN for 6 hours before the experiment was initiated. Cells that retracted remained adherent to the dishes during the 40-minute time course of this experiment. (From Ref. 48.)

tensed structures, known as tensegrity structures, to elucidate how this architecture naturally comes to express many of the seemingly complex behaviors observed in living cells undergoing shape distortion.

A. A Conceptual Analysis of Cell Deformability

It is well established on structural grounds that the CSK is an interconnected lattice consisting of discrete microfilaments, microtubules, and intermediate filaments (cf 9,31). Although much is known about molecular constituents of the adhesion complex and the CSK lattice, there is little understanding how those components function architecturally and how the CSK lattice resists shape distortion. Morphological and biophysical studies suggest that, in the living cell, microfilaments carry tensile forces even before external load is applied (9,31–36). This, in turn, causes the CSK to be initially tensed. For example, when attachments to the extracellular matrix of the endothelial cell are severed by adding tripsin, the cell rapidly retracts to a round configuration, which represents a state of minimum energy for a given volume (37). This implies that, first, in the attached (spread) cell, elastic energy is stored initially. Second, when cut across the cytoplasm by a microneedle, the living cell retracts rapidly (52).

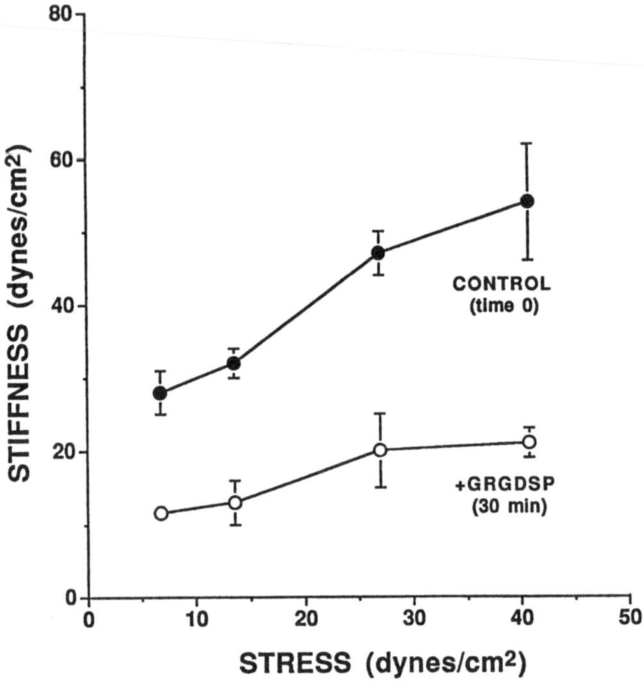

Figure 9 Effect of GRGDSP-induced cell retraction on CSK stiffness. The stiffness of adherent cells was measured using 5.5-μm diameter magnetic beads before addition of GRGDSP (control). The stiffness of the same cells was then measured again 30 minutes after addition of soluble GRGDSP (1.5 mg/mL). Cells were handled exactly as described in Figure 8. Note that both the degree of stiffening and initial stiffness (i.e., stiffness extrapolated to zero applied stress) were significantly decreased in retracted versus extended cells. (From Ref. 48.)

If, however, CSK actin filaments are first disrupted by adding cytochalasin D and then the cell is cut, retraction is inhibited. To demonstrate how the initial tension of the CSK may regulate cell ability to resist shear, we consider a microstructural approach used in the past to identify mechanisms of parenchymal deformability(23,27,28,38,39).

We view the CSK as a lattice of interconnected line elements, which are initially tensed. The total distending stress (σ) of the CSK is defined as the sum of all tensile forces transmitted by the line elements over an arbitrary transectional area per unit transectional area (A):

$$\sigma = \Sigma_{i=1}^{n} F_i \cos\theta_i / A = n\langle F\cos\theta \rangle / A, \tag{1}$$

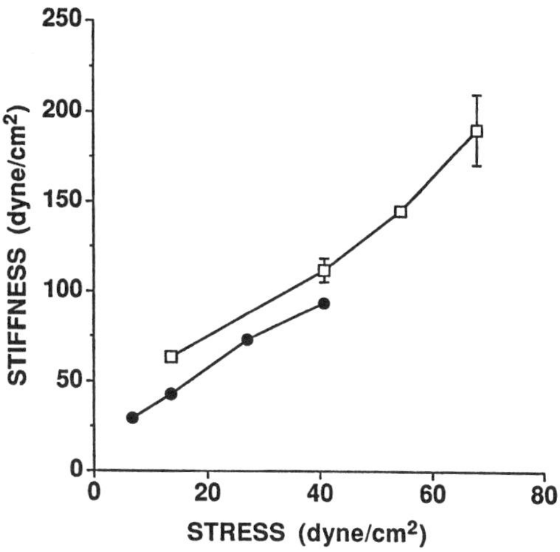

Figure 10 Cytoskeletal stiffening response of cultured pulmonary smooth muscle cells (*open squares*) and capillary endothelial cells (*closed circles*). Cells were plated in defined medium for 8 hours on similar FN-coated dishes, and increasing shear stress was applied using RGD-coated beads (5-μm diameter). Note that both cells exhibited stiffening response, although the smooth muscle cells displayed a higher initial stiffness (i.e., as determined by extrapolating the curves to zero applied stress). (From Ref. 48.)

where n is the total number of line elements transmitted across A, F_i is the force in the i-th element, θ_i is the angle between F_i and the unit outer normal to A, and $\langle\cdot\rangle$ denotes the mean value. In Equation 1, stress σ can be altered by changing n/A (i.e., spacing between the line elements), changing θ (i.e., orientation of the line elements), and changing force F in the line elements. To estimate how those mechanisms contribute to shear modulus (μ), consider a small variation ($\delta\sigma$) of σ

$$\delta\sigma = -(n\langle F\cos\theta\rangle/A)(\delta A/A) - n\langle F\sin\theta\delta\theta\rangle/A + n\langle\cos\theta\delta F\rangle/A \qquad (2)$$

The first, second, and third terms on the right hand side of Equation 2 correspond to changes in spacing, orientation, and force, respectively. Suppose that $\delta\sigma$ corresponds to a pure shear (isovolume) deformation during which A shrinks uniformly and the network extends in the direction orthogonal to A. Then $\delta A/A = -\delta s/s$, where s is a characteristic length chosen such that As = cell volume, and $\delta s/s$ is shear strain. Consider a special case of interconnectedness of line elements, which eliminates the effects of changes in orientation of the line elements and of forces they carry. Suppose that, at their junctions, the line elements run through frictionless loops and, thus, can freely slide relative to each other.

As a consequence, during pure shear deformation, the total cable length and therefore the force F in the cables does not change to the first order in strain (i.e., $\delta F = 0$). Moreover, the line elements would not rotate relative to each other, that is, $\delta\theta = 0$ (39,40). Taking these into account, it follows from Equations 1, 2, and $\delta A/A = -\delta s/s$ that $\delta\sigma = \sigma\delta s/s$. On the other hand, according to the theory of elasticity, $\delta\sigma = 2\mu\delta s/s$, where μ is shear modulus. Thus it follows that $\mu = 0.5\sigma$, that is, shear modulus is directly proportional to distending stress and does not depend explicitly on mechanical properties of individual line elements. Because of the assumptions used to derive μ, it must be taken as a lower limit (39,40).

To quantify the contributions of changes in orientation of line elements and of forces they carry, it is necessary to specify geometry or kinematics of the microstructure. For example, in a dodecahedral line element structure studied by Budiansky and Kimmel (7), this was accomplished by considering equilibrium at joints during deformation. It was found that shear modulus μ ranges from 0.5σ to 1.35σ as the line element tensile strength changes from infinitely compliant to infinitely stiff. *It is important to note, however, that μ is primarily controlled by distending stress and architectural features of the microstructure, and to a lesser degree by mechanical properties of individual line elements.* Similar dependences have been observed in isolated living cells exposed to shear stresses. Thus, there is a reason to suppose that distending stress and architecture of the CSK are the key features that underlie the ability of the cell to regulate its shape. In support of this hypothesis, the next section considers mechanical behavior of a simple tensegrity structure during uniaxial distortion as a paradigm of cellular deformability.

B. A Model of Cellular Tensegrity

As previously discussed, adherent cells display both CSK architecture and deformability that appear to conform to the architecture of tensegrity first described by Buckminster Fuller (4,9,10,12,41). In the simplest representation of tensegrity, Pugh (42) defined its structures as the interconnection of a set of isolated compression elements (e.g., struts) with a set of continuous tension elements (e.g., cables) in the aim to provide a stable volume and shape in the space. The tension element carries initial stress, conferring load-supporting capability to the entire structure. The role of compression elements is to provide initial stress in the tension elements. Together, they form a self-equilibrating, stable mechanical system.

A distinguishing characteristic of tensegrity structures is that, to resist shape distortion, they need to be initially tensed even before external loading is applied. For example, mammalian lungs can be also viewed as a tensegrity structure in which tensile forces carried by the parenchymal connective tissue systems and alveolar surface film are supported by transpulmonary pressure (i.e., the compression element in lieu of rigid struts). Another example is the spider's web in which the distending tension is provided by surrounding objects, such as tree branches, and is balanced by tensile forces in web threads. Even though they are external to the web itself, the tree branches may be viewed as compression elements in a tensegrity structure, because they are an integral part of the mechanically stable whole.

It is likely that the CSK and the extracellular matrix form a tensegrity structure (9,43). For example, the regions of the extracellular matrix that stretch between focal contacts represent local compression-resistant elements that support tension exerted by stress fibers inside the cell (9,44). Thus, cell shape stability cannot be understood unless the extracellular matrix support elements are considered as a part of an "extended CSK" (43), much like the tree branches that are required to stabilize the spider's web. In addition, within the CSK, microtubule bundles may act as compression-resistant struts and stabilize cell shape by resisting the pull of contractile microfilament lattice (32–36).

Models built of sticks and elastic strings according to the rules of tensegrity architecture qualitatively mimic many of the phenomena that have been observed in living cells, including the effect of substrate adhesion on cell shape, cell polarity, and CSK remodeling (4,9,10,43). These tensegrity structures also exhibit a stiffening response (12,45,46).

We have recently extended these qualitative notions into a formal microstructural analysis (46). For simplicity, we considered a simple tensegrity structure composed of six rigid struts interconnected with 24 linearly elastic (Hookean) cables (Figure 11) as a first step in implementing tensegrity architecture in studies of cell mechanics. Cables and struts are connected by pin joints. Cables carry initial tension balanced by compression in the struts. For convenience, the struts are assumed to be of unit length. Thus, at the reference state, the length of each cable $l_0 = \sqrt{0.375}$ and the distance between the parallel struts $s_0 = 0.5$ (47). Within the CSK, microfilaments and intermediate filaments may play the role of cables, whereas microtubules or cross-linked actin bundles may play the role of the struts (9). The internally generated initial tension in the microfilaments is provided by the actomyosin contractile apparatus.

The structure is stretched uniaxially by pulling a pair of parallel struts apart by external force T/2 applied at each endpoint of the pulled struts (not shown). The resultant pulling force is therefore T (see Figure 11). This causes changes in the distance between the pairs of parallel struts and changes in the length and orientation of the cables. From the symmetry of the structure, it follows that during uniaxial stretching, changes in length of only three distinct cables joining three distinct struts are needed to fully characterize the deformation of the structure. Relationships between lengths of these three cables and distances between the pairs of parallel struts can be obtained from geometry of

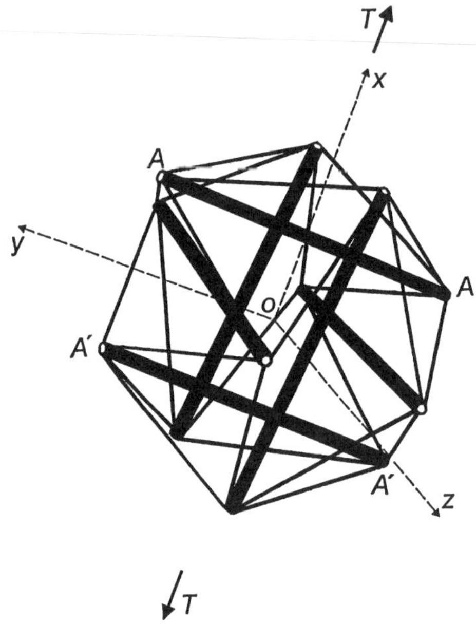

Figure 11 Six-strut tensegrity structure. Pulling forces of magnitude T/2 (not shown) are applied at each end of struts AA and A′A′, along the Ox-axis. The resultant stretching force T is indicated by the thick arrows.

the structure (46,47). From equilibrium at the junctions, a set of three equations that relate the pulling (external) force T and the forces in the cables (internal forces) are obtained. Taking into account that the force in each cable is proportional to the change in cable length (i.e., Hookean cables), and combining equilibrium equations with the equations obtained from geometry of the structure, force T is obtained as a function of change in distance between pulled struts (Δs_x).

C. Major Results from Tensegrity Analysis

A general form of T versus Δs_x relationship can be written as a product of the initial cable tension and a function that depends on the architecture of the structure (i.e., geometry of the structure and the manner in which structural elements are interconnected) as follows:

$$T = (k\Delta l_0) \times f(\Delta l_0, \Delta s_x). \qquad (3)$$

The term $k\Delta l_0$ on the right-hand side of Equation 3 equals the initial cable tension, where k is the cable stiffness and Δl_0 is the initial cable extension, that is, the difference between the cable length at the reference configuration (l_0) and its resting length. The term $f(\Delta l_0,\Delta s_x)$ is a function of Δl_0 and Δs_x (i.e., the difference in the distance between the pulled struts during and before deformation) and indicates the contribution of the architecture of the structure. The exact form of this function can be found in Stamenović et al. (46).

The initial cable tension determines the initial structural stiffness whereas architecture of the structure determines how structural stiffness changes during deformation. Structural stiffness was defined as the ratio of the stretching force to the change in the distance between pulled struts, that is, $E \equiv T/\Delta s_x$. The only parameter common in both terms on the right-hand side of Equation 3 is the initial cable extension Δl_0. Thus, the degree to which the cables are initially extended contributes to both initial structural stiffness and change of structural stiffness during deformation. On the other hand, *the cable stiffness* k *only contributes to the initial cable tension. Thus,* k *only affects the initial structural stiffness and not the change of structural stiffness during deformation.*

The above results suggest that, in order to describe cell deformability, it is not sufficient to know only mechanical properties of individual molecular components of the CSK. It is essential to understand how these components are organized architecturally.

Instructive parallels between the behavior of the six-strut tensegrity structure and observations in living cells are seen in Figure 12 , which depicts structural stiffness versus stretching force relationships obtained at different initial cable tension. The initial cable tension is varied either by varying the initial cable extension Δl_0 at a given cable stiffness k (Figure 12A), or isometrically, by varying k at a given Δl_0 (see Figure 12B). First, the tensegrity structure exhibits structural stiffness E that increases with increasing level of initial cable tension. This result is consistent with the observation that the CSK stiffness measured in living endothelial cells increases with increased cell spreading (48), which is, in turn, mediated by the CSK extension (49). Thus, it is not unreasonable to postulate higher levels of CSK tension in more highly spread cells, although this remains to be demonstrated experimentally. Furthermore, this type of response to isometric changes in the initial tension is likely to occur in airway smooth muscle cells stimulated by contractile agonists (15). Second, the tensegrity structure exhibits initial stiffness that increases with the initial tension. Interestingly, the initial CSK stiffness (i.e., the value extrapolated for CSK stiffness at zero applied stress) in spread endothelial cells has been shown to be higher than in round cells (13), a finding consistent with a possibility that the initial cell stiffness is provided by the CSK initial tension. Finally, the tensegrity structure exhibits a positive dependence of E on the applied stretching force T. This specialized form of stiffening behavior is exhibited by living cells (12,13) as

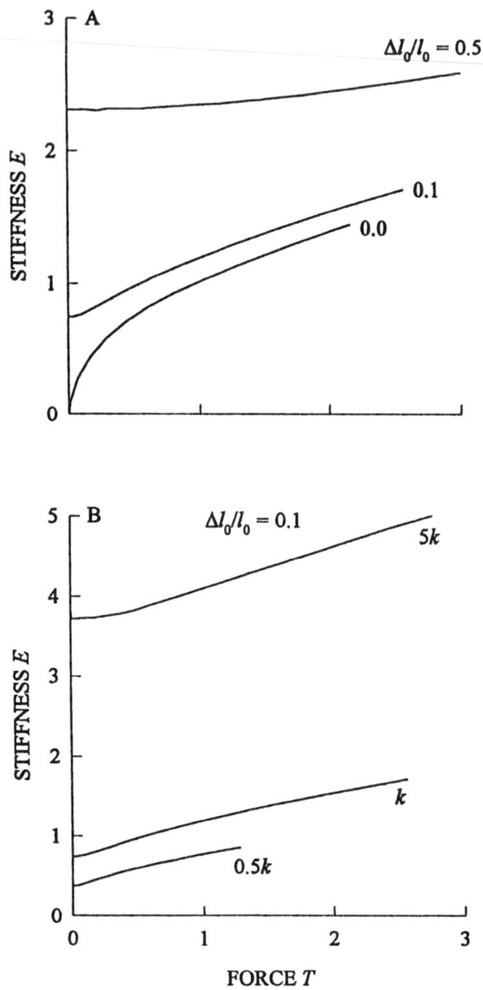

Figure 12 Plots of structural stiffness E as a function of applied stretching force T for different initial cable tension. **A**, the initial cable tension is varied by varying the initial cable extension (i.e., initial cable strain $\Delta l_0/l_0$ of 0, 0.1, and 0.5) at a unit cable stiffness k = 1. **B**, the initial cable tension is varied isometrically by varying cable stiffness (0.5k, k, 5k, k = 1) at a given initial cable strain $\Delta l_0/l_0 = 0.1$. Force is given in units of force and stiffness in unit of force/length.

well as many biological tissues (cf 19,20). Thus, our results support the concept that the distending stress and architectural features of the CSK lattice rather than the mechanical properties of its individual stress-bearing elements are the primary determinants of cell deformability. This is similar to lung parenchyma in which transpulmonary pressure and parenchymal architecture are shown to be the key determinants of the ability of the lung to resist shape distortion (1).

Despite good agreements, some of the responses of the six-strut tensegrity structure to uniaxial stretching do not correspond directly with observations in cells. For example, the structure exhibits a stiffening response that decreased with increasing initial cable extension (see Figure 12*A*). In contrast, data obtained in living endothelial cells (13) indicate that the stiffening response increases with increasing cell spreading (i.e., increasing distention). Possible reasons for this discrepancy are likely related to arbitrariness and oversimplifications of model architecture and the manner in which the model was deformed (i.e., uniaxial stretching of the model versus isovolume shear deformation of the cells). Another reason could be a neglect of some structures and mechanisms that play an important role in determining cell mechanical behavior (46).

IV. Summary

It is possible to connect some features of macroscopic behavior of the cell with the underlying micromechanics. For example, cell ability to resist distortion of shape appear to be primarily determined by the initial distending stress and architecture of the CSK lattice. Interestingly, the same underlying principles apply to lung parenchyma, as well as to many other biological systems including plant leaves, spiders' webs, and cartilage.

General description of the CSK as a discrete tensed mechanical structure agree, at least qualitatively, with data obtained from magnetic twisting cytometry. Tensegrity approach, in particular, offers the quantitative basis of several phenomena that tensegrity architecture expresses. Many of the features are also expressed in various eukaryotic cells as they resist shape distortion. This is an important finding because it has been customary to view cellular mechanics in terms of continuum mechanics (cf 50,51). Although many features of cell deformability can be described using a continuum approach, such descriptions have been based on empirical constitutive stress-strain equations. On the other hand, by considering the discrete nature of the CSK, it is possible to obtain forces and deformations that mediate cell shape distortion starting from first principles of mechanics. Nevertheless, the six-strut tensegrity structure presented here must be regarded only as a crude representation of the CSK mechanics. Even so, our analysis points to the distending stress and the architecture of the CSK as key features that might underlie the ability of a cell to regulate its shape.

Acknowledgments

This work was supported by grants from National Institutes of Health (HL-33009 and CA45548) and NASA (NAG-9-430 and NAG-9-836). Dr. Ingber is a recipient of Faculty Research Award from the American Cancer Society.

References

1. Stamenović D. Micromechanical foundations of pulmonary elasticity. Physiol Rev 1990; 70:1117–1134.
2. Davies PF, Tripathi S. Stress mechanisms in cultured cells: an endothelial paradigm. Circ Res 1993; 72:239–245.
3. Singhvi R, Kumar A, Lopez GP, Stephanopoulos GN, Wang DIC, Whitesides GM, Ingber DE. Engineering cell shape and function. Science 1994; 264:696–698.
4. Ingber DE, Folkman J. Tension and compression as basic determinants of cell form and function: utilization of a cellular tensegrity mechanism. In: Stein WD, Bronner F, eds. Cell Shape: Determinants Regulation, and Regulatory Role. San Diego, CA: Academic Press, 1989:3–31.
5. Ingber DE. The riddle of morphogenesis: a question of solution chemistry or molecular engineering. Cell 1993; 75:1249–1252.
6. Suki B, Barabási A-L, Hantos Z, Peták F, Stanley HE. Avalanches and power-law behaviour in lung inflation. Nature 1994; 368:615–618.
7. Budiansky B, Kimmel E. Elastic moduli of lungs. ASME J Appl Mech 1987; 54: 351–358.
8. Wilson TA. A continuum analysis of a two-dimensional mechanical model of the lung parenchyma. J Appl Physiol 1972; 33:472–478.
9. Ingber DE. Cellular tensegrity: defining new rules of biological design that govern the cytoskeleton. J Cell Sci 1993; 104:613–627.
10. Ingber DE, Jamieson JD. Cells as tensegrity structures: architectural regulation of hystodifferentiation by physical forces transduced over basement membrane. In: Andersson LC, Gahmberg CG, Ekblom P, eds. Gene Expression During Normal and Malignant Differentiation. London: Academic Press, 1985: 13–32.
11. Heidemann SR. A new twist on integrins and the cytoskeleton. Science 1993; 260: 1080–1081.
12. Wang N, Butler JP, Ingber DE. Mechanotransduction across the cell surface and through the cytoskeleton. Science 1993; 260:1124–1127.
13. Wang N, Ingber DE. Control of cytoskeletal mechanics by extracellular matrix, cell shape, and mechanical tension. Biophys 1994; 66:1281–1289.
14. Wang N, Planus E, Poulet M, Fredberg JJ, Barlovatz-Meimon G. The urokinase receptor mediates mechanical force transfer across the cell surface. Am J Physiol (Cell Physiol) 1995; 268:C1062–C1066.
15. Hubmayr RD, Shore SA, Fredberg JJ, Planus E, Panettieri RA, Wang N. Pharmacological activation changes stiffness of cultured human airway smooth muscle cells. Am J Physiol (Cell Physiol) 1996; 271:C1660–C1668.
16. Burridge K, Fath K, Kelly T, Nucko G, Turner C. Focal adhesions: transmembrane

junctions between extracellular matrix and cytoskeleton. Rev Cell Biol 1988; 4: 487–525.
17. Albeld SM, Buck CA. Integrins and other cell adhesion molecules. FASEB J 1990; 4:2868–2880.
18. Hynes RO. Integrins: versitility, modulation, and signaling in cell adhesion. Cell 1992; 69:11–25.
19. Fung YC. Biomechanics—Mechanical Properties of Living Tissues. New York: Springer-Verlag, 1981.
20. Mow VC, Ratcliffe A, Poole AR. Cartilage and diarthrodial joints as paradigms for hierarchical materials and structures. Biomaterials 1992; 13:67–97.
21. Frisén M, Mägi M, Sonnerup I, Viidik A. Rheological analysis of soft collagenous tissue—I. J Biomech 1969; 2:13–20.
22. McMahon TA. Muscles, Reflexes, and Locomotion. Princeton, NJ: Princeton University Press, 1984.
23. Mead J, Takishima T, Leith D. Stress distribution in lungs: a model of pulmonary elasticity. J Appl Physiol 1970; 28:596–608.
24. Lambert RK, Wilson TA. A model of elastic properties of the lung and their effect on expiratory flow. J Appl Physiol 1973; 34:34–38.
25. Fung YC. A theory of elasticity of the lung. ASME J Appl Mech 1974; 41:8–14.
26. Fung YC. Stress, deformation, and atelectasis of the lung. Circ Res 1975; 37:481–496.
27. Hoppin FG Jr., Hildebrandt J. Mechanical properties of the lung. In: West JB, ed. Bioengineering Aspects of the Lung. Vol. 3. New York: Marcel Dekker, 1977: 83–162.
28. Wilson TA, Bachofen H. A model of mechanical structure of the alveolar duct. J Appl Physiol 1982; 52:1064–1070.
29. Stamenović D, Wilson TA. A strain energy function for lung parenchyma. ASME J Biomech Eng 1985; 107:81–86.
30. Kimmel E, Kamm RD, Shapiro AH. A cellular model of lung elasticity. ASME J Biomech Eng 1987; 109:126–131.
31. Amos LA, Amos WB. Molecules of the Cytoskeleton. New York: Guilford Press, 1991.
32. Joshi HC, Chu D, Buxbaum RE, Heidemann SR. Tension and compression in the cytoskeleton of PC-12 neurites. J Cell Biol. 1985; 101:697–705.
33. Dennerll TJ, Joshi HC, Steel VL, Buxbaum RE, Heidemann SR. Tension and compression in the cytoskeleton of PC-12 neurites: quantitative measurements. J Cell Biol 1988; 107:565–674.
34. Danowski BA. Fibroblast contractility and actin organization are stimulated by microtubule inhibitors. J Cell Sci 1989; 93:255–266.
35. Kolodney MS, Wysolmerski RB. Isometric contraction by fibroblast and endothelial cells in tissue culture: a qualitative study. J Cell Biol 1992; 117:73–82.
36. Heidemann SR, Buxbaum RE. Mechanical tension as a regulator of axional development. Neuro Toxicology 1994; 15:95–108.
37. Sims JR, Karp S, Ingber DE. Altering the cellular mechanical force balance results in integrated changes in cell, cytoskeletal, and nuclear shape. J Cell Sci 1992; 103: 1215–1222.

38. Wilson TA. Mechanics of the pressure-volume curve of the lung. Ann Biomed Eng 1981; 9:439–449.
39. Stamenović D, Wilson TA. Parenchymal stability. J Appl Physiol 1992; 73:596–602.
40. Stamenović D. A model of foam elasticity based upon the laws of Plateau. J Colloid Interface Sci 1991; 145:255–259.
41. Fuler B. Tensegrity. Portfolio Artnews Annual 1961; 4:112–127.
42. Pugh A. Introduction to Tensegrity. Berkeley, CA: University of California Press, 1976.
43. Ingber DE, Dike L, Hansen L, Karp S, Liley H, Maniotis A, McNamee H, Mooney D, Plooper G, Sims J, Wang N. Cellular tensegrity: exploring how mechanical changes in the cytoskeleton regulate cell growth, migration, and tissue pattern during morphogenesis. Int Rev Cytol 1994; 150:173–224.
44. Harris AK, Wild P, Stopak D. Silicone rubber substrata: a new wrinkle in the study of cell locomotion. Science 1980; 208:177–180.
45. Thoumine O, Ziegler T, Girard PR, Nerem RM. Elongation of confluent endothelial cells in culture: the importance of fields of force in the associated alterations of their cytoskeletal structure. Exp Cell Res 1995; 219:427–441.
46. Stamenović D, Fredberg JJ, Wang N, Butler JP, Ingber DE. A microstructural approach to cytoskeletal mechanics based on tensegrity. J Theor Biol 1996; 181: 125–136.
47. Kenner H. Geodesic Math and How to Use It. Berkeley, CA: University of California Press, 1976.
48. Wang N, Ingber DE. Probing transmembrane mechanical coupling and cytomechanics using magnetic twisting cytometry. Biochem Cell Biol 1995; 73:327–335.
49. Mooney D, Langer R, Ingber DE. Cytoskeletal filament assembly and the control of cell shape and function by extracellular matrix. J Cell Sci 1995; 108:2311–2320.
50. Elson EL. Cellular mechanics as an indicator of cytoskeletal structure and function. Ann Biophys Chem 1988; 17:379–430.
51. Evans E, Yeung A. Apparent viscosity and cortical tension of blood granulocytes determined by micropipet aspiration. Biophys J 1989; 56:151–160.
52. Pourati J, Maniotis A, Spiegel D, Schaffer JL, Butler JP, Fredberg JJ, Ingber DE, Stamenović D, Wang N. Is cytoskeletal tension a major determinant of cell deformability in adherent endothelial cells? Am J Physiol (Cell Physiol) In press.

5

Dynamics of Pleural Liquid
Mechanical Factors Affecting Its Formation and Regional Distribution

STEPHEN J. LAI-FOOK and PING M. WANG

Center for Biomedical Engineering
University of Kentucky
Lexington, Kentucky

I. Introduction

The understanding of the mechanics of the pleural space has undergone considerable revision in recent years. Early studies described the origin of pleural liquid as arising from a static equilibrium between the hydrostatic and osmotic forces between pleural liquid and capillary blood. Recent studies have focused on a more complex theory of pleural mechanics that entails elements of microvascular exchange and viscous flow within the pleural space. Viscous flow concepts are treatable within the mathematical framework of fluid mechanics and lubrication theory. Indeed, lubrication of the pleural surfaces during ventilation is one of the main, if not the primary, functions of the pleural space. In this description, pleural surface pressure—the pressure caused by lung expansion opposing the recoil of the chest wall—is the independent variable that determines viscous flow within the pleural space. The presence of a thin lubricating layer of pleural liquid ensures the absence of contact between the two pleural surfaces and the identity between pleural liquid and surface pressures, a crucial assumption of viscous flow theory.

In this chapter, we review some recent studies that focus on the dynamics of pleural liquid. The net effect of a vertical gradient in pleural pressure and the force of gravity acting on pleural liquid drives a viscous flow of pleural liquid downward within the pleural space. The uniform thickness of pleural with respect to height comes about by a recirculation of pleural liquid upward along lobar margins and transversely from lobar margins toward the relatively flat costal regions of the pleural space. Ventilation and, to a lesser extent, cardiogenic motion provides an active pump for this recirculation of pleural liquid. Ventilation results in cranial-caudal gradients in lung sliding velocities and chest wall strains, which are associated with cranial-caudal gradients in pleural liquid thickness and perhaps pleural liquid filtration. These gradients are accentuated by increases in ventilation.

II. Foundations of Pleural Mechanics

A. Hydrostatic Equilibrium

Understanding of the mechanics of the pleural space has been dominated by two main viewpoints. In its earliest conception, pleural liquid was assumed to be in hydrostatic equilibrium, with pleural liquid pressure varying by 1 cm H_2O per centimeter of height, in parallel with a hydrostatic gradient in capillary pressure. Pleural liquid pressure was thought to be always lower than pleural surface pressure, the pressure expanding the lung, with the net result being the absorption of pleural liquid into pleural capillaries until contact between the two pleural membranes occurred. A contact pressure between the two pleural surfaces was thought to provide the excess force required to explain the difference between pleural liquid and surface pressures. Comprehensive reviews of the literature supporting this view have been written by Agostoni (1,2).

B. Viscous Flow—Hydrodynamic Lubrication

The second view, the one that has received more attention in recent years, assumes that pleural liquid forms a continuous, thin lubricating layer such that pleural surface pressure is identical to pleural liquid pressure. Evidence to support the latter assumption has been reviewed (3,4). Pleural surface pressure distribution is determined primarily by the matching of the lung within the chest wall, and the vertical gradient of pleural surface pressure is always less than the hydrostatic value so that there is a residual gravity force acting to drive a viscous flow of pleural liquid downward on the flat costal pleural surfaces. Ventilation and cardiogenic motion provide the energy to recirculate pleural liquid and to smooth out spatial nonuniformities in pleural liquid thickness. A recent model that falls within the context of lubrication theory has considered the buoyancy force exerted on a rigid chest wall by a rigid lung of density smaller than that of the pleural liquid (5). This model predicted a vertical gradient in pleural liquid thickness not substantiated by regional measurements of pleural liquid thickness. The model of the pleural space as a porous material (6) does not match the physical characteristics of the pleural space determined experimentally.

C. Pleural Contact and Boundary Lubrication

A critical prediction of pleural mechanics based on hydrostatic equilibrium of pleural liquid is the presence of contact between the two pleural surfaces. There is a paucity of experimental evidence that contact between the two pleural membranes ever occurs in the normal pleural space, although, in disease, such as pleural adhesions, the pleural membranes become fused. Indeed, electron microscope images of frozen cross sections of the chest wall of sheep indicate a well-defined, uniformly thick pleural liquid space (7).

Surfactant has been found in minute quantities in pleural liquid, and boundary lubrication has been proposed as a possible function for its presence (8). A similar lubrication function might be attributed to hyaluronan and glycoprotein present in pleural liquid. In our own studies, there was no region in the pleural space where the measured pleural liquid thickness was less than 5 μm, and from this consideration it is difficult to make a case for the importance of boundary lubrication. With regard to hydrodynamic lubrication in which viscous forces are important, during normal breathing at rest, hyaluronan concentration (1 μg/mL) in pleural liquid is too small to affect significantly pleural liquid viscosity (9). On the other hand, recent studies in anesthetized (9) and conscious rabbits (10) indicated an increase in pleural liquid hyaluronan concentration with ventilation, and this increase might facilitate boundary lubrication (8).

III. Spatial Gradients in Pleural Pressure

A. Pleural Liquid Pressure

There is no universally acceptable method for measuring pleural liquid pressure. The pleural space is extremely thin, ~20 μm, so that a direct measurement of pleural pressure is often invasive and requires gross distortion of the pleural space. The many conflicting results in the published literature underscore the difficulty of measuring pleural liquid pressure noninvasively.

The earliest attempts at measuring pleural liquid pressure used 1-mm diameter catheters (11). Use of rigid cannulas is a variant of this method (12,13). These methods invariably show vertical gradients (0.6–0.9 cm H_2O/cm) in pleural liquid pressure near to the hydrostatic value. The vertical pressure gradient measured with catheters and cannulas might be unrelated to pressure in the undisturbed pleural space and is most likely caused by the widened liquid column formed along the catheter or by the widened pleural space between the catheter and a lobar margin where a hydrostatic gradient exists (3,4). A hydrostatic gradient occurs in these widened spaces because viscous forces resulting from flow of pleural liquid are relatively small and the curvature of the pleural membrane adjacent to them can vary with height to balance the change in pleural liquid pressure associated with a hydrostatic gradient. For example, vertical gradients in pleural liquid pressure near to the hydrostatic value have been measured along a lobar margin in the prone position in dogs (3) where pleural surface pressure was uniform with respect to height (14,15).

Two techniques for measuring pleural liquid pressure have been developed in an attempt to avoid the distortion associated with intrapleural catheters. In the micropuncture servonulling technique, pressure is measured at the end of a micropipet of 2-to 10-μm tip diameter in conjunction with a servonulling pressure measuring system (13,16). A pleural window is made in the chest of experimental animals by dissection of intercostal muscle and endothoracic fascia until the parietal pleural membrane is exposed. The micropipet is pushed through the pleural window into the lung and slowly withdrawn until the tip is located in the pleural space. This technique has several limitations. First, the removal of intercostal muscle to make the window reduces the recoil of the chest wall locally, and thus pleural surface pressure is increased beneath the window. Accordingly, the measured pleural liquid pressure would be greater than that present if there were no pleural window. Second, there is uncertainty regarding the location of the tip of the micropipet. The tip of the micropipet is rarely observed within the pleural liquid, so that it is possible that the micropipet tip is located in the visceral or parietal pleural membrane. Finally, pleural liquid pressure by micropuncture can only be measured during apnea because ventilatory motion causes breakage of the glass micropipet.

Pleural liquid pressure measured by micropipets indicated vertical gradients in the supine rabbit to be 0.5–0.9 cm H_2O/cm, less than the hydrostatic value (13,16). The vertical gradient in pleural liquid pressure was found to be smaller in the prone than in the supine position (16). However, this result has not been confirmed by later studies (18).

The other relatively noninvasive technique, which uses a rib capsule, measures pleural liquid pressure via a liquid-filled capsule embedded in a rib (19). In this technique, a hole is drilled into a rib down to the parietal pleural membrane and a liquid-filled capsule is bonded into the hole. The parietal pleura is punctured with a needle to allow communication between the liquid in the capsule and the pleural liquid. A pressure transducer is attached to the capsule to measure pleural liquid pressure. An advantage of the rib capsule method over the micropuncture technique is that measurements can be made during ventilation. A limitation of the rib capsule technique is that measurements of pleural liquid pressure are confined to regions beneath ribs where pleural surface pressure may be lower than that in the intercostal space (20). In studies using rib capsules, vertical gradients in pleural liquid pressure were greater in the supine position (0.5–0.8 cm H_2O/cm) than in the prone position (0.2 cm H_2O/cm) in dogs (19), ponies (21), and rabbits (22). The smaller gradient in the prone rabbit has been questioned (18).

B. Pleural Surface Pressure

Many ingenious techniques have been devised to measure pleural surface pressure acting on the lung directly (1,2). In the past, direct measurements of pleural surface pressure have suffered from the same limitations as those for pleural liquid pressure. Many techniques, such as flat pleural balloons (23), are invasive so that the local recoil of the chest wall on the lung is reduced and pleural surface pressure is artifactually increased. This results in a reduction of the vertical gradient in pleural surface pressure. Other techniques, such as esophageal balloons, are limited to measurements of pleural surface pressure in the mediastinal region of the thorax so that vertical gradients of pleural surface pressure are only possible in the upright and head-down body positions (24).

Since the initial studies using radioactive xenon for lung volume imaging (25,26), there have been major advances in the estimation of pleural pressure with the advent of sophisticated lung volume imaging systems. These include computerized tomography (27) and radiographic imaging of lead beads implanted in the lung parenchyma (15). Imaging techniques are relatively noninvasive and have produced reliable measurements of spatial gradients in lung expansion from which spatial gradient of pleural pressure can be accurately inferred.

In upright humans, the vertical gradient in pleural surface pressure using the radioactive xenon technique was ~0.3 cm H_2O/cm (26,27). In the dog (15,16), the vertical gradient in pleural surface pressure measured using computerized tomography and the intraparenchymal marker technique was greater in the supine (0.8 cm H_2O/cm) than in the prone position (near 0 cm H_2O/cm), in agreement with measurements of the vertical gradient in pleural liquid pressure using rib capsules (19). In rabbits, vertical surface pressure gradients in the prone and supine body positions were similar (18), in contradiction to the vertical gradients in pleural liquid pressure measured using rib capsules (22). A small cranial-caudal gradient in pleural surface pressure in the supine dog has been measured (15).

The role of animal size on the vertical gradient in pleural pressure is still debated. Previous results (1,2) indicated that the vertical gradient in pleural surface pressure decreased with animal size, but this has not been verified by more recent results; for example, the vertical pleural pressure gradient in the supine position was as large in the pony as in the dog (19,21). Thus, body position is as important a variable as animal size in determining the vertical pleural pressure gradient. The effect of lung inflation on the vertical surface pressure gradient has also been revised recently. Recent studies have shown that lung inflation reduced the vertical pleural pressure gradient in the supine rabbit (28), contrary to previous results (29).

A result applicable to all species is that the vertical gradient in pleural pressure is always less than the hydrostatic value. This ensures that, during apnea, there is always a downward flow of pleural liquid. However, a persistent downward flow of pleural liquid is inconsistent with a pleural liquid thickness that is constant at all heights in the thorax. This paradoxical behavior served as the impetus for several studies of pleural liquid recirculation and regional pleural liquid distribution.

C. Subpleural Interstitial Pressure in the Chest Wall

Measurements of interstitial pressure in the intercostal space of the chest wall by rigid cannulas indicated a vertical gradient in liquid pressure that was less than that in the pleural liquid (14). These results point to a vertical gradient in pleural liquid filtration from the parietal pleura and chest wall (30). These predictions need to be substantiated experimentally.

D. Pleural Liquid Pressure at Lobar Margins

Although recent measurements using noninvasive techniques have shown that the vertical gradient in pleural liquid pressure is less than the hydrostatic value, there are locations in the pleural space at lobar margins where a hydrostatic gradient in pleural liquid pressure exists (31,32). Figure 1 shows the relationship between pleural liquid pressure at a lobar margin and pleural pressure on the flat costal regions with respect to height in the prone position in dogs. Note that pleural liquid pressure at the lobar margin is near 0 cm H_2O at the lung base and varies by 1 cm H_2O per centimeter of height, whereas pleural surface pressure on the flat costal surface has a constant value of –4 cm H_2O at all heights in the thorax (15). In the nondependent chest regions above 4 cm height, pleural liquid pressure at the lobar margin is more negative than the costal pleural pressure. At a lung height of 4 cm above the lung base, pleural liquid pressure at the lobar margin is equal to the costal pleural pressure. In the dependent chest regions below 4 cm height, pleural pressure in the lobar margins is greater than costal pleural pressure. Under conditions of apnea, pleural liquid in nondependent regions drains from the costal pleural surface to the lobar margins, whereas in dependent regions, pleural liquid flows from lobar margins to the costal regions. Thus, these gradients in pleural pressure can only result in a vertical gradient in pleural liquid thickness with pleural liquid thickness decreasing with height up the lung, not consistent with experimental results. However, in the nondependent chest regions, ventilation provides an active pump that causes a

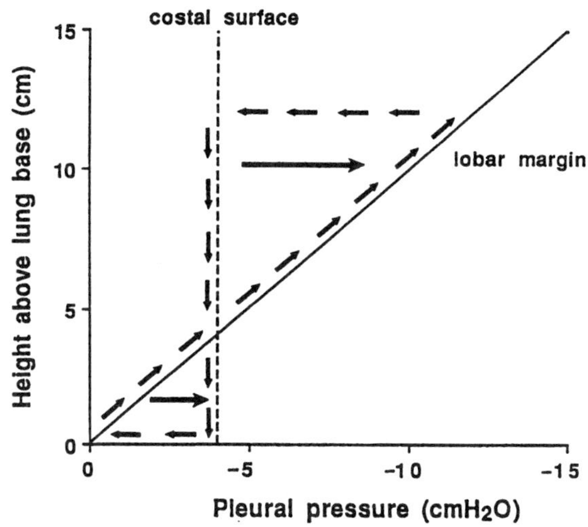

Figure 1 Pleural liquid pressure at lobar margin and costal surface versus height above lung base in the prone dog at functional residual capacity. Lobar margin pressure varies by 1 cm H_2O/cm height. Costal surface pressure is uniform with height (–4 cm H_2O). Note that above 4 cm height, lobar margin pressure is more negative than costal surface pressure. Thus, during apnea, pleural liquid flows from costal surface to lobar margin, as indicated by direction of upper long arrow. Below 4 cm height, costal surface pressure is more negative than lobar margin pressure. Thus, during apnea, pleural liquid flows from lobar margin to the costal surface, as indicated by direction of lower long arrow. Short arrows indicate pleural liquid recirculation during ventilation. Flow of pleural liquid is downward on costal surface because gravity force is greater than pleural liquid pressure gradient (zero), and is upward along lobar margins. Ventilatory pump moves pleural liquid from lobar margin to costal surface above 4 cm height and from costal surface to lobar margin below 4 cm height, in directions opposite to those of apneic conditions.

flow from the lobar margin to the costal surface that is opposite to the flow under conditions of apnea (see below).

E. Pleural Liquid Pressure in the Zone of Apposition of the Diaphragm to the Rib Cage

In the zone of apposition of the diaphragm to the rib cage, pleural liquid pressure increases with spontaneous ventilation (33–36). This behavior is similar to that of abdominal pressure but is opposite to that of pleural pressure overlying the lung, which decreases with spontaneous breathing. Thus, the vertical gradient in pleural pressure in the zone of apposition should follow the vertical gradient in abdominal pressure that is near the hydrostatic value (37). The lubrication of the pleural space in the zone of apposition needs to be examined.

IV. Modeling Recirculation of Pleural Liquid Within the Pleural Space

A model of pleural liquid recirculation has recently been proposed (38). The model consists of three elements: a gravity-dependent downward flow of pleural liquid on the flat costal surfaces, an upward flow along lobar margins, and a transverse flow from lobar margins to the flat costal surfaces (see Figure 1).

A. Gravity-Dependent Flows

The recognition that the vertical gradient in pleural pressure in all body positions was always less than the hydrostatic value has led to the conclusion that gravity must drive a downward flow of pleural liquid in the pleural space. This flow has been modeled by the following flow mechanics equation relating the downward flow (Q) of liquid between two vertical plates separated by thickness (h) with a vertical surface pressure gradient (dP/dz) (16,17):

$$\rho g - dP/dz = \nu\ Q/(Lh^3) \tag{1}$$

Where ρ is liquid density, g is gravitational acceleration, ρg is the hydrostatic gradient, ν is the liquid viscosity, and L is the transverse dimension. Although this equation represents only a rough approximation to the real situation, it illustrates the following points. First, the flow of pleural liquid is always downward if the surface pressure gradient, dP/dz, is less than the hydrostatic gradient, ρg. Second, for a constant driving pressure, the flow rate (Q) depends directly on h^3. If h is halved, Q is reduced eightfold. Thus, the flow quickly vanishes as the space thins to very small values. Moreover, in the real pleural space where the thickness might be nonuniform, the flow might be much smaller than that based on the measured thickness (39), as demonstrated in a balloon-in-cylinder model of the pleural space, in which pleural liquid thickness was two orders of magnitude smaller than that calculated using Equation 1 and the measured flow. Thus, nonuniformities in pleural liquid thickness resulting in a vanishingly small pleural liquid flow might explain, in part, why, under apneic conditions, the measured pleural liquid thickness appeared to reach a minimum value and was uniform with respect to height (40,41). A downward flow in the pleural space without any compensatory recirculation of pleural liquid should result in an increasing pleural liquid thickness with distance down the pleural space, not supported by experimental evidence. Second, in the event that the flow downward must match the net filtration rate locally, regions of the pleural space that have low filtration should have small liquid thickness, and large changes in filtration can be accommodated by relatively small changes in pleural liquid thickness.

B. Upward Flow Along Lobar Margins

Redistribution of pleural liquid from the lung bases to the upper regions of the pleural space occurs through the widened pleural space formed at lobar margins. The pleural liquid thickness profile measured by light microscopic focusing (3) is shown in Figure 2 (insert). Note that the pleural space is considerably larger immediately adjacent to the lobar margin, ~100 μm, and declines monotonically with distance from the margin, attaining a value (15 μm) measured for the costal

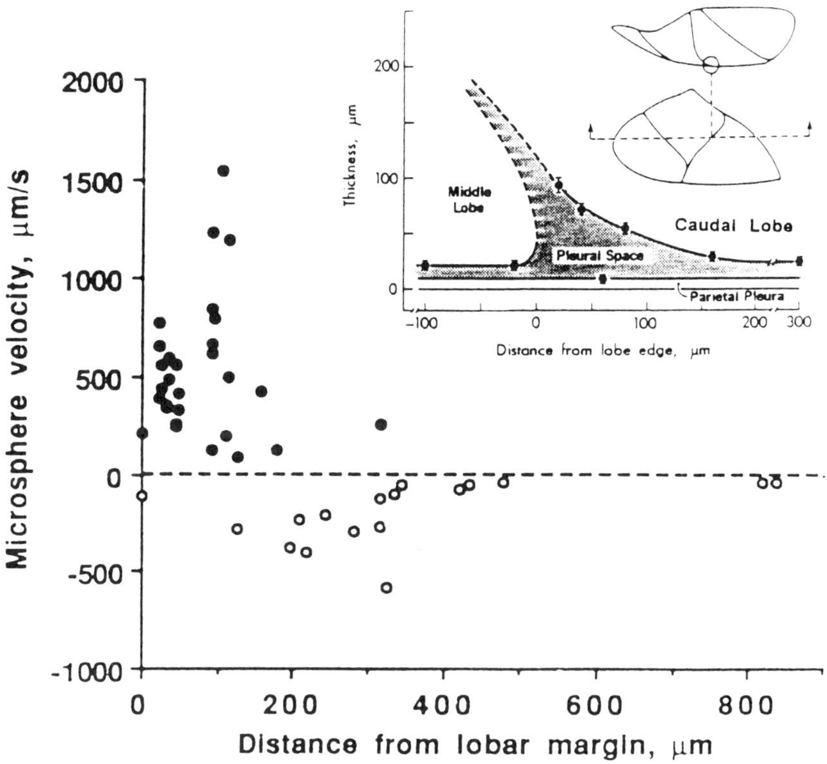

Figure 2 Upward (positive velocity) and downward (negative velocity) flow of fluorescent latex microspheres (6 μm diameter) at lobar margins caused by cardiogenic motion. Upward flow of microspheres occurred at mean distance of 78 ± 64 μm from lobar margin, whereas downward flow occurred at mean distance of 350 μm from lobar margin. (From Ref. 43.) Insert shows profile of pleural liquid thickness measured in the vicinity of a lobar margin by light microscopy in the rabbit. (From Ref. 3.)

surface (3). A similar decline in pleural liquid thickness would be expected in the pleural space around intrapleural catheter and cannulas (4). The sixfold increase in pleural liquid thickness at lobar margins ensures that, at lobar margins, viscous forces are negligible, resistance to flow is small, and the vertical gradient in pleural pressure approaches the hydrostatic value. The distribution of an injected bolus into the pleural space occurs via thc low resistance pathways at lobar margins (42). The vertical gradient in pleural liquid pressure is matched by the vertical gradient in pleural surface pressure caused by the adjustment of curvature at lobar margins according to Laplace's law.

Recent results using fluorescent microbeads (6 μm diameter) indicated that cardiogenic and ventilatory motion provides a pump that moves pleural liquid upward at lobar margins, whereas downward motion occurs distant from the lobar margin (43). Figure 2 shows the upward velocities of beads near the lobar margin resulting from cardiogenic motion compared with downward velocities of beads far from the margin measured in rabbits. The insert in Figure 2 shows pleural liquid thickness profile in the vicinity of a lobar margin measured during apnea using light microscopy (3). Note that bead motion was downward at distances greater than 200 μm from the lobar margin where the pleural liquid thickness is near the value for the flat costal region (15 μm).

C. Transverse Flows: The Ventilatory Pump

The drainage of pleural liquid from costal regions to lobar margins under apneic conditions in nondependent chest regions does not occur in vivo because there is a ventilatory pump that moves liquid from lobar margins to the flat costal surfaces. The fluid mechanics equations that describe this motion and supporting experimental evidence using a balloon-in-cylinder model of the pleural space have appeared (38). The solution of the equations shows that thickness on the flat costal surface is related to lung velocity amplitude (U) and the costal surface-to-lobar margin pressure difference (ΔP) by the following equation:

$$h = (T/\Delta P)(\nu U/T)^{2/3} \quad (2)$$

where T is tension of the visceral pleura and ν is pleural liquid viscosity. Equation 2 shows that h increases with velocity amplitude and decreases with the pressure gradient (ΔP). Measurements of pleural liquid thickness in a balloon-in-cylinder model of the pleural space in conjunction with vertical strings to simulate lobar margins have verified qualitatively the prediction from the model, as given by Equation 2. In these experiments, we used high viscosity oils (~3–10 stokes) labeled with fluorescent dye and measured thickness as a function of rotational velocity and costal surface-to-lobar margin pressure difference.

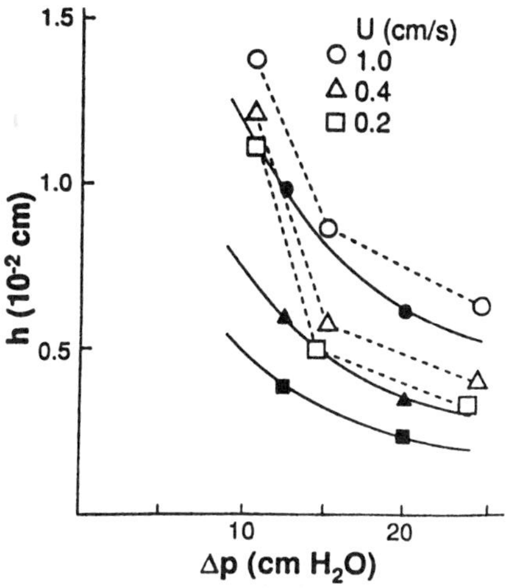

Figure 3 Pleural space thickness (h) versus costal surface-to-lobar margin pressure difference (ΔP) at three different velocity amplitudes (U) in a balloon-in-cylinder model of the pleural space. Lobar margins were simulated by vertical strings placed in the pleural space of the model. Note that qualitative agreement between theory (*full lines*) and experiment (*dashed lines*) using fluorescence labeled glycerol as pleural liquid (2.8 poise). (From Ref. 38.)

Figure 3 shows pleural liquid thickness versus costal surface-to-lobar margin pleural pressure difference measured in the pleural space model at three different velocity amplitudes. Note the qualitative agreement between the model experiments and theoretical prediction. Thickness increased with velocity amplitude and decreased with costal surface-to-lobar margin pressure difference. This behavior is qualitatively consistent with in vivo studies showing that pleural liquid thickness increases with ventilation (45). However, the scaling of h to $U^{2/3}$ predicted from Equation 2 was closely matched by some experiment conditions but not by others. For example (Figure 4), at a constant ventilation frequency, a reduction in tidal volume (V_T) from 20 mL to 6 mL resulted in the expected reduction in amplitude ($A \propto V_T^{1/3}$) and velocity ($U = 2\pi fA$) of 1.5-fold and in pleural liquid thickness of 1.3-fold. Here, changes in lung membrane tension with tidal volume were neglected. By contrast, at the constant tidal volume of 20 mL, a reduction in ventilation frequency (f) from 40 to 8 breaths/min was expected to reduce velocity by fivefold and to reduce pleural liquid thickness by 2.9-fold, much greater than the measured 40% reduction in pleural liquid thickness. It is possible that the amplitude of motion was reduced by a redistri-

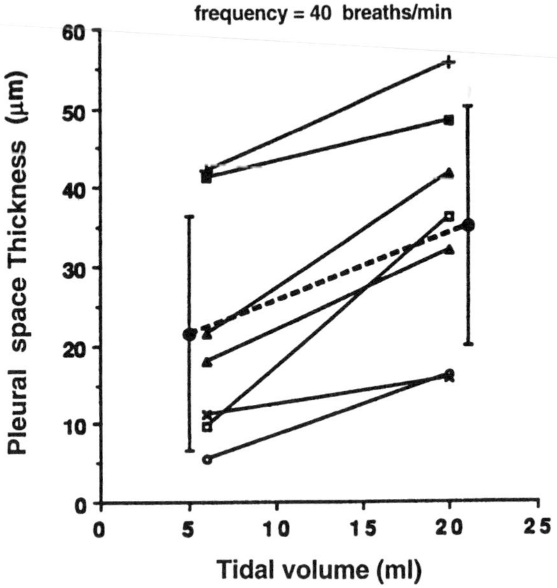

Figure 4 Effect of ventilation on pleural space thickness in rabbits. Pleural liquid thickness was measured in vivo by light emitted from the fluorescence dyed pleural liquid via a pleural window. Ventilation frequency was 40 breaths/min. Tidal volume was varied from 6 mL to 20 mL. (From Ref. 45.)

bution of the gas to apical lung regions from the caudal lung regions where pleural liquid thickness was measured.

V. Pleural Liquid Thickness

A. Measurements During Apnea

In terms of lubrication of the pleural surfaces, pleural liquid thickness is important to the evaluation of pleural contact and of the magnitude of shear stress induced during ventilation. Previous studies in several mammalian species using a variety of techniques such as light microscopic examination of frozen samples (40), electron microscopic analysis (7), and light microscopic focusing (41) indicate pleural liquid thickness to be in the range 6–30 μm during apnea. In the latter study (41), pleural liquid thickness during apnea increased with animal size. Pleural liquid thickness was independent of height in the chest except at the most dependent regions of the thorax and at the lobar margin where it was much thicker (41).

B. Effect of Mechanical Ventilation

Recent results using fluorescent imaging of pleural liquid via a pleural window in rabbits indicated that pleural liquid thickness increased with ventilation (45). In this technique, a thin transparent pleural window was made in the chest of mechanically ventilated rabbits, and a small amount of fluorescence-labeled dextran was injected into the pleural space through a rib capsule. After a period of 1 hour to allow the dye to mix with the resident pleural liquid, the fluorescent dye was measured during mechanical ventilation. Figure 4 shows pleural liquid thickness measured in the caudal region of rabbits near midchest at two different tidal volumes (6 and 20 mL) and constant ventilation frequency (40 breaths/min) in six rabbits. Pleural liquid thickness increased 40% as tidal volume was tripled at constant ventilation frequency. Pleural liquid thickness in rabbits during apnea was 11 μm and increased to 22 μm with mechanical ventilation (6 mL tidal volume and frequency 40 breaths/min). An increase in ventilation frequency from 8 to 40 breaths/min at a constant tidal volume of 20 mL increased pleural liquid thickness by 40% to 35 μm. As discussed above, this behavior is consistent, at least qualitatively, with a ventilation pump that moves liquid from lobar margins to the flat costal surfaces, opposite to the flow direction expected under apneic conditions.

C. Spatial Gradients and the Effect of Ventilation

In subsequent studies motivated by results showing a cranial-caudal gradient in albumin filtration in the chest wall (see Section VII), the thickness of the pleural space was measured using the fluorescent dye technique at three pleural windows located along the cranial-caudal dimension in anesthetized rabbits (46). Pleural windows were made at three different sites located along the cranial-caudal dimension near midchest. The results indicate that, at a ventilation frequency of 20 breaths/min and tidal volume of 20 mL, pleural liquid thickness increased with cranial-caudal distance from a mean value of ~5 μm at the second intercostal space to a value of ~30 μm at the sixth intercostal space (Figure 5). An increase in ventilation frequency from 20 to 40 breaths/min increased pleural liquid thickness only in the caudal region to ~45 μm.

D. Scaling with Body Size

Why does pleural liquid thickness increase with animal size? Under apneic conditions, pleural liquid thickness (h) increased with animal size, $h \propto M^{0.20}$, where M is body mass (Figure 6). This allometric relationship for apneic conditions was explained by a pleural liquid filtration rate that scaled with body mass. Consider the situation that pleural liquid filtration is matched to the downward flow of pleural liquid determined by the net effect of pleural surface pressure gradient and gravity, as given by Equation 1. If it is assumed that all animals

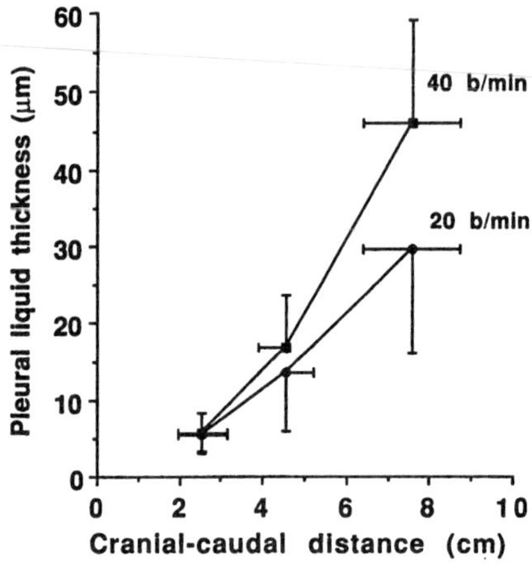

Figure 5 Pleural liquid thickness versus cranial-caudal distance from first rib measured in rabbits at ventilation frequencies of 20 and 40 breaths/min. (From Ref. 46.)

have a constant net driving pressure gradient and the downward flow of pleural liquid equals the filtration rate that is proportional to body mass, then Equation 1 reduces to: $Q \propto Lh^3$. Because transverse length, $L \propto M^{0.33}$, then $h \propto M^{0.22}$, the relationship measured in Figure 6. Thus, the increase in pleural liquid thickness with body mass measured during apnea is consistent with a filtration rate that is proportional to body mass. A pleural liquid filtration rate of 0.02 mL hr^{-1} kg^{-1} has been measured in the dog (47), sheep (48), and rabbit (49,50).

Because our studies indicated that pleural liquid thickness increased with ventilation, one might speculate that pleural liquid thickness would also increase with animal size during ventilation. The allometric relationship can be predicted with the assumption of the major factor that acts to determine pleural liquid thickness in all animals. Under apneic conditions, pleural liquid filtration rate that scales with body mass determined the increase in pleural liquid thickness with body mass. If it is assumed that during ventilation a constant shear stress in pleural liquid is the major determining factor rather than the pleural liquid filtration rate, the allometric relationship between pleural liquid thickness and body mass during ventilation is as follows.

Consider the shear stress (σ) in pleural liquid developed during ventilation as given by Newton's law of viscosity: $\sigma = \nu U/h$, where ν is pleural liquid viscosity and U is amplitude of relative velocity between the lung and chest wall. For oscillatory motion, U is the product of amplitude (A) of motion during ventilation and $2\pi f$, where f is ventilation frequency (breaths/min). If the following allometric relationships (41) are used among A, tidal volume (V_T), f, and body mass (M): $A \propto V_T^{1/3}$, $V_T \propto M$ and $f \propto M^{-1/4}$, $\sigma \propto M^{0.08}/h$. Thus, for a con-

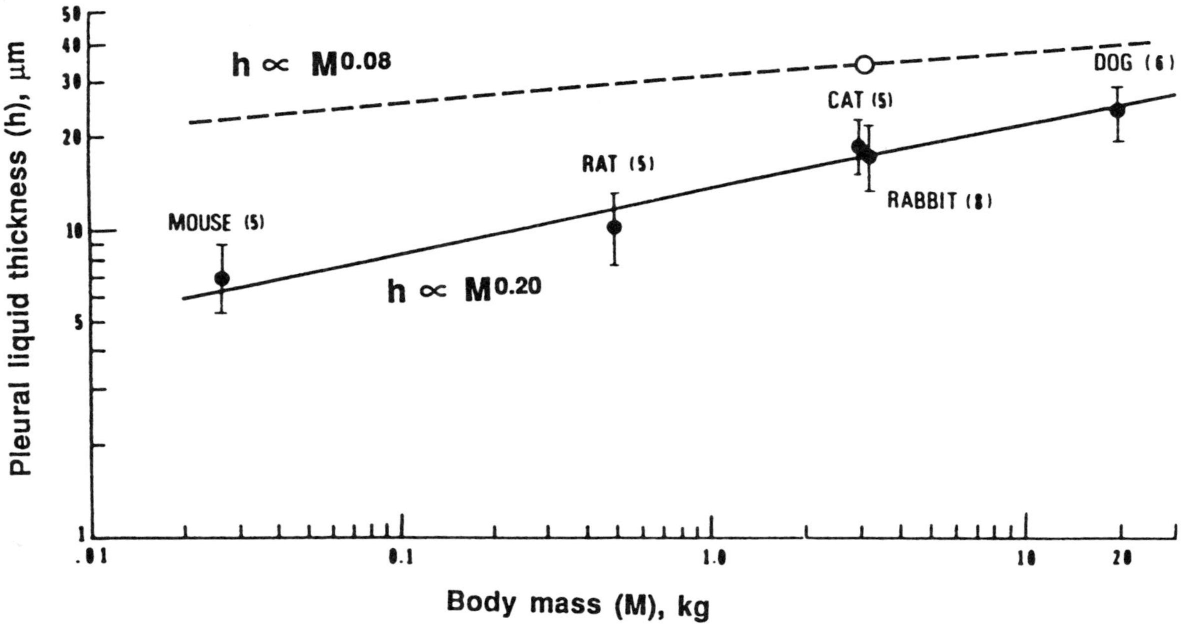

Figure 6 Pleural liquid thickness (h, μm) versus body mass (M) measured by light microscopy in five mammalian species during apnea (*full line*). Note that thickness increased with body mass during apnea: $h \propto M^{0.20}$, consistent with a pleural fluid filtration that scales with body mass. Dashed line is the allometric relationship predicted for ventilation ($h \propto M^{0.08}$) with the assumption of a constant pleural liquid shear stress, as described in the text. Point (*open symbol*) is value measured in rabbits during mechanical ventilation (45). (From Ref. 41.)

stant shear stress across species, $h \propto M^{0.08}$, that is, pleural liquid thickness should increase with body mass to the 0.08 power (see Figure 6), somewhat less than the increase based on a filtration that scales with body mass, as measured during apnea ($M^{0.20}$).

VI. Microvascular Fluid Exchange of Pleural Liquid

A. Starling and Solute Flux Equations

Pleural liquid originates from pleural capillaries through the normal processes of microvascular filtration, similar to those that occur in other organs. The Starling equation relates the filtration rate (Q) across the capillary endothelial barrier in series with the pleural membrane to the hydrostatic (P) and protein osmotic pressure (π) difference between capillary blood and pleural liquid:

$$Q_{liq} = K[(P_{pl} - P_{liq}) + \sigma_f(\pi_{liq} - \pi_{pl})] \tag{3}$$

where subscripts, pl and liq, refer to capillary blood (plasma) and pleural liquid, respectively, K is the combined endothelial/pleural membrane barrier conductivity (filtration coefficient), and σ_f is the reflection coefficient to protein. The flow of a particular solute (Q_S) is given by the solute flux equation:

$$Q_S = C_m(1 - \sigma_d)\, Q_{liq} + PS(C_{pl} - C_{liq}) \tag{4}$$

where C_m is the mean solute concentration in the membrane, σ_d is the solute drag coefficient, PS is the permeability-surface area product of the barrier, and C is the solute concentration. For the flow of a single solute, $\sigma_f = \sigma_d$. The first term on the right hand side of Equation 4 describes the solute flow resulting from convection, and the second term describes the flow resulting from diffusion.

Previous application of the Starling equation to the pleural space assumed a zero net filtration and an impermeable barrier with σ_f of 1, so the P_{liq} was much less (11 cm H_2O) than P_{pl} (1,2). More recent studies indicated a more permeable barrier and a net filtration with most of the filtration matched by lymphatic absorption. The evidence supporting a net filtration-lymphatic absorption process has been reviewed (30).

B. Permeability of the Pleural Membrane

Attempts have been made to estimate the K and PS of the pleural membrane to different size protein molecules. Experiments using pleural membrane stripped from the chest wall indicated that the pleural membrane was very permeable to protein (51–53) so that the major barrier to protein was attributed to the vascular endothelial barrier. Pleural membrane permeability measured in situ using pleural windows was 2 orders of magnitude smaller than that of stripped pleura (53).

The effect of damage to the pleural membrane during dissection on pleural liquid filtration has been reported (54).

The filtration rate of pleural liquid has been estimated by the equilibrium of radioisotopic tracers from the blood into the pleural space (47,48). Pleural filtration rates have been estimated from these and other experiments to be ~0.02 mL hr^{-1} kg^{-1} in the dog (47), sheep (48), and rabbit (49,50). Experiments using the absorption of large hydrothoraces showed a much greater absorption rate (56). Because, under these conditions, lymphatic flow can increase ~30-fold above baseline, a steady state at which filtration matches clearance is not established, and absorption of large hydrothoraces cannot provide an accurate description of filtration in the normal pleural space (30).

Pleural liquid filtration in all species occurs primarily from parietal pleural capillaries of the chest wall because its systemic circulation provides a relatively high capillary pressure (57). Reabsorption of pleural liquid may occur in the visceral pleural capillaries in the smaller animal species with a pulmonary circulation in the visceral pleura. Most of the clearance of pleural liquid occurs via lymphatic stomata in the parietal pleura (56). In sheep, the exchange vessels in the parietal pleura are 10–12 μm from the pleural space, much closer than the exchange vessels in the visceral pleura, which is located some 18–56 μm away from the pleural space (58). Also, the parietal pleural membrane is much thinner than that of the visceral pleura. Thus, pleural anatomy supports the physiological evidence that pleural liquid filtration and absorption occur via the parietal pleura (59).

C. Effect of Body Size

Experiments by Miserocchi and coworkers (60) in several mammalian species showed that the pleural-to-plasma protein concentration ratio (C_{liq}/C_{pl}) decreased with animal size. In sheep, in which the vascular supply to the visceral pleura is systemic rather than pulmonary, similar to the human, C_{liq}/C_{pl} is ~0.1 (61). This low C_{liq}/C_{pl} ratio is indicative of a microvascular barrier that is relatively impermeable to protein with a reflection coefficient σ_f approaching 1. The decrease in C_{liq}/C_{pl} with animal size has been explained on the basis of an average vascular-to-pleural hydrostatic pressure gradient that increases with animal size (60). An alternative explanation based on changes in membrane properties with animal size has been proposed (3).

D. Effect of Vascular Pressure

That an increased vascular pressure is responsible for the reduced C_{liq}/C_{pl} ratio measured with animal size is supported by two other observations. Studies in the spontaneously hypertensive rat (SHR) and its normotensive control Wisto Kyoto rat (WKY) showed that C_{liq}/C_{pl} ratio was reduced in SHR for both albumin and total protein, indicating a washdown effect caused by a higher microvascular pressure and greater filtration (62). A similar decrease in the C_{liq}/C_{pl} ratio occurred from the fetal to newborn lamb to the adult sheep as system vascular pressure increases with age (62). However, the effect of maturation on pleural membrane permeability cannot be definitely ruled out.

E. Effect of Ventilation

Preliminary studies showed that increased mechanical ventilation in anesthetized rabbits resulted in an increase in C_{liq}/C_{pl} (9,63). This suggests a change in pleural membrane permeability with ventilation, similar to the increase in pulmonary lymph-to-plasma protein concentration ratio associated with damage to the lung vascular membrane (64). The increased permeability with ventilation was associated with a greater shear stress in pleural liquid. However, in contrast to the damage to the lung vascular membrane, changes in pleural membrane permeability with ventilation would be reversible. In the preliminary studies (9,63), anesthetized rabbits were ventilated with 100% O_2 for 6 hours and the increase in protein concentration might be caused by a permeability increase caused by O_2 toxicity. More physiological experiments using conscious animals are needed before the role of ventilation in pleural filtration can be resolved.

VII. Mechanical Factors Contributing to Spatial Gradients in Pleural Liquid Filtration

A. Regional Distribution of Filtration and Absorption of Pleural Liquid

Regional absorption of pleural liquid is better understood than regional filtration. Anatomical studies in sheep (58) and rabbits (65) showed that absorption sites via lymphatic stomata are concentrated in the ventral and dorsal caudal regions of the parietal pleura of the rib cage. The visceral pleural lymphatics do not participate in pleural liquid absorption (59). The spatial distribution of lymphatic stomata has been measured in the diaphragm of rabbits (66). In sheep, lymphatic stomata have diameters of 1–3 μm and are sparsely distributed, about one every 500–1000 μm^2 of parietal pleural surface. The concentration of lymphatic stomata in the caudal regions of the pleural space was supported by studies in dogs showing lower absorption rates of radioactive tracers from apical regions than from caudal and mediastinal regions (67). It has been suggested that absorption occurred preferentially in the mediastinal regions where pleural liquid pressure was most negative (13). However, the latter measurements were done with rigid curved cannulas and there is a question of distortion of the pleural space.

The mechanism by which lymphatics absorb pleural liquid is still largely speculative. During a large hydrothorax, lymphatic absorption rates can increase up to ~30 times the normal absorption rates (30). One model assumed that the pleural liquid pressure was set by the lymphatics and that the absorption rate was determined by the pressure-volume relationship of the pleural space (68). As the volume of the pleural space was reduced, the pleural liquid pressure and the pressure gradient for lymphatic absorption decreased.

The absorption of pleural liquid by lymphatics is most likely enhanced by cardiogenic and ventilatory motion. This conclusion was reached from the following considerations. First, the distribution of lymphatic stomata, even where they are most concentrated, is sparse (58). One stomata opening of 1–3 μm in diameter is found in a surface area of 500–1000 μm^2 or a 25 × 25 μm surface area. It is unlikely that an absorption force from a lymphatic stomata on only ~1% of the pleural surface can exert a pressure acting on the entire pleural surface area. Thus, cardiogenic and ventilatory motion might act to redistribute pleural liquid from areas devoid of lymphatic stomata to the mouths of lymphatic stomata. Second, in the apical region of the pleural space, lymphatic stomata are more sparsely distributed, yet the pleural liquid pressure in the apical region is similar to that in the caudal region at the same isogravimetric plane. There appears to be no relationship between the concentration of lymphatic stomata and the regional pleural pressure as it should be if lymphatics were primarily responsible for determining pleural liquid pressure. Third, because the lymphatic stomata have diameters 1–3 μm, much smaller than the normal thickness of the pleural space, 6–30 μm, its resistance to absorption in the absence of lung motion should be more a function of the stomata geometry than of the thickness of the pleural space. The flow through the stomata should not be affected much by the changes in pleural space thickness until the pleural space thins to values comparable to the diameter of the stomata.

By contrast to the anatomical (59,65,66) and physiological (67) studies of the pleural liquid absorption sites, there is little experimental evidence for a regional distribution of pleural liquid filtration. In recent studies, we used Evan's blue dyed albumin (EBA) as a fluorescent tracer to study the regional distribution of albumin filtration in the parietal pleura and chest wall of rabbits. In these experiments, Evan's blue dye (2 mL of 1 g/dL solution) was injected into the circulation of an anesthetized rabbit breathing 100% O_2. After 6 hours of mechanical ventilation, the rib cage was isolated postmortem and fluorescent light from Evan's blue dye albumin was measured from the inner chest surface by fluorescent videomicroscopy. The results indicated a cranial-caudal gradient in albumin filtration after 6 hours of mechanical ventilation, with filtration increasing toward the caudal region (Figure 7). Albumin filtration was lowest at the cranial ribs and increased with rib number reaching a maximum at the seventh to eighth rib. This cranial-caudal distribution matched the regional distribution of lymphatic absorption sites measured anatomically (58,65) and the regional

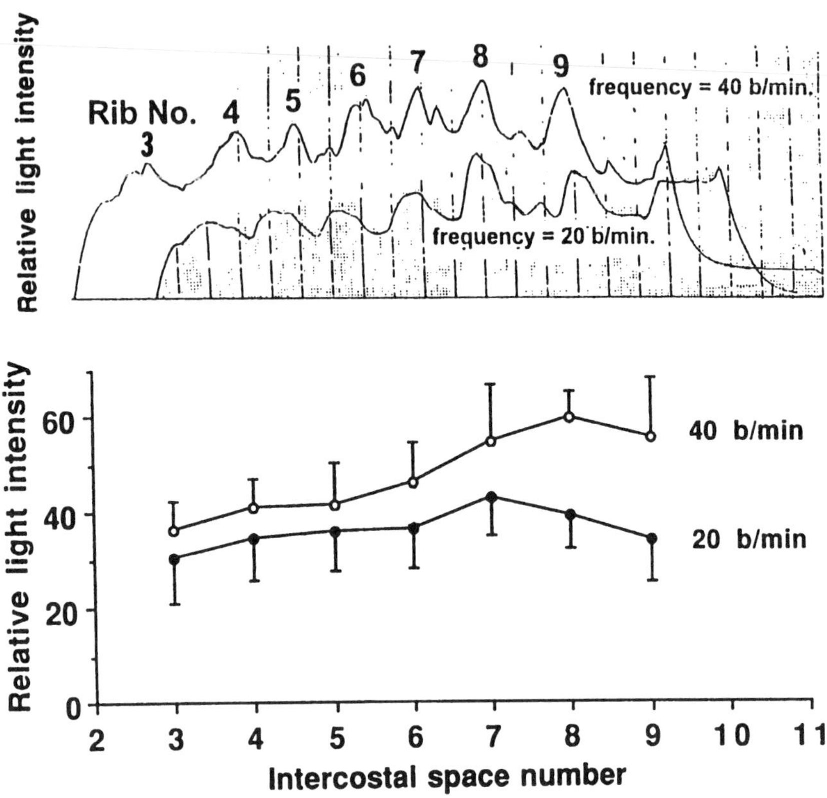

Figure 7 Fluorescent light emitted from the inner surface of the chest wall versus cranial-caudal distance at ventilation frequencies of 20 and 40 breaths/min for one animal (*top frame*). Note the cyclic variation of fluorescence with maxima associated with ribs and minima with intercostal spaces and that fluorescence increased with cranial-caudal distance. Average values (±SD, n = 3–6) for the minimum light intensity from the intercostal space versus intercostal space number are shown in bottom frame. Light intensity increased significantly with both intercostal space number and ventilation frequency. (From authors' unpublished observations.)

distribution of an absorbed bolus (67). However, in these studies, we could not separate the absorption from the filtration sites. Fluorescence images of cross sections of the frozen chest wall show that filtration was not uniformly distributed in the pleural membrane or within the chest wall (Figure 8). Filtration was greater around the ribs than in the intercostal space. Similar fluorescent images of the chest wall of FITC absorbed from the pleural liquid indicated a greater absorption in the pleural membrane overlying the intercostal muscle than overly-

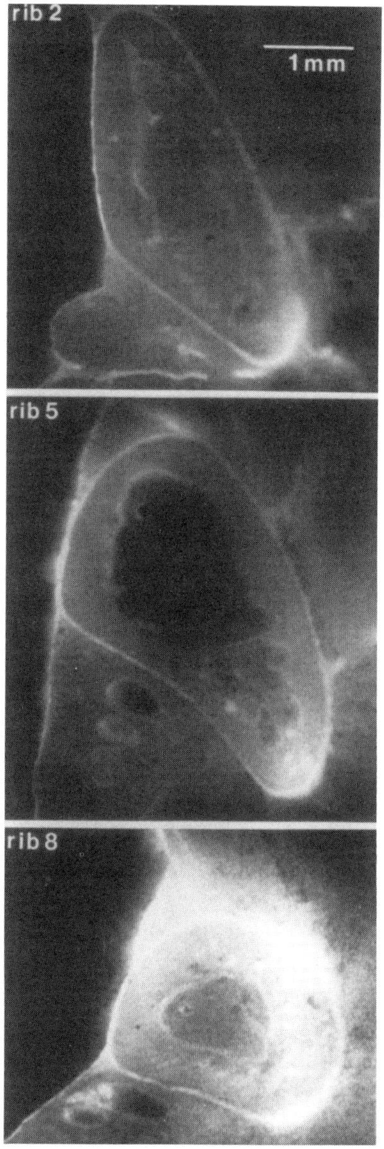

Figure 8 Fluorescent images of Evan's blue dyed albumin distribution from frozen cross sections of the rib cage (2nd, 5th, and 8th ribs) of a rabbit after 6 hours of mechanical ventilation. Parietal pleural membrane is located on the left side of each image. Cranial direction is toward the top. Evan's blue dye was injected into the circulation before the 6 hours. Note that fluorescence was greater around the ribs than in the adjacent intercostal muscle and increased with rib number. (From authors' unpublished observations.)

ing the rib (69). This is consistent with the distribution of lymphatic stomata concentrated in the intercostal pleura.

Vertical gradients in pleural filtration have been proposed because the vertical gradient in subparietal pleural interstitial pressure does not match the vertical gradient in pleural liquid pressure (70). This prediction needs to be verified experimentally.

B. Effect of Ventilation

In rabbits, an increase in mechanical ventilation for 6 hours increased the filtration of Evan's blue dyed albumin concentration from the circulation into the pleural space (63). This increase in EBA filtration was accompanied by an increase in the total protein concentration in pleural liquid (9). This indicated that pleural membrane permeability to total protein increased with the increased ventilation. However, these results were obtained in anesthetized rabbits ventilated with 100% O_2, and the effect of O_2 toxicity on membrane permeability might be a contributing factor. More definitive studies using conscious animals are needed.

C. Regional Distribution of Pleural Liquid Shear Stress and Mechanical Strain of the Chest Wall

To examine two possible reasons for the cranial-caudal gradient in filtration of Evan's blue dyed albumin measured in the parietal pleura and chest wall of rabbits and its increase with ventilation, we studied the cranial-caudal gradient in pleural liquid shear stress and mechanical strain during ventilation in rabbits. Lung motion amplitude and velocity of sliding were not uniform throughout the pleural space. There was a marked cranial-caudal gradient in velocity with values near to zero in the apical regions that increased toward the caudal regions (46). These measurements in conjunction with the measured cranial-caudal gradients in pleural liquid thickness (see Figure 5) indicated a uniform pleural liquid shear stress with cranial-caudal distance that increased with an increase in ventilation frequency from 20 to 40 breaths/min. We speculate that the increased pleural liquid filtration with ventilation was caused by a shear stress–induced increase in pleural membrane permeability. However, this cannot explain the cranial-caudal gradient in filtration because shear stress was uniform with cranial-caudal distance. The cranial-caudal gradient in filtration of albumin might be stretch-induced by the cranial-caudal gradient in mechanical strain, measured radiographically (69).

At the apical regions of the pleural space, lung relative velocity and pleural liquid thickness and local pleural liquid filtration are minimally small. Here, pleural liquid thickness might be determined by the local filtration. By contrast, in the more caudal regions where lobar margins are located and lung velocity is maximal, pleural liquid thickness might be determined by the ventilatory pump, as discussed in Section IV.

D. Spatial Distribution and Role of Microvilli

The pleural surfaces are lined by a layer of microvilli, 1–3 μm thick, depending on species (65). Microvilli are distributed in a cranial-caudal gradient with few microvilli in the apical regions and on the lung surface. The physiological importance of microvilli in relation to pleural lubrication and its role in reducing pleural liquid shear stress and in pleural liquid filtration, are unknown and need to be examined. It is of interest that microvilli are absent in the apical regions of the pleural space (65), where lung relative velocity during ventilation is minimal (46).

VIII. Summary

We have discussed some recent studies of pleural liquid dynamics both from the aspect of pleural liquid recirculation within the pleural space and of regional distribution of pleural liquid filtration and absorption. The major questions concern the mechanical factors that control pleural liquid filtration. Is there a ventilatory shear stress–induced change in pleural membrane permeability that controls filtration? In vitro studies suggest that the permeability of cultured mesothelial cells increased with shear stress (71). Do changes in mechanical strain during ventilation affect pleural liquid filtration? The importance of a regional matching of filtration to absorption relative to that of pleural liquid recirculation needs to be sorted out. The notion of a well-mixed pleural liquid space must be reconciled with a vertical gradient of absorbed protein in pleural lymphatic stomata (44). We have demonstrated a cranial-caudal gradient in filtration and absorption of pleural liquid in anesthetized rabbits ventilated with 100% O_2. These experiments need to be repeated in conscious animals. There is a need to separate the regional distribution of pleural liquid absorption from that of pleural liquid filtration. The role of boundary lubrication is an unsettled question. Mechanical ventilation has recently been found to increase hyaluronan concentration in pleural liquid (9,10) and hyaluronan might reduce pleural contact forces.

Acknowledgment

This research was supported by research grant HL 36597 from National Heart, Lung, and Blood Institute.

References

1. Agostoni E. Mechanics of the pleural space. Physiol Rev 1972; 52:57–128.
2. Agostoni E. Mechanics of the pleural space. In: Macklem PT, Mead J, eds. Handbook of Physiology. Mechanics of Breathing. Vol.III. American Physiological Society. Baltimore: Williams & Wilkins, 1986:531–560.
3. Lai-Fook SJ. Mechanics of the pleural space: fundamental concepts. Lung 1987; 165:249–267.
4. Lai-Fook SJ, Rodarte JR. Pleural pressure distribution and its relationship to lung volume and interstitial pressure. Brief Review. J Appl Physiol 1991; 70:967–978.
5. Grotberg JB, Glucksberg MR. A buoyancy-driven squeeze-film model of intrapleural fluid dynamics: basic concepts. J Appl Physiol 1993; 77:1555–1561.
6. Miserocchi G, Venturoli D, Negrini D, Gilardi MC, Bellina R. Intrapleural fluid movements described by a porous flow model. J Appl Physiol 1992; 73:2511–2516.
7. Albertine KH, Wiener-Kronish JP, Bastacky V, Staub NC. No evidence of mesothelial cell contact across the costal pleural space in sheep. J Appl Physiol 1991; 70:123–134.
8. Hills BA, Butler BD, Barrow RE. Boundary lubrication imparted by pleural surfactants and their identification. J Appl Physiol 1982; 53:463–469.
9. Wang PM, Parameswaran S, Brown LV, Lai-Fook SJ. Effect of ventilation on protein and hyaluronan concentrations in pleural liquid of rabbits (abstr). FASEB J 1996; 10:A361.
10. Wang PM, Lai-Fook SJ. Hyperventilation increases hyaluronan concentration in pleural liquid of conscious rabbits (abstr). FASEB J 1997; 11:A347.
11. Rutishauser WJ, Banchero N, Tsakiris AG, Edmundowicz AC, Wood EH. Pleural pressures at dorsal and ventral sites in supine and prone body positions. J Appl Physiol 1966; 21:1500–1510.
12. Miserochi G, Nakamura T, Mariani E, Negrini D. Pleural liquid pressure over the interlobar mediastinal and diaphragmatic surfaces of the lung. Respir Physiol 1981; 46:61.
13. Miserocchi G, Kelly S, Negrini D. Pleural and extrapleural interstitial liquid pressure measured by cannulas and micropipettes. J Appl Physiol 1988; 65:555–562.
14. Hubmayr RD, Walters BJ, Chevalier PA, Rodarte JR, Olson LE. Topographic distribution of regional lung volume in anesthetized dogs. J Appl Physiol 1983; 54: 1048–1056.
15. Hoffman EA, Ritman EL. Effect of body orientation on regional lung expansion in dog and sloth. J Appl Physiol 1985; 59:481–491.
16. Lai-Fook SJ, Beck KC, Southorn PA. Pleural liquid pressure measured by micropipettes in rabbits. J Appl Physiol 1984; 56:1633–1639.
17. Miserocchi G, Negrini D, Pistolesi M, Bellina CR, Gilardi MC, Bettinardi V, Rossitto R. Intrapleural liquid flow down a gravity-dependent hydraulic pressure gradient. J Appl Physiol 1988; 64:577–584.
18. Olson LE, Hoffman EA. Lung volume and distribution of regional air content determined by cine X-ray CT of pneumonectomized rabbits. J Appl Physiol 1994; 76: 1774–1785.

19. Wiener-Kronish JP, Gropper MA, Lai-Fook SJ. Pleural liquid pressure in dogs measured using a rib capsule. J Appl Physiol 1985; 59:597–602.
20. Hogg JC, Stein L, Martin R, Macklem PT. The interaction of the lung and chest wall in dogs. Respir Physiol 1976; 27:207–221.
21. Olson LE, Lai-Fook SJ. Pleural liquid pressure measured with rib capsules in anesthetized ponies. J Appl Physiol 1988; 64:102–107.
22. Yang Q-H, Kaplowitz MR, Lai-Fook SJ. Regional variations in lung expansion in rabbit: prone vs. supine positions. J Appl Physiol 1989; 67:1371–1376.
23. Hoppin FG Jr, Green ID, Mead J. Distribution of pleural surface pressure in dogs. J Appl Physiol 1969; 27:863–873.
24. Hyatt RE, Bar-Yishay E, Abel MD. Influence of the heart on the vertical gradient of transpulmonary pressure in dogs. J Appl Physiol 1985; 58:52–57.
25. Kaneko K, Milic-Emili J, Dolovich MB, Dawson A, Bates DV. Regional distribution of ventilation and perfusion as a function of body position. J Appl Physiol 1966; 21:767–777.
26. Milic-Emili J, Henderson JAM, Dolovich MB, Trop D, Kaneko K. Regional distribution of inspired gas in the lung. J Appl Physiol 1966; 21:749–759.
27. Hoffman EA. Effect of body orientation on regional lung expansion: a computed tomographic approach. J Appl Physiol 1985; 59:481–491.
28. Yang QH, Lai-Fook SJ. Effect of airway pressure on regional lung expansion in supine and prone rabbits. J Appl Physiol 1991; 71:76–82.
29. Agostoni E, Miserocchi G. Vertical gradient of transpulmonary pressure with active and artificial lung expansion. J Appl Physiol 1970; 29:705–712.
30. Miserocchi G. Pleural pressures and fluid transport. In: Crystal RG, West JB, et al, eds. The lung: scientific foundations. New York: Raven Press, 1991:885–893.
31. Kaplowitz MR, Lai-Fook SJ. Pressure and dimensions of pleural liquid at lobar margins of dogs and rabbits (abstr). Fed Proc 1985; 44:1027.
32. Agostoni E, Zocchi L, Agostoni PG. Pleural liquid pressure at the caudal border of the lung. Respir Physiol 1989; 75:117–128.
33. Urmey WF, DeTroyer A, Kelly KB, Loring SH. Pleural pressure increases during inspiration in the zone of apposition of diaphragm to rib cage. J Appl Physiol 1988; 65:2207–2212.
34. Agostoni E, Zocchi L, Agostoni PG, Macklem PT. Pleural pressure from abdominal to pulmonary rib cage: sweep of the lung border. Respir Physiol 1989; 75:107–117.
35. Agostoni E, Agostoni PG, Zocchi L. Pleural liquid pressure in the zone of apposition and in the lung zone. Respir Physiol 1989; 75:357–370.
36. Perez F, Fernandez P, Hernaiz MI, Jackson EG, Lai-Fook SJ, Boynton BR. Pleural pressure measured in the zone of apposition of diaphragm to rib cage in rabbits. Lung 1993; 171:345–353.
37. Loring SH, Yoshino K, Kimball WR, Barnas GM. Gravitational and shear-induced pressure gradients in the abdomen. J Appl Physiol 1994; 77:375–382.
38. Butler JP, Huang J, Loring SH, Lai-Fook SJ, Wang PM, Wilson TA. Model for a pump that drives circulation of pleural fluid. J Appl Physiol 1995; 78:23–29.
39. Lai-Fook SJ, Price DC, Staub NC. Liquid thickness vs. vertical pressure gradient in a model of the pleural space. J Appl Physiol 1987; 62:1747–1754.

40. Agostoni E, Miserocchi G, Bonanni MV. Thickness and pressure of the pleural liquid in some mammals. Respir Physiol 1969; 6:245–256.
41. Lai-Fook SJ, Kaplowitz MR. Pleural liquid thickness in situ by light microscopy in five mammalian species. J Appl Physiol 1985; 59:603–610.
42. Miserocchi G, Pistolesi M, Miniati M, Bellina CR, Negrini D, Giuintini C. Pleural liquid pressure gradients and intrapleural distribution of injected bolus. J Appl Physiol 1984; 56:526–532.
43. Wang PM, Lai-Fook SJ. Upward flow of pleural liquid near lobar margins due to cardiogenic motion. J Appl Physiol 1992; 73:2314–2319.
44. Albertine KH, Schultz EL, Wiener-Kronish JP, Staub NC. Regional differences in pleural lymphatic albumin concentration in sheep. Am J Physiol 1987; 252: H64–H70.
45. Wang PM, Lai-Fook SJ. Effect of ventilation frequency and tidal volume on pleural space thickness in rabbits. J Appl Physiol 1993; 75:1836–1841.
46. Wang PM, Lai-Fook SJ. Effect of mechanical ventilation on regional variation of pleural space thickness in rabbits. Lung 1997; 175:165–173.
47. Miniati M, Parker JC, Pistolesi M, Cartledge JT, Martin DJ, Giuntini C, Taylor AE. Reabsorption kinetics of albumin from the pleural space of dogs. Am J Physiol 1988; 255:H375–H385.
48. Weiner-Kronish JP, Albertine KH, Licko V, Staub NC. Protein egress and entry rates in pleural fluid and plasma in sheep. J Appl Physiol 1984; 56:459–463.
49. Broaddus VC, Araya M. Liquid and protein dynamics using a new minimally invasive pleural catheter in rabbits. J Appl Physiol 1992; 72:851–857.
50. Miserocchi G, Negrini D, Mariani E, Passafaro M. Reabsorption of saline-or plasma-induced hydrothorax. J Appl Physiol 1983; 54:1574–1578.
51. Kim KJ, Critz A, Crandall E. Transport of water and solute across sheep visceral pleura. Am Rev Respir Dis 1979; 120:882–892.
52. Kinasewitz GT, Groome LJ, Marshall RP, Diana JN. Permeability of the canine visceral pleura. J Appl Physiol 1983; 55:121–130.
53. Negrini D, Reed RK, Miserocchi G. Permeability-surface area product and reflection coefficient of the parietal pleura in dogs. J Appl Physiol 1991; 71:2543–2547.
54. Lai-Fook SJ, Wang PM. Effect of parietal pleural window on pleural liquid filtration in rabbits (abstr). FASEB J 1995; 9:A150.
55. Negrini D, Townsley M, Taylor AE. Hydraulic conductivity of canine parietal pleura in vivo. J Appl Physiol 1990; 69:438–442.
56. Broaddus VC, Wiener-Kronish JP, Berthiaume Y, Staub NC. Removal of pleural liquid and protein by lymphatics in awake sheep. J Appl Physiol 1988; 64:384–390.
57. McLaughlin RF, Tyler WS, Canada RO. A study of the subgross pulmonary anatomy of various mammals. Am J Anat 1961; 108:149–159.
58. Albertine KH, Wiener-Kronish JP, Staub NC. The structure of the parietal pleura and its relationship to pleural liquid dynamics in sheep. Anat Rec 1984; 208:401–409.
59. Albertine KH, Wiener-Kronish JP, Roos PJ, Staub NC. Structure, blood supply, and lymphatic vessels of the sheep's visceral pleura. Am J Anat 1982; 165:277–294.
60. Miserocchi G, Negrini D, Mortola JP. Comparative features of the Starling-lym-

phatic interaction at the pleural level in mammals. J Appl Physiol 1984; 56:1151–1156.
61. Broaddhus VC, Araya M, Carlton DP, Bland RD. Developmental changes in pleural liquid protein concentration in sheep. Am Rev Respir Dis 1991; 143:38–41.
62. Lai-Fook SJ, Kaplowitz MR. Pleural protein concentration and liquid volume in spontaneously hypertensive rats. Microvasc Res 1988; 35:101–108.
63. Wang PM, Lai-Fook SJ. Effect of ventilation frequency on fluid filtration into the pleural space of rabbits (abstr). FASEB J 1994; 8:A690.
64. Erdmann AJ III, Vaughn TR, Brigham KL, Woolverton WC, Staub NC. Effect of increased vascular pressure on lung fluid balance in sheep. Circ Res 1975; 37:271–284.
65. Wang NS. The performed stomas connecting the pleural cavity and the lymphatics in the parietal pleura. Am Rev Respir Dis 1975; 111:12–20.
66. Negrini D, Del Fabbro M, Gonano C, Kukenge S, Miserocchi G. Distribution of diaphragmatic lymphatic lacunae. J Appl Physiol 1992; 72:1166–1172.
67. Negrini D, Pistolesi M, Miniati M, Bellina R, Giuntini C, Miserocchi G. Regional protein absorption rates from the pleural cavity in dogs. J Appl Physiol 1985; 58:2062–2067.
68. Miserocchi G, Venturoli D, Negrini D, Del Fabbro M. Model of pleural fluid turnover. J Appl Physiol 1993; 75:1798–1806.
69. Lai-Fook SJ, Wang PM. Regional distribution of filtration and absorption sites of pleural liquid in parietal pleura of rabbits (abstr). FASEB J 1996; 10:A361.
70. Negrini D, Morini M, Capelli C, Miserocchi G. Gravity-dependent distribution of parietal subpleural interstitial pressure. J Appl Physiol 1985; 563:1912–1918.
71. Waters CM, Glucksberg MR, DePaola N, Chang J, Grotberg JB. Shear stress alters pleural mesothelial cell permeability in culture. J Appl Physiol 1996; 81:448–458.

6

Chest Wall Mechanics

STEPHEN H. LORING

Harvard Medical School and
Beth Israel Deaconess Medical Center
Boston, Massachusetts

JAMES P. BUTLER

Harvard School of Public Health
Boston, Massachusetts

I. Introduction

The chest wall comprises those structures that bound the lungs and move with breathing. This includes the whole trunk, although, in the traditional view of the chest wall, the back and pelvis are taken to be stationary and immobile, and the parts of the chest wall that move are thus the diaphragm (and by extension the abdominal wall) and the rib cage. In this chapter, we reexamine simplifying assumptions about the chest wall, especially those that, when viewed more realistically, lead to qualitatively different conclusions from those based on earlier assumptions. This chapter also examines ways in which variables and processes formerly considered unitary and locally determined are heterogeneous and globally determined.

II. Historical Approaches

A. Compartment Models of the Chest Wall

Fitz Rohrer, a Swiss physician and physiologist working in the early decades of this century, is credited with simplifying the respiratory system to an extent that allowed quantification of its behavior (1). By abstracting the respiratory system to a single inflatable structure, the relationship between external pressures and resultant airflow could be characterized by an equation of motion that relates the pressure differences applied to the respiratory system to the volume displacements, flows, and volume accelerations produced by those pressures (Figure 1*A*). Pressure-volume analysis of respiratory structures has dominated respiratory mechanics for most of this century.

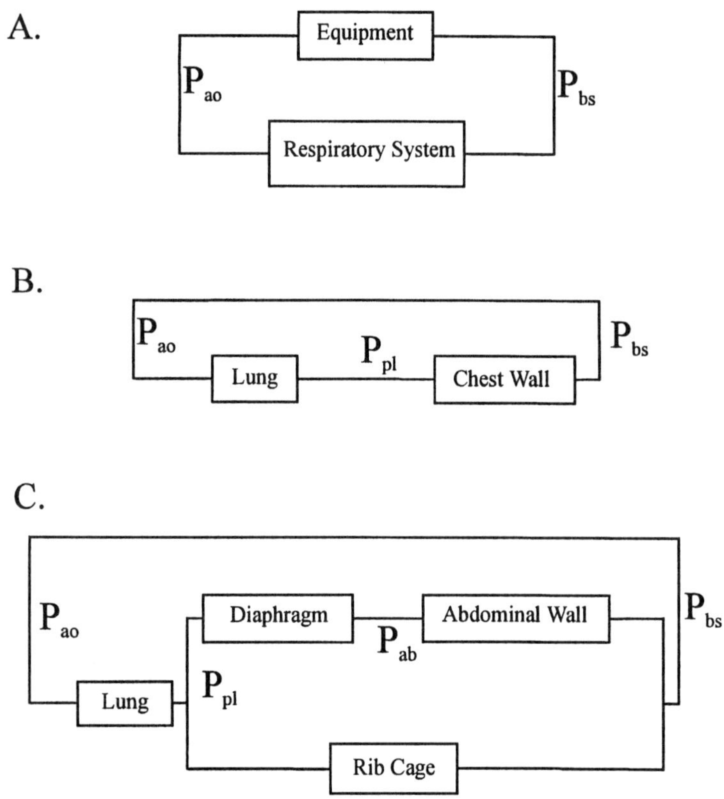

Figure 1 Schematic circuit diagrams of the respiratory system and equipment. Structures can be characterized by the relationships between the pressure difference across them and the volume displacements or flow through them. Model (**A**) allowed pressure-volume characterization of the passive respiratory system, which could be divided into lung and chest wall compartments to allow the lung to be driven by the chest wall (**B**). Agostoni and Mead later divided chest wall into rib cage and diaphragm-abdomen pathways for volume displacement (**C**). Pressures noted are at the body surface (P_{bs}), airway opening (P_{ao}), pleural space (P_{pl}), and abdominal compartment (P_{ab}).

Rohrer and later physiologists split the respiratory system into chest wall and lung, considering the chest wall as a single structure driving the lung (see Figure 1*B*). (For a review of these developments, see Ref. 2.) Pressure inflating the respiratory system could thus be expressed as the sum of transpulmonary and transthoracic pressures, and the effects of respiratory muscle contraction could be described by a quantity P_{mus}, which is the measurable difference between the pressure across a structure when muscles are activated and the pressure that would exist across that structure under conditions of muscular relaxation (at the same volume, rate of volume change, and so on). Note that P_{mus} is an indirect measure of muscle activation per se, insofar as the translation of muscle forces into induced pressure differences includes geometric features such as angles of insertion and (particularly for the diaphragm) radii of curvature, as well as changes in these angles and curvatures secondary to the activation process itself.

Still later, Agostoni and Mead (3) divided the chest wall into rib cage and diaphragm-abdomen pathways for the purpose of fractionating volume displacements (see Figure 1*C*). The conceptual division between rib cage and diaphragm-abdomen pathways was qualitatively described by noting pleural, abdominal, and transdiaphragmatic pressures in various maneuvers, but further pressure-volume analyses awaited the simplification of chest wall kinematics by Konno and Mead (4), who showed that displacements of the ventral surfaces of the chest wall in quiet breathing could be largely described with two variables, one specifying movements of the rib cage and the other movements of the mid and lower ventral abdominal wall. Their analysis conferred on the chest wall a quantitative kinematic description, with two degrees of freedom that led, like the simplifications of Rohrer, to a model mechanical system in which rib cage and abdomen each have measurable internal pressures applied to moving surfaces, which are themselves displaced by distinct muscles or groups of muscles. Goldman et al. (5) used these concepts in an analysis that yielded new understanding of the action of various respiratory muscles in quiet breathing and hyperpnea.

At this point, the major pathways for volume displacement via the rib cage and abdomen were accounted for and characterized in terms of volume and pressure, but simple assumptions concerning the action of pleural pressure on the rib cage were unable to explain the apparent inspiratory actions of the diaphragm on the rib cage. Diaphragm contraction was known to enlarge the pleural cavity, thereby lowering pleural pressure, displacing the abdominal viscera caudally and raising abdominal pressure. Goldman and Mead (6) first hypothesized that, during diaphragm contraction, the rib cage was, in effect, inflated by a pressure equal to the transdiaphragmatic pressure, an assertion consistent with their observations but difficult to justify from classical mechanics applied to the chest wall structures. However, their insight was later modified and rationalized by Loring and Mead (7) who focused on the region of diaphragmatic apposition to the rib cage. They divided diaphragmatic actions on the rib cage into three mechanical effects: 1. an expiratory effect related to the lowering of pleural pressures (note that lowered pleural pressure is inspiratory to the lung but expiratory for the rib cage), 2. an inspiratory effect related to the cephalad pull of the diaphragm at its insertions on the rib cage margin, and 3. an inspiratory effect produced by the increased abdominal pressure acting through abdominal and diaphragm-apposed portions of the lower rib cage. The latter inspiratory action was explained by an appreciation of the nature of pressures supported by or transmitted across the membrane-like diaphragm in regions of greater or lesser curvature. They argued that, in the dome of the diaphragm, where curvature is appreciable, tensions produce a substantial transdiaphragmatic pressure, whereas in the "zone of apposition" where the diaphragm is apposed to the inner surface of the rib cage, curvatures are much less pronounced, especially in the direction of principal tension (along the muscle fibers), and tensions in the diaphragm do not generate much local transdiaphragmatic pressure (Figure 2). This novel approach, later confirmed experimentally (8), allowed for a structural model of the chest wall in which anatomical features (such as the area of diaphragmatic apposition) were used to estimate mechanical consequences of muscle forces.

The role of the diaphragm-apposed region of the rib cage can be appreciated by exploring the expiratory action of abdominal muscles. Abdominal mus-

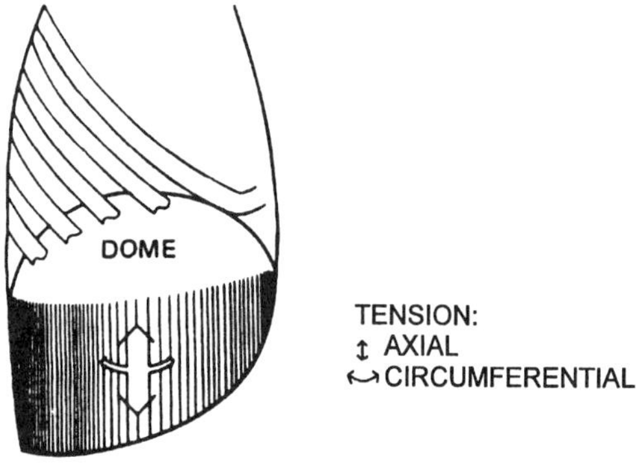

$$P_{di(ap)} = -\left(\frac{T_{ax}}{r_{ax}} + \frac{T_{cir}}{r_{cir}}\right)$$

Figure 2 Schematic illustration of the zone of apposition of diaphragm to rib cage. The law of Young and Laplace suggests that the transdiaphragmatic pressure in this region ($P_{di(ap)}$) is small because the radius of curvature in the axial direction (r_{ax}) is large and the tension in the diaphragmatic muscle in the circumferential direction (T_{cir}) is small.

cles increase abdominal pressure, which acts, via the diaphragm, to increase pleural pressure with an expiratory consequence. Additionally, the abdominal muscles pull the lower rib cage toward the pelvis, reducing thoracic volume. On the other hand, to the extent that abdominal pressure is increased, there is an expansive effect on the rib cage through the zone of apposition, with a contribution in the inspiratory direction. Thus, the net effect of abdominal muscular activation is determined by competing effects through the elevation of the diaphragm (expiratory direction) and the expansion of the rib cage through appositional pressure (inspiratory direction).

When pressure-volume analyses of the chest wall are the only tools available to explain the effects of structural elements, including muscular activation, the net effects can be described in terms of pressure differences. For example, the effects of muscular contraction on transthoracic pressures are described as P_{mus}, defined as the change in the measured transthoracic pressure from that which would have existed during muscular relaxation at the same lung volume. Other pressure-volume analyses of the chest wall have invoked special pressures, often not directly measurable, to explain effects that were due to structural and/or kinematic features of the chest wall (9–11). Other investigators have also used analogous models such as lever systems to describe thoracoabdominal mechanics (12). But increasingly, mechanical analyses of the chest wall have evolved from models consisting of compartments that are simply described by pressure-volume relationships to more complicated structural models that are more realistic and anatomically detailed. A remarkable example of such a model used for kinematic analysis is Saumarez' detailed description of rib cage motion (13). These experimental observations of the kinematics of chest wall motion are important for a variety of reasons, chiefly because they indicate the extent to which the number of degrees of freedom of motion may be reduced without loss of fidelity. That is, a structure such as the lung has, in principle, an unbounded number of ways of effecting volume changes, constrained to match the way in which its bounding container moves. If the kinematics of the rib cage and diaphragm pathways can be described in a few variables, then the net interaction of the chest wall and lung can be concomitantly simplified. For example, the observation that the rib cage is quite stiff to all but two degrees of freedom allows for considerable simplification. Similarly, the observation that the abdominal contents are approximately isovolume permits another reduction in the number of degrees of freedom. Finally, the effect of abdominal pressure on the thorax through the pathway of the zone of apposition is similarly simplified by the degree to which the rib cage in that region moves as a unit with the rest of the rib cage. Greater understanding of the kinematic detail of various parts of the chest wall has also led to graphical analyses that describe the importance of specific regions of the chest wall (11,14) and has formed the basis of more complicated models based on equilibrium equations capable of simulating chest wall behavior in a variety of circumstances (15). Finally, finite element analysis, which typically uses a large number of simultaneous equations transparent to the user and applied to numerous elemental bits of a structure, has been fruitfully applied to solve stress-strain problems in the rib cage (16,17). This approach is becoming more important in elucidating the mechanics of the diaphragm, whose complicated curvature and various material properties have discouraged analyses without great simplification of geometry (18) (see Chapter 7). With more complicated models, assumptions and boundary conditions are often critical, and great care needs to be exercised so that the findings, especially those that cannot be directly confirmed experimentally, are reasonable and solutions are unique.

B. Respiratory Muscle Actions

Whereas diaphragmatic action can often be inferred from an analysis of the transdiaphragmatic pressure and volume displacements measured at the surface, the actions of other muscles are less easy to infer from simple measurements of pressures and displacements, and they have typically been inferred from their anatomy (19). One of the earliest and most famous descriptions of respiratory muscle action was Hamberger's geometrical analysis of intercostal muscle action (20). His analysis was based on a two-dimensional parallelogram, two opposite sides of which represent the spine and the sternum, and the remaining sides, the ribs of the rib cage. This model formed the basis of current understanding of intercostal muscle action until recent three-dimensional models appeared (13,16,17,21).

A second approach to respiratory muscle function relies on the pattern of activity of the muscles during breathing and voluntary respiratory maneuvers. For example, muscles active principally during inspiration are assumed to be inspiratory. A related approach is through direct stimulation of relevant muscles to observe the mechanical results, or through prevention of contraction with other respiratory muscles to observe the reduction or augmentation of respiratory action. For example, one expects to see that, when the nerve to an inspiratory muscle is sectioned, shortening of that muscle during inhalation is reduced (or lengthening is increased) or the inspiratory tidal volume or flow rate is reduced. Numerous studies have applied these methods to establish the respiratory effects of various respiratory muscles.

III. Reexamination of Critical Assumptions

A. Pressure

Pressure-volume analyses of chest wall function have characteristically used a single pressure to represent the forces applied to surfaces of a container. This simplification has worked remarkably well, despite gravitational gradients in pressure and the presence of shear stresses. In a gas-filled cavity, without rapid or violent motions or accelerations, a single pressure would suffice to characterize the forces exerted by the gas on the surrounding walls. Gas never fills containers in the chest wall except in a pneumothorax, pneumoperitoneum, or air bubble in the stomach or other hollow viscus. In particular, the normal bounding characteristics of the chest wall include pressure gradients in the pleural liquid lining layer, which are influenced both by gravitational hydrostatic forces and by viscous pressure losses associated with pleural liquid flow. Hydrostatic pressure gradients would amount to 1 cm H_2O pressure change per centimeter of vertical height. In small animals, such gradients would be of little consequence, but in larger animals, including humans, they would not be insignificant. The interaction of hydrostatic forces and pleural liquid movement has been determined to be an important component of the pleural pressure gradient in the lung (see below and Chapter 5).

Gravitationally induced gradients of pressure have been included in some models of the chest wall, but because the vertical pressure gradients resulting from gravity are relatively constant and do not generally vary with respiration, such gradients have usually been lumped into a constant pressure offset. For example, in describing the pressure-volume characteristics of the abdominal wall, one can use gastric pressure as the relevant pressure, assuming that the abdominal wall is subjected to pressures that increase with decreasing height but that vary with time or volume displacement exactly as gastric pressure does. Similarly, pressure-volume characteristics of the lungs estimated by lower esophageal pressure is approximately valid for the lung as a whole, although the recoil pressures of the lung apices may be greater than those of the lower lobes. Gravitational gradients have been included to describe two phenomena: the direct effect of gravitational gradients on shape and displacements and the effects of immersion.

The shape of the relaxed belly wall in upright subjects was examined in detail in a treatise by Duomarco and Rimini (22) and conveyed by Agostoni and Mead (3) and others (23,24). Gravitational gradients were used to explain vertical gradients in the distribution of lung volume and ventilation by Milic-Emili and associates in their classic analysis (25), and finite element analysis has been used to explore the effects of gravity on chest wall and lung shape when pleural pressure gradients are altered by changes in body position (26). Nonlinearity of the volume-pressure characteristic of the lung and the displacement-pressure characteristic of the belly wall interact with the linear gravitational gradient in pressure to produce curvilinear vertical gradients in displacement, volume, or ventilation. For example, the shape of the relaxed belly in supine subjects, relatively flat when there is no cephalocaudal gravitational gradient, becomes curved when upright (3,24), the lower abdomen having reached a displacement at which it is relatively stiff. Similarly, the uppermost alveoli in the upright lung have reached the stiffer part of their pressure-volume characteristic, so the vertical gradient of regional lung volume should be less at the top of the lung than lower down (25).

In immersion studies, the shape and characteristics of the chest wall can be profoundly affected by the external gravitational pressure gradients (27). With immersion to the xiphoid, the belly wall becomes flat or scaphoid and extremely compliant (as it is in the supine posture) because of "cancellation" of the transmural hydrostatic pressure gradient by the external water.

It has been usual to make the simplifying assumption that the contents of the chest wall are not very shape stable and that the lung and viscera behave more or less like liquid contents in a container. However, the chest wall and its contents are sufficiently shape stable that pressure gradients often differ substantially from those predicted for a fluid-filled container. In approaching these phenomena, we discuss the support of solid objects in gravity and the effects of shape stability on pressure gradients.

B. Support of Objects in Shear

Forces applied to solids can be divided into normal forces, applied in a direction perpendicular to the surface of the object, and shear forces, applied in a direction tangential to the surface. Normal and shear stresses (force per unit area) have the same dimensions as pressure. Hydrostatic pressures exerted by fluids are normal stresses. When surfaces bounding a liquid layer slide relative to each other and when fluids flow, fluids also exert shear stress. For example, the sliding motion of the lung relative to the rib cage and to the diaphragm is associated with shear stresses on the lung. Objects in a gravitational field can be supported by shear stresses, nonuniform normal stresses, or both. The tensorial sum of shear and normal stresses plus the normal stress arising from gravity must equal zero if the object is not accelerating. For example, the cube in Figure

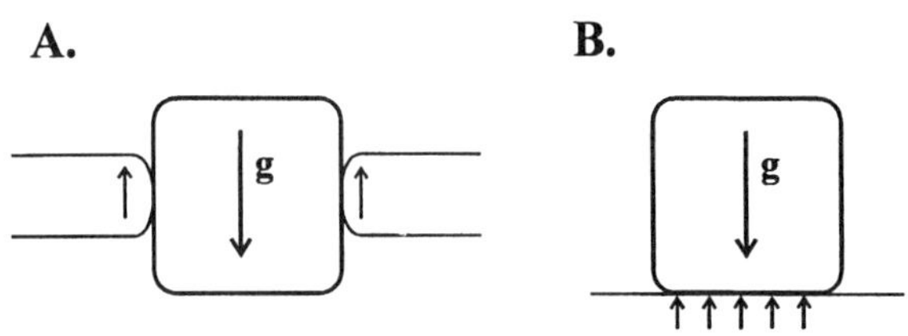

Figure 3 A cube is supported in gravity by shear stress at the sides (**A**) or by a normal stress (pressure) at its bottom surface (**B**). Arrows indicate direction and magnitude of gravitational (g), shear, and normal forces.

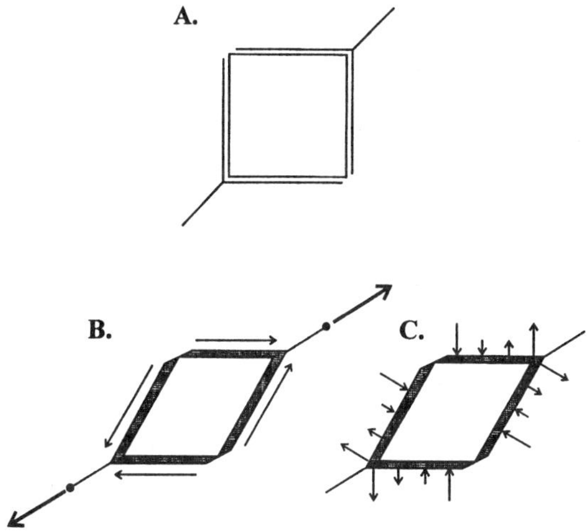

Figure 4 Equivalence of shear stress and nonuniform normal stress illustrated by distortions of the square of deformable material. An undeformed cube (**A**) undergoes similar shear deformations by traction applied to flexible but inextensible material adherent to its surfaces, which applies shear stresses (**B**), and by application of nonuniform normal stresses (**C**). (Distortions are exaggerated for illustration.)

3 can be supported by shear stresses at its sides (*A*) or by unbalanced normal stresses exerted on the bottom and/or top (*B*).

Note that there is an equivalence between the presence of pure shear stresses and nonuniform normal stresses. Thus, structures such as the lung or the cube pictured in Figure 4*A*, which can be deformed by shear stresses (see Figure 4*B*), can be viewed as equivalently distorted by the application of tensile and compressive normal stresses (i.e., nonuniform pressures) in directions 45° from the shear stress directions (see Figure 4*C*). This equivalence is important because it indicates that there may be two independent sources of isovolume distortion of the lung. One arises from the application of frank shear stresses, such as through the movement of pleural fluid associated with breathing and to a negligible extent, pleural fluid flow under gravity. The other arises from the application of nonuniform normal stresses, such as those that arise from gravitationally induced pressure gradients.

How are the viscera supported? We know that the pleural and abdominal cavities contain a small quantity of pleural or peritoneal liquid, respectively, that provides a more or less continuous layer between the surfaces of the viscera and the chest wall. For purposes of discussion, we assume that this liquid layer is continuous everywhere between the visceral surfaces and between the viscera and the epithelial lining of the chest wall cavities. Furthermore, we ignore tissue connections between the viscera and the body wall; thus, all forces acting on the visceral surfaces are, in effect, entirely transmitted by pressures and shear stresses in the liquid. If all the pressures exerted by the surfaces in the viscera were perfectly hydrostatic (i.e., exhibiting a gravitational gradient of ~1 cm H_2O/cm vertical height), the liquid would be in static equilibrium. To the extent that local pressures do not exhibit a gravitational gradient, local flows must occur, driven by departures of the local pressure gradients from hydrostatic. However, such flows are expected to be extremely small because the spaces among the viscera and between viscera and the chest wall structures are very thin (~20 μm in the pleural space), and if the period of observation is short compared with the time required for liquid to completely drain from a given region, the liquid layer will be continuous. The liquid prevents material surface-to-surface contact and thus prevents shear stresses from being statically applied by the walls of the container. Thus the viscera are supported essentially by a spatially nonuniform pressure.

In the abdomen, most of the support arises from a gravitational gradient in pressure that is nearly hydrostatic, the peritoneal liquid and the viscera having nearly equal density. By contrast, the lung has a density approximately one-fourth that of the pleural liquid, and the gravitational gradient in pleural pressure is thus far from hydrostatic on average and therefore pleural liquid flow must result. The determination of the pressure gradients from fluid flow is difficult because the fluid layers are very thin, and because of viscosity, the flows are correspondingly small. On the other hand, even a small amount of fluid flow, simply because the layer is thin, is associated with large pressure gradients, typically varying as the inverse cube of the layer thickness. The quantification of flows and pressures arising from gravitational forces and relative motions of lung and chest wall are difficult, but it appears that these effects may be important (28,29). (See Chapter 5.)

C. Uniformity of Pressure Gradients: The Abdomen

Considerable controversy has surrounded the measurement of abdominal pressures. Following the seminal work of Duomarco and Rimini (22), it was generally assumed that the abdomen was a hydrostatic system that could be modeled as a container filled with water. Investigators typically measured pressure in one part of the abdomen (or in the stomach) and assumed that pressures everywhere in the abdomen differed only according to the hydrostatic gradient. Temporal changes in pressure were usually assumed to be uniform throughout the abdomen. This model of abdominal mechanics was challenged by Decramer and colleagues (30) who reported intraabdominal pressure gradients in dogs that were not simply hydrostatic. Mead et al. (31) later explored interregional variation in pressure fluctuation in humans, finding them consistent with hydrostatic gradients when they took into account changes in height of the stomach with breathing. Loring et al. (24) studied the regional variations in abdominal pressure in dogs, concluding that shear deformation of abdominal viscera could explain those instances in which gradients in pressure were not simply hydrostatic. For illustration, they suggested a model consisting of elastic balls suspended in a liquid of equal density with a rigid container as shown in Figure 5.

Pressures in the plane of the equators of the balls along vertical and horizontal surfaces of the container are shown schematically. In Figure 5*A*, there is enough liquid surrounding the balls to prevent them from being flattened or otherwise distorted by the container. Pressures at rest are everywhere hydrostatic, exhibiting the gravitational gradient. A uniform compressive force exerted on all four walls causes a uniform increase in pressure, whereas an isovolume shape change of the container (e.g., inward displacement of the side walls and outward displacement of the top and bottom walls) that does not cause shear deformation of the balls does not affect pressure anywhere.

In Figure 5*B*, the balls are larger and there is less liquid, causing the elastic balls to be locally flattened by the container and by each other. Pressures in the large collections of liquid still exhibit a hydrostatic gravitational gradient, whereas pressures measured in the thin liquid layer between adjacent balls or between the balls and the container reflect not only gravitational gradients but also the spatially nonuniform pressures exerted by deformed elastic material. A uniform compression causes a uniform increase in pressure, whereas an isovolume shape change of the container causes local pressures to increase in regions where local deformation increases and to decrease where local deformation decreases. (We assume, here, that the balls and liquid are incompressible, that a continuous layer of liquid surrounds the balls, and that the time required for the space between them to drain dry is very long compared with the period of observation.)

Pressures within the abdomen are determined by the same three factors: gravity, uniform compression, and shear deformation. (In this analysis, we ignore inertial effects, which are probably negligible if we limit our discussion to normal breathing and other slow respiratory maneuvers in human subjects at rest. Inertia has important effects during body movements and rapid respiratory events such as forced oscillation.) Pressures within the cavities of the chest wall depend on properties of the cavities themselves, the viscera, and the liquid within the compartment as can be illustrated by reference to this model. For example, increasing the deformability and compliance of the chest wall container in Figure 5*B* would reduce the shear deformation of the balls and thus reduce the local elevations in pressure between the balls and the wall. Similarly, changing the unstressed shape of the balls to a more cubic shape would reduce local elevations in pressure between the balls and the walls substantially. Finally, increasing the viscosity of the liquid could slow the rate of relaxation of

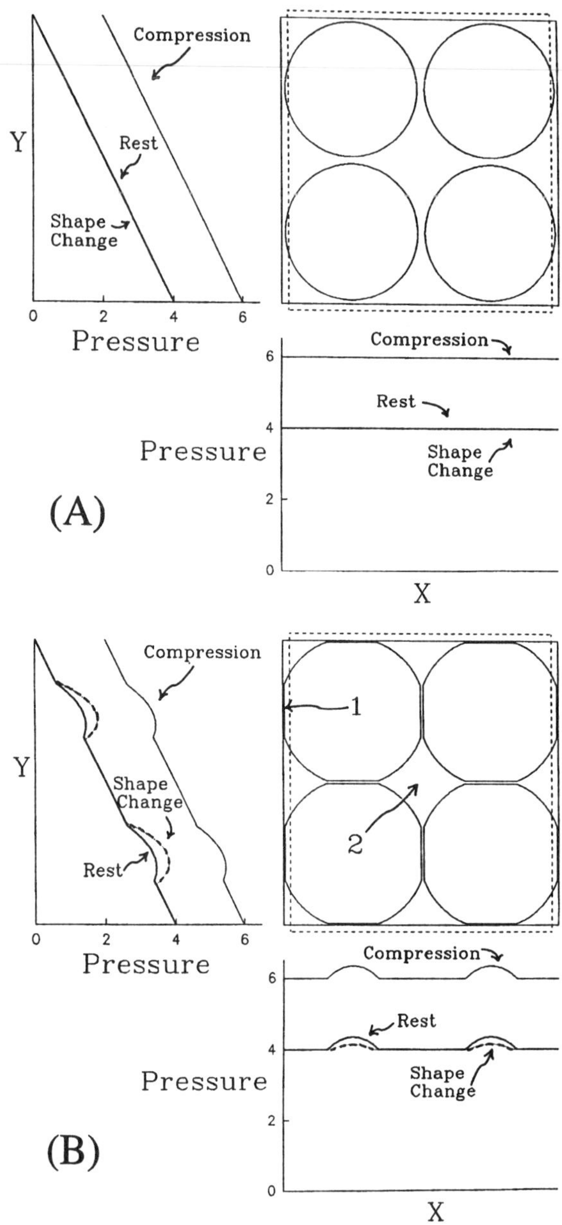
Compression
Rest
Shape Change
Y
0
2
4
6
Pressure
Compression
6
Rest
4
Pressure
Shape Change
2
(A)
0
X
Compression
1
Y
Shape Change
Rest
2
0
2
4
6
Pressure
Compression
6
Rest
4
Pressure
Shape Change
2
(B)
0
X

transient shear deformations of the viscera through redistribution of liquid within the space.

D. Shape and Pressure Distribution: Mutual Determination Versus Causation

When shape-stable solids are contained by shape-stable containers, the pressure distribution at the inner surface of the container depends on the mechanical characteristics of both structures, defined as the relationship between the shape of the structure and the forces required to achieve that shape. However, the pressure distribution can be determined from knowledge of the shape and mechanical characteristics of either structure alone. The rib cage itself, as noted above, has a shape stability conferred by its skeletal elements. Its kinematics are often described in terms of two types of rib motion: pump handle (anteroposterior) motion and bucket handle (lateral) motion (Figure 6) (32). In the abdomen, the shape stability of the liver and other organs can affect pressure gradients seen on the abdominal side of the diaphragm. The mechanical characteristics of the lung and chest wall together determine what shape the lung will assume in the chest. This shape, considering the minuscule volume of pleural liquid, is also essentially the shape of the inner surface of the chest wall. Given this shape, the distribution of pressures over the surface of the lung can be found from the mechanical characteristics of the lung or the chest wall. A simple model illustrating these ideas is shown in Figure 7. In this model, the shape of the unstressed chest wall differs from that of the unstressed lung at the same volume. When the lung is forced to conform to the chest wall, both are deformed, and the resulting pressure distribution satisfies stress equilibrium at all levels.

Figure 5 Conceptual model of abdominal container and contents. **A**, Enough liquid is present to separate neutrally buoyant elastic balls floating within it. Pressures in the plane of the equators of the balls (*left*) and lower walls of container are plotted as a function of Y- and X-coordinates, respectively. Pressures are shown at rest, during uniform compression of contents, and during isovolume shape change of container (*dashed lines*). Uniform compression causes spatially uniform increase in pressure, whereas isovolume shape change has no effect on pressure. **B**, model as above, except that there is insufficient liquid to prevent container from deforming elastic balls. Pressures at walls of container are locally increased where elastic balls are flattened. Uniform compression causes spatially homogeneous increase in pressure, whereas isovolume shape change causes local increases in pressure where elastic material is deformed further (*left*) and causes decreases in pressure where shear deformation decreases (*bottom*). (From Ref. 24.)

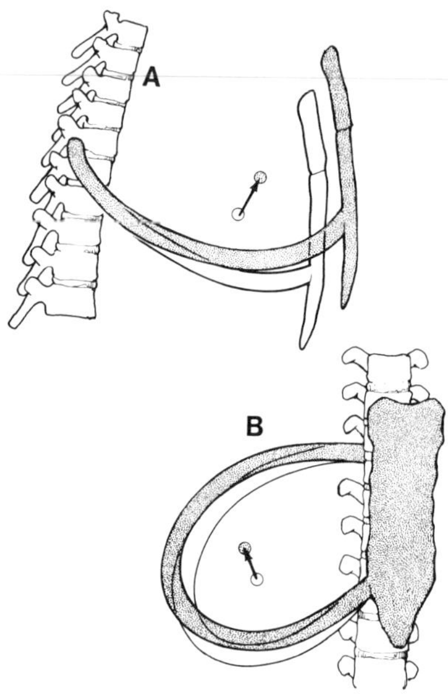

Figure 6 Motion of ribs during rib cage expansion can be characterized as a combination of pump-handle motion (**A**) and bucket-handle motion (**B**). The inspiratory pump-handle motion is rotation of the ribs about their costovertebral joints and the inspiratory bucket-handle motion is rotation of the ribs about their spinal and sternal connection. Final positions are stippled (32).

An important distinction should be drawn between the vertical pressure gradient observed at the surface of the lung and the average density of the lung. The surface pressures of the lung depend on local normal stresses, which need not reflect the vertical gradient in pressure required to support the lung hydrostatically. For example, the model lung in Figure 7 exhibits greater forces (normal stresses) at the upper surfaces than at the lower surfaces, a pressure gradient inverse to that which would be necessary to suspend the lung in fluid of equal density. Thus, the vertical gradient of pleural pressure at the boundary of the lung with the rib cage may be substantially greater or less than that predicted from lung density.

The chest, by itself, does not cause the distribution of pleural pressures or shape of the lung any more than the lung, by itself, causes the pressures or shape of the chest. One could argue that because the lung is much more deformable than the chest wall, the chest wall essentially determines the shape of the

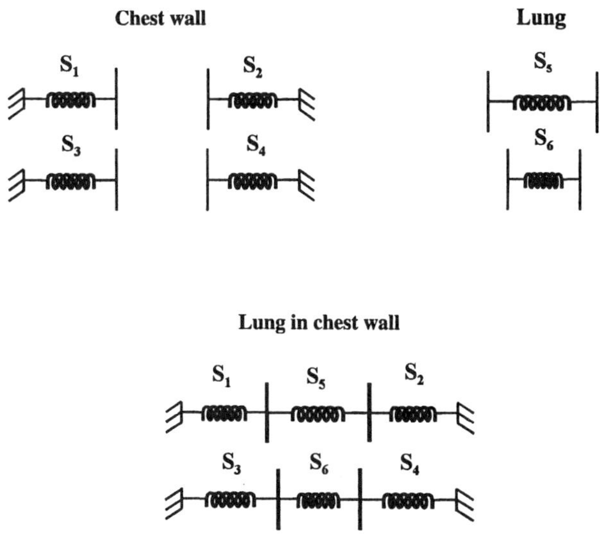

Figure 7 The chest is represented by four surfaces whose force-displacement characteristics are governed by springs S_{1-4}. Similarly, the behavior of the lungs is goverened by springs S_{5-6}. When put together, the normal force (analogous to pressure) of the lung on the chest wall is at every location equal and opposite to that of the chest wall on the lung (i.e., the forces in springs S_1, S_2, and S_5, are equal and forces in springs S_3, S_4, and S_6 are equal). The unrestrained shape of lungs, shape of the chest, and force-length characteristics of springs S_1–S_6 are sufficient to determine the final shape and forces of the assembly. Similarly, the unrestrained and final shapes of the lung and the characteristics of springs S_{5-6} or the unrestrained and final shapes of the chest and characteristics of springs S_{1-4} are sufficient to determine the forces.

combined system, and the distribution of pleural pressure is consequently determined by lung recoil properties. Similarly, one could argue that the pleural liquid, because of its small volume, has only small effects on lung and chest wall shape and the distribution of pleural pressures. However, in the mathematical sense, the pressure distribution in the space is not caused by any element in isolation. Shape and pressures are mutually determined by the characteristics of both lung and chest wall. Furthermore, the pleural liquid layer between lung and chest wall provides another way to find (determine) the pressure distribution in the pleural space—by knowing the exact geometry of the liquid layer and the flows within that layer. Thus, pressures, which can be determined from the properties and dimensions of the lung or the chest wall, can also be determined from pleural liquid geometry and dynamics.

E. Pleural Stress Jumps

The pressure in the pleural space, regardless of deviations in its hydrostatic gradient due to viscous pressure drops, is communicated to the parenchyma through the visceral pleural membrane. A basic assumption by Mead et al. (33) and in subsequent work on interdependence was that the average stress in the subpleural parenchyma is equal to pleural pressure. However, to the extent that the pleural membrane carries tension and has a nonzero mean curvature, there will be a stress jump across it, and local mean parenchymal stresses are not given simply by pleural pressure. Quantifying the contribution of the pleura to lung recoil is difficult. A major contribution to this problem was made by Hajji et al. (34), who used punch indentation tests on dog, pig, and horse lobes together with an analytical solution to an elastic half-space bound by a tensed membrane to estimate the shear modulus of the parenchyma as well as the membrane tension. Favorable comparisons were observed with isolated ablated pleural membrane specimens. Their work showed that pleural tension is not negligible. Indeed, over a wide range of lung volumes, the fraction of total incremental PdV work done by the lobe on deflation contributed by TdS work of the pleura averaged some 20%, where, P is transpulmonary pressure, T is membrane tension, and dV and dS are differential changes in lobe volume and pleural surface area, respectively. Furthermore, there was a systematic increase in T with species size; over a range of 4 to 16 cm H_2O transpulmonary pressures, T ranged from 1000 to 5000 dyne/cm in the dog to 8000 to 20,000 dyne/cm in the horse.

Although this is significant in terms of work done, the effect on local lung recoil is less clear, because the stress jump exists only by virtue of membrane curvature, and this curvature varies widely over the surface of the lobe. Thus, for example, the smooth costal surface of the dog lobe may in some locations have a radius of curvature of, say, 10 cm, which, using the above range of tensions, translates into stress jumps of 0.2–1.0 cm H_2O. That is, the parenchymal distending stress would be less by that amount. Near the lobar margins, the curvatures increase sharply, with radii of curvatures decreasing to perhaps 1 cm and with correspondingly increased values of the stress jumps. Over the diaphragmatic surface of the lobe, the curvatures are negative, and parenchymal stresses would be increased. If pleural tension were uniform, this would imply a large degree of inhomogeneity in the parenchymal stresses between these regions. Hajji et al. recognized the importance of the stress jump across the pleura and this potential origin of nonuniformity in local lung recoil, but they were careful not to attempt a direct quantification, because the degree of uniformity of T itself is unknown. Nevertheless, this remains an important and unresolved issue in current thinking about the nature of transmission of tensile forces in the lung and how pressures in the pleural space translate into parenchymal boundary conditions.

F. Shear Stresses in Deformation at the Zone of Apposition

The pleural space in the zone of apposition of the diaphragm to the rib cage exhibits pressures and pressure gradients qualitatively different from those of the remainder of the pleural space. We consider pleural pressure in the zone of apposition in static and dynamic conditions first in the region away from the cephalic margin and then in the region near the cephalic margin of the zone of apposition, and the geometry and fluid dynamics of the pleural liquid. The salient feature of this region is the sharp angle into which the margin of the lung is pulled by the divergence of the diaphragm from the rib cage wall at the edge of the free diaphragmatic dome. There being little pleural liquid to fill this space, the margin of the lung is elongated and sheared to conform to the wedge-shaped space, the elongation being associated with very low pressures at the lung apex. This explanation begs the question why the reduced pleural pressure does not draw liquid from other regions of the pleural space, thereby allowing the lung to retract and raising the pleural pressure locally. Discussion of this question is beyond the scope of this chapter, but it involves the continuous motion of the lung margin in breathing, thereby redistributing any localized liquid accumulation, and the mechanisms that maintain a relatively constant liquid volume and, more importantly, pleural liquid thickness in the pleural space (see Chapter 5 and Butler et al. [29]).

G. Coordinate Frames: How They Affect Interpretation

Kinematics of the chest wall are usually described with reference to a coordinate frame in which the back is stationary, a natural and rarely questioned result of the way human breathing is observed. The earliest quantitative kinematic observations by Konno and Mead (4) measured the displacements relative to a laboratory frame of reference of various locations on the ventral chest wall in a subject whose back was held against a stationary object. Changes in the ventral wall displacement were interpreted as changes in anteroposterior diameter. This perspective has been nearly universal and is applied in a recent study in which movements of markers on the ventral body and lateral chest wall were precisely measured in a three-dimensional system (35). In standing subjects, the anteroposterior movements of the back during breathing are probably of much lower amplitude than those of the ventral chest wall, so the usual perspective is natural and appropriate. In supine subjects, it is even more so.

Kinematic descriptions of the chest wall that involve displacement differences are independent of coordinate frame, in that anteroposterior expansion and regional volume displacements can be described with any coordinate system. However, when one ascribes the volume displacements of the chest wall compartments to a particular surface or describes the pressure-volume work done by a particular surface, the results are path dependent and thus depend on the coordinate frame of reference (Figure 8). For coordinate frame–specific analysis of volume displacements and pressure-volume work associated with various structures, see Ref. 14.

To illustrate the ways in which one can describe and attribute volume displacements and work, consider the simple two-dimensional representation of the rib cage, diaphragm, and lung shown in Figure 9. To make the analogy with three-dimensional systems more natural, consider the structures in Figure 9 to be of constant depth so that changes in area can be visualized as volume displacements. The model shows initial position (solid lines) and final position (interrupted lines) of the rib cage and diaphragm during a breath in which the rib cage moves outward and the diaphragm moves caudally in such a way that it does not change length. How much of the tidal volume is associated with rib cage displacement and how much with diaphragm motion? The question can be answered in many ways, none of which is particularly rigorous and all of which are coordinate frame–specific. Early investigators would have divided lung volume changes into displacements of the rib cage and displacements of the diaphragm-abdomen pathways. In this particular example, the rib cage, including the region below the diaphragmatic insertion, displaces 96% of the tidal volume and the remaining 4% would thus be attributed to the diaphragm. Interestingly, if one examines only the first 25% of the volume excursion, those fractions are substantially different (141% versus –41%). Mead and his followers have argued that because the rib cage actually is partly an abdominal visceral container,

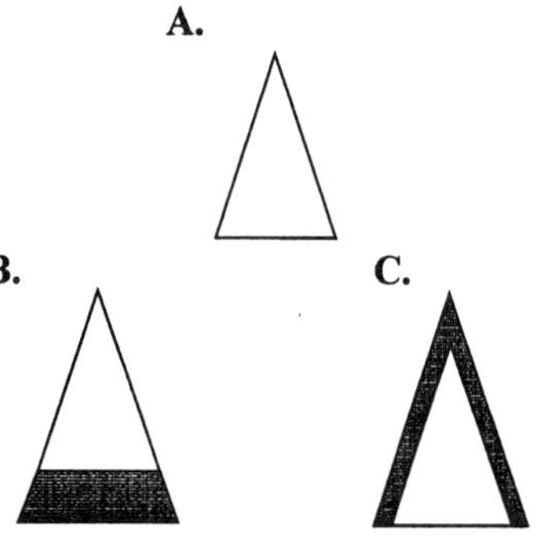

Figure 8 The triangular area (**A**) gets bigger at (**B**) or (**C**), but it is not clear which edges can be said to have swept out the additional shaded area. The contribution by any edge to area expansion (or by analogy any surface to volume expansion) depends on a frame of reference, which is arbitrary.

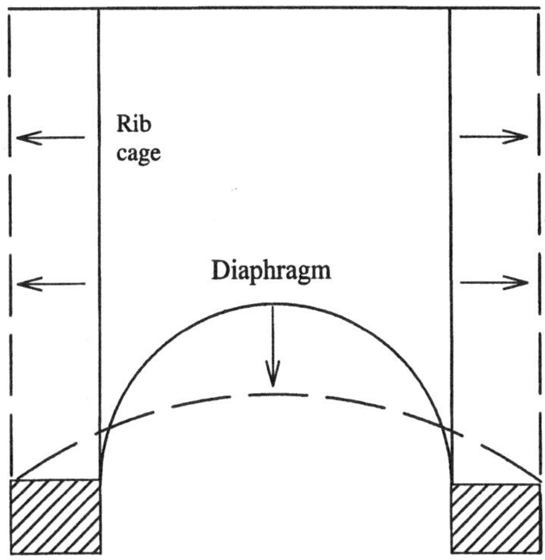

Figure 9 Two-dimensional model of a rib cage and diaphragm. The rib cage expands (*arrows*) from solid to dashed line positions by increasing its diameter, whereas the length of the diaphragm from end to end stays constant.

a large portion of the volume displaced by the rib cage is actually expanding the abdominal container (shown as the cross-hatched area in Figure 9), and the rib cage is, to this extent, an abdominal pump, not a lung pump. Using Mead's reasoning, the volume "swept out" by the rib cage–apposed portions of the lung can be compared with the volumes swept out by the diaphragm-apposed portions of the lung. That ratio is substantially different from the ratios noted above; 89% of the tidal volume is accounted for by expansion ("sweeping out") of volume by the rib cage–apposed surface of the lung and 11% is attributable to the displacement of the diaphragm-apposed portion of the lung. (For the first 25% of the excursion, those numbers are 131% and –31%.) If the lung contained within the thorax has a pressure-volume characteristic and a compliance, the pressure-volume work done by the diaphragm and rib cage during the breath described here could be calculated. The answers calculated from the volume contributions above would suggest that the diaphragm accounts for anything from 4% to 11% of the total pressure-volume work done on the lung. However, a mechanical analysis would suggest that, because the length of the diaphragm from insertion to insertion does not change during this breath, there could be no work accomplished by that structure. Thus, a real model whose characteristics and kinematics are consistent with Figure 9 would accomplish inspiration entirely by the work of the rib cage.

The model described here lacks many of the complicating features of the real rib cage and abdomen; for example, the caudal margin of the rib cage moves toward the head during inspiration, expanding the abdomen and moving the diaphragmatic insertions toward the lungs. However, the volumes swept by various surfaces always depend on what is taken to be stationary, and the attribution of pressure-volume work to motion of various surfaces of the respiratory system, although definable, is essentially arbitrary.

How, at least in principle, can the arbitrary nature of the analyses portrayed in Figure 9 be avoided? Rigorous mechanical analysis of the chest wall is possible if all of the variables relevant to a particular action are accounted for. For example, the work done on or by the diaphragm can be known by measuring tension and length of the diaphragmatic muscle because this muscle can do external work only by shortening. However, the pressure-volume work done by the diaphragm is problematic, because, as it moves, the diaphragm does work on or has work done on it by its insertions and by the chest wall deforming it in the zone of apposition. Those structures applying a force to the contracting diaphragm move it, contributing to the work done. The difficulty here is that both experimentally and conceptually, one would like to relate the forces and work done by the various muscle groups to the gross output variables such as volumes and pressures. Given the observation that only a few degrees of freedom are typically apparent (e.g., two volume pathways for lung expansion: rib cage and abdominal; a few mean pressure differences: pleural pressure on lung-apposed rib cage, transdiaphragmatic pressure on the thoracic boundary of the abdominal contents, abdominal pressure on the abdomen-apposed rib cage), this argues that such a reduction is not only possible, but desirable. On the other hand, the distributed nature of the geometric arrangement of the muscles actually effecting these pressure and volume changes makes the explicit determination of their contribution difficult.

H. Partial Systems and Complete Systems: How Conclusions Depend on What is Included

Conclusions about the function and action of parts of the chest wall depend on how much of the chest wall is included in the analysis. The analysis of the inspiratory action of the diaphragm on the rib cage illustrates this point. Mead (36) recognized two origins of this inspiratory action: 1. the action of abdominal pressure transmitted through the zone of apposition to the inner surface of the rib cage, forcing the rib cage outward, and 2. "insertional action" whereby the diaphragm pulls cephalad on its insertions with a total force (F) equal to the product of transdiaphragmatic pressure (P_{di}) and the area of the diaphragm projected on a plane perpendicular to the body axis (A_{di}). (Note that the analogous caudad pull of the abdominal wall was ignored in this analysis; see below.) Because of the articulations of the rib cage, the cephalic force has an inspiratory effect, moving the lower rib cage cephalad and outward. This analysis, formalized later (7), was internally consistent and explained experimental results. However, the treatment of the insertional force as a predictably inspiratory force was problematic for some researchers, seeming to imply that the diaphragm could "haul itself up by its bootstraps."

To illustrate how the effects of the insertional force depend on the whole respiratory system, we present this force first in relative isolation and then with progressively more of the elements and of the respiratory system, considering the respiratory actions at each step. In Figure 10*A*, the rib cage is articulated so that the ventral insertions of the diaphragm move cephalad and ventral with rib cage expansion. (The figure is drawn without an area of apposition so that insertional force is considered in isolation.) With an isometric contraction of the diaphragm, the total insertional force (F) is equal to P_{di} A_{di}, where A_{di} is the cross-sectional area of the rib cage at the insertional ring. Because this force is centered halfway between the "mobile" ventral insertion and the "fixed" dorsal insertion, it can be divided into two force vectors with amplitude $(P_{di}\ A_{di})/2$ distributed at ventral and dorsal insertions. Diaphragmatic contraction may or may not be expansive for the rib cage, however, because it is only the increase in abdominal pressure that is expansive, not the entire increase in transdiaphragmatic pressure. To the extent that P_{di} derives from a lowered pleural pressure ($P_{di} = P_{ab} - P_{pl}$), the cephalad force F at the insertions is balanced by an equal and opposite force of the transthoracic (pleural) pressure acting on the projected area of the diaphragm (A_{di}) on the cephalic rib cage, as shown in Figure 10*B*. Thus, only the abdominal component of P_{di} (i.e., P_{ab}) contributes to the expansion. These ideas are consistent with earlier analyses, although they are not always explicitly stated in them.

The analysis is not complete, however, without considering the remainder of the system—the abdomen. Here, the increase in abdominal pressure applies a force to an area of the lower abdomen (pelvis) equal to P_{ab} A_{di} in an analogous way as on the rib cage (see Figure 10*C*). Given a rigid back and pelvis, this pressure causes forces and moments in the back that resolve the imbalance of forces at the diaphragmatic insertions (see Figure 10*C*), but the effects of increasing pressure on the ventral abdominal wall are still unconsidered. What if the abdomen were accordion-like, able to withstand transmural pressures with hoop stresses while applying negligible axial tension on the rib cage margin as in Figure 10*C*? Then, increases in abdominal pressures would, through the insertional forces of the diaphragm, be expansive for the rib cage as above. But what if the abdominal wall were more membrane-like, maintaining transmural pressures by a combination of axial and circumferential stresses? There is abundant evidence that caudally directed insertional force (F_I) applied by the abdominal wall musculature could substantially cancel cephalad insertional forces of the diaphragm (see Figure 10*D*). The oblique and cephalocaudal orientation of rectus abdominis and abdominal oblique muscles suggests a significant inser-

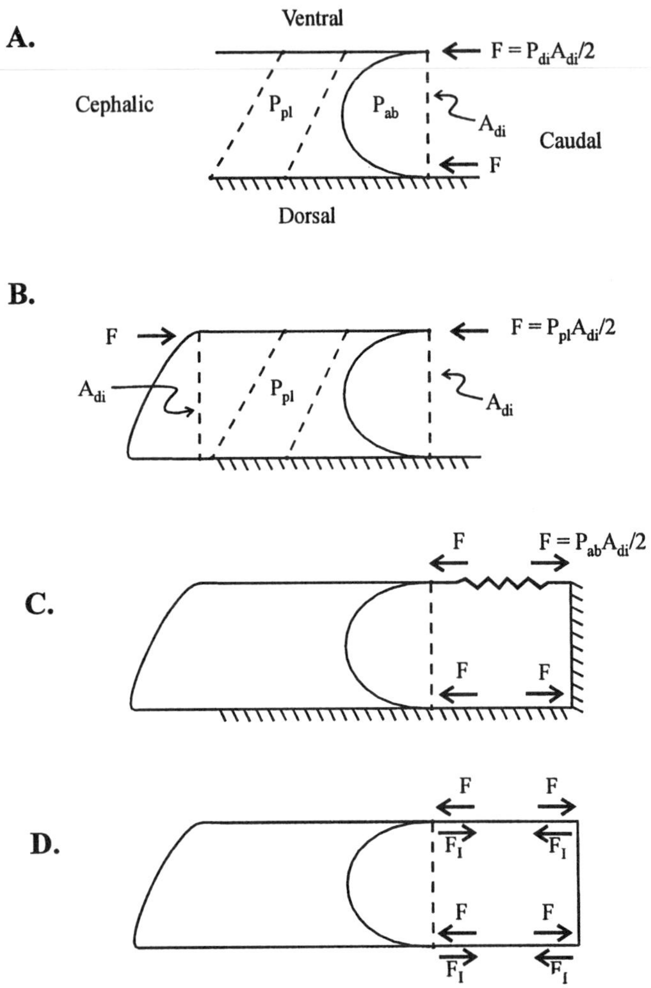

Figure 10 Progressively more inclusive model of the chest wall illustrating how inferences about the action of the diaphragm on the rib cage depends on how inclusive the model is.

tional force, and caudal movements of the rib cage margins have been demonstrated with abdominal muscle stimulation in humans (37). Moreover, pressures in the abdomen can be raised voluntarily to 150–300 cm H_2O by combined diaphragmatic and abdominal wall contractions in an expulsive maneuver in which pleural pressure does not change. This maneuver, which may produce a

30-kg cephalad insertional force at the ventral diaphragmatic insertions, typically causes no cephalad rib cage displacement, suggesting strong restraint by the abdominal wall. Thus, the insertional force, which considered in isolation is clearly inspiratory, is paired with cancelling expiratory forces that may largely or entirely eliminate its independent inspiratory action under some circumstances. Nonetheless, even though the inspiratory action of the diaphragm via its insertional forces at the rib cage margin have been well studied, a quantitative description of the combined action of the diaphragm and abdominal muscles via their rib cage insertions remains unknown.

IV. Action of Respiratory Muscles

A. Pitfalls from Observation of Muscles Acting Alone

As discussed previously, the first anatomists inferred respiratory function from muscle anatomy; their inferences were sometimes amusing but often correct. Determination of the timing of muscle contraction by palpation and later by electromyography allowed inferences about whether muscles were inspiratory or expiratory, although such evidence was not conclusive. Even muscles that are active during inspiration can be expiratory in function. For example, the abdominal wall muscles are spontaneously activated in a maximal inhalation in many subjects (38). Furthermore, a muscle need not shorten or do work to contribute to the pressure generated by a coordinated respiratory action. The most direct means of testing the action of, say, a putatively inspiratory muscle would seem to be to electrically stimulate the muscle and observe the inspiratory effects, if any, on volume, flow, or pressure. Although such experiments are straightforward in principle (although often technically difficult), the results can be hard to interpret. Consider an experiment to determine the respiratory action of intercostal muscles by De Troyer et al. (39,40). Canine external or internal intercostal muscles were electrically stimulated in one to three interspaces. The contraction of either muscle layer caused the caudal ribs to move cephalad and the cephalic ribs to move caudad. At resting lung volume, the cephalad movements of the caudal ribs were greater than the caudal movements of the cephalad ribs. Because in normal inhalation the ribs move cephalad, the "net action" of the muscles in both layers was said to be inspiratory. This was unexpected; Hamberger's two-dimensional geometrical analysis of the intercostal muscles predicted an inspiratory action for the external intercostals and an expiratory action of the internal intercostals. The apparent disagreement could be resolved by considering intercostal muscle contraction in many interspaces instead of only one to three interspaces. In a demonstration using finite element models of the canine rib cage, Loring and Woodbridge (16) reproduced De Troyer's results in a single interspace and showed that intercostal muscle activation in many interspaces produced inspiratory movements or expiratory movements depending on the muscle layer. The lesson to be learned is that the action of a particular muscle may change from inspiratory to expiratory or change in magnitude depending on which other muscles are active and how much they are involved. Put another way, the relaxed rib cage is a different mechanical system than the rib cage with coordinated inspiratory or expiratory muscle activity, with the surprising result that, for example, the respiratory action of the external intercostal muscles in a single interspace is expiratory in one system and inspiratory in the other.

Subsequently, De Troyer and colleagues explored intercostal muscle action by observing when the muscles became active in spontaneous breathing (41); by measuring the relationship between muscle shortening and muscle activation before and after local denervation of external and other intercostal muscles (42) and by measuring respiratory motion of ribs during progressive denervation of other respiratory muscles (21), showing that the external intercostal muscles had actions as had been described by Hamberger. These observations were possible because the intercostal action was studied in coordinated respiratory efforts that activated a large proportion of the inspiratory intercostal muscles.

In 1992, Wilson and De Troyer described a method, based on Maxwell's Reciprocity Theorem, for establishing the respiratory action and mechanical advantage of respiratory muscles. Theory states that the change of length of a muscle during a passive inflation with all muscles relaxed is proportional to the mechanical advantage of that muscle in converting force to inspiratory pressure. The principle was demonstrated by showing that rib displacements during a passive inflation were predictive of the pressure generated by applying forces to the same ribs in an anesthetized paralyzed dog (43). Subsequently, the dorsal external intercostals and parasternal intercostals were evaluated with Maxwell's theorem, and the muscles, when stimulated, produced respiratory pressures consistent with prediction.

B. Maxwell's Reciprocity Theorem and the Analysis of Muscles Acting Alone

Maxwell's Reciprocity Theorem as applied by Wilson and De Troyer to the problem of determining the respiratory effects of respiratory muscles states that "the effect of active muscle tension on lung volume or pleural pressure is proportional to the change of muscle length during the relaxation maneuver" (i.e., during inflation of the relaxed chest wall). The thicker the muscle, the greater the force applied, and the greater its length change, the greater its mechanical advantage. For example, an inspiratory muscle that shortens 10% during an inflation will have twice the respiratory effect of another muscle of the same mass that shortens only 5% (assuming equal activation).

Although Maxwell's theorem is physically rigorous, its application to chest wall mechanics is problematic. First, the theorem is valid only for linearly elastic systems, and the chest wall is neither perfectly linear nor perfectly elastic. The stress-strain characteristics of the chest wall are known to be nonlinear for large displacements and nonreversible for displacements of any size because of stress-strain hysteresis of tissues. More importantly, the assumption of linearity implies that the respiratory effects of different muscles are simply additive. This description of coordinated muscle activity may be formally correct as long as the active force of each muscle is taken to be the difference between the force in that muscle during activation and the force in that muscle while inactive at the same length. However, this description does not express the coupling that may affect the active forces in muscles during coordinated efforts. That is, muscle length, and hence force, may be different when the muscle is activated alone than when it is activated as part of a coordinated effort. In some situations, for example when inspiratory, expiratory, and nonrespiratory muscles are simultaneously activated in a coordinated act, Maxwell's theorem may be inadequate and misleading.

The conceptual model in Figure 11 has two muscles that pull two ribs, which are hinged at one end and restrained by springs. Each rib is connected to

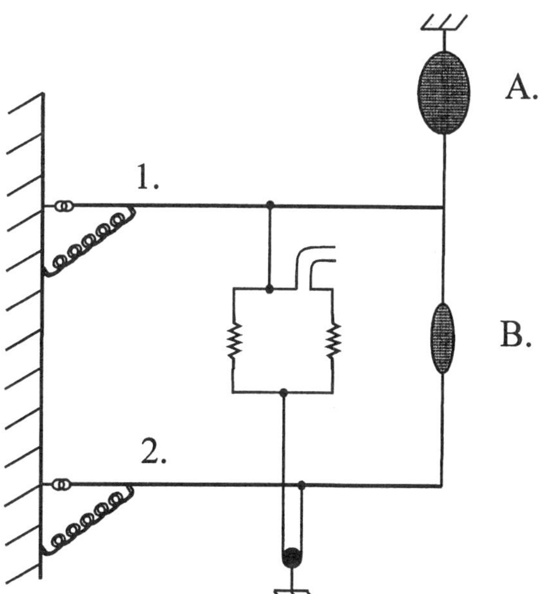

Figure 11 Conceptual model of respiratory muscle action.

a bellows, which has a length tension characteristic of a linear spring. The lower rib is connected to the bellows by a linkage so that upward motion of the rib inflates the bellows. Muscle A is connected to a stationary object at its top and to rib 1 at its bottom. Muscle B is connected between the ends of ribs 1 and 2. One can envision a coordinated contraction of the two muscles elevating both ribs and expanding the bellows. Thus, both muscles are inspiratory. Because the force applied by muscle B to the bellows is also applied to rib 1, a coordinated "inspiration" in which the ribs move equally would require that muscle A be twice as thick as muscle B (or twice as activated), as is indicated by their relative sizes.

What would Maxwell's Reciprocity Theorem say about this system and the "respiratory action" of muscles A and B? A passive inflation of this system causes the bellows to expand and both ribs rotate upward equally. There is no change of length of muscle B; muscle A shortens substantially. The prediction would be that muscle A is an inspiratory muscle and muscle B has no respiratory effect. The test of the reciprocity theorem would be to see what effect isolated contraction of muscles A and B would be. Indeed, isolated contraction of muscle B would cause an equal and opposite motion of ribs 1 and 2 and have no effect on the bellows, therefore no respiratory effect. By contrast, contraction of muscle A would cause inflation of the bellows, an inspiratory effect.

There may well be many respiratory muscles that have important functions in ventilating the respiratory system similar to that of muscle B, which do not shorten or lengthen substantially during respiratory efforts and whose respiratory function during coordinated respiratory acts cannot be directly inferred from their length changes during passive inflation.

C. A Definition of Respiratory Action in Coordinated Acts

If the action of a respiratory muscle depends on activities of other muscles, it seems reasonable to examine the muscle action during coordinated acts. In breathing, the respiratory muscles can be seen to be continuously altering pleural pressure as a means of ventilating the lungs. The sign and magnitude of the action of a given respiratory muscle depend on a number of continuously changing variables, including lung volume and the level of activity of all other active respiratory muscles. One way to define the respiratory action of a given muscle at one instant in time would be the partial derivative of pleural pressure with activation or force of that muscle, for example, $\partial P_{pl}/\partial F_i$ where P_{pl} is pleural pressure and F_i is the force developed by the ith muscle. The partial derivative is used to emphasize that the variation on the respiratory action of the muscle is defined at a particular level of activity of the muscle; such derivatives may change magnitude and even sign with changes in the level of activation as well as changes in the activity of other muscles, lung volume, and so on. In Figure

11, assuming an increase in the elastance of muscle A with activation, an increase in the activation of muscle B would be inspiratory to the bellows system during a coordinated contraction of both muscles. The determination of the respiratory function of individual muscles is a challenging task, demanding physical rigor and experimental ingenuity. The degree to which Maxwell's theorem correctly predicts muscle effects in coordinated muscular actions remains to be demonstrated.

V. Summary

Pressure-volume models of the chest wall, by simplifying chest wall anatomy and reducing stresses and displacements to a few measurable variables, have enabled great progress to be made in understanding and describing chest wall mechanics. This chapter reexamines some of the simplifications and arbitrary assumptions underlying pressure-volume analyses to include more relevant parts of a system in analyses of equilibrium and work and to recognize heterogeneity of pressure and other variables previously taken to be uniform. Future study of chest wall mechanics will rely increasingly on anatomically realistic and physically rigorous models that are less sensitive to arbitrary assumptions.

References

1. Mead J. Introduction to papers by F. Rohrer. In: West JB, ed. Translations in Respiratory Physiology. Stroudsburg: Dowden, Hutchinson & Ross, 1975:1–2.
2. Otis AB. History of respiratory mechanics. In: Macklem PT, Mead J, ed. Handbook of Physiology. Bethesda, MD: American Physiological Society, 1986:1–12.
3. Agostoni E, Mead J. Statics of the respiratory system. In: Fenn WO, Rahn H, eds. Handbook of Physiology. Washington, DC: American Physiological Society, 1964: 387–409.
4. Konno K, Mead J. Measurement of the separate volume changes of rib cage and abdomen during breathing. J Appl Physiol 1967; 22(3):407–422.
5. Goldman MD, Grimby G, Mead J. Mechanical work of breathing derived from rib cage and abdominal V-P partitioning. J Appl Physiol 1976; 41(5):752–763.
6. Goldman MD, Mead J. Mechanical interaction between diaphragm and rib cage. J Appl Physiol 1973; 35(2):197–204.
7. Loring SH, Mead J. Action of the diaphragm on the rib cage inferred from a force-balance analysis. J Appl Physiol: Respirat Environ Exercise Physiol 1982; 53(3): 756–760.
8. Urmey WF, De Troyer A, Kelly KB, Loring SH. Pleural pressure increases during inspiration in the zone of apposition of diaphragm to rib cage. J Appl Physiol 1988; 65:2207–2212.
9. Macklem PT. A mathematical and graphical analysis of inspiratory muscle action. Respir Physiol 1979; 38:153–171.

10. Macklem PT, Macklem DM, De Troyer A. A model of inspiratory muscle mechanics. J Appl Physiol 1983; 55(2):547–557.
11. Ward ME, Ward JW, Macklem PT. Analysis of human chest wall motion using a two-compartment rib cage model. J Appl Physiol 1983; 72(4):1338–1347.
12. Hillman DR, Finucane KE. A model of the respiratory pump. J Appl Physiol 1987; 63(3):951–961.
13. Saumarez RC. An analysis of possible movements of human upper rib cage. J Appl Physiol 1986; 60:678–689.
14. Mead J, Smith JC, Loring SH. Volume displacements of the chest wall and their mechanical significance. In: Lenfant C, ed. The Thorax. New York: Marcel Dekker, 1995:565–586.
15. Loring SH. Structural model of thorax and abdomen for respiratory mechanics. Mathematical Modelling 1986; 7:1083–1098.
16. Loring SH, Woodbridge JA. Intercostal muscle action inferred from finite-element analysis. J Appl Physiol 1991; 70(6):2712–2718.
17. Loring SH. Action of human respiratory muscles inferred from finite element analysis of rib cage. J Appl Physiol 1992; 72(4):1461–1465.
18. Boriek AM, Wilson TA, Rodarte JR. Displacements and strains in the costal diaphragm of the dog. J Appl Physiol 1994; 76(1):223–229.
19. De Troyer A, Loring SH. Action of the respiratory muscles. In: Macklem PT, Mead J, eds. Handbook of Physiology. Bethesda, MD: American Physiological Society, 1986:443–462.
20. Hamberger GE. De respirationis mechanismo. Iena 1727.
21. Wilson TA, De Troyer A. Respiratory effect of the intercostal muscles in the dog. J Appl Physiol 1993; 75(6):2636–2645.
22. Duomarco JL, Rimini R. La presion intraabdominal en el hombre. El Ateneo, Buenos Aires, Argentina 1947.
23. Smith JC, Loring SH. Passive mechanical properties of the chest wall. In: Macklem PT, Mead J, eds. Handbook of Physiology. Bethesda, MD: American Physiological Society, 1986:429–442.
24. Loring SH, Yoshino K, Kimball WR, Barnas GM. Gravitational and shear-induced pressure gradients in the abdomen. J Appl Physiol 1994; 77(3):1375–1382.
25. Milic-Emili J, Henderson JAM, Dolovich MB, Trop D, Kaneko K. Regional distribution of inspired gas in the lung. J Appl Physiol 1966; 21(3):749–759.
26. Ganesan S, Rouch KE, Lai-Fook SJ. A finite element analysis of the effects of the abdomen on regional lung expansion. Respir Physiol 1995; 99:341–535.
27. Reid MB, Loring SH, Banzett RB, Mead J. Passive mechanics of upright human chest wall during immersion from hips to neck. J Appl Physiol 1986; 60:1561–1570.
28. Lai-Fook SJ, Rodarte JR. Pleural pressure distribution and its relationship to lung volume and interstitial pressure. J Appl Physiol 1991; 70(3):967–978.
29. Butler JP, Huang J, Loring SH, Lai-Fook SJ, Wang PM, Wilson TA. Model for a pump that drives circulation of pleural fluid. J Appl Physiol 1995; 78:23–29.
30. Decramer M, De Troyer A, Kelly S, Zocchi L, Macklem PT. Regional differences in abdominal pressure swings in dogs. J Appl Physiol 1984; 57(6):1682–1687.
31. Mead J, Yoshino K, Kikuchi G, Barnas GM, Loring SH. Abdominal pressures

transmission in humans during slow breathing maneuvers. J Appl Physiol 1990; 68(5):1850–1853.

32. De Troyer A, Loring SH. Actions of the respiratory muscles. In: Roussos C, Macklem PT, eds. The Thorax. 2nd ed. New York: Marcel Dekker, 1994:535–563.
33. Mead J, Takishima T, Leith D. Stress distribution in lungs: a model of pulmonary elasticity. J Appl Physiol 1970; 28(5):596–608.
34. Hajji MA, Wilson TA, Lai-Fook SJ. Improved measurements of shear modulus and pleural membrane tension of the lung. J Appl Physiol 1979; 47(1):175–181.
35. Cala SJ, Kenyon CM, Ferrigno G, et al. Chest wall and lung volume estimation by optical reflectance motion analysis. J Appl Physiol 1996; 81(6):2680–2689.
36. Mead J. Functional significance of the area of apposition of diaphragm to rib cage. Am Rev Respir Dis 1979; 119:31–32.
37. Mier A, Brophy C, Estenne M, Moxham J, Green M, De Troyer A. Action of abdominal muscles on rib cage in humans. J Appl Physiol 1985; 58(5):1438–1443.
38. Mead J, Milic-Emili J, Turner JM. Factors limiting depth of a maximal inspiration in human subjects. J Appl Physiol 1963; 18(2):295–296.
39. De Troyer A, Kelly S, Zin WA. Mechanical action of the intercostal muscles on the ribs. Science 1983; 220:87–88.
40. De Troyer A, Kelly S, Macklem PT, Zin WA. Mechanics of intercostal space and actions of external and internal intercostal muscles. J Clin Invest 1985; 75:850–857.
41. De Troyer A, Ninane V. Respiratory function of intercostal muscles in supine dog: an electromyographic study. J Appl Physiol 1986; 60(5):1692–1699.
42. De Troyer A, Farkas GA. Inspiratory function of the levator costae and external intercostal muscles in the dog. J Appl Physiol 1989; 67(6):2614–2621.
43. Wilson TA, De Troyer A. Effect of respiratory muscle tension on lung volume. J Appl Physiol 1992; 73:2283–2288.

7

Diaphragm Mechanics

ALADIN M. BORIEK and JOSEPH R. RODARTE

Baylor College of Medicine
Houston, Texas

I. Introduction

The diaphragm is a thin sheet composed of a central tendon and a fringe of costal and crural muscles that extends from the central tendon to the rib cage and spine. The diaphragm has a curved shape that is essential for converting muscle tension into transdiaphragmatic pressure (P_{di}) and muscle shortening into volume displacement. Of the two muscles that comprise the diaphragm, the costal muscle is comparatively thin, and its muscle fibers extend radially from the central tendon to insert on the rib cage. The crural muscle is thicker, has a more complex criss-cross fiber arrangement, and is located next to the spine. The entire diaphragm is attached peripherally around the complete boundary of the inferior thoracic aperture. At functional residual capacity (FRC), the dome of the diaphragm is primarily composed of the central tendon, and the muscular portion is directly apposed to the inner aspect of the lower rib cage constituting the zone of apposition (ZAP).

In the following sections, models of the mechanics of the diaphragm, certain complexities of diaphragm mechanics, and current works addressing those complexities are discussed. The section on model mechanics of the diaphragm discusses the classic model and piston analogy of the diaphragm, the Whitelaw model, and some of the biophysical complexities of diaphragm modeling. The discussion of complexities of diaphragm mechanics includes the unique mechanical properties of the diaphragm and structural issues such as composition and shape. Current works describe numerous approaches to dealing with these complexities, including measuring diaphragmatic curvature, displacement and shortening of the diaphragm, and issues relating to the diaphragm as a fiber-connective tissue composite of its skeletal muscle.

II. Model Mechanics

A. Classic Model and Piston Analogy of the Diaphragm

The diaphragm was conceptualized by Loring and Mead (1) as a cylinder with muscle fibers oriented axially and therefore having no curvature along their long axis in the zone of apposition. At the junction between the lung opposed region and the zone of apposition, pleural pressure changes abruptly from abdominal pressure to pressure in the lung opposed region. With diaphragm muscle contraction, the diaphragm moves axially with a constant curvature until the zone of apposition disappears. With further muscle shortening, the radius of the curvature increases. (See figure 1.)

Kim et al. (2) used direct measurements of P_{di} and tension in dogs to compute radius of curvature from the Laplace equation. They found that radius of curvature changes little or decreases at large lung volumes rather than increasing as theory would predict. They concluded that, because curvature changed very little, the action of the diaphragm resembles that of a piston. Paiva et al. (3) measured the three-dimensional shape of the supine human diaphragm

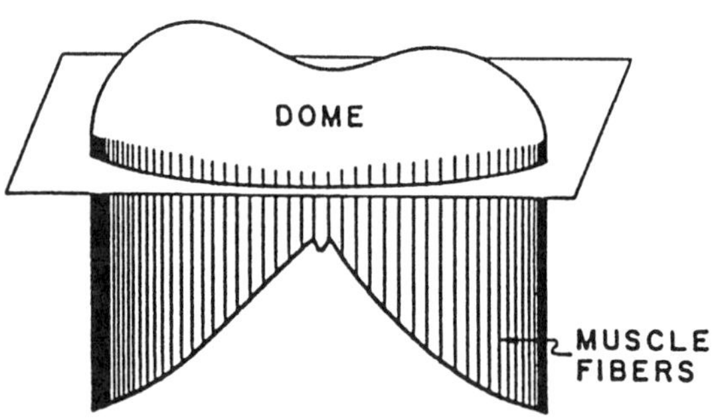

Figure 1 A schematic showing the classical model of the diaphragm. Muscle fibers are oriented along the axial direction of the cylinder. The model suggests that transdiaphragmatic pressure can be approximated by the total axial force exerted by the diaphragmatic fibers divided by the cross-sectional area of the thorax in the plane of the upper ring of the zone apposition (1).

in vivo using magnetic resonance imaging (MRI). They reasoned that lung and abdominal contents behave sufficiently like fluids so that they do not impose their shape on the diaphragm. Because the diaphragm is partly lung apposed, they concluded that it is unlikely that the diaphragm functions simply as a piston. More recent work by Gauthier et al. (4) suggested that the three-dimensional MRI data of the human diaphragm may be more accurately modeled by a "widening piston" than a simple "piston in a cylinder" model.

B. The Laplace Relation and the Whitelaw Model

For a general three-dimensional membrane, the generalized form of the Laplace equation is $\kappa_1\sigma_1 + \kappa_2\sigma_2 = \frac{P_{di}}{t}$, where P_{di} is the pressure difference across the membrane, σ_1 and σ_2 are the principal stresses in the membrane at any point *p* on the surface of the membrane, κ_1 and κ_2 are the curvatures of the membrane in the direction of principal stresses. Curvature of a membrane is, therefore, determined by P_{di}, stress, and thickness.

Whitelaw et al. (5) developed a model that presumed the diaphragm to be isotropic; that is, the material properties of the membrane were constant and independent of direction and tension was uniform, like that in a soap film. They computed the shape of a membrane with this uniform tension distribution, supported on a ring with the shape of the outline of a transverse section of the human thorax and loaded by the pressure distribution in the abdomen. The assumptions about the material properties and tension distribution may be inaccurate, but their results are nevertheless interesting. They showed that the shape of a soap film inflated from an elliptical ring that is indented across its minor axis by the spine is a double hump, like the shape of the human diaphragm.

C. Modeling Diaphragm Mechanics

When diaphragmatic muscle contracts, the diaphragm operates on the rib cage in three ways (1). First, descent of the diaphragm lowers pleural pressure (P_{pl}), which has an expiratory effect on that portion of the rib cage adjacent to the lung. Second, diaphragm contraction increases abdominal pressure (P_{ab}), which is transmitted through the apposed portion of the diaphragm to exert an inspiratory effect on the adjacent rib cage (6,7). The relative size of the lung-apposed portion of the rib cage, the ZAP of the diaphragm to the inner surface of the lower rib cage, changes with lung volume. Thus, the expiratory effect of the diaphragm increases with increasing lung volume. Third, the diaphragm has direct inspiratory actions through its chest wall insertions, elevating the rib cage (see Chapter 6).

An assumption made in investigating diaphragm mechanics is that the abdominal compartment is fluid-like, with a hydrostatic pressure gradient that is uniformly increased by diaphragm muscle contraction. If this were true and P_{pl} were uniform, then P_{di} could be adequately assessed by measuring esophageal and gastric pressures. In supine dogs, however, unless considerable volumes of fluid are instilled into the abdomen, pressure changes associated with diaphragm contraction are not uniform (8). Selective stimulation of the costal or crural diaphragm muscle causes larger pressure changes beneath the stimulated region. Furthermore, diaphragm contraction causes larger pressure changes in the cephalic than in the caudal abdomen, and the resulting pressure gradient can be sustained for a considerable time (9). Although such pressure differences are probably insignificant during measurements of maximal diaphragmatic pressure generation (10), they cannot be ignored during normal breathing.

In the classic model of the diaphragm, there is no curvature in the direction of the muscle fibers, and the model ignores curvature in the direction transverse to the muscle fibers. If the chest wall were a rigid cylinder and its radius of curvature matched the radius of diaphragm curvature, then as the diaphragm contracts and drives the lower rib cage outward, it would be constrained by the rigid cylinder of the chest wall. Therefore, $P_{di} = 0$ and $P_{pl} = P_{ab}$. This is consistent with Mead's hypothesis (11). This is also consistent with some (1,12), but not all (6), direct experimental measurements of pressures in the pleural space and in the ZAP. Urmey et al. (7) reported that changes in P_{di} in the ZAP were negligible even during large decreases in P_{pl}, providing direct experimental evidence that changes in P_{ab} is transmitted to the pleural space in the ZAP. In contrast, Macklem et al. (6) reported that P_{ab} is an important agent in displacing the lower rib cage, but during inspiratory muscle activity in the ZAP, P_{pl} may be somewhat different from P_{ab}.

Estimated measurement of P_{pl} gradients from regional lung volume distributions suggest there is a vertical gradient of P_{pl} over the dome of the diaphragm at FRC in the supine dog and little or none in the prone dog.

III. Complexities in Diaphragm Mechanics Theory

A. Anisotropic Membranes

The muscle fascicles of the diaphragm lie along curved lines, and the sheet of muscle together with the central tendon form a curved membrane. A membrane is a structure that is capable of carrying significant stresses in the plane of the membrane, but it is too thin to carry significant bending moments. Investigating diaphragm mechanics is difficult because the diaphragm has a nonlinear stress-strain law. Furthermore, the diaphragm is anisotropic; that is, the stress-strain relation along the fibers is different from that in the direction transverse to the fibers. The diaphragm has a heterogeneous structure, being composed of two different materials, the central tendon and the muscular portion.

A two-dimensional orthotropic material is defined as a material that exhibits different stiffnesses in two orthogonal directions. These two directions are along the muscle fibers and transverse to the fibers in the plane of the diaphragm. Gates et al. (13) developed a model that assumes that the diaphragm is an axisymmetrically shaped membrane of constant thickness, composed of muscle fibers that lie in the radial direction. This model suggested that the passive diaphragm in situ behaves as an orthotropic linearly elastic material for loads in the physiological range. Gates et al. arrived at the following estimates for the elastic moduli, along the fibers (E_{fiber}) and transverse to the fibers ($E_{\perp fiber}$): $E_{fiber} = 0.5 \times 10^6$ Newtons/m$^2 \pm 14\%$; $E_{\perp fiber} = 0.79 \times 10^6$ Newtons/m$^2 \pm 24\%$. This indicates a surprisingly low orthotropic ratio ($E_{\perp fiber}/E_{fiber} = 1.6$).

Boriek et al. (14) tested the hypothesis that orthotropic material properties might serve to limit the repertoire of shapes available to the diaphragm regardless of pressure distribution within the physiological range. They developed a finite element membrane model of the passive diaphragm with a hemispherical shape yet relaxed the hypothesis of homogeneous orthotropic elastic membrane used by Gates et al. Boriek et al. (14) examined the effects of an inextensible cap simulating the central tendon and orthotropic skirt (with stiffness in the direction transverse to the fibers that is greater than along the fibers) simulating the musculature of the diaphragm on the shape change of a hemispherical membrane model of the diaphragm subjected to uniform pressure loads or a hydrostatic pressure gradient. Their results demonstrated that the orthotropic muscle changed curvature less than a uniform homogeneous isotropic elastic material would when inflated. They concluded that changes of diaphragm shape are restricted because the central tendon is inextensible and the muscle is orthotropic. Although there is evidence that the diaphragm muscle is orthotropic (13,15) this seems unlikely to be a total explanation of the constancy of costal diaphragmatic shape, as discussed in Section II C.

B. Diaphragm Is Composed of Two Muscles

One complexity in understanding the mechanics of the diaphragm is that the diaphragm anatomically and functionally consists of two muscles, the costal and crural, which have different segmental and largely separate innervations (16). Relative activation of these muscles changes with posture and respiratory drive (17). If the costal and crural parts are in series, in the terminology of Macklem et al. (18), stimulation of one part would be mechanically in series: stimulation of one part of the diaphragm would stretch the other, quiescent, portion. Although this effect is seen, the stretch is less than produced by passively generated P_{di} equal to that produced when one muscle is stimulated. This observation was interpreted as meaning the costal and crural diaphragm muscles are partly in series and partly in parallel (18). The crural diaphragm muscle has no direct action on the rib cage, but merely causes descent of the dome and thus decreasing P_{pl} and increasing P_{ab}. The costal diaphragm has a similar action but also exerts direct traction on the lower ribs (19).

C. Diaphragm Shape

Another complexity is the shape of the diaphragm. The diaphragm is not an axial cylinder (20). The ring of diaphragm insertion on the chest wall is more caudal dorsally (about 30° in the dog). The left and right hemidiaphragms do not fit a single plane, but each hemidiaphragm is tilted caudally from the midline by about 10° (21). To the extent that the insertion of the diaphragm can be considered a plane, the magnitude and direction of the insertional force can be computed. The resultant force of pressure acting on a closed surface of any shape above a plane is equal to the product by the pressure and the projected area of the surface onto the plane. This force produced by P_{di} is balanced by tension of the diaphragm at its insertions on the chest wall. The mechanical advantage of the insertional force of the diaphragm is dependent on the angle between the force and the ribs. As noted above, there is a lateral component to this force, promoting a bucket handle effect. The pump handle effect would be maximal if the ribs were parallel to the ring of insertion (21).

The tilting of the ring of insertion from a transverse plane does not preclude the muscle fibers from being oriented in an axial direction with no curvature as assumed in the classic model. However, at least in the dog this is not the case; muscle fascicles in a small region of the midcostal diaphragm can be fit by a right cylinder, whose long axis is parallel to the line of insertion on the chest wall (20). Radiopaque markers were attached along three adjacent muscle bundles in the midcostal diaphragms of seven dogs. Anteriorposterior and lateral radiographic views are for a supine dog shown in Figure 2. The three dimensional positions of these markers were determined by biplane fluoroscopy. The curvature of the costal diaphragm was described by determining the best fit surface of the quadratic form $Z' = aX'^2 + bX'Y' + cY'^2$. This surface was determined so that the distance from the diaphragm to the best fit plane is a quadratic polynomial of these coordinates. Principal axes, X'' and Y'' were determined. In this description of the surface the X'' and Y'' axes lie in the directions of the principal curvatures, and the coefficients of the X'' and Y'' describe the magnitude of the two principal radii of curvature. The direction of muscle fascicles was essentially along the direction of maximum principal curvature, X'' direction, and there was essentially no curvature along Y'' (the chest wall insertion direction). Furthermore, muscle fibers lie in planes and the planes of the muscle fascicles lie perpendicular to the tangent plane of the surface. It follows that curvature of the muscle fascicles lie perpendicular to the tangent plane of the surface. It follows that the curvature of the muscle fascicles is orthogonal to the

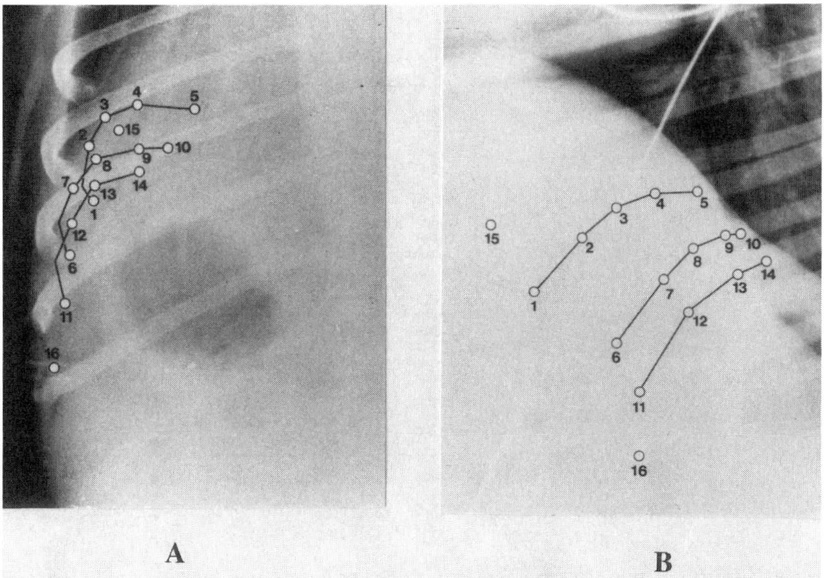

Figure 2 Radiographs of a supine dog, showing the locations of 16 metallic markers, 4–5 markers along each of the neighboring muscle fascicles, are shown at functional residual capacity with the head up. Markers 1, 11, 15, 16 were sutured along the insertion of the midcostal region of the diaphragm on the chest wall. Markers 5, 10, 14 were sutured at the origin of the three muscle fascicles on the central tendon. Markers along a muscle bundle are connected by a straight line. A, Anterioposterior view; lateral side is on left. B, Lateral view, ventral side is on right.

tangent plane of the surface at every point along the fascicle. The latter property is the defining property of geodesic (22). The properties of the muscle fascicles that Boriek et al. (20) observed in the midcostal region have functional significance. The direct contribution of muscle tension to transdiaphragmatic pressure is maximal if the muscle fascicle lies in the direction of maximal surface curvature and the direction of fascicle curvature is normal to the surface of the diaphragm (22).

The projection of the markers is plotted in Figure 3 in the coordinate system of principal curvatures. The three muscle fascicles are superimposed in this view, indicating that there is essentially no curvature in the direction orthogonal to the X″ and Z″. At all three higher lung volumes relative to end of expiration (EE), the muscle fascicles are shorter. In this projection, there is no obvious change in curvature along the muscle fascicles, whether the muscle shortens actively with an increase in muscle tension and P_{di} during spontaneous ventilation (SV) or shortens passively during mechanical ventilation (MV) with

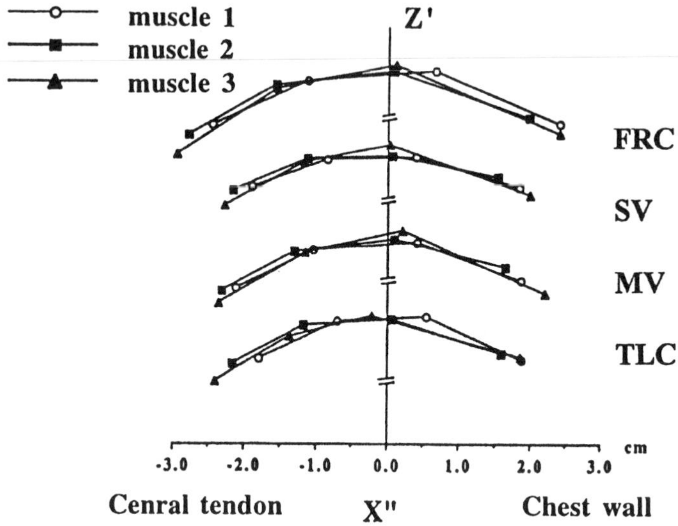

Figure 3 Examples of data on marker locations projected into the plane of maximum curvature, X″Z′ at different lung volumes are shown for a supine dog. Locations of 12 markers, 4 markers in each of the neighboring muscle bundles, are shown for each of 4 states: functional residual capacity (FRC), end of inspiration during spontaneous ventilation (SV), end of inspiration during mechanical ventilation (MV), and total lung capacity during passive inflation, the volume at an airway pressure of about 30 cm H_2O (TLC). Lines connect the markers along each muscle fascicle. The vertical axis is interrupted to allow comparisons of muscle curvature. The principal axes were determined for each condition, so rotation of the muscle fascicles around its chest wall insertion with increase in lung volume cannot be appreciated in this figure. Muscle fascicle curvature is similar at all lung volumes, with no consistent discontinuity of curvature demonstrated.

a decrease in both muscle tension and P_{di}. This figure illustrates that the muscle shortens more during SV than during MV with the same tidal volume. In this figure, principal axes were determined separately for each volume; however, the orientation of the line of insertion of the muscle on the chest wall, Y″, does not change with lung volume.

At FRC, the muscular portion of the costal diaphragm is virtually all apposed to the chest wall in the ZAP. At total lung capacity (TLC), the ZAP virtually disappears (21). There is no evidence of a discontinuity of curvature at the junction of the ZAP with the lung-apposed dome of the diaphragm. The rib cage surface appears quite straight in anterioposterior radiographs, and it is not readily apparent that at FRC the diaphragm can have a relatively uniform curvature along the muscle fascicle from origin on central tendon to insertion on chest wall. However the width of the rib cage increases with distance from the sternum in the dorsal direction. Muscle fascicles sweep laterally from their insertion on the chest wall and curve medially to insert on the central tendon. This is because the muscle fibers that run essentially in the direction perpendicular to the line of insertion on the rib cage course in a dorsal as well as cephalad direction.

D. Nonuniformity of Tension

Another degree of complexity is derived from the numerical results of a study (23) that suggested that tension in the diaphragm is nonuniform and that tension varies with location on the diaphragm surface and direction examined. As noted above, the assumption of uniform tension is compatible with the bilobed shape of the human diaphragm and the dorsal trough in the dog diaphragm.

Investigators have predicted tension in the diaphragm by using measurements of curvature from radiographic projections, providing assumptions about P_{di} gradient and making use of the Laplace law. For example, Smith and Loring (24) estimated tension of 5 and 40 g/cm in upright and supine postures, respectively. Whitelaw et al. (5) computed tension in upright humans of 10–20 g/cm. Paiva et al. predicted tensions (3) in the range of 32–54 g/cm in supine humans. There is some evidence that tension is not uniform with regard to orientation. Margulies et al. (23) used finite element analysis to compute tension from in vivo measurements of shape and P_{di} distribution of the lung apposed region of the passive diaphragm in the dog. The greatest in-plane tension was found to be essentially aligned with the direction of muscle fascicles and is two to four times larger than the tension in the direction transverse to the muscle fibers. In the central tendon of the canine diaphragm, collagen fibers have a random orientation near the midline, but, near the insertion of the muscle, collagen fibers are preferentially oriented parallel to the muscle fibers. If collagen fibers are oriented in the direction of greatest stress, this would imply that, in the muscular region of the diaphragm near the central tendon, there is greater stress along the muscle fibers than transverse to the fibers.

None of the studies discussed above considered tension in the ZAP. If the diaphragm were composed of axially oriented fibers and the thorax was cylindrical, with the same radius of curvature as a hemispherical dome, then tension in the membrane in the direction transverse to the muscle fibers would be twice the tension in the dome. Tension in the axial direction could not be defined by the Laplace equation, because there is no curvature in that direction. Furthermore, for P_{di} to be zero in the ZAP, the diaphragm would have to be constrained by the chest wall. In this situation, there could be no tension in the ZAP in the direction transverse to the muscle fibers.

As noted above, the anatomy of the dog is quite different from the classical model. Boriek et al. (20) demonstrated that there is no obvious discontinuity of curvature progressing from near the central tendon at FRC to near the chest wall at TLC, as one might expect if the edge of the ZAP moves from near the central tendon to near the chest wall. The mechanics responsible for this are not clear. It seems unlikely that there is a discontinuity of tension along the muscle fiber to match the discontinuity of pressure. Boriek et al. (14) hypothesized that the anisotropic material properties of the membranous structure of the diaphragm limit local shapes it can achieve so the diaphragm conforms to the shapes of rib cage and caudal lung. Their finite element membrane models (see Section III A.) were built to test this hypothesis. Their finding that anisotropic material properties dramatically limit the deformation of the pressurized membrane model of the diaphragm may help to explain the remarkable similarities of the shapes of the diaphragm at FRC, end inspiration, and TLC.

E. Uniaxial Versus Biaxial Load

The passive and maximally stimulated uniaxial length-tension curves of diaphragm muscle have been measured (2,25). The diaphragmatic muscle differs from other skeletal muscles in that the optimal length (L_0, at which maximum active tension occurs) is longer than the unloaded length, and active tension is maintained to shorter fractions of L_0. These data describe muscle properties under uniaxial loading.

Another complexity is that the diaphragm may be unique among skeletal muscles in that it is a single layer of muscle that supports stress in the in-plane direction transverse to the muscle fibers. Trunk skeletal muscle, such as intercostal and abdominal muscles, are in multiple muscle layers so that they can support a pressure without loading in the direction transverse to the muscle fibers, although stress has never been directly measured in these muscles. Even if stress in the diaphragm is greater parallel to the muscle fibers, there is clearly stress in the in-plane transverse direction to the fibers as well. It is likely that this transverse stress is supported by a connective tissue structure that might be different from other skeletal muscles.

Biaxial loading of the diaphragm may have important functional implications. The length-tension relationship of a homogeneous elastic material is much stiffer when subjected to a biaxial than to a uniaxial load along the muscle fibers. This is an additional complexity in relating the length-tension relationship measured in isolated diaphragm preparations relative to in vivo measurements. However, it is possible that at least the costal diaphragm is orthotropic so that length-tension relationships parallel to the muscle are independent of transverse forces in the plane of the diaphragm. In vitro measurements of passive length-tension relationships along and transverse to the costal diaphragm muscle indicate that the diaphragm is a nonlinear anisotropic material that is considerably stiffer in the direction transverse to the muscle fibers than along the fibers (26).

Limited data are available on the diaphragmatic muscle properties under biaxial loading (26). The relationship between stress in the transverse direction and the length-tension properties of the muscle in the direction of the fibers is unknown. It appears that, for the biaxial stresses that occur during mechanical ventilation and spontaneous breathing, the diaphragm is inextensible in the direction transverse to the muscle fibers direction (15). In hindsight, one might think that this property would have been anticipated by teleological reasoning. If the diaphragm were elastically extensible in the direction transverse to the muscle, then, as the muscle contracted and P_{di} and stress in the diaphragm increased, extension in the transverse fiber direction would reduce the volume displacement of the diaphragm and part of the work of muscle contraction would be expended on elastic extension in the direction transverse to the fibers.

IV. Current Works in Diaphragm Mechanics

A. Diaphragm Shape

The global shape can be computed by fitting the three-dimensional position of markers determined by a biplane videofluoroscopy to a surface using a two-dimensional spline technique (27). Contours that describe the shape of the diaphragm in a supine dog at FRC in both its passive state and during an inspiratory effort with an occluded airway at FRC, are shown in Figure 4. Lateral symmetry was assumed to generate symmetrical marker locations on the right hemidiaphragm. If the diaphragm shape were axisymmetric around the midplane of the dog, the contours would be circles with centers at the axis of symmetry. Each contour shown in Figure 4 is a constant cephalocaudal position on the surface. In each figure, the height difference between contours is 3.7 mm. With maximum inspiratory effort, marker number 2 on the ventral region of the central tendon is displaced by about 4 mm caudally whereas markers 1 and 3 on the ventral chest wall are displaced slightly caudally. The contours are straighter in the midcostal region than at the ventral and dorsal ends of the costal diaphragm, consistent with unequal principal curvatures in this region, as demonstrated previously in Figure 3. The peak of the diaphragm is closer to the ventral surface than to the dorsal surface, and there is a depression or valley in the crural region. There is a clear difference in the shape before and after inspiratory effort. After the inspiratory effort, the valley in the crural region is accentuated and the shape of the highest contour conforms generally to the shape of the central tendon.

B. Displacement and Shortening of the Diaphragm

1. Diaphragmatic Displacement

Muscle bundles of the midcostal diaphragm are shown in Fig. 5A in their plane of maximum curvature at FRC. The ζ axis in this figure is parallel to the midplane of the dog but tilted $\sim 25°$ dorsal from the axial direction. To the first

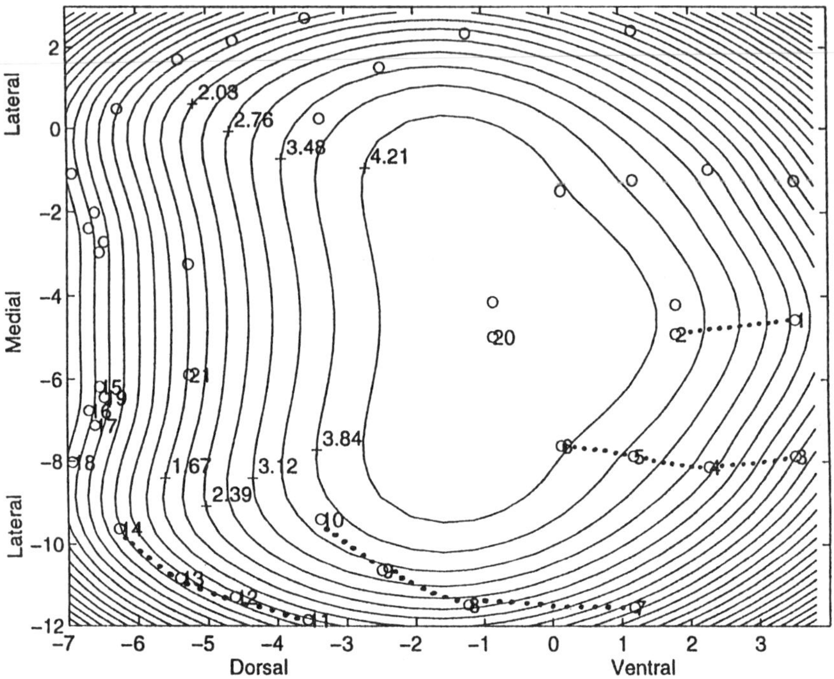

A

Figure 4 Contours that describe the shapes of the passive diaphragm, determined by a two-dimensional spline technique, are shown for a supine dog at FRC (**A**) and at end of inspiratory effort against an occluded airway at lung volume equal to FRC (**B**). Note the muscle fiber orientation (*dotted line*). Lateral symmetry was assumed to generate symmetric marker locations on the right hemidiaphragm. The isopleths are 0.37 cm apart. Note that the diaphragm has descended during inspiratory efforts. The most cephalad region of the lung-apposed surface conforms generally to the V-shape of the central tendon. The peak of the diaphragm is closer to the ventral surface than to the dorsal surface, and there is a depression or valley in the crural region. In the active state, at the end of a spontaneous inspiration, the valley in the crural region is accentuated. The depression in the crural region is more pronounced at end of inspiratory effort against an occluded airway. In the costal diaphragm, the curvature transverse to fiber direction is significantly smaller than along the fibers.

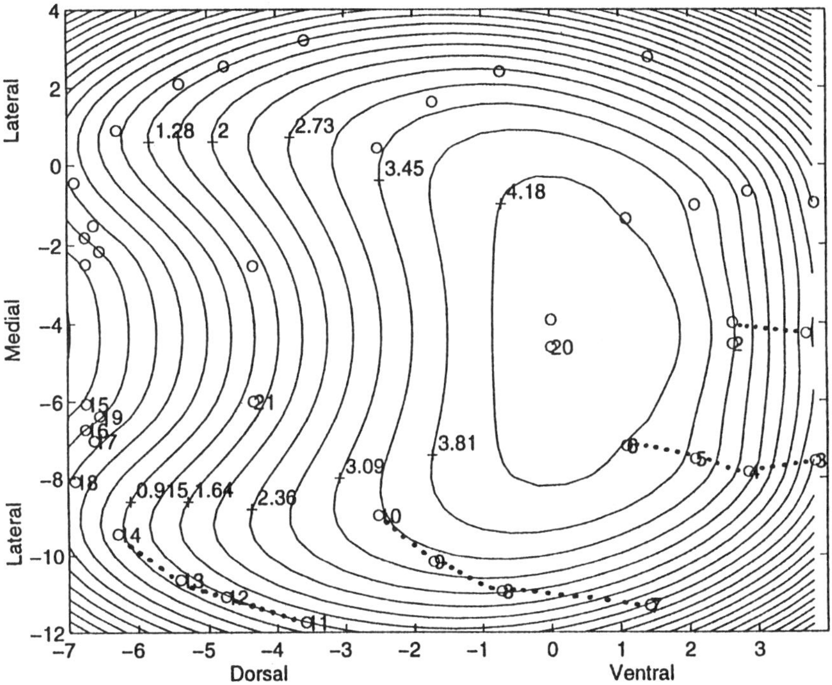

B

Figure 4 Continued

approximation the displacement of the diaphragm can be described by a simple model illustrated in Fig. 5B. In this figure markers at FRC and TLC are projected on the $\eta\zeta$. Markers at FRC are well fit by a circular arc. With inflation to TLC the markers are displaced in the plane and are still fit reasonably well by a shorter arc of a circle with the same radius. The displacements of the markers are approximately parallel and predominantly in the ζ direction. There is some lateral displacement of the chest wall that is consistent with the Loring and Mead model of inspiratory action of the diaphragm on the rib cage, but there is also a caudal displacement of the chest wall that is inconsistent with the Loring and Mead model of insertional action of the diaphragm on the rib cage (28). Because curvature changes very little with lung volume, the rotation of the muscular portion of the diaphragm in the $\eta\zeta$ plane should bring the markers inserting on the central tendon closer to the midline. However, muscle shortening is insufficient to prevent the motion of central tendon margins toward the midplane of the dog because the central tendon is extremely stiff (stresses of $\sim$50 kg/cm^2 produce <2% stretch of tendon) (29).

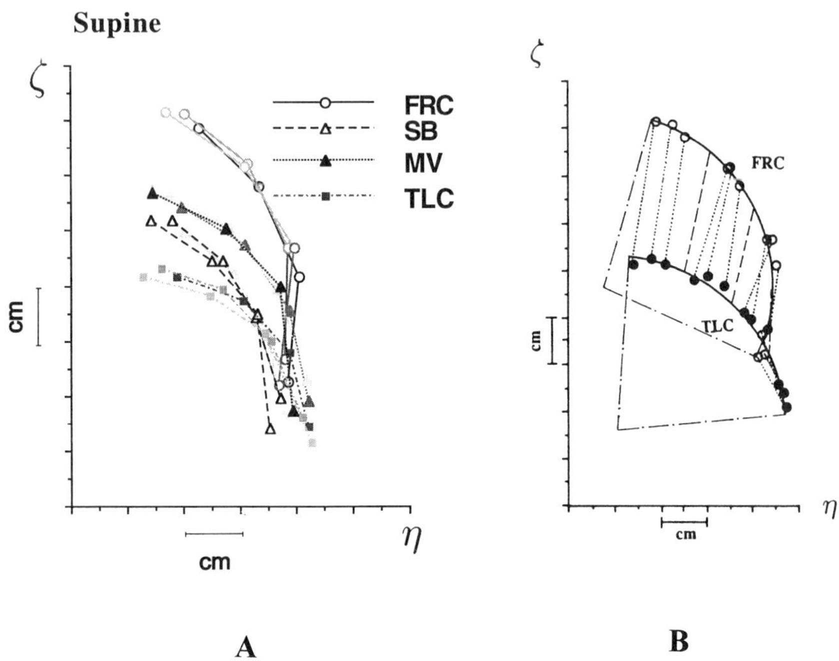

Figure 5 Example of data on marker locations projected onto $\eta - \zeta$ plane, a plane parallel to planes of muscle fascicles in a supine dog. Locations of 12 markers, 4 markers in each of 3 neighboring muscle fascicles of the midcostal region of the diaphragm, are shown for each of 4 states: functional residual capacity (FRC), end inspiration during spontaneous breathing (SB), mechanical ventilation (MV), and at total lung capacity (TLC). Lines connect the markers along each muscle fascicle. **B**. Marker locations at FRC and TLC. An arc of a circle fits data at FRC well. A shorter arc, with the same radius and with its center displaced, fits data at TLC well. Displacements of markers are shown by dotted lines.

In supine dogs, Hubmayr et al. (30) demonstrated a preferential motion of the gravitationally dependent portions of the diaphragm silhouette during SV compared with MV, which might result in a preferential ventilation of dependent lung regions, yet Sprung and associates (31) showed uniform fractional shortening. The differential displacement of the costal diaphragm, which comprises the silhouette, is due to the greater length of the dorsal muscle. The relative increase of displacement of the ventral region during MV is, however, a result of preferential shortening of the ventral costal diaphragm. In prone compared with supine dogs, motion of the diaphragm silhouette is more uniform in the prone position, but fractional shortening is not uniform, illustrating that fractional shortening is not directly coupled to regional displacement.

2. Muscle Shortening

A study of anesthetized supine dogs (32) found that muscle shortening during spontaneous breathing was 11% and 6% for the crural and costal diaphragm, respectively. These percent shortenings are a lot smaller than those shown in Figure 6. A study of chronic awake dogs (33) found that diaphragmatic tidal shortening is the same in these different portions in the right lateral decubitus standing and sitting postures during resting breathing.

The in situ force-generating capacity of the costal and crural portions of the diaphragm in anesthetized dogs was assessed, by relating in vitro contractile properties and diaphragmatic dimensions to in situ lengths (25). This study suggested that the costal diaphragm could exert 60% more tension than the crural diaphragm.

Using the marker techniques in supine dogs, Sprung et al. (30) investigated regional muscle shortening of the diaphragm from the change in length of rows extending from chest wall to central tendon relative to FRC during spontaneous and mechanical breathing. Their results showed considerable variability within and between regions of the costal diaphragm during spontaneous breathing. In contrast to studies by Newman et al. (31) and by Wakai et al. (34) using sonomicrometry, Sprung et al. (31) did not find any tendency for the crural diaphragm to shorten more than any region of the costal diaphragm.

Muscle shortening and dimensional changes in the direction transverse to the muscle fibers in the plane of the diaphragm were measured by Boriek et al. (15). They determined principal strains, that is, the strains in the orientation in which there are no shear strains. In general, principal strains with the largest

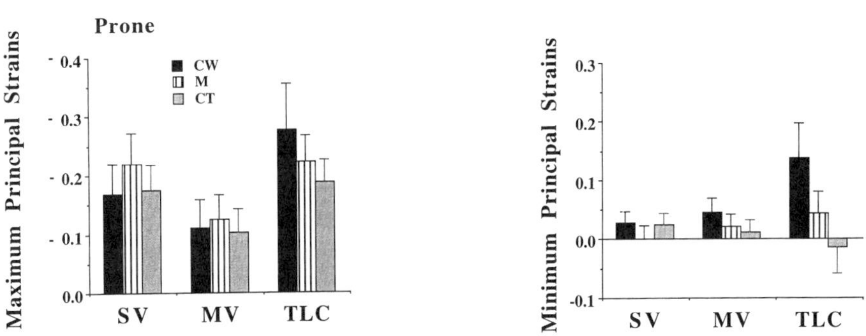

Figure 6 Principal strains E_1 (along the muscle fascicle), and E_2 (perpendicular to the muscle fascicle) in regions near the chest wall (CW), in the middle of the bundle (M), and near the central tendon (CT). Averages and standard deviation of values for all bundles in seven prone dogs are shown. At spontaneous breathing (SB), strain E_1 in the middle region is significantly different from strains near CW and CT. Strain E_2 is not significantly different from zero except near the CW at TLC.

magnitude were aligned with the direction of muscle fascicles. The data are shown in Figure 6. Muscle shortening was greater during spontaneous breathing than during MV at the same tidal volume, in agreement with the results of Sprung et al. (31). Although there was considerable variability between regions, there was no consistent difference along fascicles. Within each region, shortening was uniform along the muscle fascicles during MV. In contrast, during SV in the prone and supine positions, shortening was ~30% greater in the middle of the fascicle than near the central tendon and chest wall. This observation does not appear to be produced entirely by the connective tissue stroma because preferential length changes do not occur in the middle regions during passive shortening.

An interesting result was that the strain in the transverse direction to the costal diaphragmatic muscle fibers was very small and not statistically significantly different from zero during both passive and active inflation. If one excludes the unlikely possibility that transverse stress decreases with increasing P_{di}, the results would seem to indicate that the diaphragm behaves as an anisotropic structure; that is, its properties are dependent on position and orientation, as suggested in Section III D. Because the diaphragm is predominantly composed of parallel muscle fibers, it is not surprising that its passive material properties are anisotropic.

Skeletal muscle is incompressible and cannot change volume as it shortens. Therefore, to a first approximation, the sum of the three principal strains must be zero, and if the strain in the plane of the diaphragm transverse to the muscle fibers is negligible, as suggested in Ref. 15, this would imply that the diaphragm must thicken by about the same fraction as it shortens. Although muscle thickness could be within the resolution of ultrasound, published measures of diaphragm thickness in humans (35) report a mean increase of 2.3% in thickness per percent inspiratory capacity (IC) increase in lung volume. This value is approximately four times that predicted by Boriek et al. (15). The reason for this discrepancy is currently unknown.

C. Diaphragm as a Skeletal Muscle

1. Membrane Versus Three-Dimensional Composite Structure

It is important to differentiate the mechanics of the diaphragm as a membranous structure from the mechanical properties of the three-dimensional fiber–connective tissue composite structure of its skeletal muscle. As discussed in Section III A, the definition of a membrane in mechanics is a structure capable of carrying significant stresses in two dimensions but too thin to carry significant bending moments. When a region of muscle is activated, equilibrium length is determined by the active length-tension properties of the muscle, the load against which the muscle is working, and the degree to which the muscle is activated.

The equilibrium length of the muscle at different levels of activation determines the final shape of the diaphragm. However, the displacement of the diaphragm with changes in muscle activation is determined by the equilibrium shape of the entire membrane under the changed load and elastic properties. Margulies et al. (23) demonstrated the use of static equilibrium concept in membranes to compute the in vivo stress distribution in the diaphragm using data on its shape and a simple known transdiaphragmatic pressure distribution.

2. Effects of Muscle Lengths on P_{di}

The pressure-generating capability of the diaphragm diminishes at high lung volume and extreme muscle shortening. One possible mechanism of diaphragmatic failure as a pressure pump is that the muscle shortens to the point where it does not generate sufficient force. An alternative mechanism of diaphragmatic failure is that the diaphragm may flatten to the extent that muscle force is not transformed into pressure.

Two experimental studies have examined the relation between P_{di} and diaphragm muscle length during maximal activation by phrenic nerve stimulation (10,36). In the first study, Road et al. (10) enclosed the abdomen and lower rib cage in a rigid cast, opened the rib cage, and applied variable pressure to the abdomen through an opening in the cast. They regulated the length of the diaphragmatic muscle over the full range, from 120% to 50% of resting length. Their data demonstrated that the curve representing the P_{di} vs. muscle–length curve relationship was similar to that of muscle length–tension curve at maximum stimulation. They concluded that the shape of the diaphragm was effectively constant as the muscle shortened. This conclusion was consistent with the earlier conclusion of Kim et al. (2) who did not measure muscle length but measured both P_{di} and muscle tension versus lung volume. They found that the ratio of muscle tension to P_{di} (the effective radius of the diaphragm) was independent of lung volume. In the contrast, Hubmayr et al. (35) stimulated the phrenic nerve with the airway occluded at different lung volumes. At maximum stimulation, the muscle shortened to about the same length independent of occlusion volume, but P_{di} was much lower for occlusion at high than at low lung volume. Hubmayr et al. (36) concluded that the rate of change of P_{di} with muscle length was steeper than the rate of change of muscle tension with muscle length, and that shape change must have contributed to the decrease in P_{di} with increasing volume. In both of these studies, nonphysiological conditions were imposed. In the first, the lower rib cage was constrained; in the second, the diaphragm was activated while the intercostals were silent, and the chest wall was deformed by a paradoxical inward displacement of the upper rib cage, particularly at high P_{di}. More recently, Boriek et al. (37) reported data on the relations among muscle shape, muscle length, and lung volume at physiological states of inspiratory muscle activation in prone and supine anesthetized dogs. Their measurements include forceful inspiratory efforts at lung volumes from FRC to TLC. Their results were similar to the earlier study for quiet breathing and passive inflation (20) in that muscle fascicles of the midcostal diaphragm have the shape of circular arcs. The muscles shorten, and the arc of the muscles rotates around the line of insertion on the chest wall as the diaphragm descends, but curvature remains nearly constant. Boriek et al. (37) incorporated these observations into a kinematic model that describes muscle shortening with essentially constant curvature. From muscle curvature and values of muscle tension taken from maximal tension–length curve reported by Rochester and Farkas (25) Boriek and colleagues calculated P_{di} for maximal tension.

3. *Stress Versus Tension*

In muscle mechanics, "stress" and "tension" are often used interchangeably. When considering a membrane, tension is force per unit length and stress is tension divided by thickness. Margulies (38) reported differences in muscle thickness at different points around the circumference of the diaphragm surface. The nonuniformity of diaphragm thickness would indicate that stress in the muscle and tension in the diaphragm membrane cannot both be uniform in these different regions. In the dog, Boriek and Rodarte (39) reported essentially constant thickness along muscle fascicles of the costal diaphragm and a thickness gradient along the muscle fascicles in the crural diaphragm. If stress along a muscle is constant, then, in the crural diaphragm, tension would be nonuniform. In the costal diaphragm, the nearly constant thickness along the muscle fascicles is consistent with a nearly constant relationship between tension in the membrane and stress along the muscle fibers.

Morphometric data show the intramuscular fraction of connective tissue is relatively constant along the length of the costal of the diaphragm and that the covering membranes are a small proportion of the diaphragm thickness. The dorsal costal region of the diaphragm is significantly thinner than the rest of the costal diaphragm (36,37). Therefore, stress in the dorsal costal muscle relative to tension in that region of the diaphragm should be greater than in the middle and the ventral regions of the costal diaphragm. Furthermore, the crural diaphragm is thicker than the costal diaphragm (38,39). Therefore, by the same logic, stress in the crural muscle relative to tension should be less than in the costal region. Nevertheless, as the lung is deflated from TLC where the diaphragm should be under little or no passive stress, to FRC, where it should be under significant stress in both the supine and prone postures, there are no substantial differences in the extension of the dorsal costal or crural diaphragm regions.

In contrast to the crural diaphragm, each region of the costal diaphragm has essentially constant thickness along its muscle fascicles (39). This finding shows that a constant relationship between tension and stress is possible in the costal region. An essentially constant thickness along the course of the muscle in the costal region of the diaphragm and the likelihood of constant stress along muscle fibers suggest that there is a uniform tension in the membrane of the diaphragm in the direction of muscle fibers. In the crural diaphragm, however, the diaphragm muscle is thicker near the chest wall than near the central tendon. The crural muscle may have a stress gradient that accounts for details of diaphragmatic shape, causing the dip in the mediodorsal central tendon at lower P_{di}.

4. Muscle Fiber Architecture

An additional anatomical feature of the diaphragm may turn out to be more common in other skeletal muscles than is currently appreciated. Until recently, skeletal muscle fibers were considered to be organized in parallel, each with similar length running from origin to insertion. If muscle fibers were of different lengths, equal fractional shortening per sarcomere would produce different total shortening with the shorter muscle fascicles potentially becoming completely unloaded. A discontinuous fiber architecture is important to ensure synchronous contractions in a long muscle because myoelectrical transmission is slow, ~3 m/sec (41). Propagation of an electrical signal from the center to the ends of a 50-cm fiber should be complete within ~83 ms. Such a long delay would allow enough time for the central region near the neuromuscular junction (NMJ) to be relaxed from a single impulse before the contraction could reach the ends of the fiber. Thus, the active sarcomeres would have a huge series elastance of passive muscle and would be very ineffective at force generation (41). It has been shown that longer muscles in larger mammals are comprised of myofibers in series and that there are multiple bands of NMJ along the muscle (40).

Because the muscle in the dog and cat diaphragms is, for the most part, <6 cm in length, the efficiency advantage of serial insertion found in long skeletal muscle would not be present. However, multiple bands of NMJ were found across the diaphragmatic muscle of the dog (40) and the cat (42). Recent evidence in both species (40,42) shows that the majority of muscle fibers are nonspanning. The teleological advantage of this property is based on geometry. If the diaphragm were a flat two-dimensional membrane modeled as concentric circles, with an inner circle representing the central tendon, then the perimeter of the origin and insertion would vary inversely to the radius. If the ring were under tension, then the force applied to the origin and insertion would be equal, but the tension or force per unit length would be inversely proportional to the circumference and thus to the radius. For stress in the material to be constant, thickness would also have to increase as $\frac{1}{r}$ to balance the gradient of tension.

If, on the other hand, the diaphragm is modeled as a section of a sphere with one insertion at the equator and another half way to the pole, then even though the two perimeters are unequal, if loaded by a constant pressure, tension would be uniform because of the force supported by the curvature of the membrane. In this hypothetical model, tension would be uniform and, for stress to be uniform, thickness should be constant.

The diaphragm is not a hemisphere and the central tendon has a peculiar shape. However, the ratio of the length of the line of origin on the central tendon and the length of the line of insertion on the rib cage is ~0.62 for the costal diaphragm and ~1.2 for the crural (39). If the costal diaphragm were composed of cylindrical muscle fibers that span from origin to insertion, muscle near the central tendon region should be significantly thicker than near the chest wall. However, the thickness is essentially constant along the muscle fascicle, suggesting that muscle fibers are either conical or nonspanning (39). Single muscle fiber architecture analysis supports the latter (40). Nonspanning fibers tend to have a blunt myotendinous junction near their attachments on either the chest wall or central tendon and to have long tapered ends within the middle regions of the muscle. This fiber architecture raises interesting and unsolved questions about how stress from the contractile proteins within the muscle fiber is transmitted to the surrounding connective tissue matrix at the origin and insertion.

5. Micromechanical Inferences

Recent findings (15,26) have shown that the diaphragm under biaxial loading behaves as an anisotropic structure that has greater stiffness in the direction transverse to the muscle fibers than along the fibers, as discussed in Section III E. This observation raises the possibility that there are special structural components that are responsible for transverse inextensibility. One possibility was investigated recently by Boriek and Tidball (43), that desmin may be responsible for limiting diaphragmatic muscle strain transverse to the long axis of the myofibers. They investigated the concentration of desmin in the diaphragm and hindlimb muscles. Desmin is a transverse structural component of skeletal muscle and serves to link passive components of the myofibers to the lateral surface of muscle fibers. Desmin also links adjacent myofibrils at their Z disks into a single integrated mechanical unit. Therefore, Boriek and Tidball (43) tested the hypothesis that diaphragm muscle contains greater concentrations of desmin than hindlimb muscle by immunoblotting of muscle homogenates with antidesmin. They found that desmin concentrations are significantly higher in diaphragm than in limb musculature when values are normalized to total protein concentration or to myosin heavy chain concentration. Consequently, they concluded that desmin may be an important determinant in limiting the strain in the transverse direction to the myofibers in the diaphragm.

V. Summary

This chapter has reviewed the classic model of diaphragm mechanics and some of the biophysical complexities involved in modeling of the diaphragm, as well as a selection of the current works on diaphragm mechanics that address some of those complexities. We conclude by stressing the fact that understanding the mechanics of the diaphragm requires the realization that it is important to distinguish between the peculiar properties of the diaphragm as a unique skeletal muscle that comprises muscle fibers and connective tissue and the behavior of the diaphragm as a pressurized anisotropic membranous heterogeneous structure with a complex shape. Much recent information alters traditional thinking about the mechanics of the diaphragm. Many reliable observations seem mutually exclusive or at least difficult to reconcile with our current state of knowledge. A deeper understanding of diaphragm mechanics requires investigation of the force transmission between diaphragmatic muscle fibers and connective tissue. This will require concerted research efforts combining morphological and physiological observations of the diaphragmatic muscle. The applications of the theory of membrane mechanics and composite theory to questions of physiological interest are still in their infancy. We believe that there is indeed an exciting potential to deepen the understanding of the physiology of the diaphragmatic muscle through a rigorous mechanical and micromechanical analysis.

Acknowledgments

The authors thank Dr. Theodore Wilson for discussions of the chapter. This work was supported by the National Heart, Lung, Blood Institute Grants HL-54198 and HL-46230.

References

1. Loring SH, Mead J. Action of the diaphragm on the cage inferred from a force-balance analysis. J Appl Physiol 1982; 53:756–760.
2. Kim JA, Walter SD, Danon J, Machnach W, Sharp JT. Mechanics of the canine diaphragm. J Appl Physiol 1992; 41:369–382.
3. Paiva M, Verbanck S, Estenne M, Poncelet B, Segebarth C, Macklem PT. Mechanical implications of in vivo human diaphragm shape. J Appl Physiol 1992; 72:1407–1412.
4. Gauthier AP, Verbanck S, Estenne M, Segebarth C, Macklem PT. Three-dimensional reconstruction of the in vivo human diaphragm shape at different lung volumes. J Appl Physiol 1994; 76:495–506.
5. Whitelaw WA, Leevers AM, Road JD. Relationship among pressure, tension, and shape of the diaphragm. J Appl Physiol 1983; 55(6):1899–1905.

6. Macklem PT, Zocchi L, Agostoni. Pleural pressure between diaphragm and rib cage during inspiratory muscle activity. J Appl Physiol 1988; 65:1286–1295.
7. Urmey WF, DeTroyer A, Kelly KB, Loring SH. Pleural pressure increases during inspiration in the zone of apposition of diaphragm to rib cage. J Appl Physiol 1988; 65:2207–2212.
8. Luciano Z, Darzanity N, Newman S, Macklelm PT. Effect of hyperinflation and equalization of abdominal pressure on diaphragmatic action. J Appl Physiol 1987; 62:1655–1664.
9. Decramer M, DeTroyer A, Kelly S, Zocchi R, Macklem PT. Regional difference in abdominal pressure swings in dogs. J Appl Physiol 1984; 57:1682–1687.
10. Road J, Newman S, Derenne JP, Grassino A. In vivo length-force relationship of canine diaphragm. J Appl Physiol 1986; 60:63–70.
11. Mead J. Functional significance of the area of apposition of diaphragm to rib cage. Am Rev Respir Dis 1979; 119:31–32.
12. Loring SH, DeTroyer A. Actions of the respiratory muscles. The Thorax 1985; 29: 327–334.
13. Gates F, McCammond D, Zingg W, Dunov H. In vivo stiffness properties of the canine diaphragm muscle. Med Biol Eng Comput 1980; 18:625–632.
14. Boriek AM, Rodarte JR. Effects of transverse inextensibility and central tendon on displacement and shape of a simple diaphragm model. J Appl Physiol 1997; 82: 1626–1636.
15. Boriek AM, Wilson TA, Rodarte JR. Displacement and strains in the costal diaphragm of the dog. J Appl Physiol 1994; 76:223–229.
16. De Troyer A, Sampson AM, Sigrist S, Macklem PT. The diaphragm: two muscles. Science 1981; 213:238–239.
17. VanLunlern E, Haxhiu MA, Cherniack NS, Goldman D. Differential costal and crural diaphragm compensation for posture changes. J Appl Physiol 1985; 58:1895–1900.
18. Macklem PT, Macklem DM, DeTroyer A. A model of inspiratory muscle mechanics. J Appl Physiol 1983; 55:547–557.
19. DeTroyer A, Sampson M, Sirgist S, Macklem PT. Action of costal and crural parts of the diaphragm on the rib cage in dog. J App Phys Respirat Enviro Exercise Physiol 1984; 57:1682–1687.
20. Boriek AM, Liu S, Rodarte JR. Costal diaphragm curvature in the dog. J Appl Physiol 1993; 75:527–533.
21. Boriek AM, Rodarte JR, Margulies SS. Zone of apposition in the passive diaphragm of the dog. J Appl Physiol 1996; 81:1929–1940.
22. Angelillo M, Boriek AM, Rodarte JR, Wilson TA. Theory of diaphragm structure and shape. J Appl Physiol 1997; 83(5):1486–1491.
23. Margulies SS, Lei GT, Farkas GA, Rodarte JR. Finite element analysis of stress in the canine diaphragm. J Appl Physiol 1984; 76:2070–2075.
24. Smith JC, Loring SH. Passive mechanical properties of the chest wall. In: Handbook of Physiology. The Respiratory System: Mechanics of Breathing. Vol. 3, Bethesda, MD: American Physiological Society, 1986:429–442.
25. Rochester DF, Farkas GA. Functional characteristics of canine costal and crural diaphragm. J Appl Physiol 1988; 65:2253–2260.

26. Strumpf RK, Humphery JD, Yin FC. Biaxial mechanical properties of passive and tetanized canine diaphragm. Am J Physiol 1993; 265:H469–H475.
27. Swandell DT. Biharmonic spline interpolation. GEOS-3 Geograph Res Letters 1987; 14:139–142.
28. Wilson TA, Boriek AM, Rodarte JR. Mechanical advantage of the canine diaphragm. J Appl Physiol 1998; In Press.
29. Stromberg DD, Wiederhielm CA. Viscoelastic description of a collagenous tissue in simple elongation. J Appl Physiol 1969; 26:857–862.
30. Hubmayr RD, Rodarte JR, Walters BJ, Tonelli FM. Regional ventilation during spontaneous breathing and mechanical ventilation in anesthetized dogs. J Appl Physiol 1987; 63:2467–2475.
31. Sprung J, Deschamps C, Hubmayr RD, Walters BJ, Rodarte JR. In vivo regional diaphragm function in dogs. J Appl Physiol 1989; 67:655–662.
32. Newman SL, Road JD, Grassion A. In vivo length and shortening of canine diaphragm with body postural change. J Appl Physiol 1986; 60:661–669.
33. Fitting JW, Easton PA, Arnoux R, Guerraty A, Grassino A. Diaphragm length adjustment with body position changes in the awake dog. J Appl Physiol 1989; 66: 870–875.
34. Wakai Y, Leevers AM, Road JD. Regional diaphragm shortening measured by sonomicrometer. J Appl Physiol 1994; 77:2791–2796.
35. Wait JL, Nahormek PA, Yost WT, Rochester DF. Diaphragmatic thickness–lung volume relationship in vivo. J Appl Physiol 1989; 67:1560–1568.
36. Hubmayr RD, Sprung J, Nelson S. Determinants of transdiaphragmatic pressure in dogs. J Appl Physiol 1990; 41:2050–2260.
37. Boriek AM, Rodarte JR, Wilson TA. Kinematics and mechanics of midcostal diaphragm of dog. J Appl Physiol 1997; 83(4):1068–1075.
38. Margulies SS. Regional variation in canine diaphragm thickness. J Appl Physiol 1991; 70:2663–2668.
39. Boriek AM, Rodarte JR. Inferences on passive diaphragm mechanics from gross anatomy. J Appl Physiol 1994; 77:2065–2070.
40. Boriek AM, Miller C, Rodarte JR. Fiber architecture in the diaphragmatic muscle of dog. J Appl Physiol 1998; 84(1):318–326.
41. Loeb GE, Pratt CA, Chanaud CM, Richmond FJR. Distribution and innervation of short interdigitated muscle fibers in parallel-fiber muscle of the cat hind limb. J Morphology 1987; 191:1–15.
42. Gordon DC, Hammond CGM, Fisher JT, Richmond FJR. Muscle–fiber architecture, innervation and histochemistry in the diaphragm of the cat. J Morphology 1989; 201:131–143.
43. Boriek AM, Tidball JG. Desmin may contribute to the transverse in extensibility of the costal diaphragm in the dog. Am J Resp Crit Care Med 1995; 151(4):A585.

Part Two

AIRWAY EXCHANGE OF GAS

8

Inert Gas Exchange in the Airways

STEVEN C. GEORGE

University of California, Irvine
Irvine, California

JENNIFER E. SOUDERS and MICHAEL P. HLASTALA

University of Washington School of Medicine
Seattle, Washington

I. Introduction

The primary function of the lungs is to exchange the respiratory gases, O_2 and CO_2, between the atmosphere and the blood. However, any gas that is transported to the lung, either in the inspired air or in the blood, will exchange or interact. The overall understanding of the lungs as a gas exchanging organ has improved considerably over the past 4 decades. The dynamics of gas exchange depend strongly on the blood-gas partition coefficient (λ_b), an index of solubility. As λ_b increases, the interaction or exchange of the gas with the airways increases and the functional dead space of the lung decreases. For example, water ($\lambda_b \sim 20{,}000$ at 37°C) exchanges entirely within the airway tree as inspired air becomes fully humidified or saturated with water before entering the alveolar region. The fact that soluble gases exchange within the airways impacts several important clinical, social, and environmental areas including 1. basic understanding and treatment of airway diseases, 2. the clinical effect of inhaled environmental pollutant gases (e.g., sulfur dioxide, ketones, halogenated hydrocarbons, and aromatics), 3. alcohol breath testing and the validity of correlating blood alcohol concentration to breath alcohol concentration, and 4. monitoring of anesthetic gases and depth of anesthesia.

There are many disease processes that affect the airways including asthma, bronchitis, and bronchiectasis. Each disease has its own unique features that affect the anatomical and physiological function of the airways. For example, chronic bronchitis is associated with increased mucus production. The mucous lining of the airways is the first anatomical barrier that inhaled gases encounter; thus, one can presume that bronchitis would influence gas exchange dynamics. The most prevalent disease of the airways is asthma. The pathophysiology of asthma is complex and only partially understood. The common denominator in all cases is a hypersensitivity of the bronchial smooth muscle leading to smooth muscle contraction. This complex response of the bronchial smooth muscle is related to many factors, including the presence of inflammatory mediators, the permeability characteristics of the mucous and tissue layers, and the exchange of heat and water between the airstream and the tissue (1). The mediators responsible for acute asthma (i.e., histamine, bradykinins, leukotrienes, and prostaglandins) must diffuse from where they are released (mucosa and submucosa) to the bronchial smooth muscle. In addition, a primary therapy for acute asthma is inhaled adrenergic stimulants and glucocorticoids, which must diffuse through the mucous and tissue layers to exert the desired physiological effect. Chronic asthma is characterized by excessive mucus production, epithelial cell loss, and thickening of the basement membrane. Each of these changes may alter the diffusing properties of the tissues. This, in turn, may impact the therapeutic choice and efficacy, as well as the susceptibility to inhaled pollutants (e.g., sulfur dioxide and ozone), allergens, and exercise-induced bronchoconstriction.

Awareness of, and exposure to, pollutant and irritant gases is increasing. The inhalation of these gases can result in acute effects such as asthma or pneumonitis, as well as chronic effects such as chronic bronchitis and pulmonary fibrosis. The list of gases to which substantial segments of the population are exposed is extensive. Table 1 (2–11) includes a sampling of these gases including the blood and water solubilities at 37°C and their source or use. Absorption of these gases is primarily through the respiratory tract, and, depending on the blood solubility, absorption in the airways is likely to be substantial.

Ethanol is a highly soluble gas ($\lambda_b = 1756$ at 37°C). Recent theoretical predictions suggest that ethanol exchanges entirely within the airways (12). Alcohol breath testing has long been the standard in the field of toxicology as a means of assessing blood alcohol concentration. An implicit assumption in this method is that ethanol either does not exchange with the airways during exhalation, or that the exchange process is homogeneous within the general population. Evidence is mounting that neither assumption is valid. In fact, pretest breathing conditions, exhalation flow rate, and exhaled volume can alter breath alcohol concentration by as much as 20% (13–16). These effects can all be attributed to the substantial and complex interaction of ethanol with airways.

Table 1 Blood : Air (λ_b) and Water : Air (λ_w) Partition Coefficients of Gases at 37°C

Gas	λ_b	λ_w	Use/source	Reference
SF_6	0.009	0.001	Gas exchange physiology	Swenson et al. (2)
Nitric oxide	—	0.042	Endogenous gas	Swenson et al. (2)
Ethane	0.11	—	Gas exchange physiology	
Cyclopropane	0.6	0.24	Gas exchange physiology	Lowe and Hagler (3)
Halothane	3.0	0.86	Anesthetic	Lowe and Hagler (3)
Benzene	7.8	2.8	Solvent	Sato and Nakajima (4)
Trichloroethylene	9	—	Solvent	Sherwood (5)
Chloroform	10.3	3.8	Solvent	Larson (6)
Diethyl ether	13	12	Anesthetic	Steward et al. (7)
Toluene	15.6	2.2	Solvent	Sato and Nakajima (4)
O-xylene	31.1	2.6	Solvent	Sato and Nakajima (4)
Styrene	51.9	4.7	Solvent	Sato and Nakajima (4)
Sulfur dioxide	—	63	Combustion of fossil fuels	Perry and Green (8)
2-Hexanone	127	111	Solvent	Sato and Nakajima (4)
2-Butanone	202	254	Solvent	Sato and Nakajima (4)
Acetone	245	395	Solvent	Sato and Nakajima (4)
Ammonia	—	839	Refrigeration	Perry and Green (8)
Butanol	1,200	—	Solvent	Åstrand et al. (9)
Ethanol	1,756	2,134	Recreation, solvent	Jones (10)
2-Ethoxyethanol	22,093	23,069	Solvent	Johanson and Dynesius (11)

Finally, airway gas exchange impacts the field of anesthesiology. Analysis of inspired and expired anesthetic gases from anesthetic breathing circuits is frequently used during surgical procedures. The end-tidal levels of anesthetic gases are used to estimate depth of anesthesia and to confirm appropriate levels of anesthetic gas delivery. Many inhalational anesthetics are gases of low to intermediate solubility, which are delivered under varying conditions of inspired gas temperature, humidity, patient cardiac output and ventilatory pattern. Alterations in the end-tidal values of anesthetic agents could have implications regarding the accuracy of the instruments and thus for the quality of patient care.

The dynamics of airway gas exchange are inherently different from alveolar exchange, and current understanding of airway exchange is crude. In the airways, gas phase transport is dominated by convection and turbulent mixing, whereas diffusion is the dominant mode of transport in the alveoli. The tissue phase diffusion barrier in the airways is approximately two orders of magnitude larger and is comprised of at least 10 different cell types assembled in a very structured manner. Finally, the blood supply has a different source (systemic in nature), purpose, and structure. The goal of this chapter is twofold: 1. to outline the basic physical principles and mechanisms that govern airway gas exchange and contrast them with those of alveolar exchange, and 2. to review past experimental and theoretical work that has attempted to characterize airway gas exchange dynamics to date. In each section, emphasis is placed on gaps in current understanding of this very complex and heterogeneous phenomenon.

II. Physical Principles of Airway Gas Exchange

A. Theoretical Analysis

Exchange of an inert gas in the airways depends on physical phenomena that include the coupling of heat and mass transport, condensation, evaporation, solubility, convection, and diffusion. This section outlines these processes in the airway lumen (gas phase), mucosa (mucus and tissue), and bronchial capillary bed using a mathematical treatment. This type of approach allows one to define more easily the physical parameters that influence airway gas exchange and allows one to estimate easily their relative magnitude or importance.

Figure 1 represents a histological section of an airway in cross section with important anatomical landmarks noted. An inert gas of interest can exchange in the airways if it is either delivered in the airstream (airway lumen) or in the blood (bronchial capillary). In the lung, the important physical forces that govern the transport of a molecule include pressure gradients (convective flow), concentration gradients (diffusive flow), and intermolecular forces (which govern solubility and evaporative characteristics). The relative magnitude of each force dictates the movement. Consider the case in which the gas is delivered in the blood. During normal tidal breathing, an inert gas molecule is initially delivered to the airways by convection in the blood phase. The molecule can diffuse by random molecular motion (Brownian motion) or by turbulent mixing to another location within the capillary space, or it may dissolve in and diffuse through the surrounding tissue. Once the molecule reaches the mucus–air interface, it may evaporate and become a gas. Evaporation involves a phase change and energy transfer associated with the heat of evaporation. If evaporation occurs, the molecule may enter the airway lumen and then diffuse radially or axially, or be transported by convection to a new location within the airway. This scenario demonstrates, in a qualitative fashion, the interplay among convection, diffusion, and solubility. The forces depend strongly on time and position (axial and radial) within the airways. One approach to understanding airway gas exchange is to describe the dynamics using a mathematical treatment.

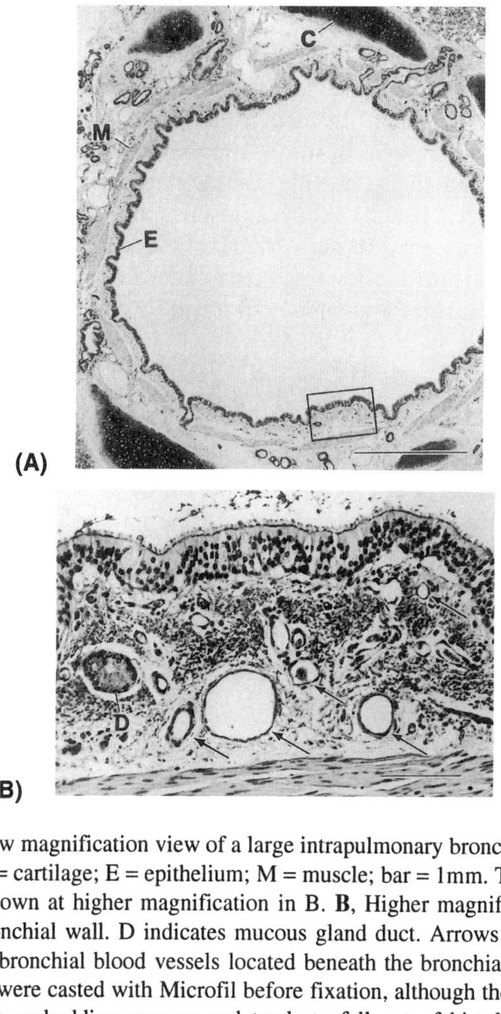

Figure 1 A, Low magnification view of a large intrapulmonary bronchus from a sheep. *Abbreviations*: C = cartilage; E = epithelium; M = muscle; bar = 1mm. The enclosed rectangular area is shown at higher magnification in B. **B**, Higher magnification view of a portion of the bronchial wall. D indicates mucous gland duct. Arrows point to some of the various sized bronchial blood vessels located beneath the bronchial epithelium. The bronchial vessels were casted with Microfil before fixation, although the casting material shrinks during the embedding process and tends to fall out of histological specimens during sectioning. Nevertheless, Microfil keeps the vessels expanded during fixation and facilitates the histological identification of blood vessels. Bar = 100 μm. (Courtesy of Daniel L. Luchtel, Ph.D.)

To provide a more quantitative approach, the histological section in Figure 1 must be simplified. Figure 2 represents a lumped or compartmental structure of the airways. The airway is divided axially into a series of control volumes, each of which has a length Δz, and radially into four compartments: 1. the airway lumen, 2. a thin layer of mucus, 3. a nonperfused tissue layer, and 4. a capillary bed. For simplicity, assume that the transport of mass is in the steady state. A detailed mathematical treatment of this model has been previously published (17). Briefly, sequential mass balances on each radial compartment result in the following expression for the steady-state flux of gas ($mL \cdot s^{-1}$) from the blood into the airstream for an airway of length L:

$$J = \frac{\dot{V}\beta_g}{A}\bar{P}_E(L) = \frac{\dot{V}\beta_g}{A}P_a\left[1 - \exp\left(-\left(\frac{\dot{V}\beta_g}{\dot{Q}\beta_b} + \frac{\dot{V}\beta_g}{D}\right)^{-1}\right)\right] \tag{1}$$

where A is the surface area (cm^2), β_x is solubility (mL gas·mL medium $^{-1}$·atm) in the gas phase (x = g) or blood phase (x = b), $\dot{Q}$ is the blood flow rate to the entire airway ($mL \cdot s^{-1}$), $\dot{V}$ is the airstream flow rate ($mL \cdot s^{-1}$), P_a is the partial pressure of the gas in arterial blood, $\bar{P}_E$ is the average partial pressure of gas exhaled from the airway at x = L, and D is the diffusing capacity of the gas in the airway (mL gas·s^{-1}·atm^{-1}). D is a combination of the diffusion-related resistances associated with the tissue, mucus, and mucus–air interface:

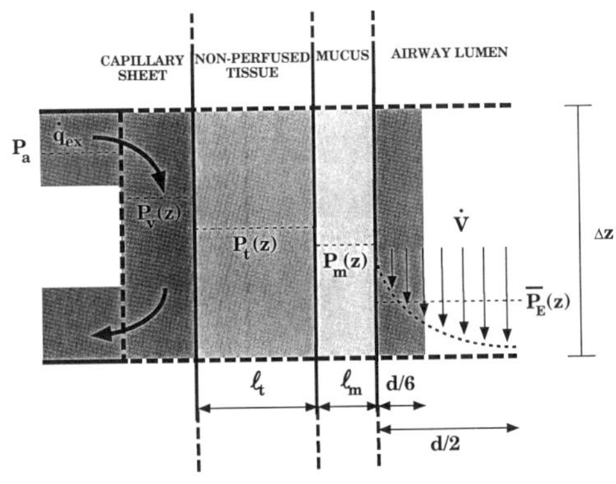

Figure 2 Sagittal section through a single control volume of the model. The horizontal dashed lines within each radial layer represent the steady-state partial pressures of an inert gas. Partial pressures within each layer are considered uniform. See text for notation. Pressure is highest in the arterial blood, then decreases relative to the resistance within subsequent layers. Airstream flow is considered laminar (*curved dashed line*). The shaded area in the lumen represents the effective gas-phase resistance resulting from molecular diffusion. The effective thickness of this gas-phase resistance is d/6 as described in the text. (From Ref. 17.)

$$D = \frac{A}{\left(\frac{\ell_t}{\mathcal{D}_t\beta_t} + \frac{\ell_m}{\mathcal{D}_m\beta_m} + \frac{1}{k\beta_g}\right)} \tag{2}$$

where $\mathcal{D}_x$ is the molecular diffusion coefficient ($cm^2 \cdot s^{-1}$) in the tissue ($x = t$) or mucus ($x = m$), ℓ_x is the thickness of the medium (cm), and k is the local mass transfer coefficient ($cm \cdot s^{-1}$), which describes empirically the rate of radial transfer at the mucus–air interface.

If the driving force for gas exchange is chosen to be the difference between the incoming arterial partial pressure and the incoming airstream partial pressure, then from Equation 1, the total resistance to tracheal gas exchange, R_{tot} ($s \cdot atm \cdot cm^2 \cdot mL\ gas^{-1}$), is given by the following expression:

$$R_{tot} = \left[\frac{\dot{V}\,\beta_g}{A}\left\{1 - \exp\left(-\left(\frac{\dot{V}\,\beta_g}{\dot{Q}\,\beta_b} + \frac{\dot{V}\,\beta_g}{D}\right)^{-1}\right)\right\}\right]^{-1}. \tag{3}$$

If $D \rightarrow \infty$ and $\dot{V} \rightarrow \infty$ in the expression for R_{tot}, then the only resistance that remains is due to the delivery rate of the gas in the blood (i.e., perfusion resistance). The perfusion-resistance, R_P, is then given by the following expression:

$$R_P = \lim_{\substack{D \to \infty \\ \dot{V} \to \infty}} R_{tot} = \frac{A}{H\,\dot{Q}\,\beta_b} \tag{4}$$

where H is a multiplier denoting the fraction of the total airway mucosal blood flow that participates in inert gas exchange. The ventilation resistance, R_V, and the molecular diffusion resistance, R_D, can be found in a similar fashion:

$$R_V = \lim_{\substack{D \to \infty \\ \dot{Q} \to \infty}} R_{tot} = \frac{A}{\dot{V}\,\beta_g} \tag{5}$$

$$R_D = \lim_{\substack{\dot{V} \to \infty \\ \dot{Q} \to \infty}} R_{tot} = \frac{A}{D} \tag{6}$$

Note from Equation 3 that R_{tot} is not a simple summation of the individual resistances. Because the driving force for gas exchange is chosen to be the difference between *incoming* partial pressures, the expression for R_{tot} includes the terms associated with the convective delivery rate of the gas in the blood and the airstream (i.e., R_P and R_V). The convective resistances are not in series with the diffusion-related resistance, and, thus, are not additive. This model provides a convenient and quantitative analysis of the physical parameters that influence airway gas exchange, and it allows one to quickly estimate the relative importance of ventilation, diffusion, and perfusion.

B. Ventilation Resistance

The ventilation resistance, as defined by Equation 5, is the resistance associated with the convective delivery or removal of the inert gas in the airstream. R_V is inversely related to the product of the mean volumetric airstream flow rate and gas-phase solubility. For most applications, non-ideal behavior in the gas phase can be neglected; therefore, β_g is identical for all gases and is equal to 1 atm^{-1} at atmospheric pressure. $\dot{V}$ progressively decreases as airway generation number increases. Thus, as the airway tree progressively bifurcates, R_V progressively increases in magnitude. Quantifying $\dot{V}$, and therefore R_V, in the airways is usually done by assuming that the airway tree has a symmetric, bifurcating structure. By using the airway dimensions (lengths and diameters) reported by Weibel (18), the magnitude of R_V can be estimated as a function of airway generation (Figure 3). Inhaled flow rate is 250 $mL{\cdot}s^{-1}$, which is an average flow rate for tidal breathing (tidal volume of 500 mL, respiratory rate of 15 breaths/

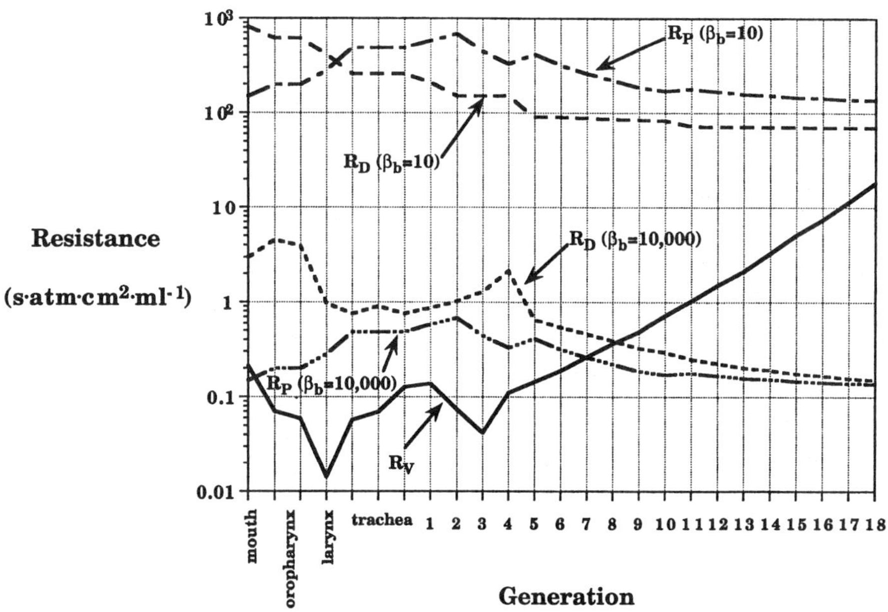

Figure 3 Theoretical resistance to airway gas exchange as a function of generation number during normal tidal breathing. R_P, R_D, and R_V are perfusion-, diffusion-, and ventilation-related resistances as described in the text. R_P and R_D are shown for two values for blood solubility, $\beta_b = 10{,}000$ and $\beta_b = 10$. The inhaled airstream flow rate is 250 $mL \cdot s^{-1}$, and other approximations associated with the calculations are outlined in detail in the text.

min). R_V is approximately constant at a value of 0.1 in the upper respiratory tract with the exception of the laryngeal region where the small diameter creates a high flow and therefore a smaller resistance. Small variations are due to variations in the diameter of the upper respiratory tract. Past the third generation, R_V progressively increases as the decrease in flow rate more than offsets the decrease in surface area.

The calculations presented in Figure 3 are for steady flow and a homogeneous branching pattern. A tidal breath, however, involves large variations in flow rate, and the branching pattern of the lung is heterogeneous in type (some are trifurcations), angle, length, and diameter. This heterogeneity in inhaled flow rate and branching pattern effectively creates a distribution of airstream flow rates across any fixed depth or axial distance into the lung. For simplicity, these effects are often neglected in the analysis of airway gas exchange dynamics, particularly the heterogeneity in branching pattern. The result is only a gross understanding of R_V and its relative impact. Future analysis must incorporate the effects of an inhomogeneous branching pattern if understanding of airway gas exchange dynamics is to improve.

C. Diffusion Resistance

The resistance to airway gas exchange associated with diffusion is the inverse of the diffusing capacity (D). D is a function of several parameters. Each can be estimated using prior experimental data or current knowledge of the physical setting. The molecular diffusion coefficient is the coefficient of proportionality in Fick's first law of diffusion. That is, the flux of a gas across a plane is proportional to the concentration gradient (more specifically, the chemical potential gradient) within the medium at the plane. Therefore, the diffusion coefficient describes quantitatively the relative ease or difficulty with which a molecule may diffuse in a specific medium. In general, the diffusion coefficient through a given tissue ($\mathcal{D}_t$) of small hydrophilic molecules (molecular weight, $M < 100$) is on the order of 10^{-6} $cm^2 \cdot s^{-1}$, and is approximately one-third of the diffusion coefficient of the molecule in water (19,20). The reduced diffusion coefficient is due partially to the increased viscosity (diffusion is inversely related to viscosity) of cytoplasm (21), but also to the presence of elastin, collagen, lipids, and other extracellular constituents.

Diffusion of larger hydrophilic molecules ($M > 100$) in the respiratory mucosa is more complex because of the organized structure of the epithelium, including the presence of the zonula occludens or tight junction (TJ). The TJ is a complex of proteins that binds tightly together the apical surface of the epithelial cells and regulates the passage of electrolytes and nonelectrolytes across the paracellular space (22). The paracellular space is a hydrophilic pathway; thus, the TJ influences the diffusing properties of large hydrophilic molecules. Several investigators have described the sieving characteristics of the epithelium as consistent with small hydrophilic "pores" (23–25). The pores represent a unique pathway for the passage of small hydrophilic molecules. The size of the pores vary among species and organ. Man et al. (24,26) estimated that the sieving characteristics of the canine trachea are consistent with heteropores, that is, two different pore populations. The first has a radius between 2 and 6 Å and comprises approximately 97.8% of the total pore surface area. The second pore is larger (radius 25 Å) and comprises the remaining 2.2% of the pore surface area. The atomic radius of a molecule, r, can be approximated by $3*M/4\pi\rho N)^{1/3}$, where ρ is the density ($g\cdot cm^{-3}$) and N is Avogadro's number. Using this approximation, the diffusion of hydrophilic molecules whose M is greater than 100 ($r \sim 3.5$ Å) is hindered because they must sift through the pores. Finally, a charged molecule has much different diffusing characteristics within the paracellular space than a polar molecule because of the presence of fixed negative charges (i.e., COO^- and PO_4^{2-}) within the tight junction (22).

As discussed, according to Fick's first law, the flux of an inert solute across a medium is proportional to the concentration gradient. If the medium is homogeneous, then the flux is inversely proportional to the thickness of the medium. In our analysis of airway gas exchange, this effect is reflected in the thickness of the tissue and mucous layers. Because the bronchial circulation is delivered by discrete capillaries that have a distribution of distances from the airway lumen, ℓ_t is difficult to quantitate, and, as yet, there is limited information. Gastineau et al. (27) reported the thickness of the bronchial epithelium in humans using surgical specimens. The measurements did not include the subepithelial tissue, and all of the bronchioles (approximately generations 11–18) were lumped into a single unit. However, Souders et al. (28) measured the distance that 15 μm fluorescent microspheres lodged in the canine trachea. The geometric mean distance was approximately 125 μm, which is approximately 15 μm greater than the thickness of the epithelium. Therefore, a reasonable estimate of the tissue barrier thickness is to add 15 μm to the epithelial thickness data from Gastineau et al. (27).

The thickness of the mucous layer may be even more difficult to quantitate. Because of its fluid-like nature and the fact that it is the immediate source of water for humidification of the inspired air, ℓ_m is constantly changing from breath to breath. ℓ_m is commonly reported to be approximately 10 μm (29); however, the mucous layer is difficult to capture in its in vivo state. In addition, a second function of the mucus is to act as a carrier of particulate matter from the periphery of the lung to the upper airways and oropharynx. Thus, the total volume of mucus in the peripheral airways should be approximately equal to that in the upper airways. In light of the increasing lumenal surface area as the airways branch, ℓ_m is likely to be a strong function of axial position. It has been reported that the mucous layer is, in fact, discontinuous in the peripheral airways

(30). One method of estimating ℓ_m is to assume a thickness of 10 μm in the trachea. Then, scale ℓ_m in each subsequent airway generation such that the volume of mucus in each generation is equal to that in the trachea. Because the mucous layer is the first line of defense against inhaled foreign gases and particulate matter, a more sophisticated in vivo description would provide important insight into gas exchange dynamics.

The local mass transfer coefficient, k, describes the interphase transport of gas between the mucus and air. It is analogous to the local heat transfer, h. k and h are related by the Chilton-Colburn analogy (31). k includes the resistance associated with evaporation and molecular diffusion across an effective unstirred boundary layer near the airway lumen wall. There is extensive literature devoted to developing empirical relationships for k when flow is either laminar or turbulent. The most common form for the relationship is $Sh = K(Re)^a (Sc)^b$, where Sh is the Sherwood number ($kd/\mathcal{D}_g$), d is the diameter of the airway and $\mathcal{D}_g$ is the gas phase diffusion coefficient), Re is the Reynolds number (dimensionless number representing the ratio of convective to viscous forces), Sc is the Schmidt number (dimensionless number representing the ratio of viscous to diffusive forces), and K is a proportionality constant. The analogous relationship for h involves the Nusselt number, Nu (hd/k), where k is the thermal conductivity of the medium ($J \cdot cm^{-1} \cdot s^{-1} \cdot °C$), $Nu = K(Re)^a (Pr)^b$, and Pr is the Prandtl number (dimensionless number representing the ratio of viscous to diffusive energy forces).

Several groups of investigators have studied the dependence of either Nu or Sh on Re. Hanna and Scherer (32,33) measured mass transfer coefficients in a cast model of human airways from the nasal vestibule to the distal trachea. Values for K (K_{insp} and K_{exp} are the constants of proportionality for inspiration and expiration, respectively) and the exponent "a" are summarized in Table 2 (32,34). Johnson and Linderoth (35) studied the heat transfer coefficient in the main stem and lobar bronchi of dogs during inspiration. Nuckols (36) used a physical model of bifurcating pipes (three consecutive generations) to simulate expiration. Thus, for branching or intrathoracic airways, the following relationships have been proposed for Sh:

$$Sh = 0.259^* (RE)^{0.785} (Sc)^{0.333} \quad \text{(inspiration)} \tag{7}$$

$$Sh = 0.0512^* (Re)^{0.751} (Sc)^{0.333} \quad \text{(expiration)} \tag{8}$$

Ingenito (34) proposed a slightly different correlation in studies of heat transfer coefficients in the upper airways. Ingenito's correlation was of the form $Sh = K^*(Re^*Sc)^a$. The coefficients K and "a" were determined experimentally in cadaveric nasal cavities and are summarized in Table 2. Then, using a model of airway heat transfer and measured intrathoracic airstream temperatures down to the fifth generation, Ingenito proposed the following relationship for Sh in branching or intrathoracic airways:

Table 2 Parameters in Empirical Correlations for Heat and Mass Transfer Coefficients

	K_{insp}		K_{exp}		a_{insp}		a_{exp}
Anatomical location	Hanna[a]	Ingenito[b]	Hanna[a]	Ingenito[b]	Hanna[a]	Ingenito[b]	Hanna[a]
Nasal vestibule	0.056	0.148	0.017	0.330	0.856	0.625	0.984
Nasal cavity (to turbinates)	0.056	0.116	0.017	0.274	0.856	0.744	0.984
Nasal cavity (turbinates)	0.129	0.021	0.039	0.178	0.856	1.129	0.984
Nasopharynx (proximal)	0.064	0.057	0.0207	0.413	0.856	0.937	0.984
Nasopharynx (distal)	0.032	0.00026	0.0098	0.0000551	0.856	1.459	0.984
Oropharynx	0.046	—	0.0153	—	0.856	—	0.984
Hypopharynx	0.076	—	0.0254	—	0.856	—	0.984
Larynx	0.046	—	0.0146	—	0.856	—	0.984
Trachea (proximal)	0.032	—	0.0103	—	0.856	—	0.984
Trachea (distal)	0.045	—	0.0148	—	0.856	—	0.984

[a]Soruce: Ref. 32.
[b]Source: Ref. 34.

$$Sh = 0.227 * (Re * Sc)^{0.668} \quad \text{(inspiration)} \tag{9}$$

$$Sh = 0.209 * (Re * Sc)^{0.668} \quad \text{(expiration)} \tag{10}$$

Tsu et al. (37) compared the performance of the correlations proposed by both Hanna and Ingenito in a model of simultaneous heat and mass transfer. The model matched mean intra-airway temperature profiles (38) better when the correlation of Ingenito was used. These experimental studies did not include any data past the fifth generation and the range of Re spanned approximately 300–2500. Thus, it is difficult to extrapolate the empirical correlations into the lower airways where much smaller flows ($Re < 1$, Figure 4) have a large impact on flow patterns and hence, k.

Laminar flow in tubes occurs for approximately $Re < 2100$. Flow constrictions (e.g., in the larynx) and bifurcations in the airway tree induce turbulent mixing in the upper airways. Thus, empirical correlations for k are most useful in the upper airways. However, as the linear velocity of the airstream slows as a result of progressive bifurcations, the dominant type of flow is laminar. As flow enters a tube with a velocity distribution other than that of steady laminar flow, a specific length of the tube must be traversed by the flow before the parabolic velocity profile is established. The length is referred to as the entrance length, L_e. An estimate L_e is $0.035*Re*d$ (39). At approximately the fifth generation, L_e is approximately 7% of the length of the airway based on the mean inspiratory flow rate of 250 $mL \cdot s^{-1}$ and the airway dimensions of Weibel (18). For distal generations, L_e becomes progressively smaller. For fully developed laminar flow through a hollow tube, an analytical expression for k can be de-

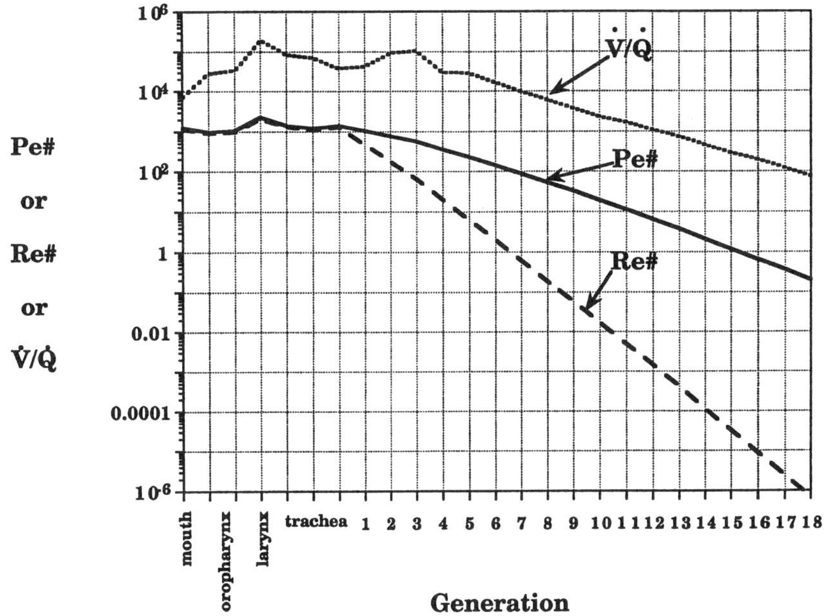

Figure 4 Peclet number (Pe), Reynolds (Re) number, and the ventilation to perfusion rate ratio ($\dot{V}/\dot{Q}$) as a function of generation number during normal tidal breathing. The inhaled airstream flow rate is 250 $mL \cdot s^{-1}$, and other approximations associated with the calculations are outlined in detail in the text.

rived, which is independent of Re and Sc and given by $(6D_g)/d$ or $Sh = 6$ (17). Thus, the best estimate for k is to use the empirical correlations in the upper airways (i.e., through generation 5); then, for generations 5–18, use the laminar flow relationship $[k = (6D_g)/d]$. This estimate of k is consistent with the range of Re (300–2500) and generation number (extrapulmonary airways through generation 5) used to develop the empirical correlations. This is a crude estimate of k, especially in the distal airways where heterogeneous branching patterns affect k. A greater knowledge of k in the smaller airways is a prerequisite for understanding small airway gas exchange.

The final terms in the expression for the diffusing capacity are the solubilities in the respiratory tissue and mucus. Because mucus is comprised of >95% water (40), there is little information on the solubility of gases in mucus. The solubility properties of mucus are almost exclusively assumed to be identical to those for water, for which there is substantial information. There is a significant amount of data on the solubility of a variety of gases in many tissue types

(3,41–47). For example, Perbellini et al. (46) measured the tissue : air partition coefficients of nine industrial aliphatic hydrocarbons in seven different tissues including the lung. The limitation in studies of this type is that the lung is homogenized, or ground into a slurry. Thus, the measured partition coefficient describes the entire lung and gives no information on the specific tissue types within the lung including the respiratory mucosa. More recently, George et al. (19) measured the tissue : saline partition coefficient of three compounds (ethanol, methyl ethyl ketone, and 2-ethoxyethanol) in the respiratory mucosa of the dog trachea. The technique is relatively simple and may prove useful in future studies of respiratory mucosal solubility.

Using the approximations described above and approximating the solubility of a gas in mucus and tissue as equal to that in blood, an estimate for R_D can be made as a function of axial position (see Figure 3). Two values of β_b are shown, and it is evident that R_D is a strong inverse function of β_b in the upper respiratory tract and upper airways (Equations 2 and 6). For a blood solubility of 10,000, a point is reached at approximately generation 8, where R_D, R_V, and R_P are the same magnitude. For airways distal to this point, R_V is the dominant resistance due to very slow airstream flow rates. For an intermediate solubility gas ($\beta_b = 10$), R_D is much larger than R_V throughout the airway tree. Even at generation 18, where the airstream flow rate is approximately 0.001 $mL \cdot^{-1}$, R_V is still an order of magnitude smaller that R_D.

D. Perfusion Resistance

As was the case with the ventilation-related resistance, the resistance to gas exchange associated with perfusion is a convective resistance. R_P is inversely related to the product of the total blood flow rate to the airway and the solubility in the blood. However, unlike R_V, the solubility in the medium (i.e., blood) depends strongly on the inert gas. β_b has been measured for a wide range of gases in a wide range of species including human, dog, and rabbit (44,45,48). Table 1 summarizes the value for β_b for several gases of interest at 37°C, some of which are discussed in greater detail in Section III. The blood flow rate to the airways, called the bronchial circulation, has been studied extensively. Although there are several thorough reviews of the bronchial circulation (49,50), the important features and several new pieces of information particularly relevant to airway gas exchange are discussed. The bronchial circulation is systemic in nature, that is, it arises from the left side of the heart and is saturated with oxygen. The primary function of the bronchial circulation is to supply oxygen and nutrients to the airway tissue, including the epithelium, as well as to assist in the heating and humidification of inhaled air (51). The flow rate of the bronchial circulation is extremely difficult to measure because it arises from multiple arterial sources along the aorta and supplies not only the airways but also the mediastinal lymph nodes, visceral pleura, lower esophagus, and the vasa vasorum of the pulmonary arteries and veins (52). The technique used most commonly in humans is to measure the blood flow returning to the left side of the heart during total cardiopulmonary bypass (53–55). This technique has been under a variety of pathophysiological conditions. Under normal conditions, the blood flow rate of the bronchial circulation is between 20 and 40 $mL \cdot min^{-1}$ or 0.5%–1.5% of cardiac output (52).

More recently, the use of fluorescent microspheres have been used as a marker of bronchial blood flow in animals. Souders et al. (28) used fluorescent microspheres to measure the tracheal blood flow in dogs and reported a value of 0.013 $mL \cdot s^{-1}$, which is in good agreement with data of Baile et al. (56) who reported a value of 0.025 $mL \cdot s^{-1}$ in the trachea and main stem bronchi of dogs using radioactive microspheres. Bernard et al. (57) quantified for the first time the axial distribution of bronchial blood flow per unit volume of tissue in dogs. The normalized blood flow (per unit volume of tissue) was inversely related to airway diameter. As airway generation increases, the blood flow per unit volume of tissue increases. The following relationship was reported:

$$\dot{Q}(x) = v_t(x)\overline{\dot{Q}}F(x) \tag{11}$$

where $v_t(x)$ is the volume of tissue (cm^3) in airway x, F(x) is a weighting factor given by Bernard et al. (57), and $\dot{Q}$ is the mean control volume blood flow on a unit volume of tissue basis. These parameters are defined by the following relationships:

$$v_t(x) = \pi d \ell_t(x) \Delta z \tag{12}$$

$$F(x) = 0.19 + (2.8) \exp(-0.51d(x)) \tag{13}$$

$$\overline{\dot{Q}} = \frac{\dot{Q}_{tot}}{V_t} \tag{14}$$

where d(x) is the airway diameter (mm), $\dot{Q}_{tot}$ is the total blood flow to all airways, and V_t is the total volume of tissue in all airways. This information is critical to the understanding of airway gas exchange in that R_P is inversely related to blood flow rate.

If blood flow to the trachea is fixed at 0.013 $mL \cdot s^{-1}$ (28) and the blood flow to the remaining airways is calculated using the distribution function of Bernard et al. (57), the magnitude of R_P can be estimated as a function of β_b in a fashion similar to that done for R_D and R_V (see Figure 3). R_P goes through a maximum value at generation 2. This is due to the fact that the blood flow to an airway depends on the blood flow per unit volume of tissue (which increases with decreasing airway diameter) multiplied by the volume of the tissue (which decreases with decreasing airway diameter). As solubility increases, R_P becomes smaller in absolute magnitude because R_P is inversely related to β_b (see Equation

4); it is also smaller relative to R_D. The relative contribution of the mucus–air interface (i.e., k) to R_D increases as solubility increases. Thus, over much of the airway tree, R_P is the largest resistance for intermediate gases, but R_D becomes the largest resistance for highly soluble gases.

Despite all that is known about the bronchial circulation, several important characteristics of the bronchial circulation have yet to be described. As discussed earlier, the part of the bronchial circulation that exchanges gas with the airstream consists of discrete capillaries. The capillary bed has been described qualitatively in several species including dog, sheep, guinea pig, and rat (58–61). Laitinen et al. attempted to quantify the density (capillaries·cm^{-3}) of capillaries in the respiratory mucosa of dogs (60), but this study did not label the capillaries in any fashion before fixation. Thus, the number of capillaries perfused at systemic pressure may be quite different. In addition, there is no information describing the distribution of distances that the capillaries are from the lumen, and whether or not this distribution is a function of axial position in the airway tree. The future success and validity of airway gas exchange modeling depend on this information.

E. Axial Diffusion

The mathematical analysis in Section II A neglects axial diffusion in all of the radial compartments. This assumption is valid in the tissue and mucous layers because radial gradients are, in most cases, much larger than axial gradients. However, in the gas phase, this assumption breaks down in the smaller airways when convective transport decreases and the relative magnitude of diffusive transport increases. A simple technique to estimate the relative importance of the convective and diffusive transport is to calculate the Peclet number, or Pe. Pe is a dimensionless number that represents the ratio of convective velocity to diffusive velocity. For transport in a cylinder, Pe is equal to the following:

$$\mathrm{Pe} = \frac{\dot{u}}{\mathcal{D}_g/d} = \frac{4\,\dot{V}}{\pi d \mathcal{D}_g} \tag{15}$$

where $\dot{u}$ is the mean linear velocity of the gas phase (cm·s^{-1}), and $\mathcal{D}_g$ is the molecular diffusion coefficient of the inert gas in the gas phase. When Pe is equal to 1, convective and diffusive velocity are equal. Using the airway dimensions of Weibel and assuming a mean inspired and expired flow rate of 250 mL·s^{-1} (based on a respiratory rate of 15 breaths/min^{-1}, and a tidal volume of 500 mL), the Pe can be calculated for each axial position in the airways (see Figure 4). It is evident that at approximately generation 15, Pe is equal to 1. In reality, one should not neglect axial diffusion once the Pe becomes less than ~5, which occurs at approximately generation 13. Between generations 13 and 18, both convection and diffusion must be considered, and after generation 18, diffusion dominates and convection may be neglected.

F. Energy Transport

The transport of energy is coupled with the transport of mass and can only be truly neglected under specific conditions. For example, when the inspired air is fully warmed to body temperature and saturated with water, the latent energy transport (that associated with the condensation and evaporation of the inert gas) is likely to be negligible. However, if the inspired air is cold and dry, there is likely to be a substantial amount of latent energy transport resulting from the evaporation of water and of sensible heat transport resulting from the temperature gradient between the inspired air and the mucosa. This transport of energy influences the temperature of the mucous and tissue layers, which subsequently affects the solubility and diffusivity of the inert gas in these media. For example, the solubility of ethanol in blood and water is an exponential function of temperature (10) and the diffusivity is empirically proportional to temperature (21).

The coupled transport of heat and mass in the airways has been addressed in several mathematical models (32,37,62,63). Unfortunately, the set of equations that describe this phenomenon must be solved numerically and are not conducive to the type of analysis presented in Section II A. However, if the transport of mass is neglected and focus is solely on the transport of sensible heat, a set of equations analogous to that presented in Section II A leading to the following expressions can easily be derived:

$$R_{P,h} = \frac{A}{\dot{Q}\,\tilde{C}_{P,b}} \tag{16}$$

$$R_{V,h} = \frac{A}{\dot{V}\,\tilde{C}_{P,g}} \tag{17}$$

$$R_{D,h} = \frac{A}{D_h} \tag{18}$$

$$D_h = \frac{A}{\left(\dfrac{\ell_t}{\alpha_t\,\tilde{C}_{P,t}} + \dfrac{\ell_m}{\alpha_m\,\tilde{C}_{P,m}} + \dfrac{1}{h}\right)} \tag{19}$$

where $R_{P,h}$, $R_{V,h}$, and $R_{D,h}$ are the resistance to heat transfer associated with perfusion, ventilation, and diffusion, respectively, under steady-state conditions. D_h is the total diffusing capacity for sensible heat in an airway ($J \cdot s^{-1}$), $\tilde{C}_{P,x}$ is the constant pressure volumetric heat capacity ($J \cdot {}^\circ C^{-1} \cdot mL^{-1}$) of blood ($x = b$), tissue ($x = t$), or mucus ($x = m$), and α_x is the thermal diffusivity ($cm^2 \cdot s^{-1}$) of tissue ($x = t$) and mucus ($x = m$). This exercise is useful in determining the parameters necessary to understand heat transport in the airways as well as the relative magnitudes of each resistance under specific conditions. There is substantial knowledge about several of these parameters. For example, the thermal diffusivity of tissue is approximately 1.5×10^{-3} $cm^2 \cdot s^{-1}$ (64), and a good estimate of the heat capacity of tissue, mucus, and blood is that of water, which is well characterized. As in the case with mass transfer, much less is known about the heat transfer coefficient, especially in the smaller airways, although this is not as critical because most heat transfer occurs in the upper airways. Heterogeneous branching patterns introduce mixing patterns that affect the transport coefficients. A thorough study of this phenomena is necessary to further current understanding of heat and mass exchange in the smaller airways.

III. Experimental and Theoretical Evidence of Airway Gas Exchange

For purposes of clarity, the effects of solubility on inert gas exchange in the airways is broken down into three sections, based on λ_b. Gases with $\lambda_b > 100$ are defined as high solubility gases; those with $1 \leq \lambda_b \leq 100$ are defined as intermediate solubility gases; and gases with $\lambda_b < 1$ are defined as low solubility gases. We examine how the general principles of gas exchange apply to gases of a given solubility using the theoretical development of Section II, then explore some specific examples of gases that have been studied both experimentally and theoretically.

A. High-Solubility Gases ($\lambda_b > 100$)

As seen in Figure 3, diffusion-related (R_D) and perfusion-related (R_P) resistances are the dominant resistances to the exchange of a highly soluble gas (λ_b = 10,000) at the mean ventilation flow rate of tidal breathing. R_D is the dominant resistance in the upper respiratory tract where the tissue thickness is the largest (approximately 500 μm in the oral and nasal cavities). In the intrapulmonary airways, R_D remains the largest resistance, although R_P is closer in magnitude because both ℓ_t and $\dot{Q}$ become smaller. The pattern of the relative magnitudes of R_P and R_D is similar for all gases. As blood solubility increases, the capacity for the blood to transport the gas increases (thus, R_P decreases), but so too does the capacity for the gas to diffuse through the tissue (R_D decreases as β_b and β_t are closely correlated). This pattern is modified only by the relative magnitude of the resistance associated with diffusion across the mucus–air interface (see Figure 3).

Davidson and Schroter (65) developed a general model of gas absorption in the airways during inhalation. In other words, the inhaled airstream is the source of the gas. They made many assumptions about the lung to make the governing equations more tractable, such as assuming a fully developed laminar flow in each airway (similar to that made in the model development in Section II regarding k). The model made some useful predictions including that the axial concentration profile of a gas in the airstream is a function of solubility (in this case water solubility). Their model predicted that, for $\lambda_w = 500$, the inhaled gas is nearly completely desorbed by the ninth generation (Figure 5). The concentration of the gas in the airstream at the ninth generation was approximately 2%–5% of the inhaled concentration.

Davies (66) studied the exchange behavior of low-solubility foreign gases that contaminate inhaled air and are desorbed to the respiratory tract by diffusion through the surfaces of the airways. Davies noted that inhaled foreign gases or vapors have a very small mass, which means that inertial impaction and sedimentation are not causes of deposition. Transport of gas molecules from the inhaled air to the walls of the airways (desorption) occurs solely by diffusion. For diffusive transport to take place from the lumen of an airway to the wall, a substantial radial concentration gradient is essential. If the concentration of molecules entering the airway is high, it is possible to saturate the surface of the airway so that the concentration of the foreign gas near the surface builds up and diffusion slows down. This may result in the inhaled gas being desorbed in the upper airways at the commencement of exposure, but penetrating deeper into the lungs as the walls of the upper airways become saturated and cease to absorb the molecules. Davies surmised that if *all* contaminant molecules that

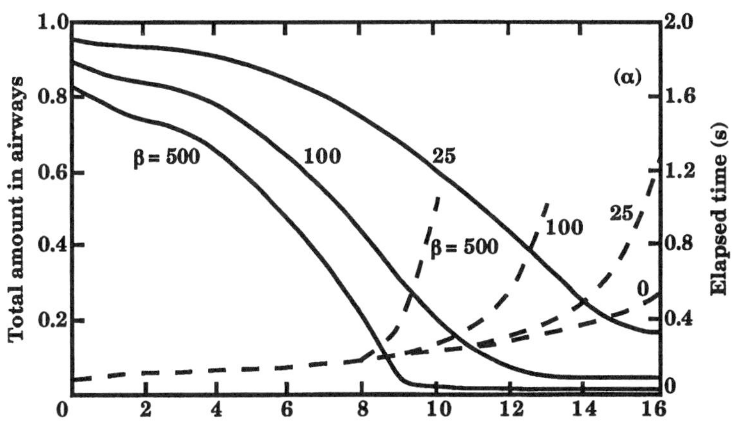

Figure 5 The amount of solute in all airways of the branching-lung model, expressed as a fraction of the initial amount injected at the model entrance, is calculated when the solute center of mass has reached the end of a generation. It is plotted versus generation number (*solid lines*), with the dashed lines representing the corresponding elapsed time. The simulations correspond to the inhalation of a solute pulse at a constant flow rate F of 20 L/min, with $\mathcal{D}_1 = 0.1$ cm^2/s, $\mathcal{D}_2 = 10^{-5}$ cm^2/s, and b = 1.1, for solubility coefficients β = 25, 100, 500. Poiseuille flow in each airway is assumed and the solute distribution is taken to be initially zero in the tissue and radially uniform in the gas. (From Ref. 65.)

struck the surfaces were eliminated (i.e., for highly soluble gases), no gas would penetrate beyond the dead space of the lungs and none would enter the alveolar region. Elimination at the wall would depend strongly on the solubility of the foreign molecules or on chemical fixation to the airway surface. For turbulent or plug flow of a highly soluble gas, Davies' model predicted that, during inspiration, complete desorption would occur by the end of the intrasegmental bronchi (fourth generation).

In general, the exchange of gas with the airways is proportional to the total resistance associated with exchange. Figure 3 and Equations 2–6 show that the higher the solubility, the greater the relative exchange in the airways. To illustrate this concept, experimental and theoretical studies documenting the gas exchange behavior of specific highly soluble inert gases can be reviewed and applied to the predictions of the mathematical model presented in Section II.

1. Water ($\lambda_b \approx 20{,}000$ at 37°C)

It has been known for some time that the airways participate in the exchange of heat and moisture. It has been noted from experimental measurements (1,38,67,68) that inspired air is warmed and humidified because heat and water diffuse from the mucosa of the airways (absorbed by the airstream) as a result of temperature and water vapor pressure gradients that exist. During expiration, the gradients are reversed, and heat and water diffuse back to the airways (desorption). Figure 6 is the experimental data from Ray et al. (68) that represents the water vapor concentration in the airways of intubated dogs down to 6 cm distal to the carina. The data represent three different breathing conditions in which respiratory rate and tidal volume were varied between 8.5 and 26 breaths/ min^{-1} and 200 and 600 mL, respectively. Water vapor concentration increases as the airstream moves distally into the lung, demonstrating the absorption of water from the airways. During exhalation, water vapor concentration decreases as the airstream moves toward the mouth, demonstrating the desorption of water from the air to the airways.

This process is not restricted to the upper airways, but rather it has been shown to involve the entire tracheobronchial tree. As the need to condition more air is increased by either raising the minute ventilation or lowering the temperature of the inspired air (thereby lowering water content), the point at which the inspirate reaches a local equilibrium with the temperature and water vapor pressure of the airway wall moves progressively deeper into the lungs (see Figure 6). Under extreme conditions, such as the inhalation of frigid air at a minute ventilation of 50 $L \cdot min^{-1}$, the transfer of heat and water vapor persists in airways less than 2 mm in diameter (67). However, even under these conditions, the exchange of water is complete before the inspired air reaches the alveoli (69).

Hanna and Scherer developed a model of simultaneous heat and water

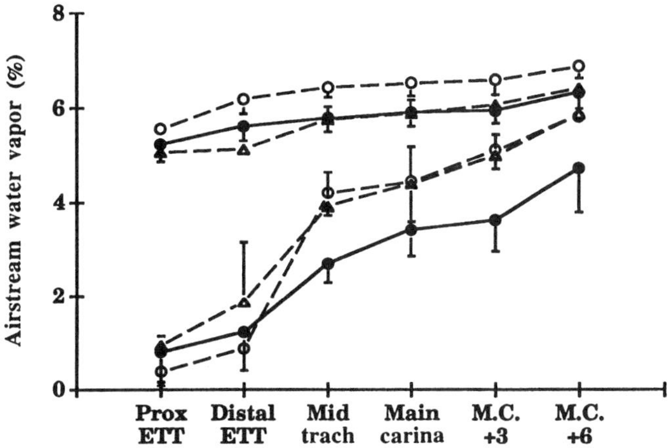

Figure 6 Inspiratory (lower group of three lines) and expiratory (upper group of three lines) extremes of airstream water vapor versus airway location during three different breathing conditions: m, RR = 8.5 br•min^{-1}, TV = 600; 1, RR = 26.3 br•min^{-1}, TV = 600; Δ, RR = 25.7 br•min^{-1}, TV = 200. Means ± SD (among animals) are shown. *Abbreviations*: Prox ETT = proximal tip of endotracheal tube; Mid-trach = midtrachea; MC +3 = 3 cm distal to main carina; MC +6 = 6 cm distal to main carina. (From Ref. 68.)

exchange (33) and implemented their empirical correlations for the heat and mass transfer coefficient. They predicted that inspired air is 75% saturated by the end of the nasal cavity and completely saturated by approximately the fifth airway generation. They used the temperature of the capillary bed as a free model parameter to match the experimental water vapor data of several different investigators (70,71).

Tsu et al. (37) developed a mathematical model to describe the dynamics of heat, water, and soluble gas exchange with the airways. This model was a fundamental advancement in the modeling and understanding of water vapor exchange because it was the first model to incorporate the following: 1. a mucous layer that would expand or contract with either condensation or evaporation, respectively, and 2. the secretion of fluid from the tissue to the mucus with liquid evaporation from the airway surface. For instance, the model predicted that during oral breathing of room air at rest, the greatest amount of conditioning of the inspired air occurs in the trachea and large bronchi, whereas the smaller bronchial airways participate in the conditioning process to a lesser degree, with water exchange complete at approximately the sixth generation. There is also a tradeoff between the increased heat and water recovery afforded by a thicker mucosal layer and a decreased ability to exchange water, resulting in deeper penetration of cooler, drier air into the lungs.

Tsai et al. (72) modeled the exchange of heat and water in the trachea alone and focused on the *radial* concentration profile of water. The fundamental advancement in modeling water exchange was the addition of a blood flow rate. This differs substantially from the model of Tsu et al. (37), who assumed a uniform radial concentration profile within the airway lumen and an infinite blood flow. They concluded that the thickness of the tissue layer and the blood flow rate influence the radial concentration profile. This result is consistent with the analysis in Section II A.

2. *Ethanol ($\lambda_b \approx 1800$ at 37°C)*

Although λ_b of ethanol is much less than that of water, ethanol has been shown through experimental studies and theoretical modeling to exchange entirely within the bronchial tree. Tsu et al. (69) demonstrated that alcohol arriving at the mouth following a tidal breath comes primarily from the mucous layer of the airways and not the alveoli. Inspired air absorbs alcohol from the mucous layer in a bimodal axial distribution until reaching approximately the 12th–15th airway generation, where the air reaches a local equilibrium with the partial pressure of ethanol in the mucus (Figure 7). During exhalation, a portion of the ethanol absorbed by the airstream on inspiration is desorbed to the mucous layer. The amount of desorption depends on breathing pattern such as the breathing frequency.

George et al. (12) further tested and validated the model by collecting exhaled ethanol profiles from human subjects. The subjects inhaled to total lung capacity (TLC) and exhaled at a constant controlled rate, using both rapid and

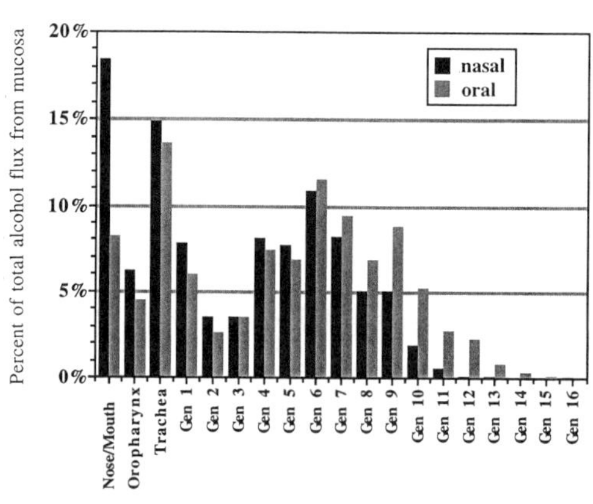

Figure 7 Axial distribution of alcohol flux from the airway mucosa. Data are shown for both nasal and oral breathing conditions. (From Ref. 69.)

slow exhalation rates. In these experiments, it was noted that the only dead space for ethanol in the exhalate was apparatus dead space. Thus, the anatomical dead space for ethanol was effectively nonexistent and the exchange of ethanol occurred throughout the respiratory tree. The shape of the exhaled ethanol profile was found to be strongly dependent on the diffusing capacity of ethanol in the bronchial mucosa. Therefore, the exchange of ethanol must be limited, at least in part, by diffusion. Using the preexisting model to fit the experimental data, George et al. (12) predicted that the diffusing capacity of ethanol in the nonperfused tissue layer of the airways, D_t, is only 8% of a predicted diffusing capacity that assumes a maximal surface area, and diffusing properties equivalent to that of water. The reduced diffusing capacity has a profound effect on the distribution of alcohol flux between the airway lumen and the mucous layer.

During inspiration, the airstream absorbs ethanol from the surrounding mucus and tissue. During exhalation, a portion of the ethanol absorbed on inspiration is desorbed back to the mucous layer. The amount of ethanol desorbed depends on the partial pressure difference (driving force) of ethanol between the airstream and the mucous layer. The reduced diffusing capacity of ethanol in the airway mucosa retards the diffusion of ethanol from the bronchial circulation through the tissue. Thus, during exhalation, the partial pressure of ethanol in the mucus is reduced, which increases the driving force for desorption. Increasing the desorption of ethanol during exhalation decreases the partial pressure of ethanol in the exhaled airstream.

Because ethanol is exchanged primarily across the airway mucosa, conditions that alter the temperature and water content of the airways influence the exhaled ethanol concentration. It has been known for some time that body temperature alters the end-tidal ethanol concentration by more than ±20% (73,74). In addition, ambient temperature (75) and breathing pattern (76) can alter the exhaled ethanol concentration. The combined effects of airway temperature and humidity have also been demonstrated by Ohlsson (16) in a study comparing single breath exhalations to the breath alcohol concentration measured with isothermal rebreathing, which conserves both the heat and water content of inspired gas. In this study, breath ethanol was found to vary no more than ±10% of the blood ethanol level when isothermal rebreathing was employed. George et al. (13) later used mathematical modeling to predict that the effects of pretest breathing maneuvers on end-tidal ethanol concentration were due primarily to changes in the axial profile of ethanol content in the mucous lining of the airways, rather than to changes in temperature.

3. *Acetone ($\lambda_b \approx 340$ at 37°C)*

Acetone, although still highly soluble, is a less soluble gas than either water vapor or ethanol. Although the studies of water vapor and ethanol have shown their exchange to be primarily limited by diffusion, the exchange of acetone might be limited both by perfusion and diffusion. This could influence the degree of acetone exchange that would occur across the airways.

One of the earliest models of airway gas exchange was proposed by Dubois and Rogers (77) in 1968. Although the complexity of their model was limited by a lack of computing speed and additional knowledge about the physical environment of the airways (e.g., bronchial capillary bed structure, tissue thickness), the model provided pioneering insights into the factors that affect airway gas exchange, in particular, the effect of blood solubility. They predicted that the desorption rate of inhaled acetone would be approximately three orders of magnitude larger than cyclopropane and five orders of magnitude larger than SF_6. This difference is proportional to the difference in blood solubility (see Table 1).

The fact that acetone exchanges with the airways has been known for some time. Schrikker et al. (78) studied the wash-in and wash-out of several highly soluble gases, including acetone, to assess the excretion of such gases by the lung. The acetone wash-out curve showed that the volume of gas expired before the beginning of the phase II slope was considerably smaller than it was for other less soluble gases, including CO_2 (Figure 8). During the wash-out, the phase II slope for acetone was negative for the first few breaths, and then became positive, but still remained lower than the slopes for less soluble gases.

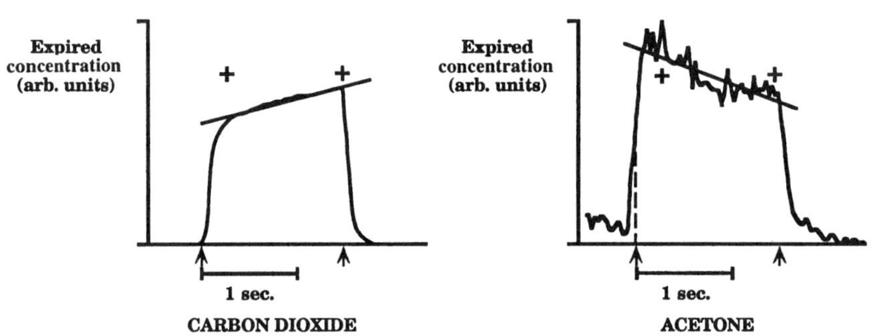

Figure 8 Concentration-time curves for CO_2 and acetone recorded simultaneously. In both figures, the first arrow indicates the beginning of phase II for CO_2, and the second arrow points to the end of expiration. Similarly, the first plus sign refers to the time at which 20% of the time interval between the two arrows has elapsed, and the second plus sign coincides with the end of expiration. The slope of the alveolar plateau is then calculated from the relative change in the concentration during the time interval determined by the two plus signs. These recordings concern the first expiration during wash-out in an experiment with a workload of 100 W. The slope for CO_2 is +11.7% per second and for acetone −20.9% per second. (From Ref. 78.)

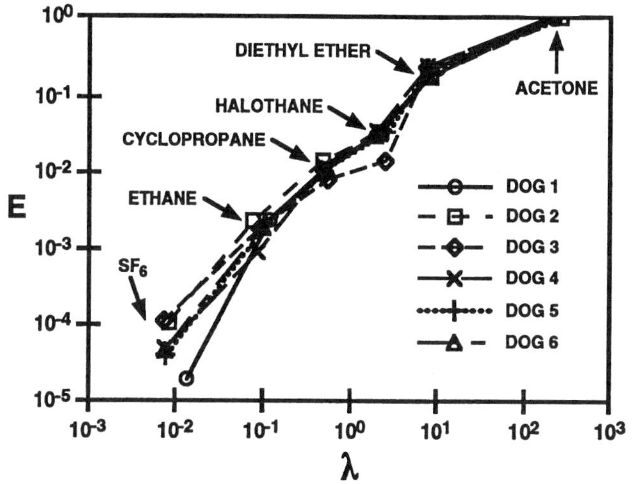

Figure 9 Relationship between inert gas partition coefficient (λ_b) and excretion (E) in group 1 dogs infused with six inert gases of various molecular weights and solubilities. Data are presented in a double-log manner to highlight differences between gases and dogs that would not be readily evident in conventional semilog plot normally used to present data in the multiple inert gas elimination technique. (From Ref. 2.)

The authors concluded that these two observed effects demonstrate that acetone in the expired air must originate from the epithelial tissue lining the conducting airways. A later study (79) also demonstrated that, for high solubility gases in general, gas exchange in the airways cannot be ignored for highly soluble tracer gases. In addition, dead space ventilation depends on λ_b, such that the value of the measured dead space is not unique. Therefore, the dead space value measured with highly soluble gases does not apply to that measured using other, lower solubility gases.

Because these results indicated that gases with solubilities comparable to acetone might be exchanged entirely across the airways, and because the ethanol studies indicated that such airway gas exchange would likely be diffusion-limited, Swenson et al. (2) examined the diffusion-related differences in inert gas elimination across the trachea using a spectrum of six gases (the gases used in the multiple inert gas elimination technique, or MIGET [80]) ranging from very low solubility (sulfur hexafluoride, $\lambda_b \approx 0.01$) to acetone. The excretion (defined as the partial pressure of the gas in expired air divided by the partial pressure of the gas in the mixed venous blood) of the six gases including acetone is shown in Figure 9. The magnitude of airway gas exchange is a strong positive function of blood solubility. The excretion of acetone was approximately 0.8, demonstrating a substantial exchange at a $\dot{V}/\dot{Q}$ of approximately 80. The possibility of a perfusion limitation to airway gas exchange was examined later by Souders et al. (28).

Theoretically, if a gas with a high solubility such as acetone is exchanged entirely or nearly entirely across the airways, then the excretion of that gas will be nearly 1.0 and should not be substantially altered by an increase in blood flow through the bronchial circulation. This hypothesis was tested by Souders et al. (28) using the in situ dog trachea experimental preparation of Swenson et al. (2). Blood flow to the trachea was altered pharmacologically and measured with 15-μm fluorescent microspheres, and the excretion of the six MIGET gases was assessed. They reported a significant perfusion limitation to gas exchange across the trachea (i.e., the excretion of the gas was a function of blood flow). The magnitude of the response of each gas to changes in bronchial blood flow was similar (Figure 10). These experimental results were analyzed using the

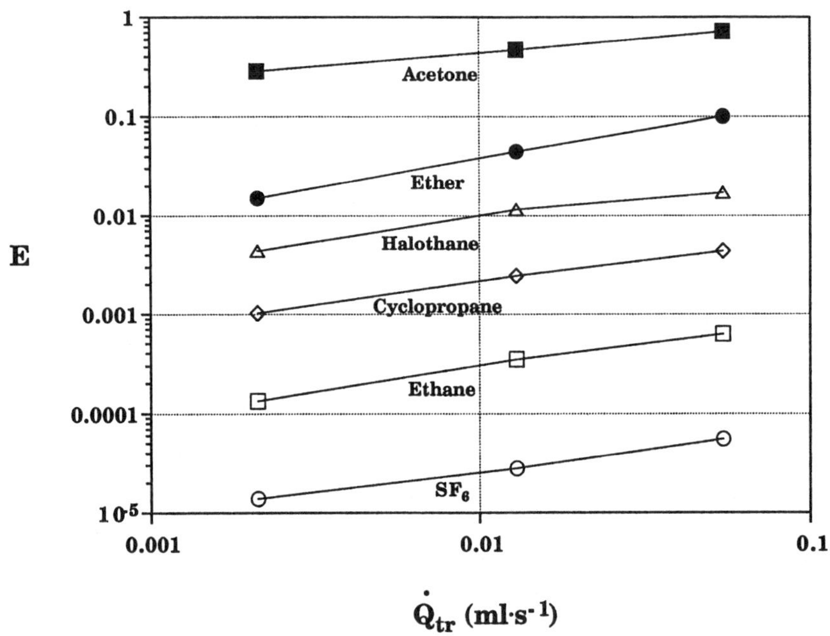

Figure 10 Relationship between excretion (E) and blood flow to the trachea as measured with 15-μ fluorescent microspheres. Excretion values are mean values from eight dogs. Gases of different solubility respond similarly to changes in blood flow. As blood flow increases, the excretion of a gas increases, indicating that airway gas exchange is limited in part by perfusion from the bronchial circulation. (From Ref. 28.)

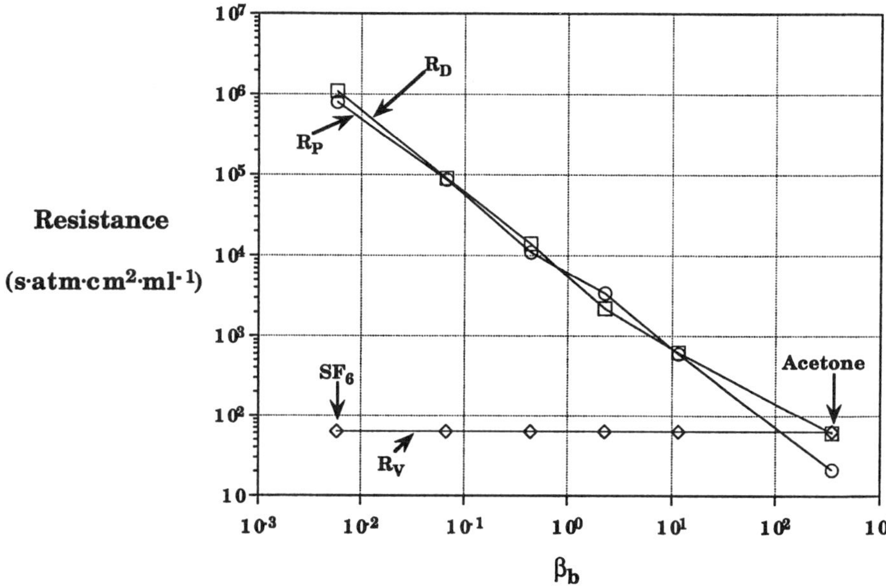

Figure 11 Theoretical resistance to airway gas exchange as a function blood solubility for the steady-state exchange of the six MIGET gases across a trachea at the baseline blood flow rate (0.013 $mL \cdot s^{-1}$) and a ventilation flow rate of 1 $mL \cdot s^{-1}$). R_P, R_D, and R_V are perfusion-, diffusion-, and ventilation-related resistances as described in the text.

model presented in Section II A (17). The airway exchange of gases whose blood solubilities span the range of the MIGET gases ($0.01 < \lambda_b < 300$) have a similar response to changes in blood flow because the resistance to exchange in the tissue layer has a similar functional dependence on the blood solubility. Both R_P and R_D are inversely related to solubility (either blood or tissue). Because tissue and blood solubility are closely correlated, both R_P and R_D decrease a similar magnitude in response to an increase in solubility. In contrast, the ventilation resistance is independent of tissue and blood solubility; thus, as λ_b becomes large, the relative magnitude of R_V increases. This model analysis of airway gas exchange shows that acetone was the only gas (28) that was sensitive to all three resistances to gas exchange (i.e., perfusion-, diffusion-, and ventilation-related resistances; Figure 11).

B. Intermediate Solubility Gases ($1 \le \lambda_b \le 100$)

As λ_b decreases, the interaction of a gas with the airways decreases. For intermediate solubility gases, we would hypothesize that the pulmonary exchange is a combination of airway and alveolar exchange. For $\beta_b = 10$, Figure 3 demonstrates that, although R_D is the largest resistance in the upper airways (due to the thick tissue barrier), R_P is the largest resistance over the remaining airway tree. This reversal (compared to $\beta_b = 10{,}000$) is due to decreasing relative magnitude of the resistance associated with mucus–air interface, which is independent of β_b. For $\lambda_w = 25$, the model of Davidson and Schroter (65) predicts that the concentration of a gas in the ninth generation is approximately 65% (as opposed to 2%–5% for $\lambda_w = 500$) of the inhaled concentration and decreases to approximately 25% by generation 16.

R_P and R_D are the dominant resistance for intermediate solubility gases in the airways (see Figure 3). A substantial amount of exchange of intermediate gases is likely to occur in the respiratory bronchioles, the transition region of the lung between the airways and alveoli. Assumptions in the model development break down in this region (e.g., neglecting axial diffusion or the extrapolation of the mass and heat transfer coefficient correlations) and thus it is difficult to quantify the relative magnitudes of R_P, R_D, and R_V for these gases in the region of the lung where the greatest exchange occurs. However, there is a substantial volume of literature devoted to the experimental study of intermediate solubility gases in the airways. By combining the insight into airway gas exchange provided by the model with the experimental results, we can begin to understand the parameters that control intermediate solubility gas exchange.

1. Ethyl Acetate ($\lambda_b \approx 75$ at 37°C)

Two studies by Schrikker et al. (78,79) examined the exchange of this intermediate solubility gas across the airways. The first study looked at wash-in and wash-out of ethyl acetate (among other gases) to study the effects of solubility on excretion of these gases. The more soluble the gas, the more rapidly it appeared on exhalation, and, therefore, the measured dead space for a gas was smaller as its solubility increased. The authors surmised that the early appearance of more soluble gases during exhalation meant that these exhalation profiles originated from the epithelial tissue lining the conducting airways. The observed differences between the excretion values of the various soluble tracer gases implied that dead space ventilation depends on λ_b; in other words, the value of the measured dead space is not unique. The dead space observed with ethyl acetate was larger than that of acetone but less than that of diethyl ether. This is consistent with increased interaction of a gas with the airways as solubility increases.

2. Ether ($\lambda_b \approx 10$ at 37°C)

The airway exchange dynamics of several ethers have been studied. Wanner et al. (81) studied the uptake of dimethyl ether ($\lambda \approx 9$) in the airways of sheep and determined that this uptake was a function of the bronchial blood flow. Dahl et al. (82) studied sites of propyl ether uptake in dogs ($\lambda \approx 10$) as compared to the uptake of several other gases. Propyl ether was one of the compounds with the lowest solubility and showed virtually no uptake in the nasal cavity, increasing uptake in the airways with increasing airway generation, and 47% of its total uptake occurring in the airways. Schrikker et al. (78), studying wash-in and wash-out of several gases, discovered that diethyl ether ($\lambda \approx 12$) was exchanged in part across the airways and in part through alveolar gas exchange. Although the measured dead space was larger than that measured by acetone or ethyl acetate, it was still smaller than the volume of the airways, indicating a significant amount of airway exchange.

Diethyl ether is one of the six MIGET gases and was thus included in the studies of Swenson et al. (2) and Souders et al. (28). Figures 9 and 10 demonstrate a substantial exchange of diethyl ether in the airways that is dependent on the blood flow rate (excretion approaches 0.1 at high blood flow rates).

3. *Halothane ($\lambda_b \approx 3$ at 37°C)*

As one of the MIGET gases, the exchange of halothane was also studied in these latter two experiments. Halothane is a gas of intermediate solubility, but differs from many of the other gases that have been studied because of its larger size (molecular weight of halothane = 197, as compared with diethyl ether, which has a molecular weight of 74). When Swenson et al. (2) observed the excretion of six inert gases of varying solubility across the canine trachea, they noted that the excretion of higher molecular weight gases like halothane were depressed more than anticipated on the basis of their solubilities (see Figure 9). This result suggested a molecular weight dependence to airway gas exchange. This was examined further in the same study (2) by observing the behavior of three additional gases of nearly equal intermediate solubilities, which differed in molecular weight (MW): acetylene, MW = 26; Freon-22, MW = 86.5; and isoflurane, MW = 185. The authors observed an MW dependence in the excretion of these gases, confirming the concept that gas exchange across the airways is diffusion limited.

C. Low-Solubility Gases ($\lambda_b < 1$)

Although the magnitude of the exchange of low-solubility gases in the airways is negligible compared with alveolar exchange, under specific conditions a non-negligible (from a physiological standpoint) amount of exchange can occur. This exchange can be measured and can shed insight into airway exchange dynamics, in general. In addition, the exchange of *endogenous* low solubility gases such as nitric oxide (NO) with the airways can have physiological sequelae. As was the case with intermediate solubility gases, R_P and R_D are the dominant resistances (see Figure 3) in the airways because of the low solubility (Equations

2–6). There is a significant volume of literature devoted to the experimental study of low solubility gases in the airways and the lungs, in general, primarily because oxygen is a low solubility gas.

1. Nitric Oxide ($\lambda_b \approx 0.042$ at 37°C)

The dynamics of NO exchange in the airways and the lung, in general, differs substantially from the gases presented thus far because of two factors: 1. NO is produced endogenously by the cells of the lung, and 2. NO is chemically reactive. The exchange of reactive gases is presented in greater detail in Chapter 9; however, the endogenous production of a gas by the lungs is somewhat unique (CO_2 is another example). Because of the enormous interest in NO and its physiological functions in the lung, a brief description of its exchange properties is presented.

NO is synthesized in vivo from enzymatic degradation of L-arginine to L-citrulline. The enzyme is nitric oxide synthase (NOS), whose activity has been identified in a variety of pulmonary cells present in the airways, including macrophages (83), neutrophils (84), mast cells (85), fibroblasts (86), vascular smooth muscle cells (87), endothelial cells (87), and bronchial epithelial cells (88) (see Figure 1). Each of these cell types represents a possible source of NO in the exhaled breath. Several groups of investigators have measured the concentration of NO in the exhaled breath both as a mixed expired concentration as well as dynamically, providing evidence for a baseline production of NO in vivo.

Borland and Higenbottam (89) measured mixed expired and alveolar samples of NO from normal humans and reported values ranging 8–15 ppb. Persson et al. (90) recorded exhalation profiles of both carbon dioxide and NO in humans at rest, following a breathhold, following hyperventilation, and during exercise. Breathholding significantly increased the peak value of NO from 3 ppb to more than 100 ppb following a 60-second breathhold. Hyperventilation had essentially no effect on exhaled NO. Although NO concentration decreased during exercise, the production rate increased. In addition, the NO profile had a significantly different shape when compared with CO_2. The phase III slope of NO was negative, yet the dead space calculations for both NO and CO_2 were essentially identical. This same laboratory next measured exhalation NO profiles in three different groups of human subjects: 1. controls, 2. treated asthmatics (either β_2-agonists or corticosteroids), and 3. smokers. All exhalation profiles were preceded by a 15-second breathhold. The shape of the exhalation profile again demonstrated a precipitous decrease in the concentration of NO during phase III. In addition, peak levels in asthmatics were increased (59 ppb) and decreased in smokers (15 ppb) when compared with controls (39 ppd). They concluded the following: 1. exhaled NO is produced in small airways (i.e., terminal and respiratory bronchioles) of the lung, 2. NO may act as an endogenous bronchodilator in an inflammatory disease such as asthma, and 3. smoking may destroy NO-producing cells and/or downregulate the production of NO because of the high concentration of NO in cigarette smoke (91).

Kharitonov et al. (92) measured the exhalation profiles of NO in normal humans, untreated asthmatics, asthmatics treated with β_2-agonists, and asthmatics treated with corticosteroids. They demonstrated that peak values of exhaled NO did not differ significantly in normals (80 ppb) and asthmatics treated with corticosteroids (101 ppb). However, asthmatics treated with β_2-agonists or untreated had a significantly higher level (283 ppb). Inhalation of L-NMMA, a specific inhibitor of NOS, significantly reduced peak exhaled NO concentrations, and ambient levels of NO had no effect on exhaled levels. This study concluded that exhaled NO is from an endogenous source in the lung and that exhaled levels in asthmatics are significantly higher because of the inflammatory nature of this disease. It has been previously demonstrated that inflammatory cytokines from inflammatory cells can induce NOS in airway smooth muscle cells (93).

Schedin et al. (94) attempted to quantify the relative contribution of the upper and lower airways to exhaled NO. They studied a series of different populations including patients with a chronic tracheostomy, anesthetized patients, intensive care patients, and nasal NO from normal volunteers. Exhaled levels from the nasal cavity were substantially larger than those from the lower airways. The estimated production rate of NO from the nasal cavity ($8–10 \times 10^{-9}$ $mol \cdot min^{-1}$) was approximately an order of magnitude larger than that of the lower airways (0.8×10^{-9} $mol \cdot min^{-1}$). The physiological significance of nasal NO production is unknown.

The apparent discrepancies among several of the studies that have measured exhaled NO is attributed to the use of different protocols as well as different analytical techniques. It is apparent that the production of NO within the entire respiratory tree is heterogeneous and depends on several factors including 1. axial position within the respiratory tract, 2. exercise level, 3. presence of inflammatory diseases such as asthma, 4. use of antiinflammatory mediators, and 5. chronic inhalation of tobacco smoke.

The low solubility of NO limits the exchange of exogenous NO in the airways. However, because the cells of the airways produce NO, this represents an additional means for a gas to "exchange" in the airways. The model development in Section II A is inadequate to analyze NO because it does not contain any production or consumption parameters. Current knowledge of the exchange dynamics of NO is in its infancy, and much more sophisticated modeling and experimentation is needed.

2. *Cyclopropane ($\lambda_b \approx 0.629$ at 37°C), Ethane ($\lambda_b \approx 0.111$ at 37°C), and Sulfur Hexafluoride (SF_6, $\lambda_b \approx 0.009$ at 37°C)*

Swenson et al. (2) and Souders et al. (28) have provided the only direct experimental evidence that low solubility gases exchange in the airways. The data from Swenson et al. (2) is shown in Figure 9 and demonstrates that, under baseline blood flow conditions to the trachea, the excretion of a gas from the trachea at a $\dot{V}/\dot{Q}$ of approximately 80 is a strong function of blood solubility and is nonzero for low solubility gases such as cyclopropane, ethane, and SF_6. Thus, although the magnitude of gas exchange in the airways for low solubility gases is small, it is a measurable quantity. The data from Souders et al. (28) is shown in Figure 10 and demonstrates the blood flow dependence of airway gas exchange for low solubility gases. The blood flow dependence can be understood by looking at the values of R_P, R_D, and R_V for the six MIGET gases in Figure 11. For low solubility gases, R_P and R_D have the same magnitude; thus, changes in blood flow affect the flux of gas across the airway wall and hence the excretion. The range of $\dot{V}/\dot{Q}$ attained by Souders et al. (28) would be found in approximately generations 14–18 during normal tidal breathing (see Figure 4). In the trachea, $\dot{V}/\dot{Q}$ is much larger (approximately 50,000); however, this increase is due primarily to an increase in $\dot{V}$. The relative magnitudes of R_D and R_P in trachea at a $\dot{V}/\dot{Q}$ of 50,000 are still comparable.

IV. Summary

The airways are a complex and heterogeneous (in structure and function) component of the lungs. Because of their anatomical location (i.e., in between the alveoli and the atmosphere), the airways cannot avoid participating in gas exchange. Mathematical modeling and experimentation have provided important insight into the factors that control the relative magnitude of airway gas exchange compared with alveolar exchange.

The model presented in Section II demonstrates that, under most conditions, the greatest single factor affecting airway gas exchange is the solubility of the gas in water, tissue, and blood. As solubility increases, the resistance to airway gas exchange decreases because the blood can deliver more gas to the airways and the capacity for the gas to diffuse through the tissue and mucus increases. Thus, the relative amount of airway exchange increases as solubility increases. The model also identifies additional parameters that can have a significant impact on gas exchange, depending on such factors as disease and breathing frequency. For example, a disease such as asthma can cause thickening of the respiratory mucosa, which subsequently increases the diffusion-related resistance. Breathing frequency alters the flow rate of gas, and, hence, impacts the resistance associated with the mucus–air interface. This can affect airway gas exchange in the distal airways for highly soluble gases.

In general, experimental and theoretical studies of airway gas exchange have led the scientific community to several important conclusions. The dead space of the lung is not unique, but depends on the gas used in the measurement. This may impact the interpretation of MIGET studies, which frequently calculate the lung dead space based on the measured retention and excretion of higher solubility gases (ether and acetone). The absorption of pollutant gases by lung is heterogeneous and depends strongly on the solubility of the gas. Thus, exposure to certain highly soluble gases may involve uptake strictly through the bronchial circulation. Teratogenic levels of certain gases may need to be recalculated when taking into account the possibility that these substances may be concentrated in the airway mucosa. Therapeutic drugs that have a pulmonary route of delivery or that act upon the airways (i.e., asthma medications) may be able to be designed to take advantage of the characteristics of airway gas exchange. A highly soluble drug with a large diffusing capacity that exchanges entirely across the bronchial circulation would concentrate more of the molecules at the specific site of action. Because of the high solubility of ethanol, breath ethanol measurements depend strongly on the physical environment of the airways and the breathing technique.

Although much is known about airway gas exchange, there remain substantial gaps in current knowledge. Of particular importance is knowledge of small airway exchange. A large number of important gases in the intermediate solubility range have a substantial exchange in the small airways and the respiratory bronchioles. Current knowledge of the circulations (bronchial and pulmonary) needs to improve before we can adequately understand this exchange process. In addition, there is essentially no information about the nature of the mucus–air interface in this region. Both modeling and experimentation will play large roles in future understanding of the very important and complex physiology of airway gas exchange.

References

1. McFadden ER. Respiratory heat and water exchange: physiologic and clinical implications. J Appl Physiol 1983; 54:331–336.
2. Swenson ER, Robertson HT, Polissar NL, Middaugh ME, and Hlastala MP. Conducting airway gas exchange: diffusion related differences in inert gas elimination. J Appl Physiol 1992; 72:1581–1588.
3. Lowe HJ, Hagler K. Gas chromatography in biology and medicine. Porter, ed. London: 1969; 86–104.
4. Sato A, Nakajima T. Partition coefficients of some aromatic hydrocarbons and ketones in water, blood and oil. Br J Industr Med 1979; 36:231–234.

5. Sherwood RJ. Ostwald solubility coefficients of some industrially important substances. Br J Industr Med 1976; 33:106–107.
6. Larson CO. Uptake and distribution of anesthetic agents. In: Papper and Kitz, eds. New York: McGraw-Hill, 1963:5–16.
7. Steward A, Allot PR, Cowles AL, Mapleson WW. Solubility coefficients for inhaled anaesthetics for water, oil, and biological media. Br J Anaesthesiol 1973; 45: 282.
8. Perry RH, Green DW. Perry's Chemical Engineers' Handbook. New York: McGraw-Hill, 1984.
9. Åstrand I, Ovrum P, Lindqvist T, Hultengren M. Exposure to butyl alcohol uptake and distribution in man. Scand J Work Environ Health 1976; 3:165–175.
10. Jones AW. Determination of liquid/air partition coefficients for dilute solutions of ethanol in water, whole blood, and plasma. J Anal Toxicol 1983; 7:193–197.
11. Johanson G, Dynesius B. Liquid/air partition coefficients of six commonly used glycol ethers. Br J Industr Med 1988; 45:561–564.
12. George SC, Babb AL, Hlastala MP. Dynamics of soluble gas exchange in the airways: III. Single exhalation breathing maneuver. J Appl Physiol 1993; 75:2439–2449.
13. George SC, Babb AL, Hlastala MP. Modeling the concentration of ethanol in the exhaled breath following pre-test breathing maneuvers. Ann Biomed Eng 1995; 23: 48–60.
14. Jones AW. Effects of temperature and humidity of inhaled air on the concentration of ethanol in a man's exhaled breath. Clin Sci 1982; 63:441–445.
15. Jones AW. How breathing technique can influence the results of breath-alcohol analysis. Med Sci Law 1982; 22:275–280.
16. Ohlsson J, Ralph DD, Mandelkorn MA, Babb AL, Hlastala MP. Accurate measurement of blood alcohol concentration with isothermal rebreathing. J Stud Alc 1990; 51:6–13.
17. George SC, Souders JE, Babb AL, Hlastala MP. Modeling steady state inert gas exchange in the canine trachea. J Appl Physiol 1995; 79:929–940.
18. Weibel E. Morphometry of the Human Lung. New York: Springer Verlag, 1963.
19. George SC, Babb AL, Deffebach ME, Hlastala MP. Diffusion of non-electrolytes in the canine trachea: effect of tight junction. J Appl Physiol 1996; 80:1687–1695.
20. Krogh A. The rate of diffusion of gases through animal tissues, with some remarks on the coefficient of invasion. J Physiol 1919; 52:391–408.
21. Wilke CR, Chang P. Correlation of diffusion coefficients in dilute solutions. Am Inst Chem Eng J 1955; 1:264–270.
22. Schneeberger EE, Lynch RD. Structure, function, and regulation of cellular tight junctions. Am J Physiol 1992; 262:L647–L661.
23. Hingson DJ, Diamond JM. Comparison of nonelectrolyte permeability patterns in several epithelia. J Membrane Biol 1972; 10:93–135.
24. Man SFP, Hulbert WC, Mok K, Ryan T, Thomson ABR. Effects of sulfur dioxide on pore populations of canine tracheal epithelium. J Appl Physiol 1986; 60:416–426.
25. Wangensteen OD, Schneider LA, Fahrenkrug SC, Brottman GM, Maynard RC.

Tracheal epithelial permeability to nonelectrolytes: species differences. J Appl Physiol 1993; 75:1009–1018.
26. Man SFP, Thomson ABR. Nonelectrolyte permeability of canine tracheal epithelium. J Appl Physiol 1981; 51:363–368.
27. Gastineau RM, Walsh PJ, Underwood N. Thickness of the bronchial epithelium with relation to exposure to radon. Health Phys 1972; 23:857–860.
28. Souders JE, George SC, Polissar NL, Swenson ER, Hlastala MP. Tracheal gas exchange: perfusion-related differences in inert gas elimination. J Appl Physiol 1995; 79:918–928.
29. Luchtel DL. The mucous layer of the trachea and major bronchi in the rat. Scanning Electron Micr 1978; 2:1089–1098.
30. Sleigh MA, Blake JR, Liron N. The propulsion of mucus by cilia. Am Rev Respir Dis 1988; 137:726–741.
31. Chilton TH, Colburn AP. Mass transfer (absorption) coefficients: prediction from data on heat transfer and fluid friction. Industr Eng Chem 1934; 26:1183–1187.
32. Hanna LM, Scherer PW. Measurement of local mass transport coefficients in a cast model of the human upper respiratory tract: J Biomech Eng 1986; 108:12–18.
33. Hanna LM, Scherer PW. A theoretical model of localized heat and water vapor transport in the human respiratory tract. J Biomech Eng 1986; 108:19–27.
34. Ingentio EP. Respiratory fluid mechanics and heat transfer.
35. Johnson CE, Linderoth LS. Deep diving respiratory heat and mass transfer. School of Engineering, Duke University, 1976.
36. Nuckols ML. Heat and water vapor transfer in the human respiratory system at hyperbaric conditions. 1981.
37. Tsu ME, Babb AL, Ralph DD, Hlastala MP. Dynamics of heat, water, and soluble gas exchange in the human airways: I. A model study. Ann Biomed Eng 1988; 16: 547–571.
38. McFadden ER, Pichurko BM, Bowman HF, Ingenito E, Burns S, Dowling N, Solway J. Thermal mapping of the airways in humans. J Appl Physiol 1985; 58:564–570.
39. Bird RB, Stewart WE, Lightfoot EN. Transport Phenomena. New York: John Wiley & Sons, 1960.
40. Lopez-Vidriero MT, Das I, Reid LM. Respiratory defense mechanisms. Brain, Proctor, Read, eds. New York: Marcel Dekker, 1977:289–356.
41. Cander L. Solubility of inert gases in human lung tissue. J Appl Physiol 1959; 14: 538–540.
42. Carles AC, Kawashiro T, Piiper J. Solubility of various inert gases in rat skeletal muscle. Pflugers Arch 1975; 359:209–218.
43. Gargas ML, Burgess RJ, Voisard DE, Cason GH, Andersen ME. Partition coefficients of low-molecular-weight volatile chemicals in various liquids and tissues. Toxicol Appl Pharmacol 1989; 98:87–99.
44. Meyer M, Tebbe U, Piiper J. Solubility of inert gases in dog blood and skeletal muscle. Pflugers Arch 1980; 384:131–134.
45. Ohta Y, Ar A, Farhi LE. Solubility and partition coefficients for gases in rabbit brain and blood. J Appl Physiol 1979; 46:1169–1170.

46. Perbellini L, Brugnone F, Caretta D, Maranelli G. Paritition coefficients of some industrial aliphatic hydrocarbons (C5-C7) in blood and human tissues. Br J Industr Med 1985; 42:162–167.
47. Young IH, Wagner PD. Solubility of inert gases in homogenates of canine lung tissue. J Appl Physiol 1979; 46:1207–1210.
48. Wagner PD, Naumann PF, Laravuso RB. Simultaneous measurement of eight foreign gases in blood by gas chromatography. J App Physiol 1974; 36:600–605.
49. Deffebach ME, Charan NB, Lakshminarayan S, Butler J. The bronchial circulation: small, but a vital attribute of the lung. Am Rev Respir Dis 1987; 135:463–481.
50. Laitinen LA, Laitinen A. The bronchial circulation. Butler, ed. New York: Marcel Dekker, 1992:79–106.
51. Solway J. Airway heat and water fluxes and the tracheobronchial circulation. Eur Respir J 1990; 3:608s–617s.
52. Agostoni P, Godden DJ, Baile EM. The bronchial circulation. In: Butler, ed. New York: Marcel Dekker, 1992:181–196.
53. Agostoni PG, Arena V, Biglioli P, Doria E, Sala A, Susini G. Increase of alveolar pressure reduces systemic-to-pulmonary bronchial blood flow in humans. Chest 1989; 96:1081–1085.
54. Baile EM, Ling H, Heyworth J, Hogg JC, Pare PD. Bronchopulmonary anastomotic and noncoronary collarteral blood flow in humans during total cardiopulmonary bypass. Chest 1985; 6:749–754.
55. Deal CW, Louis E, Kerth WJ, Osborne JJ, Gerbode F. Bronchopulmonary precapillary blood flow during cardiopulmonary bypass. Am Heart J 1968; 75:43–48.
56. Baile EM, Nelems HMB, Schulzer M, Pare PD. Measurement of regional bronchial arterial blood flow and bronchovascular resistance in dogs. J Appl Physiol 1982; 53:1044–1049.
57. Bernard SL, Glenny RW, Polisar N, Luchtel DL, Lakshminarayan S. Distribution of pulmonary and bronchial blood supply to airways measured by fluorescent microspheres. J Appl Physiol 1996; 80:430–436.
58. Charan NB, Turk GM, Dhand R. Gross and subgross anatomy of bronchial circulation in sheep. J Appl Physiol 1984; 57:658–664.
59. Hughes T. Microcirculation of the tracheobronchial circulation. Nature 1965; 205: 425–426.
60. Laitinen A, Laitinen LA, Moss R, Widdicombe JG. Organisation and structure of the tracheal and bronchial blood vessels in the dog. J Anat 1989; 165:133–140.
61. Sobin SS, Frasher WG, Tremer HM, Hadley GG. The microcirculation of the tracheal mucosa. Angiology 1963; 14:165–170.
62. Ingenito EP, Solway J, McFadden ER, Pichurko BM, Cravalho ER, Drazen JM. Finite difference analysis of respiratory heat transfer. J Appl Physiol 1986; 61: 2252–2259.
63. Saidel GM, Kruse KL, Primiano FP. Model simulation of heat and water transport dynamics in an airway. J Biomech Eng 1983; 105:189–193.
64. Newman WH, Lele PP. A transient heating technique for the measurement of thermal properties of perfused biological tissue. J Biomech Eng 1985; 107:219–227.
65. Davidson MR, Schroter RC. A theoretical model of absorption of gases by the bronchial wall. J Fluid Mech 1983; 129:313–335.

66. Davies CN. Absorption of gases in the respiratory tract. Ann Occup Hyg 1985; 29: 13–25.
67. McFadden ER, Jr. Heat and water exchange in human airways. Am Rev Respir Dis 1992; 146:S8–S10.
68. Ray DW, Ingenito EP, Strek M, Schumacker PT, Solway J. Longitudinal distribution of canine respiratory heat and water exchanges. J Appl Physiol 1989; 66: 2788–2798.
69. Tsu ME, Babb AL, Sugiyama EM, Hlastala MP. Dynamics of soluble gas exchange in the airways: II. Effects of breathing conditions. Respir Physiol 1991; 83:261–276.
70. Cramer I. Heat and moisture exchange of respiratory mucous membranes. Ann Otol Rhinol Laryngol 1957; 66:327–343.
71. Inglestedt S. Studies on the conditioning of air in the respiratory tract. Acta Otolaryngol Suppl 1956; 131: – .
72. Tsai CL, Saidel GM, McFadden JER, Fouke JM. Radial heat and water transport across the airway wall. J Appl Physiol 1990; 69:222–231.
73. Fox GR, Hayward JS. Effect of hypothermia on breath-alcohol analysis. J Forens Sci 1987; 32:320–325.
74. Fox GR, Hayward JS. Effect of hyperthermia on breath-alcohol analysis. J Forens Sci 1989; 34:836–841.
75. Schoknecht G, Hahlbrauck B. Detection of extraneous gases in breath alcohol analysis. Blutalkohol 1992; 29:193–204.
76. Mulder JA, Neuteboom W. The effects of hypo- and hyperventilation on breath alcohol measurements. Blutalkohol 1987; 24:341–347.
77. Dubois AB, Rogers RM. Respiratory factors determining the tissue concentrations of inhaled substances. Respir Physiol 1968; 5:34–52.
78. Schrikker ACM, de Vries WR, Zwart A, Luijendijk SCM. Uptake of highly soluble gases in the epithelium of the conducting airways. Pflugers Arch 1985; 405:389–394.
79. Schrikker ACM, de Vries WR, Zwart A, Luijendijk SCM. The excretion of highly soluble gases by the lung in man. Pflugers Arch 1989; 415:214–219.
80. Wagner PD, Saltzman HA, West JB. Measurement of continuous distributions of ventilation-perfusion ratios: theory. J Appl Physiol 1974; 36:588–599.
81. Wanner A, Barker JA, Long WM, Mariassy AT, Chediak AD. Measurement of airway mucosal perfusion and water volume with an inert soluble gas. J Appl Physiol 1988; 65:264–271.
82. Dahl AR, Snipes MB, Gerde P. Sites for uptake of inhaled vapors in beagle dogs. Toxicol Appl Pharmacol 1991; 109:263–275.
83. Jorens PG, VanOverveld FJ, Bult H, Vermeire PA, Herman AG. L-arginine-dependent production of nitrogen oxides by rat pulonary macrophages. Eur J Pharmacol 1991; 200:205–209.
84. Rimele TJ, Sturm RJ, Adams LM, Henry DE, Heaslip RJ, Weichman BM, Grimes D. Interaction of neutrophils with smooth muscle: identification of a neutrophil-derived relaxing factor. J Pharmacol Exp Ther 1988; 245:102–111.
85. Bissonnette EY, Hogaboam CM, Wallace JL, Befus AD. Potentiation of tumor necrosis factor-a-medicated cytotoxicity of mast cells by their production of nitric oxide. J Immunol 1991; 147:3060–3065.

86. Jorens PG, VanOverveld FJ, Bult H, Vermeire PA, Herman AG. Synergism between interleukin-1 beta and interferon-gamma, an inducer of nitric oxide synthase, in rat lung fibroblasts. Eur J Pharmacol 1992; 224:7–12.
87. Busse R, Mulsch A. Induction of nitric oxide synthases by cytokines in vascular smooth muscle cells. Fed Exp Biol Soc Lttr 1990; 275:87–90.
87. Ignarro LJ, Byrns RE, Buga GM, Wood KS. Endothelium-derived relaxing factor from pulmonary artery and vein possesses pharmacologic and chemical properties identical to those of nitric oxide radical. Circ Res 1987; 61:866–879.
88. Kobzik L, Bredt D, Lowenstein C, Snyder SH, Drazen JM, Sugarbaker D, Stamler JS. Nitric oxide synthase in human and rat lung. Am J Respir Cell Mol Biol 1993; 9:371–377.
89. Borland C, Cox Y, Higenbottam T. Measurement of exhaled nitric oxide in man. Thorax 1993; 48:1160–1162.
90. Persson MG, Wiklund NP, Gustafsson LE. Endogenous nitric oxide in single exhalations and the change during exercise. Am Rev Respir Dis 1993; 148:1210–1214.
91. Norman V, Keith CH. Nitrogen oxides in tobacco smoke. Nature 1965; 205:915–916.
92. Kharitonov SA, Yates D, Robbins RA, Logan-Sinclair R, Shinebourne EA, Barnes PJ. Increased nitric oxide in exhaled air of asthmatic patients. Lancet 1994; 343: 133–135.
93. Nakayama DK, Geller DA, Lowenstein CJ. Cytokines and lipopolysaccharide induce nitric oxide synthase in cultured rat pulmonary artery smooth muscle. Am J Respir Cell Mol Biol 1992; 7:471–476.
94. Schedin U, Frostell C, Persson MG, Jakobsson J, Anderson G, Gustafsson LE. Contribution from upper and lower airways to exhaled endogenous nitric oxide in humans. Acta Anaesthesiol Scand 1995; 39:327–332.

9

Kinetic Determinants of Inhaled Reactive Gas Absorption

AKHIL BIDANI and EDWARD M. POSTLETHWAIT

University of Texas Medical Branch
Galveston, Texas

I. Introduction

Pollutant gases such as ozone (O_3), nitrogen dioxide (NO_2), and sulfur dioxide (SO_2), undergo reactive absorption at specific sites within the tracheobronchial tree. O_3 is a ubiquitous oxidant pollutant produced from reaction between nitrogen oxides and volatile organic compounds, which are emitted from anthropogenic and natural sources (1). O_3 reacts with a broad spectrum of biomolecules and, thus, can be toxic to humans, animals, and vegetation (2). On the other hand, NO_2 is produced primarily from spontaneous oxidation of its precursor, nitric oxide (NO), and occurs predominantly as a consequence of high temperature combustion processes. There is the potential of intrapulmonary generation of gas-phase NO_2 during therapeutic inhaled nitric oxide (NO) administration. NO_2 exists as a free radical and, therefore, like O_3, initiates an exposure-induced oxidative stress (3). Both of these oxidants have been implicated as major potential contributors to environmentally induced lung disease. SO_2 is also derived from combustions (sulfure-containing fuels) but is less chemically reactive and exhibits substantially greater aqueous solubility than either O_3 of NO_2 (4). Upon inhalation, SO_2 induces bronchoactivity, especially in those individuals with hyperactive airways.

This brief review summarizes a few of the important conceptual building blocks that are necessary to investigate the determinants of inhaled reactive gas absorption. We reserve the word reactive for inhaled gases that react primarily (if not exclusively) with the airway and aveolar epithelium. Both CO_2 and O_2 also undergo complex reactions in blood, but these are not the focus of this review. Interested readers are referred to other sources for those gases (5–7). This review of reactive gas absorption relies heavily on the previous work of Miller and coworkers (8–12), Overton and coworkers (13–16), Hanna et al. (17), Seinfeld (18), and Ultman and coworkers (19–21). In this chapter, physicochemical properties and their relationship to tissue dose (Section II) are discussed. The effect of phase-equilibria on reactive gas absorption (Section III) is discussed, followed by a summary of the effects of reaction kinetics on mass transfer (Section IV). In Section V, some lumped and distributed mathematical models of upper and lower airways reactive gas absorption are summarized. In Section VI, the use of mathematical models in the interpretation of selected experimental studies of reactive gas absorption is reviewed. In Section VII, an innovative method to noninvasively estimate reactive gas absorption in humans is presented (21). In Section VIII, the most important issues related to inhaled reactive gas absorption are summarized. A list of symbols is provided as Table 1.

II. Gas Physicochemical Properties and Tissue Dose

Inhaled reactive gases have the potential to cause abnormalities in biochemical, functional, and structural properties of the airway epithelium. The nature of injury depends on the mechanism of interaction of the inhaled gas with the target tissues whereas the extent of injury depends on the local concentration of the inhaled toxicant gas. When a toxic gas is inhaled, its transport through the highly branched tracheobronchial tree results in a unique distribution of concentration within the airways based on the ratio of regional delivery of the inhaled gas to the local rate of gas uptake (19,20). Unlike most of the respiratory gases that interact minimally with the airway epithelium and flux across the alveolar-capillary barrier, inhaled reactive gases can undergo complex biochemical interactions with the airway lining liquid and are thus locally quenched. Even though the quantitation of respiratory gas flux is possible from measurements of the rate of uptake into blood or excretion from blood, toxic inhaled gases interact primarily with the airway and alveolar epithelium, so that there is no simple effluent stream to monitor the rate of inhaled gas uptake by the pulmonary tissues.

The determination of the appropriate definition of dose from which to establish the dose–biological response is fundamental to the assessment of envi-

Table 1 List of Symbols

Symbol	Definition
a	airway perimeter
A_C	Cross-sectional area
$C_{AG\infty}$	Bulk gas-phase concentration of A
$C^*_{AG\infty}$	Gas-phase concentration of A in the liquid-phase that would be in equilibrium with the bulk gas-phase partial pressure, $p_{AG\infty}$
C_{AGi}	Interfacial gas-phase concentration of A
$C_{AL\infty}$	Bulk liquid-phase concentration of A
d	Tube diameter
D_{AG}	Gas-phase diffusion coefficient of A
D_{AL}	Liquid-phase diffusion coefficient of A
D_{Ar}	Diffusion coefficient of reacted species A
D_{LNO_2}	Overall diffusing capacity for NO_2
F_{PA}	Fractional penetration of A
H_{SO_2}	Henry's law constant for SO_2
$\bar{H}_{SO_2}$	Modified Henry's law constant for SO_2
$\tilde{H}_{SO_2}$	Dimensionless capacitance coefficient for SO_2
k_{rA}	Reaction rate constant for A
k_{mGA}	Gas-phase mass transfer coefficient for A
k_{mLA}	Liquid-phase mass transfer coefficient for A
K_{mGA}	Overall gas-phase mass transfer coefficient for A
K_{mLA}	Overall liquid-phase mass transfer coefficient for A
K_{mNO_2}	Overall mass transfer coefficient for NO_2
$\bar{K}_i$	Equilibrium constant for species i
L	Tube length
M_A	Rate of mass transfer of A
N_{Da}	Damkohler number
N_{Ha}	Hatta number
N_{Pe}	Peclet number
N_{Re}	Reynolds number
N_{Sc}	Schmidt number
N_{Sh}	Sherwood number
p_{SO_2}	Partial pressure of SO_2
$p_{AG\infty}$	Bulk gas-phase partial pressure of A
p_{AGi}	Interfacial gas-phase partial pressure A
$P_{AL\infty}$	Bulk liquid-phase partial pressure of A
$p^*_{AL\infty}$	Gas-phase partial pressure of A that would be in equilibrium with the bulk liquid-phase concentration, $C_{AL\infty}$
R	Universal gas constant
S	Surface area for gas absorption
T	Absolute temperature
U_A	Uptake coefficient for A
α	Physical solubility coefficient

(continued)

Table 1 Continued

β_{SO_2}	Reactive capacitance coefficient for SO_2
δ_G	Gas-phase interfacial film thickness
δ_L	Liquid-phase interfacial film thickness
ξ	Dimensionless reaction enhancement factor
$\eta_{R,E}$	Dimensionless external reaction effectiveness factor
ϕ	Fractional flux (mass transfer flux in the presence of reaction/mass transfer flux in the absence of reactions)
Γ	Dimensionless radial mass-transfer parameter

ronmental risk assessment and to evaluate the biological effects attributable to inhaled airborne toxicants. Although some data relate pollutant gas exposure to biological response, the critical relations between exposure and dose, and dose and response are less well defined. This is primarily because it has been problematic to quantify pollutant inhaled gas dose accurately. Dose could be expressed in various ways: the total mass of ozone absorbed by the total respiratory tract or specific regions within the respiratory tract, or the amount of ozone absorbed per unit of lung surface area, volume, or target cell. One approach has been to calculate dose based solely on exposure parameters, neglecting gas absorption by the respiratory tract. One such calculated parameter is the cumulative dose, which is useful for animal studies because it is based on the product of inhaled gas concentration and exposure time (22). Another parameter is the effective dose, which is more accurate because it accounts for breathing pattern. Effective dose is expressed either as the product of inhaled gas concentration in the air being breathed, volume of air inhaled in 1 minute of ventilation (minute ventilation), and exposure time (23), or as a mathematical function that gives these factors different weights (24,25). It is also necessary to estimate tissue dose from inhaled dose. A straightforward approach is to determine the distribution of the absorbed mass along the respiratory tract surface and to correlate this dose with the regional biological response. At present, however, air sampling measurements within the confined space of the lung are limited to the larger proximal airways of humans, and functional changes as indicators of response (such as airway hyperreactivity) are difficult to localize to a specific lung region or, as in peripheral airways, are often difficult to detect.

The dose of a reactive inhaled gas to the target tissues in the respiratory tract is dependent on several factors: 1. the ambient reactive gas concentration; 2. the amount of inhaled gas inspired into the respiratory tract during exposure; 3. the amount of inhaled reactive gas absorbed in the mouth, nose, and airways upstream of the target tissues; 4. the amount of reactive gas absorbed in the lower airways and acini; 5. the amount of reactive gas that reacts with the mucus and surfactant overlying the target tissues; and 6. the amount of reactive gas and reactive products that ultimately reach and react with the target cells. The first two factors can be quantified with reasonable accuracy. The challenge has been to accurately quantify the latter four factors. Among these, accurate measurements of the regional distribution of reactive gas absorption within the respiratory tract have remained a challenging but critical step in determining the dose of inhaled reactive gas and its relationship to lung injury.

A complete description of mass transport of an inhaled reactive gas consists of three main elements: the mass conservation equation, rate equations for diffusion and chemical reaction with appropriate coupling, and thermodynamic phase-equilibrium expressions. Our review of reactive gas absorption relies heavily on the vast body of engineering and related literature (26–34) wherein sophisticated analytical methods exist for analysis of the complex interactions among convective, diffusive, and reactive processes. Application of the principles of fluid mechanics, transport phenomena, and reaction engineering is necessary for the quantitative delineation of the rate-limiting steps in reactive gas absorption in the lungs.

III. Effect of Ionic Equilibria on Reactive Gas Absorption

The equilibrium between physically dissolve gas and its partial pressure is represented by the Henry's law coefficient for physical solubility, H (or alternatively by the Bunsen solubility coefficient, α). Table 2 lists the Henry's law coefficients of some selected gases in water at 25°C. These values reflect only the

Table 2 Henry's Law Coefficients for Selected Respiratory and Toxicant Gases (Dissolved in Water at 25°C)

Species	H (M/atm)
O_2	1.3×10^{-3}
NO	1.9×10^{-3}
O_3	9.4×10^{-3}
NO_2	1.0×10^{-2}
CO_2	3.4×10^{-2}
SO_2	1.24
HNO_2	49.0
NH_3	62.0
H_2O_2	7.1×10^{4}
HNO_3	2.1×10^{5}

physical solubility of each gas, regardless of the subsequent fate of the dissolved gas. Several of these species, once dissolved, either undergo acid-based equilibrium reactions or react with biological substrates. The relevant principles of phase equilibria as they relate to dissolution of nonreactive gases in solution have been discussed in Chapter 8. Here, the focus is on the effect of ionization reactions on gas solubility (18,35,36). Chemical reaction equilibria impose additional constraints on aqueous concentrations of a dissolved species. As an example, consider the absorption of SO_2, which results in the following equilibria:

$$SO_2(g) + H_2O \rightleftarrows SO_2 \cdot H_2O \tag{1}$$

$$SO_2 \cdot H_2O \rightleftarrows H^+ + HSO_3^- \tag{2}$$

$$HSO_3^- \rightleftarrows H^+ + SO_3^{--} \tag{3}$$

with the equilibrium constants ($\overline{K}$'s) defined as

$$\overline{K}_{hs} = \frac{[SO_2 \cdot H_2O]}{p_{SO_2}} \tag{4}$$

$$\overline{K}_{s1} = \frac{[H^+]\,[HSO_3^-]}{[SO_2 \cdot H_2O]} \tag{5}$$

$$\overline{K}_{s2} = \frac{[H^+]\,[SO_3^{--}]}{[HSO_3^-]} \tag{6}$$

The concentration of the dissolved species are given by

$$[SO_2 \cdot H_2O] = \overline{K}_{hs}\, p_{SO_2} \tag{7}$$

$$[HSO_3^-] = \frac{\overline{K}_{s1}\,[SO_2 \cdot H_2O]}{[H^+]} = \frac{\overline{K}_{hs}\,\overline{K}_{s1}\,p_{SO_2}}{[H^+]} \tag{8}$$

$$[SO_3^{--}] = \frac{\overline{K}_{s2}\,[HSO_3^-]}{[H^+]} = \frac{\overline{K}_{hs}\,\overline{K}_{s1}\,\overline{K}_{s2}\,p_{SO_2}}{[H^+]^2} \tag{9}$$

The additional relationship among the concentration of the ions in solution is that of electroneutrality:

$$[H^+] = [OH^-] + [HSO_3^-] + 2[SO_3^{--}] \tag{10}$$

Using the equations for $[OH^-]$, $[HSO_3^-]$, and $[SO_3^{--}]$ and the equilibrium constant for dissociation of water (K_w) in Equation 10 yields the following:

$$[H^+] = \frac{\overline{K}_w}{[H^+]} + \frac{\overline{K}_{hs}\overline{K}_{s1}p_{SO_2}}{[H^+]} + \frac{2\overline{K}_{hs}\overline{K}_{s1}\overline{K}_{s2}p_{SO_2}}{[H^+]^2} \tag{11}$$

which may be written in terms of $[H^+]$ as

$$[H^+]^3 - (\overline{K}_w + \overline{K}_{hs}\overline{K}_{s1}p_{SO_2})\,[H^+] - 2\overline{K}_{hs}\overline{K}_{s1}\overline{K}_{s2}p_{SO_2} = 0 \qquad (12)$$

For a given temperature, which determines the values of $\overline{K}_w$, $\overline{K}_{hs}$, $\overline{K}_{s1}$, $\overline{K}_{s2}$, and p_{SO_2}, $[H^+]$ (or pH) can be determined from Equation 12. Once $[H^+]$ is known, all the other concentrations can be calculated from Equations 8 and 9. The total concentration of SO_2 in solution, including physically dissolved SO_2 and that in the form of HSO_3^- and SO_3^{--} is given by

$$[SO_2]_{total} = [SO_2 \cdot H_2O] + [HSO_3^-] + [SO_3^{--}] \qquad (13)$$

The total cconcentration of SO_2 ($[SO_2]_{total}$) can be related to the partial pressure of SO_2 by

$$[SO_2]_{total} = \overline{K}_{hs}p_{SO_2}\left(1 + \frac{\overline{K}_{s1}}{[H^+]} + \frac{\overline{K}_{s1}\overline{K}_{s2}}{[H^+]^2}\right) \qquad (14)$$

Because $\overline{K}_{hs}$ is identical to the Henry's law coefficient H_{SO_2}, one can express $[SO_2]_{total}$ in terms of a modified Henry's law coefficient, $\overline{H}_{SO_2}$:

$$[SO_2]_{total} = \overline{H}_{SO_2}p_{SO_2} \qquad (15)$$

$$\overline{H}_{SO_2} = H_{SO_2}\left(1 + \frac{K_{s1}}{[H^+]} + \frac{K_{s1}K_{s2}}{[H^+]^2}\right) \qquad (16)$$

Because by Equation 16, $\overline{H}_{SO_2}$ is always greater than H_{SO_2}, it can be seen that the total amount of SO_2 always exceeds that predicted by Henry's law alone. This example illustrates the ability of a reversible chemical reaction to increase the absorptive capacity of an aqueous solution for a soluble gas. It can also be noted that $[SO_2]_{total}$ is quite pH dependent.

Alternatively, one can express $[SO_2]_{total}$ as the sum of the physically dissolved SO_2 and that in the reacted forms:

$$[SO_2]_{total} = [SO_2]_{phys\ sol} + [SO_2]_{reacted} \qquad (17)$$

Based on Equation 17, it is possible to define a reactive capacitance coefficient (β_{SO_2}):

$$\beta_{SO_2} = \left(\frac{d[SO_2]_{reacted}}{dp_{SO_2}}\right) = H_{SO_2}\left(\frac{\overline{K}_{s1}}{[H^+]} + \frac{\overline{K}_{s2}}{[H^+]^2}\right) \qquad (18)$$

or, alternatively, a dimensionless capacitance coefficient ($\tilde{H}_{SO_2}$):

$$\tilde{H}_{SO_2} = \left(\frac{\overline{H}_{SO_2}}{H_{SO_2}}\right) = 1 + \frac{\overline{K}_{s1}}{[H^+]} + \frac{\overline{K}_{s2}}{[H^+]^2} \qquad (19)$$

Figure 1*A* illustrates the aqueous concentration of $[SO_2]_{total}$, $[HSO_3^-]$, and $[SO_2]$ plotted against the partial pressure of SO_2. These concentrations were

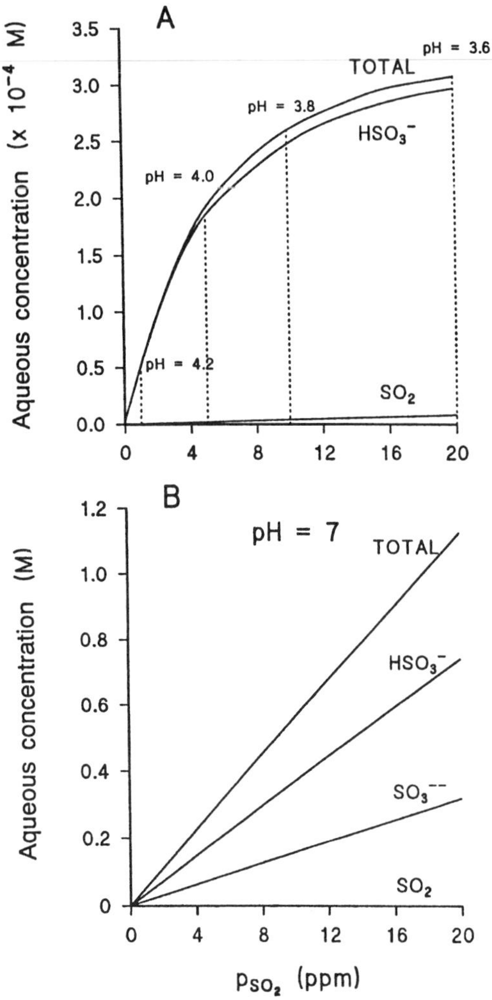

Figure 1 Relationship between total SO_2 content and SO_2 partial pressure (p_{SO_2}) at 37°C in pure water. **A**, Variable solution pH (near-zero buffer capacity). **B**, pH maintained at 7.0 (infinite buffer capacity).

obtained for each p_{SO_2}, by first estimating $[H^+]$ using Equation 12. This $[H^+]$ was then used to estimate $[SO_2]_{total}$ and $[HSO_3^-]$. Figure 1*A* indicates that there is a dramatic decline in pH of the unbuffered solution during SO_2 absorption. Mucus and epithelial tissues are expected to have significant nonbicarbonate buffer capacity because of the presence of proteins and phosphate. This high buffer capacity would aid in blunting the pH change associated with SO_2 absorption. For the hypothetical case of "perfect buffering," so that pH is maintained at 7.0, there is dramatic increase in the predicted absorptive capacity over the same range of p_{SO_2} (see Figure 1*B*), an almost 1000-fold increment in $[SO_2]_{total}$. These calculations suggest that the in vivo SO_2 dissociation curve is very sensitive to the nonbicarbonate buffer capacity of the relevant compartment.

IV. Effect of Reaction Kinetics on Mass Transfer

A. Overall Mass Transfer Coefficient

Mass transfer across the interfaces between gases and liquids can be described using a two-film model (gas-film and liquid-film) (27–29,32,34). The rate of mass transfer of gas "A" through the gas-side film is

$$\dot{M}_{AG} = k_{mAG}\, S(C_{AG\infty} - C_{AGi}) = \left(\frac{k_{mAG}}{RT}\right) S\,(p_{AG\infty} - p_{AGi}) \tag{20}$$

where k_{mAG} is the gas-phase mass transfer coefficient, S is the surface area for gas absorption, R is the universal gas content, T is the absolute temperature, $p_{AG\infty}$ is the bulk-phase partial pressure, and p_{AGi} is the interfacial partial pressure. Similarly, the rate of mass transfer through the liquid-side film is given by

$$\dot{M}_{AL} = k_{mAL}\, S\,(C_{ALi} - C_{AL\infty}) \tag{21}$$

At steady state, $\dot{M}_{AG} = \dot{M}_{AL}$:

$$\dot{M}_{A} = \left(\frac{k_{mAG}}{RT}\right) S\,(p_{AG\infty} - p_{AGi}) = k_{mAL}\, S\,(C_{ALi} - c_{AL\infty}) \tag{22}$$

The overall rate of steady-state interfacial gas transfer can be expressed as

$$\dot{M}_{A} = K_{mAG}\, S\left(p_{AG\infty} - \frac{C_{AL\infty}}{H_A}\right) = K_{mAL}\, S\,(H_A p_{AG\infty} - C_{AL\infty}) \tag{23}$$

where K_{mAG} and K_{mAL} represent the overall gas-phase and liquid-phase mass transfer coefficients and are defined as

$$K_{mAG} = \frac{1}{\left(\frac{RT}{k_{mAG}}\right) + \left(\frac{1}{k_{mAL}H_A}\right)} \tag{24}$$

$$K_{mAL} = \frac{1}{\left(\frac{RTH_A}{k_{mAG}}\right) + \left(\frac{1}{k_{mAL}}\right)} \tag{25}$$

It is customary to rewrite Equation 23 as

$$\dot{M}_A = K_{mAG}\, S\, (p_{AG\infty} - p^*_{AL\infty}) = K_{mAL}\, S\, (C^*_{AG\infty} - C_{AL\infty}) \tag{26}$$

where ($p^*_{AL\infty}$) is the partial pressure of A in the gas-phase that would be in equilibrium with the bulk liquid concentration, $C_{AL\infty}$; and ($C^*_{AG\infty}$) is the concentration of A in the liquid-phase that would be in equilibrium with the bulk gas-phase pressure of A, $p_{AG\infty}$.

Equations 24 and 25 can often be simplified for systems in which most of the mass transfer resistance lies in either the gas-phase interfacial film or the liquid-phase interfacial film. When solute gas A is very soluble in the liquid-phase (i.e., H_A is very large), then $1/(k_{mAL}\, H_A) \rightarrow 0$, and $K_{mAG} = k_{mAG}/(RT)$. For this case, the overall rate of interfacial transfer is determined by the gas-phase mass transfer coefficient, and the overall rate of gas uptake is said to be *gas-phase limited*. On the other hand, when A is very insoluble (i.e., H_A is very low), $1/(k_{mAL}\, H_A) \gg (RT)/k_{mAG}$ and $K_{mAG} = k_{mAL}$. Therefore, for this case, the overall rate of interfacial transfer is determined by the liquid-phase mass transfer coefficient, and the overall rate of gas uptake is said to be *liquid-phase limited* (28,29,32,34).

B. Reactivity of Inhaled Gases

For purposes of modeling pollutant gas uptake, Dahl (37) has suggested that inhaled gases can be divided into three categories based on their chemical properties. This classification is based on the free energy (ΔF) of the appropriate reactions of the inhaled with biological constituents. For a reaction such as

$$A + B \rightleftarrows C + D \tag{27}$$

the equilibrium constant, $\overline{K}$, is given by

$$\overline{K} = \left(\frac{[C]\,[D]}{[A]\,[B]} \right) \tag{28}$$

The free energy of the reaction (ΔF, kcal/mol) is related to the equilibrium constant $\overline{K}$ by

$$\Delta F = -(RT)\,(\log_e \overline{K}) \tag{29}$$

For $\Delta F = 3$ kcal/mol, $\overline{K} = 0.0077$, indicating that ~99% of the reactants (A and B) are present at equilibrium. Conversely, if $\Delta F = -3$ kcal/mol, $\overline{K} = 130$, indicating that only 1% of the reactants (A and B) are present at equilibrium (37).

According to this scheme (37), the first category is that of stable molecules. These can be defined as compounds for which the free energy of a chemical reaction that occurs in a physiological system is greater than 3 kcal/mol. For such gases, at thermodynamic equilibrium, less than 1% are present as products and thus are unlikely to produce significant toxic products. The second category is that of reactive gases. These are gases that have both free energies of reaction of less than −3 kcal/mol and half-times for uncatalyzed chemical reactions in physiological systems of 10 minutes or less. Less than 1% of a reactive gas remains unreacted at thermodynamic equilibrium. The third category contains metabolizable gases. These are gases for which $\Delta F < -3$ kcal/mol, but that have half-times for uncatalyzed chemical reaction in physiological system of >10 minutes. For these cases, uncatalyzed reactions are so slow that they would behave like stable gases were it not for enzyme-catalyzed reactions (37).

C. Kinetic Analysis of a Surface Interfacial Reaction

In this discussion, we consider the case in which a gas-phase species "A" undergoes reaction at the gas-liquid interface. Because the reaction occurs at the surface rather than in the bulk liquid-phase, the rate of the reaction (r_{Ai}) must be expressed in terms of *moles reacted per unit area of surface per unit time*. For a first order surface reaction:

$$-r_{Ai} = k_{rA}\, S\, C_{AGi} \tag{30}$$

where the first order rate constant, k_{rA}, has the dimensions of length per unit time, instead of time^{-1} for a first order homogeneous reaction.

For a steady state, the rate of diffusive mass transfer, $\dot{M}_A$, from the bulk gas-phase across the gas-phase boundary layer, characterized by a gas mass transfer coefficient, k_{mGA}, must equal the rate of the surface reaction ($\dot{M}_A = -r_{Ai}$):

$$k_{mGA}\, S\, (C_{AG\infty} - C_{AGi}) = k_{rA}\, S\, C_{AGi} \tag{31}$$

The steady-state rate of mass transfer can be expressed in terms of an overall gas-phase mass transfer coefficient, K_{mGA}:

$$\dot{M}_A = K_{mGA}\, S\, C_{AG\infty} \tag{32}$$

$$K_{mGA} = \left(\frac{1}{\dfrac{1}{k_{mGA}} + \dfrac{1}{k_{rA}}} \right) \tag{33}$$

Equation 33 can be used to evaluate the relative importance of the gas mass transfer coefficient and the first order reaction rate constant for such in-series processes. For very fast reactions, $k_{rA} \gg k_{mGA}$, and the following is obtained:

$$\dot{M}_A \approx k_{mGA}\, S\, C_{AG\infty} \tag{34}$$

The overall rate of gas uptake can only be increased by increasing the rate of mass transfer (i.e., increasing either mass transfer coefficient or the bulk gas-phase solute concentration). This is then a *mass transfer–limited* process.

For very slow reactions, $k_{rA} \ll k_{mGA}$, and Equation 32 reduces to:

$$\dot{M}_A \approx k_{rA}\, S\, C_{AG\infty} \tag{35}$$

In this instance, the overall process is *reaction rate limited.* The overall rate of gas uptake in such a case can be enhanced by an increase in the reaction rate, such as by an elevated temperature.

Effectiveness factors have been used in the engineering literature to quantify the effects of microtransport on observed rates of reaction (26,30,31). The *external reaction effectiveness factor*, $\eta_{R,E}$, defines ratio of the *observed rate* of surface reaction to the *intrinsic reaction rate* in the absence of mass transfer limitations:

$$\eta_{R,E} = \left(\frac{\text{observed rate of surface reaction}}{\text{intrinsic rate of surface reaction}} \right) \tag{36}$$

The external reaction effectiveness factor thus lies between zero (severe mass transfer limitations) and 1 (no mass transfer limitation). For the first order surface reaction, Equation 30 represents the observed rate and Equation 35 the intrinsic rate. The dimensionless external effectiveness factor for A is thus

$$(\eta_{R,E})_A = \left(\frac{k_{mGA}}{k_{mGA} + k_{rA}} \right) \tag{37}$$

Another important dimensionless number used in the analysis of surface reactions is the *Damkohler number* (26,27,34), N_{Da}, defined as

$$N_{Da} = \left(\frac{\text{rate of reaction}}{\text{rate of mass transfer by molecular diffusion}} \right) \tag{38}$$

For a first order surface reaction and gas-phase film-diffusion model, the Damkohler number is given by

$$N_{Da} = \left(\frac{k_{rA}\, C_{AG\infty}}{k_{mGA}\, C_{AG\infty}} \right) = \left(\frac{k_{rA}}{k_{mGA}} \right) \tag{39}$$

Combining Equation 36 and Equation 39 yields the following relationship between the external effectiveness factor and the Damkohler number:

$$\eta_{R,E} = \left(\frac{1}{1 + N_{Da}} \right) \tag{40}$$

Thus, when the process is mass transfer limited (i.e., $k_{rA} \gg k_{mGA}$), N_{Da} is large and the effectiveness factor, $\eta_{R,E}$, approaches zero. At the other extreme, when the process is reaction rate limited (i.e., $k_{rA} \ll k_{mGA}$), N_{Da} is small and the effectiveness factor approaches 1.

D. Simplified Analysis of Interfacial Gas Transfer with Surface Chemical Reaction

To gain insight into the role of an irreversible chemical reaction on diffusive fluxes across a gas–liquid interface, we consider the example of diffusion of gas "A" from the bulk gas-phase ("G∞") to a gas-liquid interface ("i"), where the physically dissolved gas may either undergo an irreversible reaction to product "B" or diffuse into the bulk liquid phase ("L∞").

$$\mathrm{A(G\infty)} \xrightarrow[k_{mG}]{\text{diffusion}} \mathrm{A(i)} \tag{41}$$

$$\mathrm{A(i)} \xrightarrow[k_{r}]{\text{reaction}} \mathrm{B(i)} \tag{42}$$

$$\mathrm{A(i)} \xrightarrow[k_{mL}]{\text{diffusion}} \mathrm{A(L\infty)} \tag{43}$$

The gas and liquid phases are considered well mixed with bulk phase concentrations of $[A]_{G\infty}$ and $[A]_{L\infty}$, respectively. The change from $[A]_{G\infty}$ to $[A]_i$ occurs across a very thin gas film of thickness (δ_G) near the interface. Similarly, the change from $[A]_i$ to $[A]_{L\infty}$ occurs across a very thin liquid film of thickness (δ_L) near the gas–liquid interface. The diffusive fluxes from the bulk gas- and liquid-phase to the interface are given by

$$\dot{M}_{AG,diff} = \frac{D_{AG}}{\delta_G RT} S\,(p_{AG\infty} - p_{AGi}) = \left(\frac{k_{mGA}}{RT}\right) S\,(p_{AG\infty} - p_{AGi}) \tag{44}$$

$$\dot{M}_{AL,diff} = \frac{D_{AL}}{\delta_L} S\,(C_{ALi} - C_{AL\infty}) = S\,k_{mLA}\,(C_{ALi} - C_{AL\infty}) \tag{45}$$

In Equations 44 and 45, k_{mGA} and k_{mLA} represent film mass trasnfer coefficients, $k = D/\delta$, and S represents the interfacial surface area. The rate of the first order irreversible interfacial reaction can be represented in terms of a first order reaction rate constant, k_{rA}, as

$$\dot{M}_{Ai,react} = k_{rA}\,S\,C_{ALi} \tag{46}$$

At steady state, by mass balance $\dot{M}_{AG,diff} = \dot{M}_{AL,diff} + \dot{M}_{Ai,reac}$, so that the steady-state rate of mass transfer, using Henry's law ($C_{Li} = H\,p_{Gi}$), is given by

$$\dot{M}_A = \frac{S\,H_A\,p_{AG\infty}(k_{mLA} + k_{rA}) - S\,k_{mLA}\,C_{AL\infty}}{1 + \left(\frac{H_A R\,T}{k_{mGA}}\right)(k_{rA} + k_{mLA})} \tag{47}$$

For the case when $k_{mGA} \gg k_{mLA}$, k_{rA} and $C_{AL\infty} = 0$:

$$\dot{M}_A = S\,H_A\,(k_{rA} + k_{mLA})\,p_{AG\infty} \tag{48}$$

Thus, a plot of $\dot{M}_A$ versus $p_{AG\infty}$ should be a straight line with slope = S H_A (k_{rA} + k_{mLA}). For the cases when $k_{rA} \gg k_{mGA}$, k_{mLA}, or when $k_{mLA} \gg k_{mGA}$, k_{rA} and $C_{AL\infty}$ = 0:

$$\dot{M}_A = S\left(\frac{k_{mGA}}{RT}\right)p_{AG\infty} \tag{49}$$

For this case, a plot of $\dot{M}_A$ versus $p_{AG\infty}$ should be a straight line with slope = S $k_{mGA}/(RT)$.

E. Gas-Liquid Mass Transfer with Bulk Liquid-Phase Chemical Reaction

If it is assumed that the gas-phase resistance is negligible, then for diffusion of species A across a liquid film into the bulk liquid-phase, we evaluate the steady-state profile of A in the liquid film (thickness δ_L) in the absence and presence of a first order irreversible chemical reaction (28–32,34). A mass balance yields the following second order differential equation (30,31,34):

$$D_{AL}\left(\frac{d^2\,C_{AL}}{d\,x^2}\right) = k_{rA}\,C_{AL} \tag{50}$$

where k_{rA} is a first order reaction rate constant, and D_{AL} is the diffusion constant in the liquid-phase. The appropriate boundary conditions for this case are

$$C_{AL} = C_{ALi} \text{ at } x = 0;\ C_{AL} = C_{AL\infty} \text{ at } x = \delta_L \tag{51}$$

where C_{ALi} represents the surface concentration of A (in equilibrium with the gas-phase), and $C_{AL\infty}$ represents the bulk liquid-phase concentration of A, and δ_L is the thickness of the liquid film. The final solution is (34):

$$\left(\frac{C_{AL}}{C_{ALi}}\right) = \frac{1}{\sinh(s\delta_L)}\left[\frac{C_{ALi}}{C_{AL\infty}}\sinh\left(s\delta_L\,\frac{x}{\delta_L}\right) + \sinh\left(s\delta_L\left(1 - \frac{x}{\delta_L}\right)\right)\right] \tag{52}$$

where s is defined as

$$s = \sqrt{\frac{k_{rA}}{D_{AL}}}$$

The corresponding equation to describe the concentration profile in the absence of a chemical reaction is given by

$$C_{AL} = C_{ALi} - (C_{ALi} - C_{AL\infty})\left(\frac{x}{\delta_L}\right) \tag{53}$$

Thus, in the absence of a chemical reaction, the concentration profile is a straight line with a constant slope $(=(C_{ALi} - C_{AL\infty})/\delta_L)$. In the presence of a chemical reaction ($k_{rA} > 0$), the concentration profile is curvilinear (Figure 2). Comparison of these concentration profiles indicates that the effect of the chemical reaction is to steepen the concentration gradient within the liquid film and thus increase the flux of gas into the liquid–gas interface. The flux of gas into the liquid is

$$\dot{M}_A = -D_{AL}\, S\left(\frac{dC_{Ai}}{dx}\right)_{x=0} = (s\, D_{AL}\, S)\,\frac{C_{Ai}\cosh(s\delta_L) - C_{A\infty}}{\sinh(s\delta_L)} \tag{54}$$

If one defines the liquid mass transfer coefficient, $k_{mL}(=D_{AL}/\delta_L)$, then one can formulate the dimensionless Hatta number (N_{Ha}) (26,33):

$$N_{Ha} = (s)\,(\delta_L) = \frac{\sqrt{k_{rA}\, D_{AL}}}{k_{mLA}} \tag{55}$$

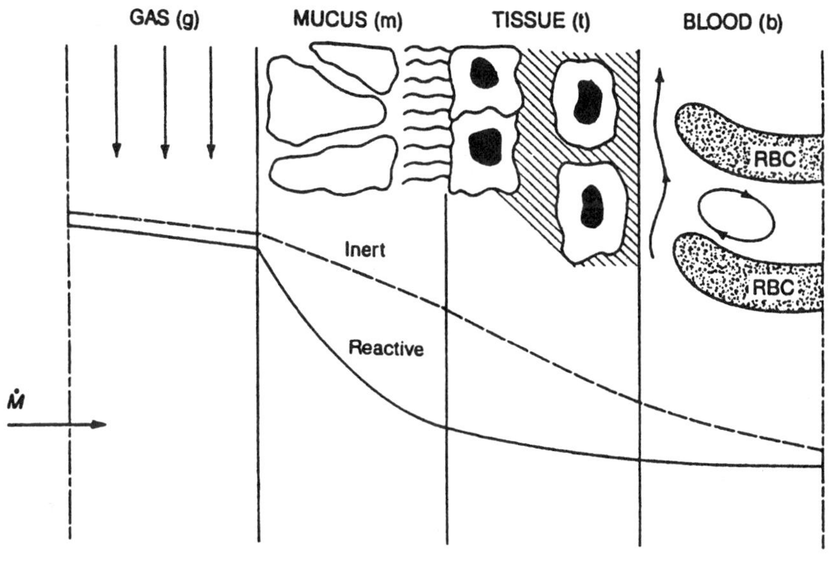

Figure 2 Schematic representation of the four-layer model of diffusion across the bronchial wall. The blood layer is represented as a continuous planar diffusion barrier, and, in vivo, the bronchial capillaries are sparsely distributed throughout the tissue layer. (From Ref. 20.)

The Hatta number is used to quantify flux enhancement at the gas–liquid interface when reaction accompanies mass transfer. It is analogous in function to the Thiele modulus in fluid–solid systems (27,28,30–32) and incorporates the mass transfer coefficient as well as the diffusion constant and the reaction rate constant. Thus, by explicitly incorporating the liquid mass transfer coefficient, k_{mLA}, the Hatta number includes the effects of all the three interacting processes, namely liquid-phase diffusion, reaction within the liquid-phase, and interphase mass transfer. The larger the Hatta number, the faster the reaction rate relative to the rate of mass transfer. Extremely fast reactions are characterized by $N_{Ha} > 3$, whereas extremely slow reactions are characterized by $N_{Ha} < 0.3$. Substituting the equation for Hatta number (Equation 55) in Equation 54, we obtain the expression for mass transfer flux in the presence of chemical reaction:

$$(\dot{M}_A)_{\text{with reaction}} = \frac{k_{mLA}\, S\, N_{Ha}}{\tanh(N_{Ha})}\left(C_{ALi} - \frac{C_{AL\infty}}{\cosh(N_{Ha})}\right) \tag{56}$$

In the absence of a chemical reaction:

$$(\dot{M}_A)_{\text{without reaction}} = k_{mLA}\, S\, (C_{ALi} - C_{AL\infty}) \tag{57}$$

For the special case in which bulk concentration is zero (i.e., $C_{AL\infty} = 0$), one can define another useful dimensionless ratio known as the *reaction-enhancement factor*, ξ (30,31,34):

$$\xi = \left(\frac{\dot{M}_{\text{with reaction}}}{\dot{M}_{\text{without reaction}}}\right) = \frac{N_{Ha}}{\tanh(N_{Ha})} \tag{58}$$

The enhancement factor ξ relates the gas flux that occurs in the presence of reaction to that which occurs in the absence of reaction. In equation 58, as the Hatta number increases, $\tanh(N_{Ha}) \rightarrow 1$, and the enhancement factor approaches the value of the Hatta number itself.

F. Overall Mass Transfer Coefficients in the Presence of Chemical Reactions

Ultman (20) has provided a summary of the phenomenological equations necessary to estimate individual mass transfer coefficients for different kinetic and flow conditions (Table 3). For mass transfer across an airway segment (or alveolar capillary barrier), there are four major barriers to be considered: gas phase ("G"), the mucus layer ("Mu") (or surfactant-hypophase); lung tissue ("T") (incorporating the epithelium, interstitium, and the endothelium), and blood ("B") (see Figure 2). Because gas tensions at air/mucus, mucus/tissue, and tissue/blood are unknown, it is necessary to compute overall uptake from gas-phase partial pressure, p_{AG}, and blood gas tension, p_{AB}. The rate of steady-state inert gas ab-

Table 3 Mathematical Relationships for Individual Mass Transfer Coefficients

Condition	Mass Transfer Coefficient, k_m
Stationary barrier of thickness δ	
Nonreactive gas	$\left(\frac{D_A}{\delta}\right)$
Reactive gas at equilibrium	$\left(\frac{D_A}{\delta}\right)+\left(\frac{\beta_A D_{Ar}}{H_A\delta}\right)$
Reactive gas, first order kinetics	$\left(\frac{D_A N_{Ha}}{\delta}\right)$
Boundary-layer diffusion in tube of diameter d and length L	$\left(\frac{D_A}{\delta}\right) c\,(N_{Re})^m (N_{Sc})^n \left(\frac{d}{L}\right)$

sorption is a function of the overall mass transfer coefficient, K_{mA}, and the overall driving force $(p_{AG} - p_{AB})$:

$$\dot{M}_A = K_{mA}\, S\, (p_{AG} - p_{AB}) \tag{59}$$

Because the four mass transfer resistances are in series, the overall mass transfer coefficient is related to the sum of the resistance offered by each barrier:

$$K_{mA} = \frac{1}{\left(\frac{RT}{k_{mA}}\right)_G + \left(\frac{1}{H_A k_{mA}}\right)_{Muc} + \left(\frac{1}{H_A k_{mA}}\right)_T + \left(\frac{1}{H_A k_{mA}}\right)_B} \tag{60}$$

Because K_{mA} is a harmonic mean, its value is determined by the phase having the smallest mass transfer conductance ($=H_A \cdot k_{mA}$), or the largest mass transfer resistance ($=1/(H_A \cdot k_{mA})$). For species that undergo chemical reaction, the flux is progressively reduced by the fractional conversion. To account for chemical reactions, say, in mucus and tissue, one can use a flux fraction, ϕ, to weigh the respective mass transfer resistance (20):

$$K'_{mA} = \frac{1}{\left(\frac{RT}{k_{mA}}\right)_G + \left(\frac{1}{H_A k_{mA}}\right)_{Muc} + \left(\frac{\phi_m}{H_A k_{mA}}\right)_T + \left(\frac{\phi_m \phi_t}{H_A k_{mA}}\right)_B} \tag{61}$$

where the fractional flux ϕ (<1) increases the value of the overall mass transfer coefficient for a reactive gas relative to that for an inert gas (see Equation 61).

Using this formulation, Ultman (20) has estimated the individual mass transfer coefficients for all phases—gas, mucus, and tissue—as well as the overall mass transfer coefficients for SO_2 and O_3. The results of these calculations for SO_2 and O_3 are shown in Figure 3. Whereas the overall mass transfer coefficients for O_3 are higher than those for SO_2, the individual barrier conductance and the overall conductance ($=H \times k_m$) would be much higher for SO_2 than for O_3 because $H_{SO_2} \approx 160\ (H_{O_3})$. These results suggest that SO_2 should be almost completely absorbed within the upper airways, whereas O_3 absorption would be expected to be most significant in the distal conducting airways and proximal respiratory zone. A comparison of the values of the mass transfer conductance ($H_A \cdot k_{mA}$) indicates that the limiting resistance is in the gas and tissue layers for SO_2 and in the mucous layers for O_3. These calculations suggest that mucus provides a protection to the underlying tissues for an irreversibly reactive gas such as O_3. Increments in gas flow, which would minimize gas phase resistance, would be predicted to enhance SO_2 absorption but have relatively little effect on O_3 uptake.

V. Predictions of In Vivo Reactive Gas Absorption Using Mathematical Models

The quantitative description of inhaled gas uptake necessitates use of appropriate mass conservation continuity equations and inclusion of the discrete transport and reaction mechanisms in four compartments: gas, liquid lining, tissue, and blood. An integral part of the modeling process is the selection of physical and mathematical assumptions to make the problem tractable. Selection of a suitable model must be justified within the context of the purpose it is to serve and the data required for its validation. A common simplification is to ignore spatial variations in species concentration in one or more dimensions. Another useful approach is the use of lumped mass transfer coefficients to quantitate interphase mass transfer. These two approaches can help reduce the three-dimensional convective-transport problem into a more tractable one-dimensional differential description. The advantage of the latter approach is that it allows the results to be expressed in terms of one or more dimensionless parameters that provide an intuitive character to the predictions. The governing material-balance equations for such lumped compartmental models are ordinary differential equations, which renders them more amenable to numerical or analytical solution. Because of their nature, such lumped models cannot realistically incorporate detailed effects of geometry or fluid dynamics.

Distributed-parameter models, which include spatial variations in concentration, are governed by partial differential equations. Use is made of effective diffusion coefficients, D_{eff}, to account for gas mixing and dispersion along the aiways. The advent of high-speed computers and efficient techniques of numerical integration allows one to embark on the ambitious task of retaining the

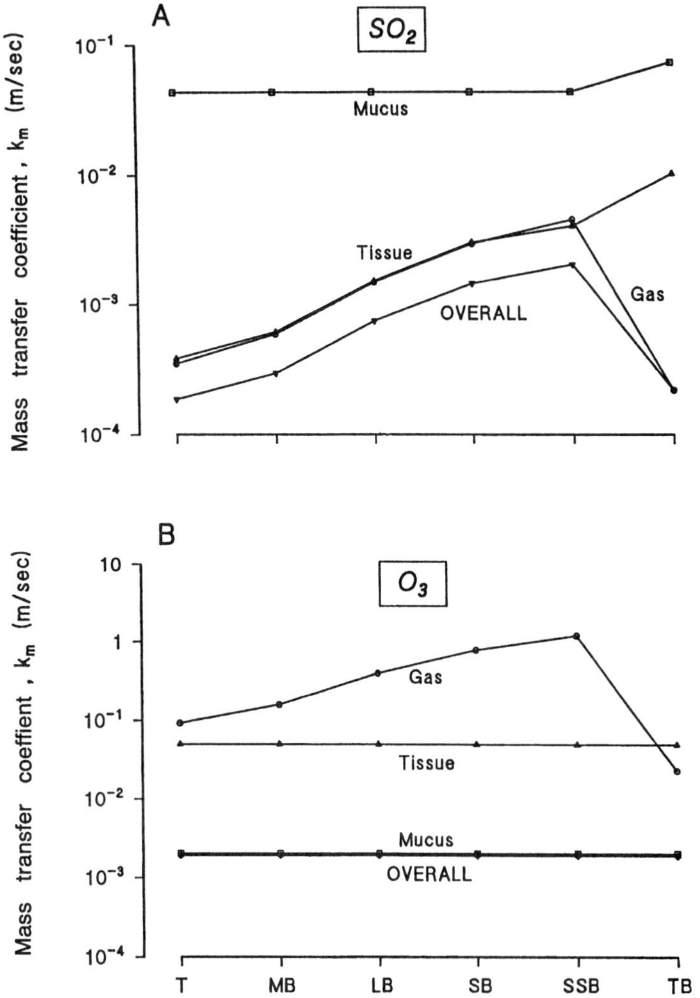

Figure 3 Estimated values for the individual (mucus, gas, and tissue) and overall mass transfer coefficients for SO_2 (**A**) and O_3 (**B**). *Abbreviations*: T = trachea; MB = main bronchi; LB = lobar bronchi; SB = segmental bronchi; SSB = subsegmental bronchi; TB = terminal bronchioles. (Adapted from Ref. 20.)

analytical complexities, but the results are often difficult to interpret unless a formal sensitivity analysis is included. These latter models require adequate quantitative description of the anatomical branching of the tracheobronchial airways; Weibel's model (38) is the most widely used. Such models have the advantage of predicting system behavior.

A. Model of Nasal Gas Absorption

An excellent example of the benefits of model simplification is the work of Aharonson et al. (39), who developed a steady-state one-dimensional model of nasal gas uptake. These authors modeled the nose as a tortuous conduit surrounded by a combined mucous-tissue layer that is surrounded by a sheath of capillaries. Neglecting longitudinal mixing in the gas stream, a steady-state mass balance equation was written for a differential length, dy, of the nasal airway:

$$\left(\frac{\dot{V}}{RT}\right)\frac{d(p_A)_G}{dy} = -K_{mGA}(y)\, a(y)\, [(p_A)_G - (p_A^*)_B] \tag{62}$$

where the overall mass transfer coefficient for interfacial transfer between the gas-phase and blood, K_{mGA} (y) and airway perimeter a(y), are both functions of longitudinal position, y. $\dot{V}$ is the volumetric flow rate, and $(p_A)_G$ and $(p_A^*)_B$ represent the partial pressure of solute gas in the airway and the blood, respectively. By assuming that the gas tension, $(p_A^*)_B$, in blood is negligible, this ordinary differential equation may be integrated from the airflow inlet to the outlet:

$$\frac{(p_A)_{Go}}{(p_A)_{Gi}} = \exp\left(-\frac{K_{mGA}(S)\,RT}{\dot{V}}\right) \tag{63}$$

where $(K_{mGA})(S)$ is the value of $K_m(y)$ a(y) integrated over the length of the nasal airway. If one defines R_U as reactive uptake coefficient ($=K_{mGA}(S)RT$), and fractional penetration, F_{pA}, as $(p_A)_{Go}/(p_A)_{Gi}$, then

$$F_{pA} = \exp\left(-\frac{R_U}{\dot{V}}\right) \tag{63}$$

This equation is similar to that derived by Kleinman (40) to model gas uptake in the nasal and oral routes. Changes in R_U may reflect changes in the mass transfer coefficient K_{mGA} or those in surface area, (S). The estimated values of F_{pA} from the data of Frank et al. (41) and Yokoyama and Frank (42) on the nasal uptake of SO_2 and O_3 are shown in Figure 4. Using Equation (63), Aharonson et al. (40) found R_U to increase with flow rate for both SO_2 and O_3. This increment in R_U (and K_{mGA}), was most likely due to decrease in the gas-phase mass transfer resistance ($1/k_{mGA}$).

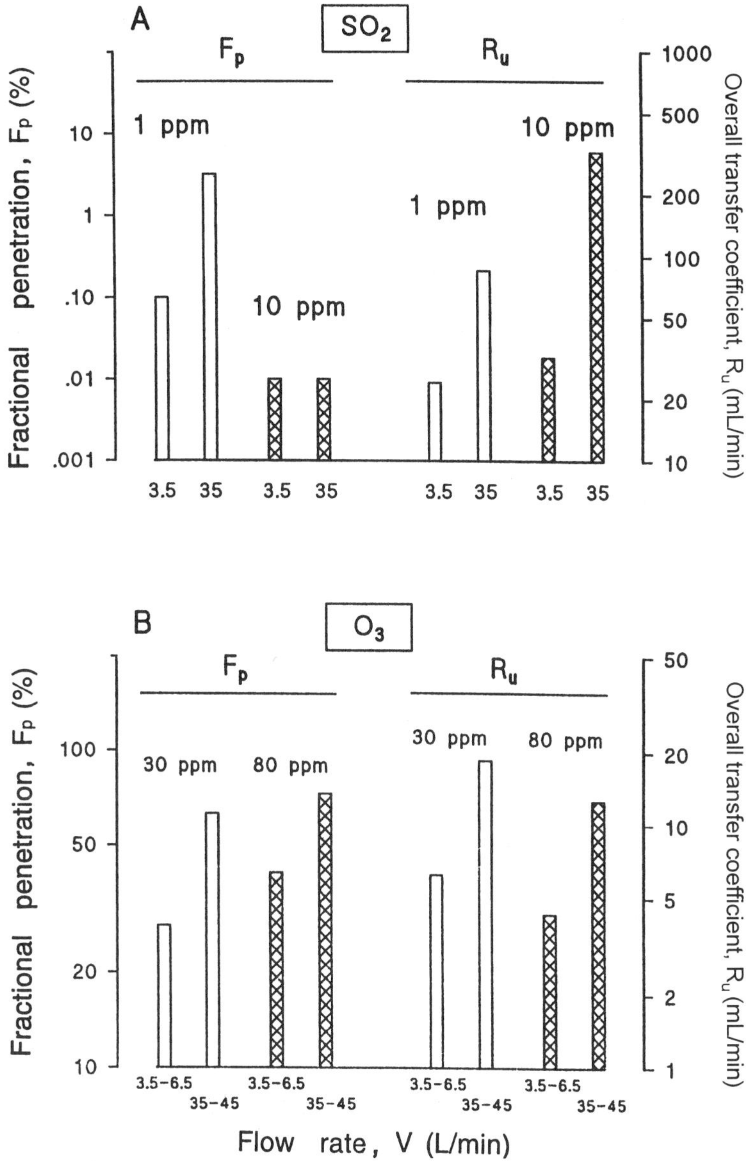

Figure 4 Estimated values for the penetration fraction (F_p) and the overall transport coefficient (R_u). (Adapted from Ref. 17.)

B. Distributed Parameter Models

McJilton et al. (43) apparently developed the first distributed-parameter model of reactive gas uptake, beginning with a mass balance on a differential section of the airway lumen:

$$\left(\frac{A_c}{RT}\right)\left(\frac{\partial p_{AG}}{\partial t}\right) = -\left(\frac{\dot{V}}{RT}\right)\left(\frac{\partial p_{AG}}{\partial x}\right) + \left(\frac{1}{RT}\right)\frac{\partial}{\partial x}\left(D_{AG}A_c\frac{\partial p_{AG}}{\partial x}\right) = a\left(\frac{\dot{M}_A}{S}\right) \quad (64)$$

where p_{AG} represents the partial pressure averaged over the cross-sectional area A_c available for flow, a is the perimeter available for gas absorption, and both A_c and a are increasing functions of axial distance x. S is the surface are for gas absorption. In Equation 64, the first term represents species accumulation, the second-term net rate of input of species A by gas bulk flow, the third term the longitudinal (axial) diffusional rate of transport of A, and the last term the rate of uptake of A from the lumen across the gas–liquid interface.

In solving Equation 64, McJilton et al. (43) used a finite-difference algorithm in which respiratory air flow, $\dot{V}$, varied in a sinusoidal manner, and in which the airways were divided into 25 longitudinal zones corresponding to the 23 generations of Weibel's model (38). Each airway zone was assumed to be bounded by a tissue layer coated with an inner liquid film of either mucus (in the conducting zones) or surfactant (in the respiratory zones). The principal assumptions in absorption between the gas, liquid, and tissue layers were that the diffusion resistance of the gas phase boundary layer was negligible, transport through the liquid layer could be considered as steady-state diffusion, and chemical reactions were assumed to occur exclusively at the liquid–tissue interface, where pollutant was instantaneously consumed. Because there is no accumulation or depletion of pollutant within the liquid film, the influx of pollutant across the airway lumen is identical to the tissue dose in this model. Because it was assumed that pollutant concentration is negligible at the liquid–tissue interface, the uptake flux, M_A/S, could be expressed at the product of the diffusive conductance of the liquid film, $(H_A \cdot k_A)$, with the partial pressure in the airway lumen, p_{AG}. McJilton et al. (43) assumed a liquid film thickness of 10 μm in upper airway generations, 3–5 μm in the alveolar ducts, and 0.3 μm in the alveoli. Predicted values of the local dose, expressed as mass absorbed per unit bronchial surface area per breath, are shown in Figure 5*A*, for O_3 and SO_2. It is predicted that the O_3 dose is uniformly distributed within the conducting airway segments and then declines sharply in the distal air spaces distal to the 20th model segment. For SO_2, a much more soluble gas, the uniform portion of the dose distribution is predicted to be at a higher level and begins to decline sharply beyond the 10th model segment.

To overcome one of the major shortcomings of the McJilton model (43) of localizing chemical reactions at the liquid–tissue interface and ignoring reaction

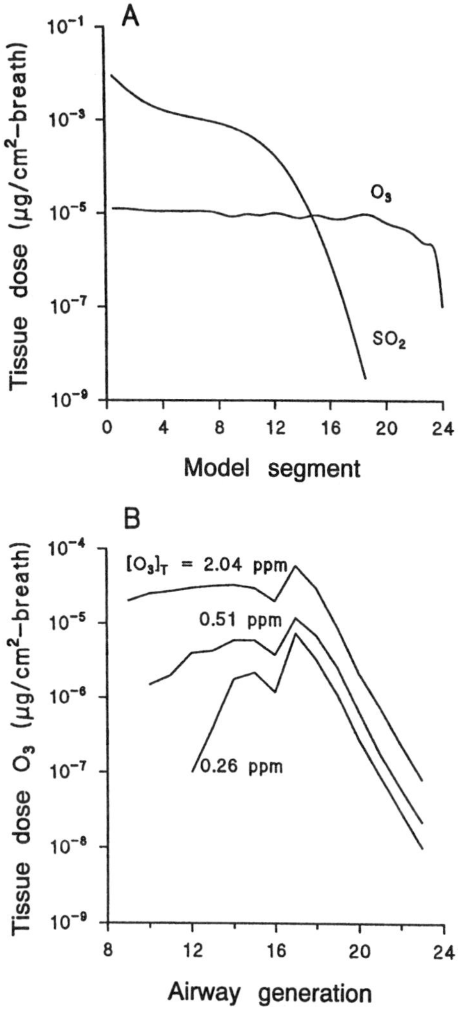

Figure 5 **A**, Tissue dose distribution in the airways for SO_2 and O_3 predicted by the McJilton model (43). Input parameters for these computations: Inhaled concentration = 1000 μg/m^3, tidal volume = 500 mL, and breathing frequency = 15 breaths/min. (Redrawn from Ref. 20.) **B**, Tissue O_3 dose distribution in man for various tracheal ozone concentrations predicted by the Miller et al. (8) model (tidal volume = 500 mL; respiratory rate = 15). (Redrawn from Ref. 8.)

limitations, Miller et al. (8) developed a distributed parameter model of O_3 uptake wherein the site of chemical reactions of O_3 were localized to the mucous layer. In particular, these authors (8) modeled the mucous layer as a stagnant barrier into which O_3 diffuses in from the airway lumen to react with reactive biological substrates, diffusing in from the underlying tissue compartment. At the reaction plane where O_3 and reactive substrates meet, it was assumed that these are instantaneously consumed by chemical reaction. The depth of penetration of this reaction plane within mucus was determined by the rate of O_3 absorption relative to the rate of reactive substrate supply to this reaction plane. Other modifications in the Miller et al. (8) model included the use of a mass transfer coefficient, k_m, and a mixing coefficient to include radial and axial transport in the airways. Miller et al. (8) also used the Weibel model (38) of the branching airways. The tissue doses predicted by the Miller et al. model (8) increased from a value of zero in the trachea, where the reaction plane cannot completely penetrate the thick mucous layer, to a maximum value in the 17th generation where the mucous layer is the thinnest (see Figure 5*B*). In more distal airway generations, the dose declined because absorption was spread out over the rapidly increasing surface area. Despite the marked decline in tissue dose per unit surface area from the conducting airways to the respiratory zone, the total mass of O_3 absorbed was predicted to be five times that absorbed in the conducting airways (8).

In an extension of their previous model, Miller et al. (9) and Overton et al. (14) incorporated the finite rate of O_3 reaction in surfactant, tissue, and blood, as well as in mucus. The bronchial wall was modeled as stagnant mucus overlying bronchial tissue. Similarly, the respiratory zone was modeled as a series of stagnant surfactant, tissue, and stationary blood layers. Quasi–steady-state transport by simultaneous diffusion and chemical reaction was assumed to occur within each layer. First order reaction kinetics were assumed. The equations of this model were linear; therefore, when normalized to the tracheal concentration, the predicted O_3 dose distributions were independent of the tracheal concentration.

Dose was defined as the quantity of O_3 absorbed or reacted per unit surface area per unit time ($\mu g \cdot cm^{-2} \cdot min^{-1}$). Because of the linearity of the system (the computed results are proportional to the inhaled tracheal concentration), dose was normalized to the input tracheal concentration. The uptake or absorption of O_3, as a result of chemical reactions in any compartment, is the dose of that compartment (e.g., mucus dose, tissue dose, blood dose). Net dose is the sum of the liquid, tissue, and blood compartment doses. This model was used by Miller et al. (9) and Overton et al. (14) to determine the sensitivity of the compound dose distribution to several parameters, including the gas-phase mass transfer coefficient, the axial dispersion coefficient, the mucous reaction rate constant, and the minute volume of breathing. The model predictions were insensitive to the gas-phase mass transfer coefficient. Similarly, the magnitude of the longitudinal mixing coefficient had little effect on O_3 uptake.

Miller et al. (9) and Overton et al. (14) examined the sensitivity of the model predicitons to the assumed value the mucous reaction rate constant, k_r. They varied k_r from 0 (no reactions) to 10 times the reference value 1198 sec^{-1} (Figure 6). The no-reaction curves correspond to the case in which there is only physical absorption in the mucous lining. The net does of O_3 is plotted against the generation number in Figure 6*A*. Generations 0 to 16 correspond to the tracheobronchial or mucus-lined region of the lung in their model. At generation 16–17, the predicted net dose declined sharply for the subsequent generations. Differences in net dose resulting from varying reaction rate constant k_r were greatest in the region of the lung near the trachea and they decrease with higher generation numbers as one moves distally into the lung. In the region of generations 17–23, the net doses were similar, regardless of the value for k_μ, with a maximal difference of a factor of 2. Figure 6*B* illustrates the effect of the mucous reaction rate constant on the tissue dose. By contrast to the tracheobronchial net dose (see Figure 6*A*), the predicted tissue dose increased as the reaction rate, k_r, decreased. This is because liquid layer reactions reduce the quantity of O_3 available to react with tissue. The tissue dose was much more sensitive to mucous reactions than was net dose. For example, in the trachea, the tissue dose for no reaction and the tissue dose for twice the reference value differed by a factor of 1000. All curves increased in going from the trachea to the 15–17 generations, where they peaked and then decreased in subsequent generations. With no reactions in the liquid lining, the peak tissue dose occurred in generation 15. As k_r increased, the peak tissue dose shifted to the 17th generation. For all regions, the peak tissue dose decreased with increasing k_r; however, the tissue dose in the pulmonary region differed by no more than a factor of 2 (as in the case of net dose in Figure 6*A*). Furthermore, in the pulmonary region, the tissue dose and the net dose (for the same k_r) were essentially the same. The predicted tissue dose was a few percent lower than the net dose, the difference being due primarily to O_3 uptake in blood.

Figure 7 summarizes the results of Miller et al. (9) and Overton et al. (14) on the predicted O_3 uptake resulting from different mucous reaction rate constants in the different lung regions and compartments. These data are the percentage of mass of O_3 taken up by a given compartment. This percentage is based on the total mass inhaled, which was nearly constant 87.4%–91.5%. However, the distribution of the fractional uptake was dependent on the value of the mucous reaction constant. As k_r increased, the pulmonary uptake decreased because of greater fractional absorption in the tracheobronchial region. The surfactant compartment was predicted to absorb less then 0.2% of the inhaled O_3. The blood compartment was predicted to absorb more but had a minor role in the quantity absorbed ($\leq$2.4%).

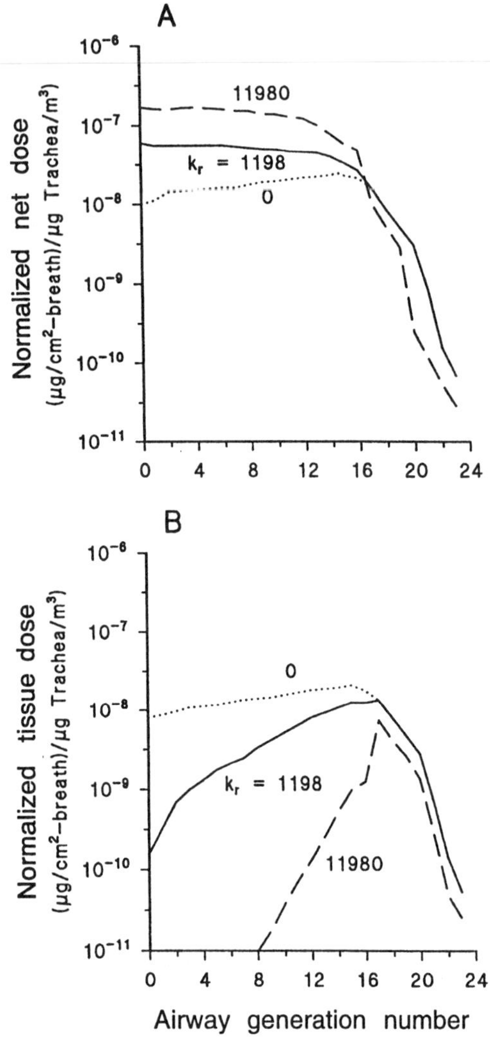

Figure 6 Predicted net O_3 dose (**A**) and tissue O_3 dose (**B**) versus generation number for several values of the mucus reaction-rate constant (k_r). The reference value is $k_r = 1198\ sec^{-1}$. The dose ($\mu g/cm^2$-breath) can be calculated by multiplying ordinate values by the tracheal concentration ($\mu g/m^3$). (Note generation 0–16: mucus-lined tracheobronchial region; generation 17–23: surfactant-lined pulmonary region.) (Redrawn from Ref. 9.)

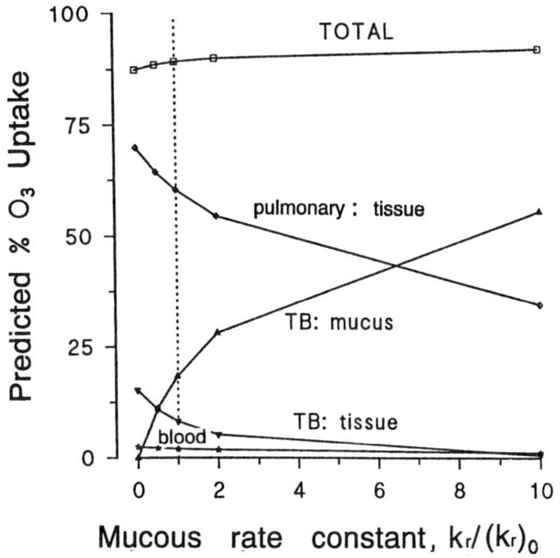

Figure 7 Regional O_3 uptake versus normalized mucus rate constant (k_r). *Abbreviations*: tb = tracheobronchial. (Adapted from Ref. 9.)

There was minimal effect on tissue dose as the surfactant rate constant was varied from its nominal value ($k_\sigma = 21.4$ sec^{-1}) to a value 10 times this number (9). Changing the thickness of the surfactant layer from the reference values of 1.25, 1.0, and 0.5 μm in generations 17, 18, and 19 (representing the respiratory bronchioles) to a common value of 0.125 μm led to an increase in the peak tissue dose at generation 17 to be greater by a factor of 3 (9). These results would indicate that the surfactant layer thickness may play an important role in protecting the underlying alveolar epithelium.

Grotberg et al. (44,45) noted several limitations in the previous models (8,9,14). They pointed out that previous models (8,9,14) simulated ozone transport in airways using a one-dimensional flow model. The gas-phase was simulated by two sequential steps: axial dispersion and radial diffusion. The axial dispersion coefficient was based on data of Scherer (46) that was derived from experiments that have zero wall flux. Sankarsubramanian and Gill (47) had previously shown that dispersion coefficients can differ by an order of magnitude of mass transfer occurs at the gas–wall interface. In addition, the dimensionless mass transfer coefficients (*Sherwood number*, or N_{Sh}) used in previous studies (8,9,14) were assumed to be the same for all airway generations, which did not allow for the variety of transport regimens within the lung. In the Grotberg model (44,45), transport of the toxic gas in the airways was governed by the convection-diffusion processes in the gas (subscript G) and the liquid (subscript

L) phases. Several major assumptions were imposed and these may be summarized as 1. the flow and concentration fields are quasisteady; 2. the process is axisymmetric; 3. the breathing pattern is a square wave; 4. ozone reacts instantaneously and irreversibly with the mucous reactants; 5. the mucous reactant flux is constant in a given airway generation; 6. no interfacial resistance to ozone transfer occurs; 7. the tissue has a large capacity to absorb O_3 so that the ozone concentration is always zero at the liquid–tissue interface; 8. the entrance concentration is uniform; 9. the liquid lining layer is stationary; 10. the airway dimensions depend on the tital volume; and 11. the liquid lining satisfies a thin film approximation. For a representative airway, these authors modeled a finite length tube (length L; radius r_a) consisting of a cylindrical liquid shell. In cylindrical coordinates (r, Θ, z) the dimensionless quasi–steady-state mass balance equation for the toxic gas in the gas phase was as follows:

$$N_{Pe}\, \nabla(C_G \cdot \vec{U}) = \nabla^2 C_G \text{ for } 0 \le z \le \lambda,\ 0 \le r \le r_l \tag{65}$$

where C_G is the concentration of toxic species in gas-phase, $\vec{U}$ is the gas-phase velocity vector, $\lambda = L/r_a$; $r_L = 1_{-\varepsilon}$ (the position of the gas–liquid interface); $\varepsilon = \delta_L/r_a$; r_a is airway radius and δ_L = liquid layer thickness. Similarly, the mass balance for the liquid phase was given by the continuity equation:

$$\left(\frac{\partial^2 C_L}{\partial y^2}\right) + \left(\frac{\varepsilon}{r_L + \varepsilon y}\right)\left(\frac{\partial C_L}{\partial y}\right) + \varepsilon^2\left(\frac{\partial^2 C_L}{\partial z^2}\right) = 0 \text{ for } 0 \le z \le \lambda,\ 0 \le y \le \delta_R(z) \tag{66}$$

The gas–liquid interface was located at $y = 0$ and the liquid–tissue interface at $y = 1$. These authors modeled the kinetics of the reaction of O_3 with mucous reactants as instantaneous, similar to Overton et al. (14). For instantaneous kinetics, the reaction surface is located at $y = \delta_R(z)$. The corresponding mass balance for the reactants was expressed as

$$\left(\frac{\partial^2 C_R}{\partial y^2}\right) + \left(\frac{\varepsilon}{r_L + \varepsilon y}\right)\left(\frac{\partial C_R}{\partial y}\right) + \varepsilon^2\left(\frac{\partial^2 C_R}{\partial z^2}\right) = 0 \text{ for } 0 \le z \le \lambda,\ \delta_R(z) \le y \le 1 \tag{67}$$

where C_R is the concentration of reactants. Grotberg et al. (44,45) defined as a dimensionless radial mass transport parameter, Γ, as follows:

$$\Gamma = \left(\frac{D_L}{D_G H_{O_3} \varepsilon}\right) \tag{68}$$

that represents the ratio of the gas-phase diffusion resistance to the liquid-phase diffusion resistance, with ε representing the ratio of liquid layer thickness to airway radius (=δ/a). Γ is larger for smaller ε (relatively thinner liquid layer), smaller H (larger liquid solubility), and larger (D_L/D_G) (relatively larger liquid diffusivity). Because (D_L/D_G) is approximately 10^{-4}, Γ is small. However if ε is very small or if H is very small, Γ may be large. For ozone and the typical liquid lining thickness of healthy animals, $\Gamma < 0.06$ for all cases, and, for most airways, $\Gamma < 0.01$ (44,45). On the other hand, for SO_2, $\Gamma \gg 1$ (44,45).

Grotberg et al. (44,45) applied the model to the full tracheobronchial tree for different flow regimens as determined by the Peclet number ($N_{Pe} = Ur_a/D_G$), where U is the characteristic fluid velocity, r_a is the airway radius, and D_G is the gas-phase diffusivity. Asymptotic methods were used in regions of the tracheobronchial tree, where $N_{Pe} \ll 1$ and $N_{Pe} \gg 1$. Specification of the tidal volume (V_T) and respiratory rate allowed calculation of the Peclet number for each airway generation ("i"), ($(N_{Pe})_i = U_i(r_a)_i/D_G$). Values for airway diameters, lengths for each airway generation, were taken from Weibel's data. Thickness of the liquid lining (δ_L) were taken from data of Overton et al. (14). Ozone diffusivity in gas-phase, D_G, was taken as 0.195 cm^2/s and the liquid diffusivity was estimated as 1.61×10^{-5} cm^2/s. Henry's law coefficient was taken as $\hat{H} = 7$ g/mL (air)/g/mL (water). Inlet ozone concentration was taken as 1 ppm ($=1.886 \times 10^{-9}$ g/mL), and the kinematic viscosity of air, ν, 0.15 cm^2/s. Values of the mucous production rates and mucous reactant concentrations were taken from Miller et al. (9). Using these numbers, the value of the dimensionless absorption parameter, Γ, was estimated at 3.54×10^{-3}.

The rate of ozone absorption ($\dot{M}^*$, gm/s), was normalized to the mass flux of ozone at the tracheal inlet. Thus, absorption in the ith generation, was expressed as $\dot{M}_i = \dot{M}^*/(r_T D_G C_T)$, where r_T represents the tracheal radius and C_T is the O_3 concentration at the tracheal inlet. The fractional uptake in each generation was defined as, $\phi_i = \dot{M}_i^*/(\pi r_T^2 U_T C_T)$. Finally, the tissue dose of O_3 was defined as, $(\text{Dose})_i = \dot{M}_i^*/S_i$, where S_i is the total surface area of generation "i."

In Figure 8*A*, the airway concentrations are shown for various values of the radial transport parameter, Γ. Given a base set of data, which result in a distribution of Γ_i for the airways, the curves in Figure 8 were obtained at multiples of Γ (0.5, 1, or 2). The greatest decrease in concentration occurs between generations 14 and 20, and, as Γ increases for any airway in this region, the concentrations are lowered. The absorption as a function of airway generation is shown in Figure 8*B*. The predicted absorption increased as Γ increased for generations proximal to generation 18. As a consequence, generations beyond 18 were predicted to have decreasing absorption for increasing Γ. Figure 8*C* indicates that the tissue dose also experiences a maximum at generation 17, and the curves cross at generation 18 as in Figure 8*B*. Two values of N_{Pe} were chosen to correspond to the calculations of Miller et al.: 1. $(N_{Pe})_T = 500$ for respiratory rate (RR) = 15/min and $V_T = 500$ mL and 2. $(N_{Pe})_T = 2300$ for RR = 20.3/min and $V_T = 1750$ mL. In Figure 9*A*, it can be seen that, for an increase in $(N_{Pe})_T$, the absorption is not significantly different for generations proximal to 15, but that it is significantly increased for generations 17 and beyond. In addition, the maximal absorption shifts from generation 17 to generation 18.

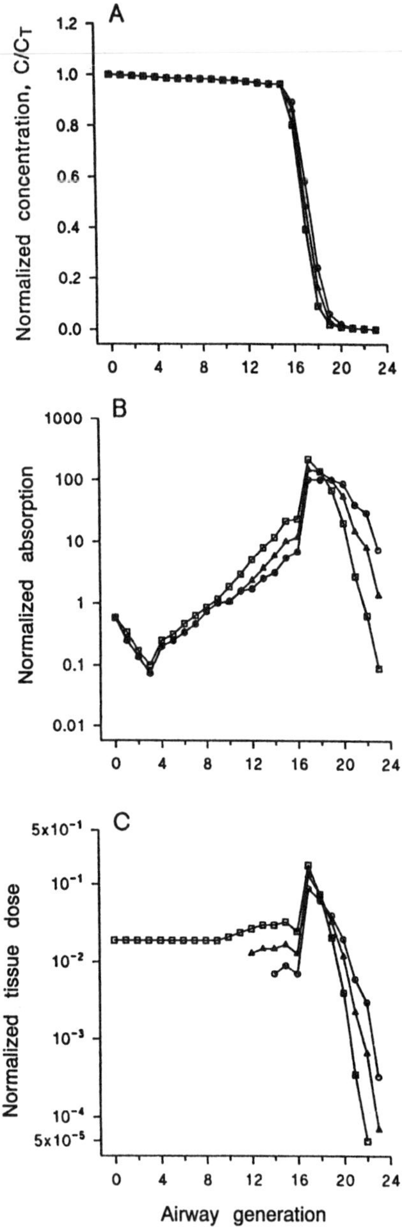

Figure 8 Computed normalized airway ozone concentration (**A**), normalized ozone absorption (**B**), and normalized tissue O_3 dose (**C**) profiles versus generation number for three values of the dimensionless parameter Γ. ($\Gamma = 0.5$ (O), $\Gamma = 1.0$ (Δ), $\Gamma = 2.0$ ($\square$). (Redrawn from Ref. 45.)

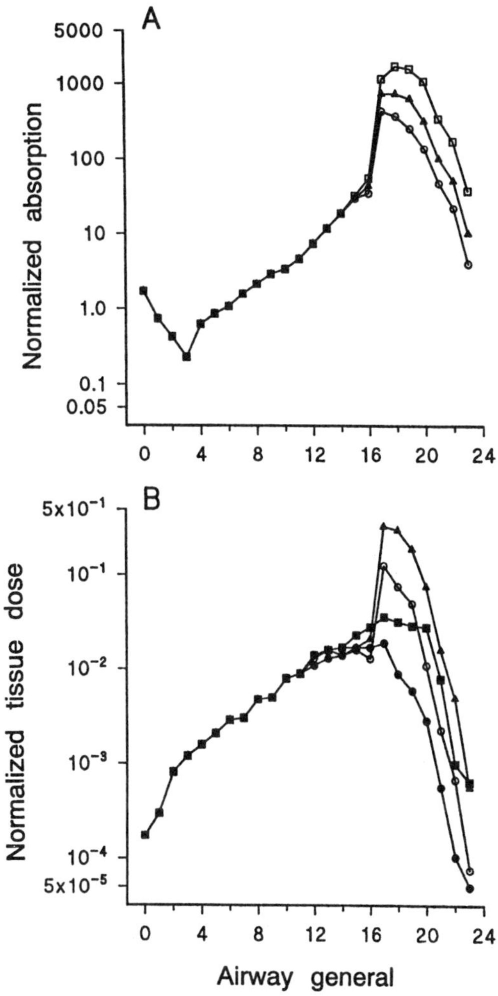

Figure 9 **A**, Computed fractional uptake of ozone versus generation number for three values of the tracheal Peclet number [$N_{Pe} = 500$ (○), $N_{Pe} = 990$, and $N_{Pe} = 2300$ (Δ)]. (**B**) Computed tissue ozone dose profile versus generation number for two values of the tracheal Peclet number [$N_{Pe} = 500$ (○) and $N_{Pe} = 2300$ (Δ)] computed by Grotberg et al. (45) compared with the predictions of Miller et al. (9) [$N_{Pe} = 500$ (●) and $N_{Pe} = 2300$ (▲)]. (Redrawn from Ref. 45.)

Comparison of the tissue dose to that obtained by Miller et al. (9) is shown in Figure 9*B*. The relative changes in dose are different between the two models. More striking are the differences in the absolute value of tissue dose, which are approximately an order of magnitude higher at generation 17 with this model for $(N_{Pe})_T = 2300$.

The model of Grotberg et al. (44,45) predicts significantly higher ozone doses to the tissues than those predicted previously (8,9,14). Grotberg et al. (44,45) ascribed this difference to two major factors: 1. Miller et al. (9) used an average Sherwood number of 8 to calculate all the mass transfer coefficients, whereas the Grotberg model (44,45) accounts for the expected differences in the Sherwood number for different airway generations, and 2. The use of relatively more sophisticated approach to alveolated surface modeling in the low Peclet number region (44,45).

C. Effect of Ventilatory Inhomogeneities on Tissue Dose

Most previous models used symmetric lung anatomies in which all possible pathways from the airway opening to the alveolar sacs were geometrically identical and received an equal fraction of the inspired gas. This idealization, although simplifying the computation of serial variations in O_3 dose, precludes the evaluation of the effect of parallel inhomogeneities in ventilation on tissue dose.

Within any given airway generation, substantial inhomogeneities exist in the lengths of individual conducting airways. To evaluate the effect of path length on regional dosimetry, Overton and Graham (16) used one-dimensional convection-dispersion and multiple path anatomical models for the rat lung. Whereas they observed that, in general, dose declined distally, within any given airway generation there was substantial path length–dependent variation in dose (Figure 10*A*), suggesting that equivalent length path models do not accurately predict the extent of airway surface dose inhomogeneities.

Mercer et al. (48) used three-dimensional reconstructions of distal rat lungs to determine the distribution of gas volumes within individual ventilatory units. In their analysis of ventilatory unit volume effects on the dose of inhaled O_3, they observed that the larger gas exchange units ventilated by more proximal airways receive a dose (per unit surface area) twofold greater than the average. Furthermore, there was substantial variation in O_3 uptake among the proximal segments of the ventilatory units (see Figure 10*B*).

VI. Interpretation of Experimental Data on Gas Absorption Using Mathematical Models

A. Reactive Gas Absorption in Isolated Trachea

Ben-Jebria et al. (49) characterized the absorption of sulfur-dioxide (SO_2) into excised porcine tracheae by a step-response method in which SO_2 outlet concen-

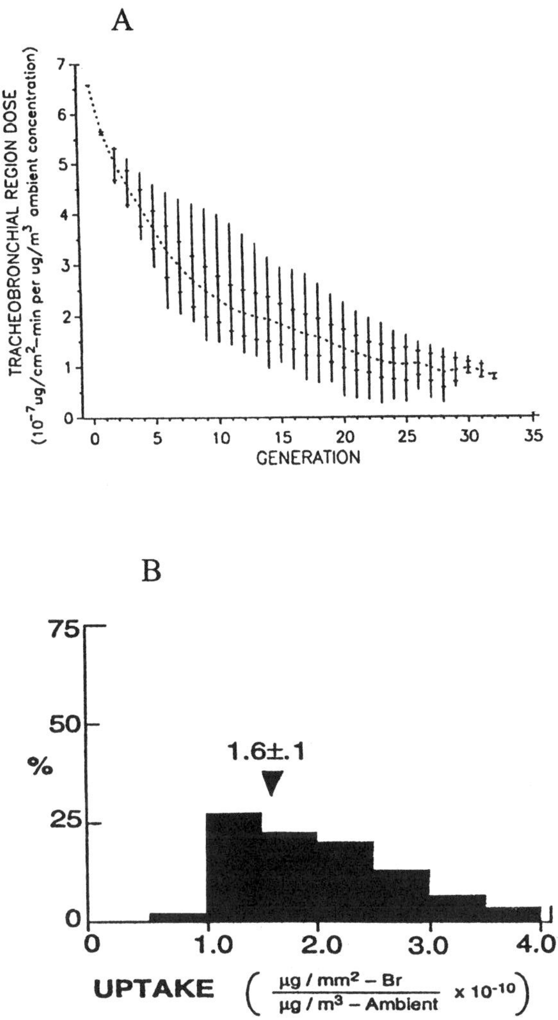

Figure 10 **A**, Predicted tracheobronchial region airway dose (flux divided by exposure concentration) versus generation number. The mean dose per generation is denoted by the dashed line; vertical lines indicate the predicted range of doses, and the horizontal bars ± one standard deviation from the mean. Generation 0 represents trachea. (From Ref. 16.) **B**, Distribution of ventilatory unit ozone uptake: model predictions for variations in proximal alveolar region uptake by different ventilatory units. A functionally significant fraction of the ventilatory units (corresponding to larger gas exchange units ventilated by more proximal airways) is predicted to receive a ≥ twofold uptake per unit surface area than the average. (From Ref. 48.)

trations were monitored during a 30-minute interval following introduction of inlet concentrations of 0.1–0.6 ppm SO_2 at steady air flows of 2.7–11.0 L/min. These data were analyzed using a diffusion-reaction theoretical model incorporating three independent parameters: a gas-phase mass transfer coefficient, a tissue-phase diffusivity × solubility product, and a tissue-phase reaction constant.

In the *diffusion-reaction model*, the dissociation of SO_2 in aqueous solution is represented primarily by Equation 9. At a pH of 7.0, the equilibrium constant for reaction (9) is so large that the ratio of $[HSO_3^-]$ to $[SO_2]$ is greater than 100,000 : 1, and SO_2 is transported through the aqueous phase primarily as HSO_3^-. In a well-buffered system, variations in pH are small, and the chemical equilibrium between the gas and aqueous phases can be expressed by a linear equation:

$$[HSO_3^-] = \beta_{SO_2} (p_{SO_2}) \tag{69}$$

where β_{SO_2} is the effective solubility coefficient for SO_2 ($=10^{pH}\overline{K}_{s1}\overline{K}_{s2}$). As SO_2 penetrates into tissue from its site of formation at the gas-tissue interface, HSO_3^- may undergo irreversible reactions with biochemical substrates. If it is assumed that the transport of HSO_3^- in tracheal tissue is by one-dimensional diffusion with simultaneous first order chemical reaction in a planer slab, the governing continuity equation is given by (27)

$$\left(\frac{\partial[HSO_3^-]}{\partial t}\right) = (D_{HSO_3^-})\left(\frac{\partial^2[HSO_3^-]}{\partial z^2}\right) - k_r\,[HSO_3^-] \tag{70}$$

where $D_{HSO_3^-}$ is the effective binary diffusion coefficient of HSO_3^- in tissue, and k_r is a first order reaction rate constant for the chemical reaction between HSO_3^- and biochemical substrates. The overall mass transfer coefficient was defined as the diffusion-flux normalized by the driving force between bulk gas-phase and deep tracheal tissue ($=p_{SO_2}$):

$$K_{mG} = -(D_{HSO_3^-})\left(\frac{R\,T}{p_{SO_2}}\right)\left(\frac{\partial[HSO_3^-]}{\partial z}\right) = 0 \qquad \text{at } z = 0 \tag{71}$$

The solution to Equation 70 subject to the initial condition and boundary conditions (Equation 71) may be written as

$$K_{mG} = \frac{k_{mG}}{(1-\theta)}\left[\exp\left(\frac{1}{\theta} - 1\right)\operatorname{erfc}\sqrt{\left(\frac{k_r t}{\theta}\right)} + \sqrt{\theta}\operatorname{erf}\sqrt{k_r t} - \theta\right] \tag{72}$$

where θ is a dimensionless group:

$$\theta = \frac{k_r(D_{HSO_3^-})}{k_{mG}/(\beta_{SO_2}RT)^2}$$

According to Equation 72, K_{mG} will decay in an exponential manner from a starting value of $K_{mG} = k_{mG}$ at $t = 0$ to a smaller asymptotic value (49):

$$K_{mG} = \left(\frac{1}{\dfrac{1}{k_{mG}} + \dfrac{1}{(\beta_{SO_2} RT)\sqrt{k_r D_{HSO_3^-}}}} \right) \tag{73}$$

Equation 72 indicates that, initially, when tissue is free of HSO_3^-, diffusion is controlled by the gas-phase diffusion resistance alone. Subsequently, HSO_3^- forms at the gas–tissue interface and penetrates deeper into tissue, causing a progressive increase in the overall diffusion resistance until a steady state is reached (in approximately 10 minutes). At this final steady state, Equation 72 indicates that the overall gas-phase mass transfer resistance ($1/K_{mG}$) is the sum of individual resistances, resulting from the gas phase ($1/k_{mG}$) and that due to the tissue phase ($1/[\beta_{SO_2}RT(k_rD_{HSO_3})]$) (see Equation 73).

Because of the time-dependent nature of the underlying absorption process, it was possible to separate K_{mG} into the contributions of gas-phase and tissue-phase diffusion resistances (49). The effects on K_{mG} of different airflows from 2.7 to 11.0 L/min and different inlet SO_2 concentrations of 0.12–0.59 ppm were studied. Values of k_{mG} were found to be proportional to the convective gas flow. This indicates that radial transport occurred through a boundary layer whose thickness was diminished by increments in axial velocity. The estimated value of $k_r = 0.0017$ sec^{-1} was approximately 1 million smaller than the rate constant predicted when ozone reacts with mucus (9), indicating that SO_2 is a relatively unreactive gas. On the other hand, the estimated value of $D_{HSO_3}(\beta_{SO_2} RT)^2 = 0.28$ m^2/s was about six times larger than the corresponding value for O_3 dissolved in water (49), probably because of the relatively high solubility of SO_2. The effect of a large solubility is to reduce the importance of the diffusion resistance in tissue compared to that in the gas-phase. In particular, Ben-Jebria et al. (49) computed that the percentage of steady-state diffusion gas-phase resistance increased from 15% to 41% as convective flow decreased from 11 to 2.7 L/min (Figure 11).

B. Kinetics of Gas Absorption in Isolated Lungs

Despite the well-documented limitations (e.g., time constraints to preparation stability, edema formation, loss of innervation and lymph flow, differential loss of bronchial perfusion), isolated lung preparations offer a number of distinct investigational advantages for characterizing the determinants of reactive gas absorption. Isolated lungs represent a biologically relevant model, which maintain intact air space surface and tissue compartments and enable reproducible control of reactive gas delivery and physiological parameters to an extent that can often not be achieved in whole animal preparations (e.g., tidal and functional

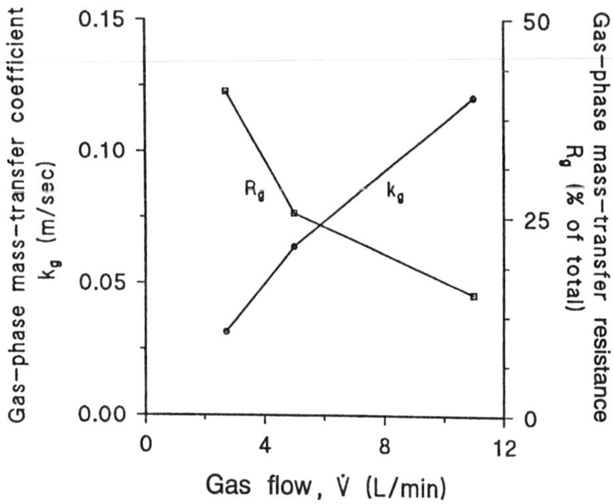

Figure 11 Estimated values for the gas-phase mass transfer coefficient (k_g) and gas-phase mass transfer resistance (R_g) as a function of gas flow (V) for SO_2 absorption in excised porcine trachea. (Adapted from Ref. 49.)

residual capacity [FRC] volumes, ventilation frequency, perfusion status and perfusate constituents, and temperature). Furthermore, studies can be performed under either steady-state or non–steady-state (transient) conditions wherein the reactive gas is inspired at a constant rate or made the limiting reagent via rebreathing of respiratory gases from a closed compartment, respectively. The general utility of the isolated lung for gas absorption kinetics has been described elsewhere (50). We have used an isolated rat lung model to investigate the determinants of gas absorption in the lower respiratory tract. Admittedly, although these studies are limited in their ability to provide site-specific absorption rates, they do permit evaluation of the role of global parameters such as perfusion, ventilation, and temperature.

In the isolated perfused rat lung when a steady-state exposure regimen is initiated, the absorption of inhaled O_3 and NO_2 rapidly reached a constant rate that was maintained for at least 60 minutes (51,52). O_3 was more efficiently scrubbed from inspired air than NO_2, with the fractional uptake of $O_3 \approx 95\%$, and that for $NO_2 \approx 70\%$. Absorption rates were proportional to inspired dose rates (i.e., $[NO_2 \text{ or } O_3]_i \cdot V_t \cdot f$) for both O_3 and NO_2 (Figure 12). In general, this held true across varying combinations of inspired concentration, tidal volume, and ventilation frequency. During steady-state exposures, absorption of O_3 and NO_2 was independent of vascular perfusion (51,52) and demonstrated tempera-

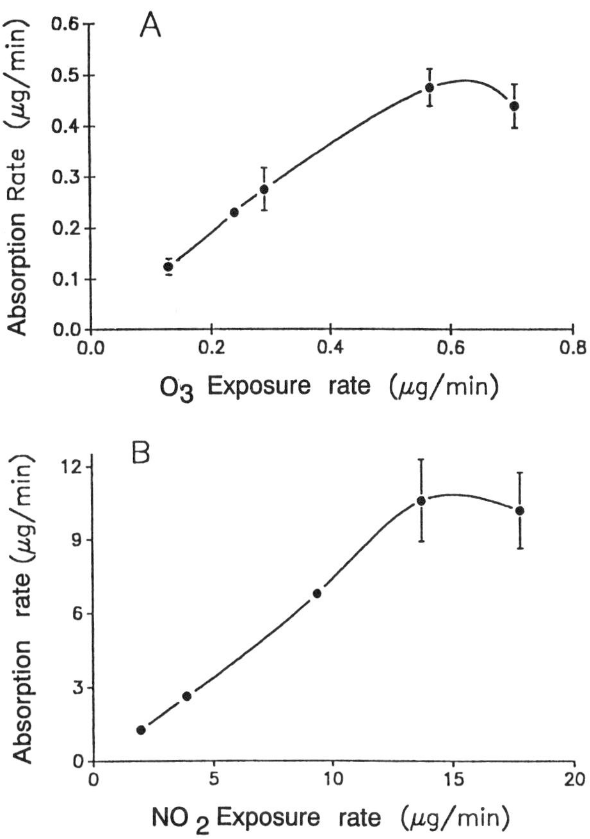

Figure 12 The relationship between the O_3 (**A**) and NO_2 (**B**) inspired exposure rate and the respective absorption rates in isolated rat lungs. Nonperfused lungs were exposed to the respective gases under quasi–steady-state conditions. Exposure rate was altered via inspired concentration ($[O_3]_i = 0.5$–3.0 ppm; $[NO_2]_i = 10$–106 ppm). V_t (≈ 2.5 mL), FRC (4 mL), and f (50/min) were fixed. (O_3 data from Ref. 52 and NO_2 data from Ref. 51.)

ture dependence. If the temperature of the exposure system (i.e., isolated lung and inspired gases) was increased, a concomitant increase in fractional uptake was noted (51,52).

To investigate the overall kinetics of NO_2 absorption, we adapted the isolated lung preparation to study the non–steady-state absorption of NO_2 (53). Via subatmospheric ventilation, nonperfused lungs rebreathed NO_2 from a closed space (exposure vessel) such that changes in the intravessel pressures could be equated to tidal volume, V_t. As with steady-state exposures, fractional uptakes were stable over exposure time. By determining the time-dependent change in $[NO_2]_G$, we characterized the kinetics of NO_2 uptake within the lung. NO_2 absorption displayed first order kinetics with respect to NO_2 when $([NO_2]_g)_0 \leq 11$ ppm. Analogous to the formulation used for the physiological measurement of carbon monoxide diffusing capacity (D_{LCO}) (7), for a first order process, the time course of change in partial pressure of NO_2 can be expressed in terms of an overall diffusing capacity for NO_2 (D_{LNO_2}):

$$\frac{(p_{NO_2})_G}{(p_{NO_2})_{G0}} = \exp\left[-\left(\frac{D_{LNO_2}(RT)}{V_G}\right)t\right] \tag{74}$$

where V_G is the volume of the closed NO_2 vessel. A plot of $\ln[(p_{NO_2G})/(p_{NO_2G})_0]$ versus time yielded a straight line with slope = (D_{LNO_2} (RT)/V_G)). Substituting the appropriate parameter values, we obtain $D_{LNO_2} = 0.12$ mL NO_2/((min)(mm Hg)) = 1.8×10^{-3} μmol/((min)(ppm)). One can relate D_{LNO_2} to an overall mass transfer coefficient, K_{mNO_2}, by

$$D_{LNO_2} = K_{mNO_2} \cdot S \cdot H_{NO_2} \tag{75}$$

Based on a surface area $S = 0.4\ m^2$ suggested by Miller (8) for Sprague-Dawley rats, we obtain $K_{mNO_2} = 1.94 \times 10^{-3}$ cm/s. This nominal value for K_{mNO_2} must be interpreted cautiously. Because the true surface area for gas absorption in our experiments is not precisely known, the calculated value of K_{mNO_2} does not represent a true mass transfer coefficient. When compared under equivalent conditions, the diffusing capacity for O_3 (D_{LO_3}) was approximately three times greater for O_3 than NO_2. These results are consistent with the greater reactivity of O_3 and suggest that O_3 may be absorbed at sites more proximal than the predominant site for NO_2 absorption.

C. Kinetics of Gas Absorption in Model Biological Systems

To investigate the reactivity of biological substrates present in the lining fluid of airway and alveolar epithelium, we measured the in vitro kinetics of gas absorption in model biological systems. A simplified exposure system was employed, which incorporated a glass exposure vessel, constant gas inflow, a planar gas–liquid interface, and an aqueous-phase contained in the bottom of the vessel. Absorption was quantified by determining the rate of disappearance of gas-phase O_3 or NO_2. The model biochemical reduced glutathione (GSH), which is present in high concentration within pulmonary epithelial lining fluid (ELF) and reacts rapidly with both NO_2 and O_3, and bronchoalveolar lavage fluid (BALF), as a model of ELF, were studied (54–56). The concentration of ELF constituents within the BALF was increased by sequentially using the BALF recovered from one lung to subsequently lavage a second and/or third lung [e.g., $(BALF)_{x2}$].

Minimal gas-phase disappearance of either NO_2 or O_3 occurred during exposure of water or buffer alone. Importantly, the presence of aqueous-phase reactive substrates (GSH or BALF) greatly increased removal of NO_2 or O_3 from the gas-phase. NO_2 uptake demonstrated a nonlinear aqueous-phase substrate concentration dependence in model (GSH) (Figure 13*B*) and biological (BALF;

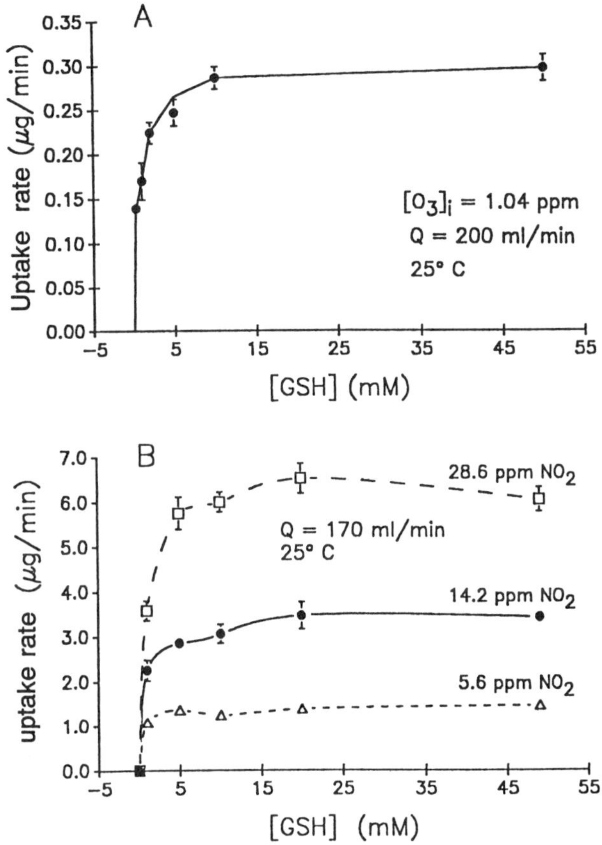

Figure 13 The effect of aqueous substrate concentration on in vitro O_3 (**A**) and NO_2 (**B**) absorption. Solutions of reduced glutathione were exposed under well-mixed, steady-state conditions (constant inflow rate) to either 1 ppm O_3 or 5.6–28.6 ppm NO_2 in air. Absorption was determined from the difference between exposure vessel inflow and exit concentrations. In both cases, absorption was highly dependent on the GSH concentration and reached a saturation rate between 5 and 10 mM GSH. (For **A**, data are from Ref. 58; for **B**, data are from Ref. 54.)

not shown) systems with the overall rate of gas-phase disappearance saturable by high concentrations of aqueous reactants. The observed dependence of the rate of gas-phase NO_2 disappearance (r_{NO_2}), on $[NO_2]_G$ and aqueous concentrations of GSH may be represented by a Michaelis-Menten relationship:

$$r_{NO_2} = \frac{(V_{max})^{NO_2}\,[GSH]}{(\overline{K}_{GSH} + [GSH])} \tag{76}$$

where $\overline{K}_{GSH}$ is the Michaelis-Menten K_m for GSH and $(V_{max})^{GSH}$ is related to $[NO_2]_G$ by an overall mass transfer coeficient, $K_m^{NO_2}$, by

$$(V_{max})^{NO_2} = (K_m)^{NO_2}\,S\,H_{NO_2}\,(p_{NO_2})_G \tag{77}$$

A plot of $(V_{max})^{GSH}$ (obtained from Figure 13*B*) versus $(p_{NO_2})_G$ yields $(K_m^{NO_2}\,S\,H_{NO_2}) = 0.21$. Using a Langmuir plot (29) of $([GSH]/r_{NO_2})$ versus [GSH] yields, $\overline{K}_{GSH} = 0.01$–$0.06$ mM. Combining Equations 76 and 77 gives the final expression:

$$r_{NO_2} = \frac{(0.21)\,(p_{NO_2})_G\,[GSH]}{(\overline{K}_{GSH} + [GSH])} \tag{78}$$

O_3 absorption displayed similar absorption properties (see Figure 13*A*). Similar to observations made in the isolated lung, under equivalent exposure conditions, absorption by both GSH and BALF was proportionally greater for O_3 than NO_2. A concomitant increase in the net flux of NO_2 into GSH and BALF solutions occurred with increasing temperature, contrary to what would be expected if the uptake was solely due to pure physical solubility. Fractional uptake of both O_3 and NO_2 by GSH displayed a nonlinear dependence on aqueous phase pH (Figure 14) with absorption clearly dependent on the presence of reduced moieties.

Under fixed aqueous-phase conditions, NO_2 disappearance from the gas-phase exhibited first order kinetics with respect to NO_2 for both GSH and BALF when the initial NO_2 concentration was ≤ 10 ppm (55). The presence of a significant interfacial mass transfer resistance was inferred from the increment in the rate of NO_2 disappearance during combined stirring of the bulk phase and gas–liquid interface during both steady-state and transient exposure conditions (Figure 15). In examining these data, we make the assumption that the reaction of NO_2 with aqueous GSH occurs at the surface itself, similar to chemical reactions of reactive gases at a catalyst surface in chemical reactors. For such surface reactions, our previous method (outlined in Section IV D) can be applied. The initial rate of NO_2 uptake during unstirred conditions, $(r_{NO_2})_0^u$, can be represented as

$$\left(\frac{(r_{NO_2})_0^u}{S}\right) = K_{mNO_2}\,([NO_2]_{G0}) \tag{79}$$

where k_{mNO_2} represents the overall mass coefficient and is defined as

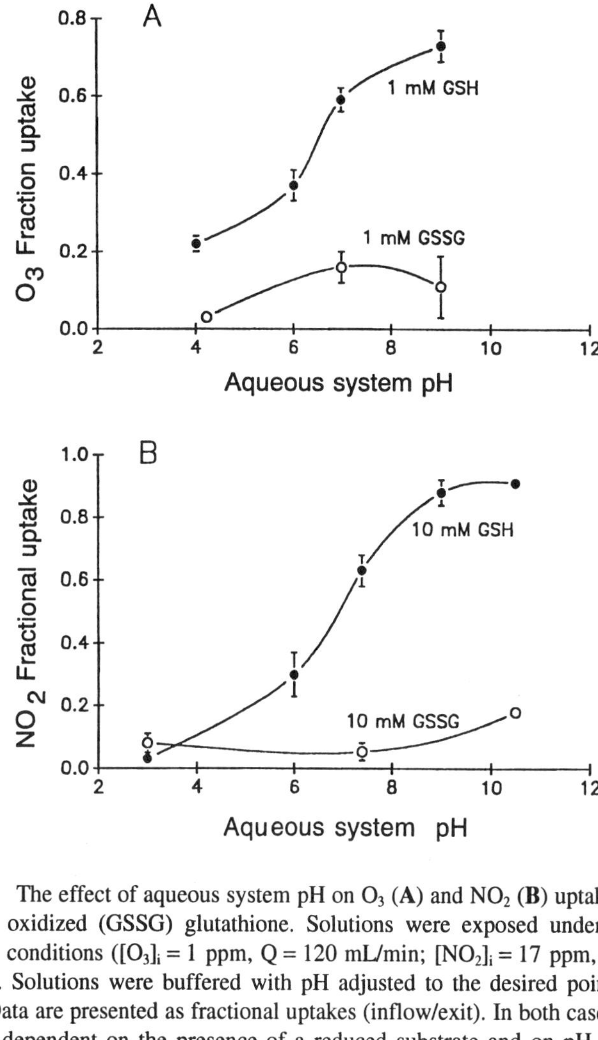

Figure 14 The effect of aqueous system pH on O_3 (**A**) and NO_2 (**B**) uptake by reduced (GSH) and oxidized (GSSG) glutathione. Solutions were exposed under well-mixed, steady-state conditions ($[O_3]_i = 1$ ppm, Q = 120 mL/min; $[NO_2]_i = 17$ ppm, Q = 170 mL/min; 25°C). Solutions were buffered with pH adjusted to the desired point just before exposure. Data are presented as fractional uptakes (inflow/exit). In both cases, absorption was highly dependent on the presence of a reduced substrate and on pH. (For **A**, data are from Ref. 58; for **B**, data are from Ref. 54.)

$$K_{mNO_2} = \left(\frac{(k_{mG})_{NO_2} (k_r)^{NO_2}}{(k_{mG})_{NO_2} + (k_r)^{NO_2}} \right) \tag{80}$$

Over the linear range $NO_2 < 10$ ppm, K_{mNO_2} can be obtained from Figure 15, as 0.0245 (cm/s). If it is assumed that during stirred conditions the gas-phase mass transfer resistance is negligible, then for the stirred conditions, the overall mass

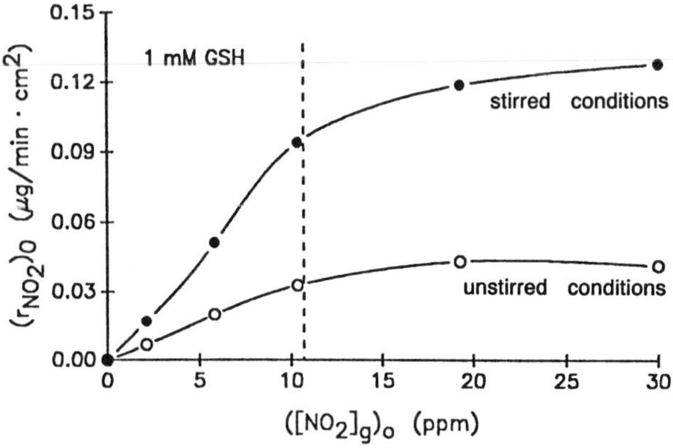

Figure 15 The initial rate of NO_2 gas-phase disappearance by GSH under both stirred and unstirred conditions. 1 mM GSH (pH 7.4) was exposed under transient conditions (25°C) and the initial rates determined from the relationship $r_0 = k\cdot([NO_2]_g)_0$. Stirring induced a significant augmentation in the initial absorption rates. Regardless of stirring conditions, the initial rates saturated above 10.5 ppm $([NO_2]_g)_0$. (From Ref. 57.)

transfer coefficient $K_{mNO_2} = k_r^{NO_2}$, and can be estimated from Figure 15 as 0.090 (cm/s). Using these values of $(k_r)^{NO_2}$ and K_{mNO_2} in Equation 80, we estimate $(k_{mG})_{NO_2} = 0.033$ (cm/s). Based on these estimates of $(k_r)^{NO_2}$ and $(k_{mG})_{NO_2}$, one can estimate the Damkohler number, N_{Da} as 2.7 and effectiveness factor, η as 0.27, using Equations 37 and 38, respectively. These results suggest that, under the conditions of our experiments, NO_2 uptake is gas-phase mass transfer limited. Also, it must be emphasized that the estimate of the reaction rate constant is probably an underestimate, because even under stirred conditions there is likely to be some residual gas-phase mass transfer resistance. Nevertheless, these calculations provide a reasonable example of using mass transfer principles in the presence of chemical reaction, as outlined earlier in Section IV.

A number of studies have suggested that the reactions of NO_2 and O_3 with biological substrates in the epithelial lining fluid occur at the interface itself (56). To investigate this hypothesis, an aqueous film was mimicked by placing filter paper into the bottom of an exposure vessel (57). When the filter paper was minimally wetted using GSH or BALF solutions, the kinetics of NO_2 gas-phase disappearance were analogous to observations with bulk aqueous systems. An additional exposure system, incorporating dual gas chambers separated by a barrier membrane, was used to study NO_2 transmembrane transport. Addition of NO_2 to the gas-phase on one side of a water-wetted barrier did not restrict, compared to dry conditions, NO_2 or O_2 transport across the barrier into the opposing gas chamber. However, if the porous barrier was wetted with GSH or

BALF, whereas O_2 transfer was unaffected, transmembrane movement of NO_2 was significantly restricted, even though the barrier pores were substantially larger than the molecular radius of the NO_2. Presumably, reactive substrates within the aqueous film surrounding the pores reacted with the NO_2, preventing its transmembrane transport. Based on these observations, it is postulated that it is not NO_2 per se but rather its aqueous substrate-derived reaction products that must initiate the processes that lead to cellular injury (57,58).

VII. Noninvasive Measurement and Analysis of Reactive Gas Absorption in Humans

Perhaps the most elegant and innovative application of the principles of mass transfer and mathematical modeling is that by Hu et al. (59) who have developed an innovative fast-responding ozone measurement system to noninvasively measure the absorption of inhaled ozone in different regions of the respiratory tract of healthy adult males. In this method, a small volume of O_3 is rapidly introduced into an inhaled airstream, and the O_3 concentration is continuously monitored at the airway opening throughout the remainder of the inspiration and the following expiration (59). The absorption of O_3 during this single breath is then computed as the difference between the integrals of inspired and expired O_3 concentration data. Moreover, O_3 absorption can be mapped as a function of V_P (the airway volume to which a bolus would penetrate if there were no absorption) by using data from a series of test breaths in which bolus injection occurs at a different time during each inhalation.

To simulate the bolus experiment, a mathematical model was formulated wherein the lung was considered as a symmetrically branching structure in which the longitudinal distribution of ozone concentration and absorption are the same along all possible airway paths from the airway opening to the alveolar sacs. It was also assumed that O_3 reacts so rapidly in mucus and tissue that its absorption rate is proportional to the local gas-phase concentration of O_3. For the case of steady flow through a straight tube, it can be shown that the fraction of entering O_3 that exits the tube is given by (59):

$$1 - \Lambda = \exp\left(-\frac{K_m a \Delta V}{\dot{V}}\right) \tag{81}$$

where Λ is the amount of O_3 absorbed relative to the amount of O_3 in an entering bolus; $\dot{V}$ is the volumetric gas flow rate, and ΔV is the tube volume. Equation 81 is valid for any shape of the entering bolus. In the derivation of Equation 81, it was assumed that ($K_m a$) is constant, that the back pressure of the solute from the tube wall is negligible, and that axial convection is much greater than axial dispersion.

To apply this theory to the experimental data, Hu et al. (59) visualized the tracheobronchial system as a series of compartments, each of which behaves as a separate tube. Longitudinal position within this multicompartmental model was specified by a volume coordinate, V_P corresponding to the penetration of a bolus beyond the O_3 sampling point at $V_P = 0$ during inhalation. Ozone uptake (Λ) was expressed as the amount of O_3 absorbed during a single breath relative to the amount in the inhaled bolus. Measurements of Λ were correlated with the penetration volume (V_P) of the bolus into the respiratory tract. Values of V_P less than 70 mL were considered to be associated with the upper airways, values between 70 and 180 mL were associated with the lower conducting airways, and values greater than 180 mL were associated with the respiratory air spaces.

During quiet oral breathing, Λ increased smoothly with V_P, with 50% of the inhaled O_3 absorbed in the upper airways and the balance absorbed within the lower conducting airways. This compares favorably with the previous results that 40.4% of continuously inhaled O_3 is removed by the extrathoracic airways (60). The effect of increasing the respiratory flow, as might be associated with exercise, was to shift the Λ-V_P distribution distally so that significantly less O_3 was absorbed in the upper airways and more reached the respiratory air spaces. Compared with oral breathing, nasal breathing caused a proximal shift in the Λ-V_P distribution to the extent that absorption in the upper airways increased from 50% to 80%. This trend, previously noted in dogs (42), is likely the result of the large surface : volume ratio, intense flow patterns, and ample supply of mucous substrates in the nose. Therefore, as exercise intensity increases, the lower conducting airways and respiratory air spaces may become more susceptible to O_3 damage because of normal changes in breathing from nasal to oral and increases in respiratory flow. The peak O_3 concentration of an inhaled bolus did not have a significant effect on the Λ-V_P distribution. This would imply that the diffusion and chemical reaction processes dictating O_3 absorption are linear.

The overall mass transfer resistance, ($1/K_m$), was equated to the sum of the individual mass transfer resistances through the gas boundary layer, ($1/k_{mG}$), and the liquid-lining layer, λ/k_{mL} (21,59), where k_{mG} and k_{mL} are the individual mass transfer coefficients in the gas and liquid-lining layers, respectively, and λ is an equilibrium partition-coefficient defined as the molar concentration of O_3 in air relative to that in mucus or surfactant ($=1/\hat{H}$). The liquid-phase mass transfer coefficient, k_{mL}, would be expected to depend on the diffusion and reaction dynamics within the liquid-lining layer but be independent of the gas flow. Hu et al. (59) related k_{mG} to the gas flow rate by a power-law equation of the form $k_{mG} = mV^n$, where m and n were empirical constants whose value depend on the geometry of the gas–liquid interface and the nature of convective gas flow (laminar versus turbulent).

The strong dependence of ($K_m a$) on respiratory flow (Figure 16*A*) indicates that the diffusion resistance of the gas boundary layer was an important determi-

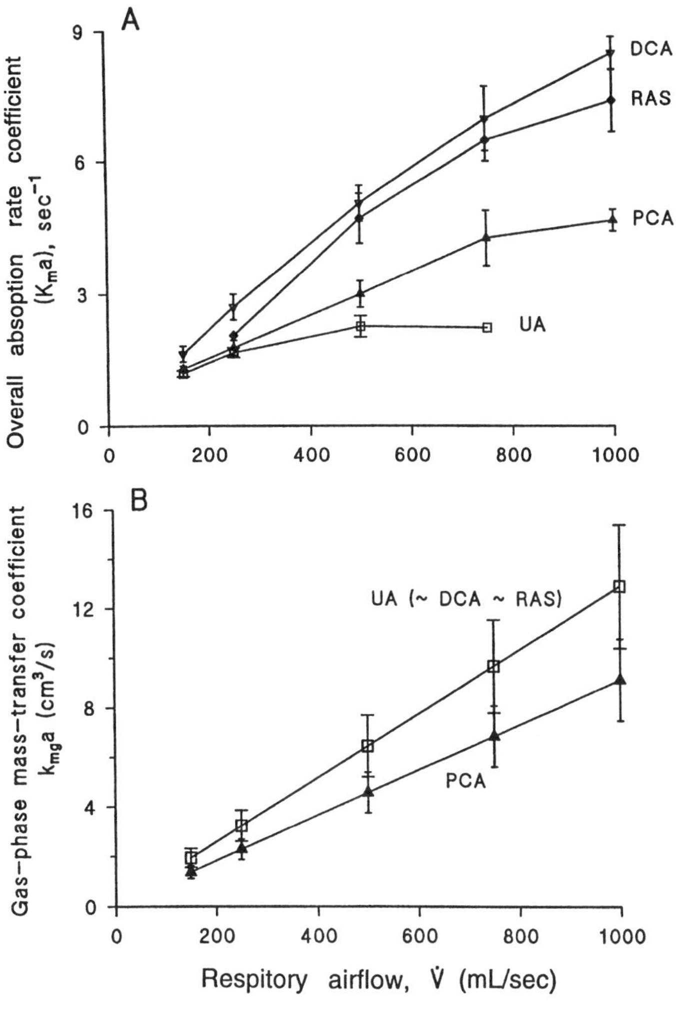

Figure 16 Overall absorption rate coefficient ($K_m a$) and gas-phase mass transfer coefficient as a function of air flow (V) in the four-compartmental model of Hu et al. (59) for analyzing ozone absorption by the human lung. *Abbreviations*: UA = upper airways; PCA = proximal conducting airways; DCA = distal conducting airways; RAS = respiratory airspaces. (Adapted from Ref. 20.)

nant of O_3 absorption in these experiments. Increments in gas flow resulted in an increase in the gas-phase mass transfer coefficients (see Figure 16*B*). From the values of the overall mass transfer coefficient and the gas-phase mass transfer coefficient, the liquid-phase mass transfer coefficient, k_{mL}/λ, was estimated for the various compartments (Figure 17). This increasing importance of the gas diffusion resistance with distal penetration into the airways would be expected because the gas velocity progressively decreases as the airways subdivide.

To further examine the importance of the liquid-phase mass transfer resistance, it was assumed that, as O_3 diffuses through the liquid-lining layer, it undergoes a first order homogeneous chemical reaction with biochemical substrates (21,59), for which the conventional diffusion-reaction theory for formulating k_{mL} (33) was used.

$$\left(\frac{k_{mL}}{\lambda}\right) = \sqrt{k_r D_L}\,\coth\left[\left(\delta\sqrt{\frac{k_r}{D_L}}\right)\right]/\lambda \qquad (82)$$

where coth is the hyperbolic cotangent function, k_r is the reaction rate constant, D_L is the diffusion constant in the liquid-phase, and δ is the thickness of the liquid-lining layer. Assuming that D_L is relatively constant throughout the liquid lining layer, Equation 82 predicts that k_{mL} increases as δ decreases or as k_r increases. However, according to Figure 17, k_{mL}/λ progressively decreased as

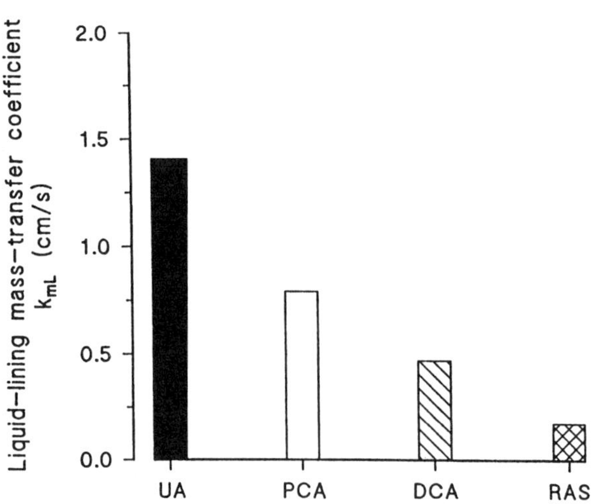

Figure 17 Liquid-lining mass transfer coefficient (k_{mL}) for the four-compartmental model of Hu et al. (59) for analyzing ozone absorption by the human lung. *Abbreviations*: UA = upper airways; PCA = proximal conducting airways; DCA = distal conducting airways; RAS = respiratory airspaces. (Adapted from Ref. 21.)

the bolus penetration increased and, consequently, as the liquid lining layer decreased in thickness. Based on these data, it was concluded that the reactivity of the liquid lining layer must decrease between the mouth and the peripheral airways (21,59). To quantify this trend, the values of k_r in the mucous layer were computed from the k_{mL}/λ, by approximating $\lambda = 0.69$ and $D_L = 2.7 \times 10^{-5}$ cm/s by their aqueous values (9), and by making the reasonable assumption that $\delta > 0.2$ µm in all conducting airways. These calculations yielded a value for k_r of 7.3×10^6, 2.3×10^6, and 8.2×10^5 s^{-1} in the mucous lining of the upper airway, conducting airways proximal (CAP), and conducting airways distal (CAD) compartments, respectively (21,59).

Based on their cumulative data, Ultman and Ben-Jebria (21) and Hu et al. (59) concluded that the large majority of inhaled O_3 does not reach the respiratory zone during quiet breathing. However, an elevated respiratory flow concomitant with exercise would deliver O_3 to the alveolar region. Moreover, because the nose is more efficient at O_3 uptake than the mouth, oral breathing would result in a deeper penetration of O_3 than nasal breathing. During diffusion through the mucous blanket, while en route to underlying epithelium, O_3 undergoes a chemical reaction with biochemical substrates; the rate constant of this reaction is on the order of 1 million reciprocal seconds. Because of this very rapid rate, the diffusion resistance through mucus is relatively low, and the larger diffusion resistance through the respired gas boundary layer is an important determinant of the net rate of O_3 absorption.

VIII. Summary

In comparison with calculated estimates of dose, mathematical dosimetry models offer a more comprehensive approach to defining pollutant tissue dose to the respiratory tract. These models generally have two components. The first is to determine the regional distribution of the inhaled pollutant gas in the respiratory tract. Mathematical expressions or equations are used to describe the transport of inhaled gas by convection (bulk transport), or by longitudinal and radial diffusion. With these equations it is possible to analyze how the pollutant gas is transported within the respiratory tracts of humans and animals, and how its transport is altered by changing breathing patterns. The second component is to determine how much inhaled gas is absorbed by the mucus in the airways and the surfactant in the alveoli, and how much then moves by convection and diffusion through these fluid layers to react with the underlying respiratory tissues. This final quantity is the tissue dose of the inhaled gas that is the most useful value for exposure-dose-response relations.

The dosimetric models of Miller and coworkers (8,9,14) and Grotberg and coworkers (44,45) used different approaches to describe ozone transport and absorption in an idealized human lung. The idealized model (38) portrays the lung as a symmetrically branching network with 24 generations of airways. Each generation consists of only one type of airway, which is located at the same volumetric depth in the lungs. For example, the trachea is generation 0 and the terminal bronchioles are at generation 16. Despite their theoretical differences, all the models predict that, for resting breathing, the tissue doese increases gradually from the trachea to a maximum value at generation 17, which corresponds with the respiratory bronchioles where the mucus-covered conducting airways lead into the surfactant-covered gas-exchange tissues in the acinus (i.e., respiratory bronchioles, alveolar ducts, alveolar sacs, and alveoli). At deeper generations within the acinus, tissue dose decreases markedly. At the acinar entrance, the liquid lining layer is thin and the cross-sectional surface area of the lung starts to expand to promote gas transport to the lung surface. Both of these factors work to increase the dose of ozone to the local tissues. Even though the conducting airways absorb a large fraction of ozone fairly evenly over their length, the relatively thick mucous layer provides protection to the underlying airway epithelium. Therefore, the tissue dose increases appreciably only where the covering layer becomes thinner in the terminal portions of the conducting airways. It is significant that the highest tissue dose predicted by the models is at the acinar entrance because this region corresponds to the primary site of tissue damage found in animals exposed to ozone (61–63). The relationship of pollutant concentration, barrier thickness, and site of lung injury is shown schematically in Figure 18 (10). The three mathematical dosimetry models predicted different patterns and magnitudes of tissue dose in humans. Miller et al. (8,9) predicted that a broad region of high tissue dose extends from generation 11 (terminal bronchi) to generation 18 or 19 (respiratory bronchioles). In contrast, Grotberg and coworkers (44,45) predicted a sharp peak of tissue dose from generation 17 (maximum) to 19, with the maximum dose at generation 17 being almost one order of magnitude greater than that predicted by Miller and coworkers (8,9).

When tidal volume and breathing frequency are increased to represent exercise, the models predict that tissue dose increases dramatically in the respiratory bronchioles at the acinar entrance and in the distal acinar generations but that dose to the airway epithelium is either the same as resting breathing (8,9,44,45) or only modestly increased despite a lower absorption per breath because of the greater number of breaths taken per unit of time (15). Overton and Graham (15) predicted that, during maximal exercise, ozone absorption for the total lung increases with age ranging from 87% for 2-year-old children to 93% for adults; the respective values for acinar absorption are 78% for 2 year olds and 90% for adults.

It is important to consider the chemical reaction kinetics between inhaled reactive gases and biomolecules within the mucus and surfactant in order to

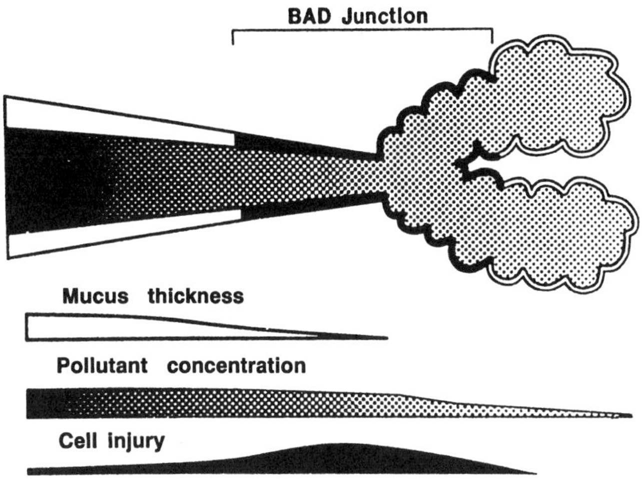

Figure 18 Schematic of the relationship between pollutant concentration, mucous thickness, and the site of inhaled oxidant-inducing lung injury. *Abbreviations*: BAD junction = bronchoalveolar duct junction. (From Ref. 11.)

assess tissue dose accurately. For a highly reactive gas such as ozone, for example, it may be inadequate to consider only the portion of the absorbed ozone that may escape reacting with substrates and penetrates through the mucus and surfactant, as was done in the dosimetric models described above. It is possible that ozone reacts partially or completely with glycoproteins, unsaturated lipids, proteins, and other constituents at the surface of the mucous and surfactant layers to form products, such as aldehydes and hydrogen peroxide, which are themselves reactive. These reaction products may, in turn, initiate a cascade of chemical reactions that produce other reactive products that ultimately come in contact with and damage tissues (64). Ozone or NO_2 and its reactive products can react with the lipid membranes of cells, causing lipid peroxidation and the production of free radicals, which then go on to cause further damage. Protection of the tissues from O_3 or NO_2 also depends on variations in the thickness and completeness of the fluid layers: the mucus may be 20 μm thick in the upper airways and decrease to about 0.1 μm in the small airways; surfactant may be only 0.1 μm in the alveoli (9).

Chemical reactions provide an added level of complexity to the task of estimating the distribution and absorption of an inhaled reactive gas. Thus, there is need for quantitative characterization of the kinetic reactivity of specific reactive substrates within the biological elements in mucus, tissue, and cells. This new information on specific kinetic parameters for biological substrates needs to be fully accommodated in mathematical dosimetry models. Improved quantitative description of mass transfer of inhaled reactive gases through individual diffusion barriers, particularly the mucous layer, bronchial wall, and the alveolar-capillary network is necessary. There is a need to incorporate both ventilatory and perfusion inhomogeneities in mathematical models so as to expand their applicability. For example, heterogeneities in lung geometry and airway mechanics might induce parallel inhomogeneities in the dose delivered to the distal airways. Thus, individuals with underlying disease may be at risk of regional lung damage at an inhaled dose, which might be safe for individuals with anatomically normal lungs. Furthermore, recent studies have demonstrated that exposure time may also variably influence mass transfer rates (65), which may stem from exposure-induced alterations in the physicochemical properties of the lung lining layer (e.g., reactive substrate concentrations). Because of the large parameter set necessary for a realistic quantitative description, it is vital that mathematical models be subjected to a rigorous formal parameter sensitivity analysis to allow delineation of the crucial parameters and rate-limiting steps in the overall gas absorption. Using consistent experimental protocols, total uptake of selected pollutants should be measured in different animal species and then used to develop rules for extrapolation. Specifically, the uptake rate should be correlated using known interspecies differences in lung volume, surface area, respiratory rates, and rate-limiting mass transfer coefficients within the framework of an appropriate mathematical model. An adequate quantification of the magnitude and site of pollutant reactive gas absorption is an interdisciplinary problem requiring the modeling skills of engineers, as well as biological expertise of biochemists, toxicologists, and physiologists.

Acknowledgments

This work was supported through funds provided by NIH grant HL54696, the UTMB Biomedical Engineering Center, and the Constance Marsili Schafer Endowed Research Fund.

References

1. U.S. Environmental Protection Agency. Air Quality Criteria for Ozone and Related Photochemical Oxidants EPA/600/AP-93/004cF, 1996. Volume III.
2. Lippman M. Health effects of troposheric ozone: review of recent research findings and their implications to ambient air quality standard. J Expos Anal Environ Epidemid 1993; 3:103–129.
3. Schlesinger RB. Nitrogen oxides. In: Lippman M, ed. Environmental Toxicants: Human Exposures and Their Health Effects. New York: Van Nostrand Reinhold, 1992:412–453.

4. Lippman M. Sulfur oxides—acidic aerosols and SO_2. In: Lippman M, ed. Environmental Toxicants: Human Exposures and Their Health Effects. New York: Van Nostrand Reinhold, 1992:543–574.
5. Bidani A, Crandall ED. Quantitative aspects of capillary CO_2 exchange. In: Chang HK, Paiva M, eds. Respiratory Physiology. An Analytical Approach. New York: Marcel Dekker, 1989:371–419.
6. Bidani A. Analysis of abnormalities of capillary CO_2 exchange in vivo. J Appl Physiol 1991; 70:1686–1699.
7. Wagner PD. Diffusion and chemical reaction in pulmonary gas exchange. Physiol Rev 1977; 57:62–71.
8. Miller FJ, Menzel DB, Coffin DL. Similarity between man and laboratory animals in regional pulmonary deposition of ozone. Environ Res 1978; 17:84–101.
9. Miller FJ, Overton JH, Jaskot RH, Menzel DB. A model of the regional uptake of gaseous pollutants in the lung. I. The sensitivity of the uptake of ozone in the human lung to lower respiratory tract secretions and exercise. Toxicol Appl Pharmacol 1985; 79:1–27.
10. Miller FJ, Graham JA. Research needs and advances in inhalation dosimetry indentified through the use of mathematical dosimetry models of ozone. Toxicol Lett 1988; 44:231–246.
11. Miller FJ, Smolko Ed, Crapo JD. Extrapolation modelling: advancements and research issues in lung dosimetry. In: Crapo JD, Miller FJ, Smolko ED, Graham JA, Hayes AW, eds. Extrapolation of Dosimetric Relationships for Inhaled Particles and Gases. San Diego: Academic Press, 1989:3–14.
12. Miller FJ, Overton JH, Kimbell JS, Russell ML. Regional respiratory tract absorption of inhaled reactive gases. In: Gardner DE, Crapo JD, McClellan RO, eds. Toxicology of the Lung. 2nd ed. New York: Raven Press, 1993:485–525.
13. Overton JS. Physiochemical processes and the formulation of dosimetry models. J Toxicol Environ Health 1984; 13:273–299.
14. Overton JH, Graham RC, Miller FJ. A model of the regional uptake of gaseous pollutants in the lung. II. The sensitivity of ozone uptake in laboratory animal lungs to anatomical and ventilatory parameters. Toxicol Appl Pharmacol 1987; 88:418–432.
15. Overton JH, Graham RC. Predictions of ozone absorption in human lungs from newborn to adult. Health Physics 1989; 57:29–36.
16. Overton JH, Graham RC. Simulation of the uptake of a reactive gas in a rat respiratory tract model with an asymmetric tracheobronchial region patterned on complete conducting airway cast data. Comput Biomed Res 1995; 28:171–190.
17. Hanna LM, Frank R, Scherer PW. Absorption of soluble gases and vapors in the respiratory system. In: Chang HK, Paiva M, eds. Respiratory Physiology: An Analytical Approach. New York: Marcel Dekker, 1989:277–316.
18. Seinfeld JH. Atmospheric Chemistry and Physics of Air Pollution. New York: John Wiley & Sons, 1986:197–272.
19. Ultman JS. Gas transport in the conducting airways. In: Engel LA, Paiva M, eds. Gas Mixing and Distribution in the Lung. New York: Marcel Dekker, 1985:63–136.
20. Ultman J. Transport and uptake of inhaled gases. In: Air Pollution, the Automobile, and Public Health. Health Effects Institute. Washington, DC: National Academy Press, 1988:323–366.

21. Ultman JS, Ben-Jebria A. Noninvasive determination of respiratory ozone absorption: development of a fast-responding ozone analyzer. Health Effects Institute Research Report #39. Cambridge, MA: Health Effects Institute, 1990.
22. Gelzleichter TR, Witschi H, Last JA. Concentration-response relationships of rats to exposure to oxidant air pollutants: a critical test of Haber's law for ozone and nitrogen dioxide. Toxicol Appl Pharmacol 1992; 65:73–80.
23. Silverman F, Folinsbee LJ, Barnard J, Shepard RJ. Pulmonary function changes in ozone: interactions of concentration and ventilation. J Appl Physiol 1976; 41: 859–864.
24. Folinsbee LJ, Drinkwater BL, Bedi JF, Horvath SM. The influence of exercise on the pulmonary function changes due to exposure to low concentrations of ozone. In: Folinsbee LJ, Borgia JF, Drinkwater BL, Gliner JA, Bedi JF, eds. Environmental Stress: Individual Human Adaptations. New York: Academic Press 1978:124–145.
25. Adams WC, Savin WM, Christo AE. Detection of ozone toxicity during continuous exercise via the effective dose concept. J Appl Physiol 1981; 51:415–422.
26. Astarita G. Mass Transfer with Chemical Reaction. New York: Elsevier, 1967.
27. Bird RB, Stewart WE, Lightfoot EN. Transport Phenomena. New York: John Wiley & Sons, 1960.
28. Cussler EL. Diffusion: Mass Transfer in Fluid Systems. New York: Cambridge University Press, 1984.
29. Doran PM. Bioprocess Engineering Principles. New York: Academic Press, 1995.
30. Fogler HS. Elements of Chemical Reaction Engineering. Englewood Cliffs, NJ: Prentice Hall, 1992.
31. Froment GF, Bischoff KB. Chemical Reactor Analysis and Design. New York: John Wiley & Sons, 1990.
32. Hines AL, Maddox RN. Mass Transfer: Fundamentals and Applications. Englewood Cliffs, NJ: Prentice Hall, 1985.
33. Hobler T. Mass Transfer in Absorbers. New York: Pergamon Press, 1966.
34. Weber WJ, DiGiano FA. Process Dynamics in Environmental Systems. New York: John Wiley & Sons, 1996:503–567.
35. Clever HL, Battino R. The solubility of gases in liquids. In: Dack MRJ, ed. Solutions and Solubilities. Techniques in Chemistry, Vol. 8. New York, John Wiley & Sons, 1975:380–441.
36. Mackay D, Shiu WY. A critical review of Henry's law constants for chemicals of environmental interest. J Phys Chem Ref Data 1981; 10:1175–1195.
37. Dahl AR. Contemporary issues in toxicology: dose concepts for inhaled vapors and gases. Toxicol Appl Pharmacol 1990; 103:185–197.
38. Weibel ER. Morphometry of the Human Lung. New York: Academic Press, 1963.
39. Aharonson EF, Menkes H, Gurtner F, Swift DL, Proctor DF. Effect of respiratory airflow rate on removal of soluble vapors by the nose. J Appl Physiol 1974; 37: 654–657.
40. Kleinman MT. Sulfur dioxide and exercise: relationships between response and absorption in upper airways. J Air Pollution Control Assoc 1984; 34:32–37.
41. Frank NR, Yoder RE, Brain JD, Yokoyama E. SO_2 (^{38}S labeled) absorption by the

nose and mouth under conditions of varying concentration and flow. Arch Environ Health 1969; 18:315–322.

42. Yokoyama E. Frank R. Respiratory uptake of ozone in dogs. Arch Environ Health 1972; 25:132–138.
43. McJilton C, Thielke J, Frank R. Ozone uptake model for the respiratory system (abstr A33). San Francisco, CA: American Industrial Hygiene Association Conference, 1972:20.
44. Grotberg JB. Gas absorption in pulmonary airways at low Peclet number. J Biomech Eng. 1990; 112;177–182.
45. Grotberg JB, Seth BV, Mockros LF. An analysis of pollutant gas transport and absorption in pulmonary airways. J Biomech Eng 1990; 112:168–176.
46. Scherer PW, Shendalman LH, Crenne NM, Bouhuys A. Measurement of axial diffusivities in a model of the bronchial airways. J Appl Physiol 1975; 38:719–726.
47. Sankarsubramanian R, Gill WN. Unsteady convection diffusion with interphase mass transfer. Proc R Soc Lond Series A, 1973; A333:115–119.
48. Mercer RR, Anjilvel S, Miller FJ, Crapo JC. Inhomogeneity of ventilatory unit volume and its effects on reactive gas uptake. J Appl Physiol 1991; 70:2193–2205.
49. Ben-Jebria A, Full AP, DeMaria DD, Ball BA, Ultman JS. Dynamics of sulfur dioxide absorption in excised porcine tracheae. Environ Res 1990; 53:119–134.
50. Postlethwait EM, Bidani A. In-vitro systems for studying respiratory system toxicology. In: Roth RA, ed. Comprehensive Toxicology. Vol. 8. Toxicology of the Respiratory System. New York: Permagon, 1997.
51. Postlethwait EM, Bidani A. Reactive uptake governs the pulmonary airspace removal of inhaled nitrogen dioxide. J Appl Physiol 1990; 68:594–603.
52. Postlethwait EM, Langford SD, Bidani A. Determinants of inhaled ozone absorption in isolated rat lungs. Toxicol Appl Pharmacol 1994; 125:77–89.
53. Postlethwait EM, Langford SD, Bidani A. Kinetics of NO_2 airspace absorption in isolated rat lungs. J Appl Physiol 1992; 73:1939–1945.
54. Postlethwait EM, Langford SD, Bidani A. Reactive absorption of nitrogen dioxide by pulmonary epithelial lining fluid. J Appl Physiol 1990; 69:523–531.
55. Postlethwait EM, Langford SD, Bidani A. Interfacial transfer kinetics of NO_2 into pulmonary epithelial lining fluid. J Appl Physiol 1991; 71:1502–1510.
56. Kanofsky JR, Sima PD. Reactive absorption of ozone by aqueous biomolecule solutions: Implication for the role of sulfhydryl compounds as targets for ozone. Arch Biochem Biophys 1995; 31:52–56.
57. Postlethwait EM, Langford SD, Bidani A. Transfer of NO_2 through pulmonary epithelial lining fluid. Toxicol Appl Pharmacol 1991; 109:464–471.
58. Langford SD, Bidani A, Postlethwait EM. Ozone reactive absorption by pulmonary epithelial lining fluid constituents. Toxicol Appl Pharmacol 1995; 132:122–130.
59. Hu S-C, Ben-Jabria A, Ultman JS. Longitudinal distribution of ozone absorption in the lung: quiet respiration in healthy subjects. J Appl Physiol 1992; 73:1655–1661.
60. Gerrity TR, Weaver RA, Berntsen J, House DE, O'Neil JJ. Extrathoracic and intrathoracic removal of O_3 in tidal-breathing humans. J Appl Physiol 1988; 65:393–400.
61. Mellick PW, Dungworth DL, Schwartz LW, Tyler WS. Short term morphological

effects of high ambient levels of ozone on the lungs of rhesus monkeys. Lab Invest 1977; 36:82–90.

62. Stephens RJ, Sloan MF, Evans MJ, Freeman G. Early response to low levels of ozone. Am J Pathol 1974; 74:31–58.
63. Hatch GE. Comparative biochemistry of airway lining fluid. In: Parent RA, ed. Treatise on Pulmonary Toxicology. Vol. I. Comparative Biology of the Normal Lung. Ann Arbor, MI: CRC Press, 1992:617–632.
64. Pryor WA. How far does ozone penetrate into the pulmonary air/tissue boundary before it reacts? Free Rad Biol Med 1991; 12:83–88.
65. Asplund PT, Ben-Jebria A, Rigas ML, Ultman JS. Longitudinal distribution of ozone absorption in the lung: effect of continuous inhalation exposure. J Appl Physiol. In press.

10

Gas and Particle Transport in the Lung

CHANTAL DARQUENNE

University of California, San Diego
La Jolla, California

MANUEL PAIVA

Université Libre de Bruxelles
Brussels, Belgium

I. Introduction

Study in the fields of gas and particle transport in the lung has proceeded in parallel, with very limited cross-fertilization. Here, we focus on particle dispersion through the bronchial tree, showing that much can be learned from each field in terms of experimental techniques, model simulations, and understanding of mechanisms. Particle deposition is discussed in detail in Chapter 12, and gas exchange in the airways and O_2 and CO_2 diffusion through the alveolar capillary membrane are excluded in this discussion. These subjects are dealt with in several chapters of this book. Furthermore, we have also excluded discussion of charged and nonspherical particles (e.g., fibers).

The classical work of Altshuler et al. (1) was aimed at answering the question: "What information on the mixing of pulmonary flow is contained in the measurements of exhaled aerosol?" The authors pioneered the use of aerosol inspirations and the comparison of aerosol and gas concentrations during a subsequent breath as a new tool to investigate pulmonary ventilation. The measurement of nitrogen concentration with a rapid gas analyzer, after an inspiration of oxygen, the so-called single breath wash-out, was first performed by Fowler (2) one decade earlier. The attempts to understand the observed nitrogen expired concentration profile have stimulated much of the research in gas mixing and ventilation in the lung.

One of the characteristics of both gas molecules at normal pressure and inhaled particles is that binary molecular and particle interactions can be neglected. For gases, this corresponds to the classical approximation leading to the ideal gas law. For spherical particles, the approximation leads to Stokes-Einstein equation for Brownian motion. Theoretically, a direct consequence of these principles is that two independent experiments should give similar results: 1. the tidal inspiration of inert gas or aerosol, followed by the measurement of the expired concentration, or 2. a succession of inspired boluses, such that its sum equals the tidal inspiration. Theoretically, much more information is obtained from the bolus-expired concentrations. Bolus of radioactive xenon was first used by Dollfuss et al. (3) to measure regional lung ventilation. Inspiration of bolus of an inert gas (argon) at different preinspiratory lung volumes was first described by Cumming et al. (4). Heyder and Davies (5) and Muir et al. (6) performed aerosol bolus experiments. The development of this technique during the past years is associated with the production of monodisperse aerosols. Bolus (particle or inert gas) testing is the focus of this chapter.

II. Concepts

A. Definitions

Vocabulary used by researchers working in different fields is not always the same. The following are concepts and definitions used in this discussion:

Aerodynamic (equivalent) diameter: Diameter of a unit density (g/cm^3) sphere, which would undergo sedimentation at the same velocity as the particle in question.

Aerosol: A gas (usually air) in which particles are suspended. Therefore, it consists of two phases: a gas and a particle phase.

Axial (or longitudinal) dispersion: Mixing process resulting from nonuniformities in the axial velocity profiles and the molecular diffusivity. It can be quantitatively described by the sum of an effective (or apparent) diffusion coefficient characterizing convective mixing (K_{cv}) and the binary molecular diffusion coefficient (D): $K = K_{cv} + D$.

Axial streaming: Dispersion with particles confined to their streamlines.

Brownian motion: Random motion of particles whose size and mass are much larger than those of the host medium molecules. The particle diffusion (Brownian diffusion) flow is also described by Fick's law.

Bulk (or piston or plug) flow: Hypothetical movement of all gas species at the mean velocity of the airstream.

Convective (or bulk) mixing: All mechanisms, except molecular or Brownian diffusion for molecules and particles, respectively, that are involved in the irreversible transfer of matter (turbulent mixing is a particular case of convective mixing).

Diffusion front: Quasistationary gas concentration profile within airways during inspiration at constant flow.

Fick's law of diffusion: The mass flux (quantity of a substance per unit of area and time) is equal to the diffusion coefficient times the concentration gradient (concentration per unit of length).

Particle recovery: Ratio of the particle number concentration in (or a given fraction of) the exhaled volume and the particle concentration in the inhaled aerosol.

Peclet number (Pe): $Pe = ud/D$, where u is the mean convective velocity, d the diameter of a duct of circular cross section, and D the molecular diffusion coefficient.

Reynolds number (Re): $Re = ud/\nu$, where u is the mean convective velocity, d the diameter of a duct of circular cross section, and ν the kinematic viscosity (viscosity divided by fluid density).

Sedimentation velocity: Mean settling velocity at which a particle falls under gravitation.

Streamline: Curve, tangent in each point to the mean molecular velocity.

Taylor dispersion (or Taylor-Aris dispersion): Axial dispersion (k) of a constituent of diffusion coefficient D for fully developed laminar flow with mean velocity u in a duct of constant cross section radius r in the limit where a mean distance L is covered and the following condition holds: $4\ L/r \gg u\ r/D$. Then $k = D + r^2u^2/48D$ (7–9).

B. Mechanisms of Particle Transport

Usually, in the inhaled air, particles are suspended and carried with the bulk flow through the respiratory tract. If all inhaled particles would be carried along air streamlines, they would behave like a nondiffusing, nonabsorptive gas. However, particle trajectories differ from air streamlines because of forces acting upon the particles. The efficiency of particle transport across the streamlines and consequently toward airway and parenchymal surfaces is considered in this section. Efficiency depends mainly on the size of the particles.

Particles larger than approximately 0.1 μm in diameter settle across streamlines under the action of gravity. According to Stokes' law, particles sediment with a velocity as follows:

$$V_S = \frac{\rho_p g d_p^2}{18\mu} \qquad (1)$$

where ρ_p and d_p are particle density and diameter, respectively, g is gravitational acceleration, and μ is air viscosity. It follows that the probability of deposition by sedimentation increases with increasing particle size and density. The probability of deposition also increases with increasing residence time of the particles in the respiratory tract.

Particles larger than approximately 1.5 μm in diameter carry sufficient mass to be also transported by the action of inertial forces. The displacement of the particles resulting from this mechanism is usually expressed as a function of the Stokes' number, which is defined by

$$Stk = \frac{\rho_p d_p^2 u}{18\mu d} \tag{2}$$

where u is the mean air velocity in an airway with a diameter d. The efficiency of inertial transport increases with increasing particle size and density.

Another particle transport mechanism is due to Brownian motions. It is effective for particles smaller than approximately 1 μm in diameter. The diffusion rate is proportional to the diffusion coefficient D_B that can be calculated from the following equation:

$$D_B = \frac{ckT}{3\pi\mu d_p} \tag{3}$$

where c is the Cunningham correction factor (10) that accounts for the decreased air resistance caused by slippage when the diameter of the particle (d_p) comes close to the mean free path of gas molecules, k is the Boltzmann's constant, T is the absolute temperature, and μ is the dynamic viscosity of air. The efficiency of the diffusional particle transport increases with decreasing particle size. However, it is orders of magnitude lower than molecular diffusion.

Particles of unit density in the size range 0.4–0.5 μm diameter present minimum intrinsic mobility and consequently their intrapulmonary trajectories have the smallest differences with the air streamlines. This is why these spheres can be considered a nondiffusing gas and used to probe convective mixing. This is also why these spheres are those of minimum deposition in the human respiratory tract. Deposition for particles smaller than 0.4–0.5 μm diameter increases with decreasing particle size because of diffusional transport. For particles larger than 0.4 μm in diameter, deposition increases with increasing particle size because of gravitational and inertial transport.

Diffusional and gravitational particle transport are time-dependent mechanisms, whereas inertial particle transport is a velocity-dependent mechanism. Therefore, particle deposition in the extrapulmonary and large intrapulmonary airways is governed by inertial transport. In these airways, the bulk flow velocity is large enough for exposing particles to sufficiently large inertial forces. But the residence time of the particles carried with the bulk flow through these airways is too short for an appreciable contribution of gravitational and diffusional transport onto the airway surfaces. Toward the periphery, the bulk air flow velocity decreases and, at the same time, the time available for gravitational and diffusional particle transport increases so that the contribution of inertial transport to the overall transport decreases and particle transport is governed by the time-dependent mechanisms, sedimentation and diffusion.

Intrapulmonary particle deposition is discussed in detail in Chapter 12.

III. Gas and Particle Transport in the Healthy Lung

Conducting airways, acini, and alveoli are not only structural entities but they also correspond to a logical functional separation for the simultaneous study of gas-particle transport. This chapter shows that 1. in the conducting airways, the transport of gas or particles is almost identical, 2. the acinar branching is determinant for gas (not particle) transport and mixing, and 3. within one alveolus, it is necessary to describe particle transport, whereas gas diffusion can be considered as instantaneous.

A. Transport and Mixing in the Conducting Airways

Before an inspired molecule of oxygen reaches an alveolus and the lung capillaries, it has to flow through the conducting airways, whose volume approaches 175 cm^3 in humans (11). This volume was derived from a hyperinflated cadaveric lung, and the mean value for normal subjects is slightly smaller. Most of what is known about gas mixing in the alveolar zone of the lung results from studies with inspired inert gases, whose concentrations are measured in the subsequent expirations. Therefore, any inference on mixing in the lung periphery depends on knowledge of gas transport in the conducting airways.

Altshuler et al. (1) demonstrated that convection contributes to gas transport from tidal air to lung air. They used particles of about 0.5 μm diameter as a tracer of mass movement of the air in which they were suspended. Because these particles behave as a "nondiffusing" gas, their transport from tidal air to lung air is an indication for the convective exchange (mixing) of tidal and lung air. The researchers showed that particles inhaled in a single breath are not only exhaled with the tidal air but also with lung air. During tidal breathing, particles remain suspended in lung air at the end of each exhalation and are thus transported deeper into the lungs during subsequent inhalations.

One of the most detailed descriptions of gas transport in the conducting airways was given in 1985 by Ultman, where an extensive reference list can be found. This chapter focuses on more recent literature and discussion is limited to normal breathing. For an inspiratory mouth flow of 0.4 L/s, Reynolds number (Re) decreases from approximately 3000 at the glottis to 1 at the level of terminal bronchioles. This calculation is usually performed based on the symmetrical 23-generation Weibel model (11), and the asymmetry of real lung introduces some variability on Re. The longitudinal molecular or particle flow ($\dot{V}_T$) in the airways can be expressed as the sum of bulk transport and longitudinal mixing, which is mathematically written as a generalization of Fick's law of diffusion (12):

$$\dot{V}_T = C\dot{V} - A(K_{cv} + D)\frac{\partial C}{\partial x} \tag{4}$$

where C is the cross-sectional (A) averaged particle or gas fraction, $\dot{V}$ the volumetric flow, $C\dot{V}$ the bulk transport, x the distance measured in the flow direction, D the molecular diffusion coefficient, and K_{cv} the longitudinal dispersion coefficient associated to convective mixing.

Chemical engineers have extensively used the so-called impulse response theory to study the dynamics of chemical processes within tubes. Adapted to the study of gas and particle mixing within the bronchial tree, this technique consists of a bolus (inert gas or particles) inspiration, followed by the measurement of its concentration during the subsequent expiration. A first quantitative description of axial dispersion was given by Scherer et al. (13) based on the dispersion of benzene in a five-generation model of the bronchial tree. These authors have suggested the following equation for the axial dispersion coefficient

$$K_{cv} = \gamma u d \tag{5}$$

where K_{cv} is the effective diffusivity, u the mean axial velocity, d the airway diameter, and γ equals 1.08 for inspiration and 0.37 for expiration. Haselton and Scherer (14) explained convective mixing based on irreversibilities in axial streaming caused by the difference in shape between the velocity profiles during inspiration and expiration (15).

The first quantitative evaluation of axial dispersion in pulmonary airways was given by Ultman et al. (16). These authors performed experiments in which the subjects inhaled He and SF_6 bolus and measured the dispersion or volume variance σ^2 of their expired concentrations (Figure 1). The inspired bolus were followed by a given volume of air up to the end of the inspiration (penetration

Figure 1 Bolus-response data for a healthy male subject at a constant respiratory flow of 0.4 L/s. The progressive spreading of the expired SF_6 distribution is shown at penetrations of 80 mL (**A**), 135 mL (**B**), and 205 mL (**C**). The dashed lines demark the end of inspiration. The relationship between volume variance σ^2 and bolus penetration $\overline{V}$ is given (**D**) for both He (closed circles) and SF_6 (closed triangles). (From Ref. 16.)

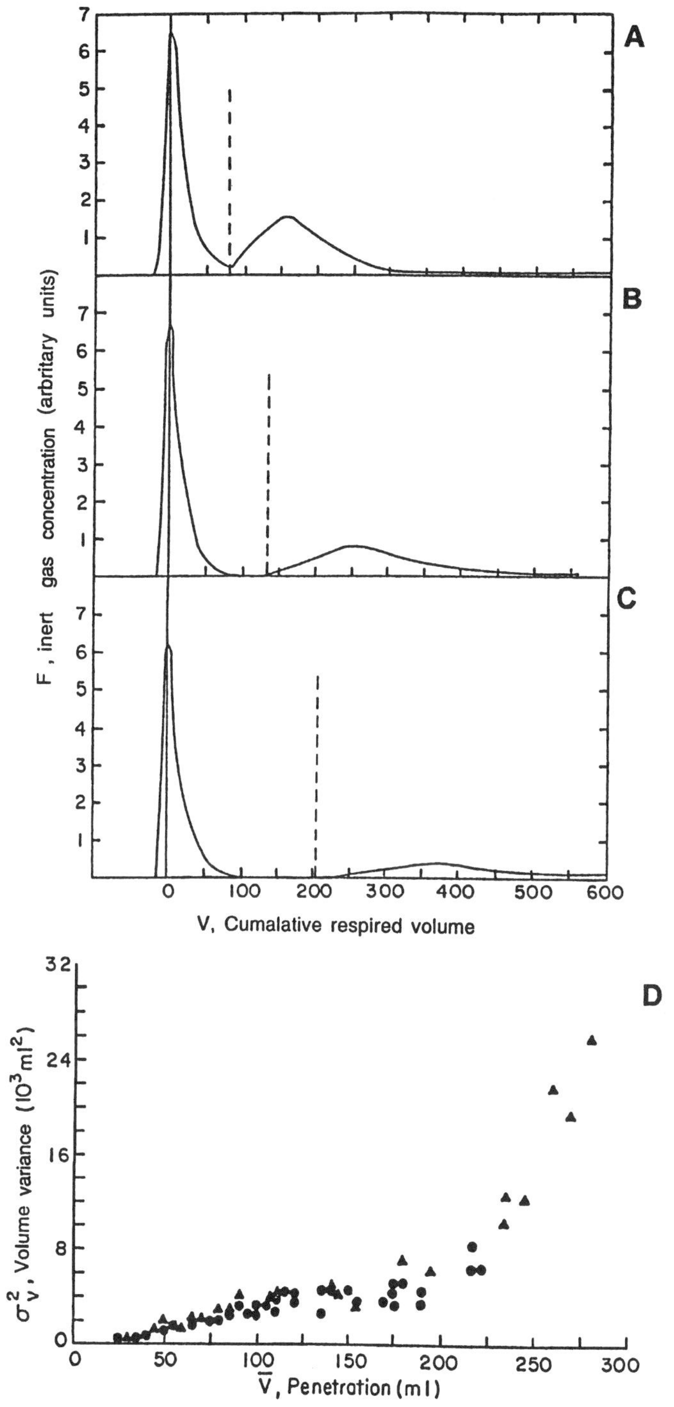

A
B
C
D
F, inert gas concentration (arbitrary units)
V, Cumalative respired volume
σ_v^2, Volume variance (10^3 ml^2)
$\bar{V}$, Penetration (ml)

volume) and an expiration at constant flow. The lower panel of Figure 1 represents both He and SF_6 volume variances:

$$\sigma^2 = \sigma^2_{ex} - \sigma^2_{in} \tag{6}$$

as a function of the (inspired) bolus penetration volumes. σ^2_{ex} and σ^2_{in} are the variances of the expired and inspired distributions, respectively. A remarkable result of this study was that, for bolus penetrations smaller than 150 mL, σ^2 was virtually identical for He and SF_6. This result did not support Taylor type of dispersion, in which a dependence on molecular diffusion is expected. Subsequent studies by the same group (12) are compatible with the following expression for convective mixing:

$$K_{cv} = 0.167\ ul \tag{7}$$

where u is the mean axial velocity and l the length of the corresponding branch of the bronchial tree. Here, the numerical factor is the same for inspiration and expiration and corresponds to axial streaming for fully developed laminar flow in a duct of length l (12). However, Equation 7 is only valid for Pe (d/l) > 200 (negligible radial diffusion), where d is the airway diameter. For He and SF_6 during quiet breathing, this corresponds to the first three or four generations of the bronchial tree (12). For particles, because Brownian diffusion is so small, Pe (d/l) is larger than 200 in almost all the bronchial tree.

Although it is tempting to consider a potential role of Taylor dispersion in the airways, both theoretical (17) and experimental results (18) suggest that its effect, if any, is very small. This is not surprising in view of the extraordinary complexity of flow in the airways including secondary flows at the bifurcations. Although Taylor dispersion probably does not apply directly for mixing in the lung, it gives an upper limit for axial dispersion to which results can be compared.

During recent years, measurements performed simultaneously with gases and aerosols increased current understanding of convective mixing in the conducting airways. Although the experiments were performed in (mechanically ventilated) dogs airways (19), the general conclusions derived from Figure 2 are most probably also valid in humans. These authors used the bolus technique with monodisperse particles with an aerodynamic diameter of 0.86 μm but with 2% He and 2% SF_6 (plus 79% N_2 and 17% O_2) in the bolus. The penetration volumes ranged from 35 to 155 mL. Schulz et al. (19) computed the volumetric half-widths instead of variance differences (See Equation 6). For aerosol concentration measurements, the half-width presents the advantage of decreasing the errors caused by a large noise for small concentrations. It is defined as the width of the bolus (in mL) between the two points of one-half the maximum concentration. Up to a volume penetration of 150 mL, bolus dispersion was almost the same as previously shown by Ultman in humans. However, more

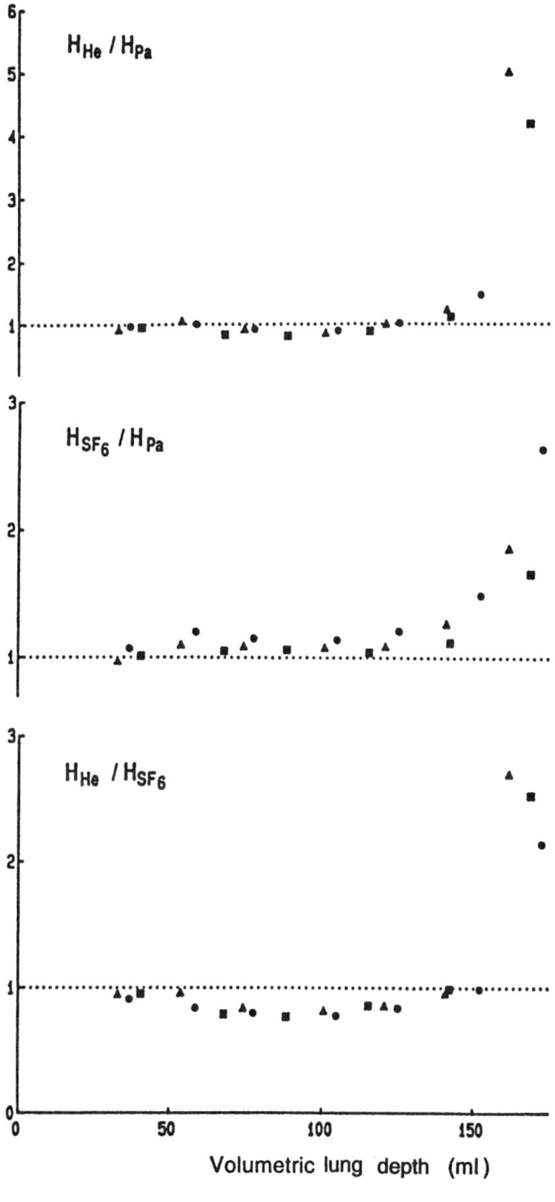

Figure 2 Ratios of bolus half-widths of He and particles (H_{He}/H_{Pa}), SF_6 and particles (H_{SF_6}/H_{Pa}), and He and SF_6 bolus (H_{He}/H_{SF_6}) plotted versus volumetric lung depth. Individual values for all three dogs are given. (From Ref. 19.)

importantly, the dispersion was also almost the same for aerosols, whose diffusion coefficient is about five to six orders of magnitude smaller than for He and SF_6.

To evaluate a potential role of sedimentation, Schulz et al. (19) performed additional measurements with particles with an aerodynamic diameter of 2.38 µm. In these particles, the settling velocity and displacement by inertial forces are 7.7 times larger than for 0.86-µm particles and no systematic differences were found. These results strongly support convective mixing as the only relevant mixing mechanism in the conducting airways, confirming and extending the results obtained by Ultman et al. (16) with He and SF_6. Both Ultman et al. (16) and Schulz et al. (19) have shown minor differences between He and SF_6, which can be explained by a small Taylor dispersion effect.

Previous results also have a major consequence in the quantitative description of gas and aerosol transport and mixing in the conducting airways when they are modeled by a symmetrical structure like the classical Weibel model (11): the following transport equation can be used:

$$\frac{\partial C}{\partial t} = K\frac{s}{S}\frac{\partial^2 C}{\partial x^2} + \frac{1}{S}\frac{\partial (sK)}{\partial x}\frac{\partial C}{\partial x} - \frac{\dot{V}}{S}\frac{\partial C}{\partial x} - \frac{L}{S} \tag{8}$$

with

$$K = D + K_{cv} \tag{9}$$

where C is the gas or aerosol concentration as a function of time (t) and position (x) along the airway. K is the axial diffusivity, D the molecular diffusion coefficient, and K_{cv} the effective diffusion coefficient characterizing convective mixing. s and S are the total cross-sectional area of the airways alone, and the total cross section of airways plus alveoli. In the conducting zone of the lung (no alveoli) $S = s$. $\dot{V}$ is the flow rate ($\dot{V} = Su$, where u is the mean axial velocity in the airway) and L is the deposition term. For aerosols, D is the Brownian diffusion coefficient, which can be neglected, except in the alveoli. An equation equivalent to Equation 8 was first used in the early 1970s (20,21), with $L = 0$ to describe inert gas transport and mixing in the human lung.

Equation 8, which is only valid in a symmetrical structure rests also in the very important implicit assumption bound to any one-dimensional analysis: radial diffusion is instantaneous and therefore velocity and concentration are uniform over the cross section of the airways. Mean axial velocity refers to the velocity of a hypothetical bulk flow. Even with these limitations, the observation of a similar dispersion of gases and aerosols in the conducting airways is the best validation of its use in simulations of transport of molecules or particles in that region. Taulbee and Yu (22) were the first to use Equation 8 for the complete bronchial tree and, subsequently, Taulbee et al. (23) incorporated Equation 5 for dispersion. These authors have found a good agreement between simulations and experiments. Although they have focused more on aerosol deposition from the analysis of single breaths, they have found that convective mixing in the conducting airways plays a relatively minor role in the overall mixing process.

A critical analysis of the use of Equation 8 in the simulation of aerosol transport and deposition published recently (24) has shown the limitations of this equation to study aerosol deposition, particularly for tidal breaths. However, the computation of aerosol dispersion has shown a surprising good agreement with experiments, which may be partially due to the use of Equation 7 for dispersion. These authors confirmed the finding by Taulbee et al. (23) that, for tidal breaths with full inhalation of aerosols, the dispersion in the conducting airways play a minor role on deposition. However, bolus experiments are much more sensitive to dispersion than single breaths, particularly in the oral-laryngeal path (25). Darquenne and Paiva (24) have also shown that aerosol deposition is a very insensitive index. Indeed, for a given particle diameter, aerosol deposition is almost identical for very different parameters of the model. This is one of the reasons for the increasing interest in other variables derived from bolus experiments. In a recent study, Darquenne et al. (26) compared numerical simulations and experiments for bolus tests. The experiments were performed with 0.87-μm diameter particles on 10 healthy subjects for penetration volumes up to 1500 mL. The numerical data were obtained by solving Equation 8 in a trumpet model of the lung based on data of Haefeli-Bleuer and Weibel (11,27). The computations agreed reasonably well with the experiments. The authors also tested the sensitivity of the simulations to different parameters. Simulated dispersion appeared to be insensitive to altered values of the deposition term (L in Equation 8) whereas it was largely affected by modified values of the convective mixing coefficient (Equation 7) in the alveolar zone of the lung. By the incorporation of different dispersion coefficients and using parameter fitting, one can expect to shed light on convective mixing mechanisms in the conducting airways. To our knowledge, this approach has not been attempted yet, although the recent work of Batycky and Edwards (28) may be a first step in that direction.

B. Intra-Acinar Transport

The acinus is defined as the largest parenchymal lung unit of which all airways are alveolated (27). It starts with the first respiratory bronchiole and contains all generations out to the periphery. The terminal bronchiole (last nonalveolated unit) is sometimes considered as part of the acinus. For a symmetrical structure, this would only decrease the number of acini by a factor of two. However, in the real asymmetrical lung, the two definitions are not trivially related. In humans, more than 95% of the lung volume is peripheral to the respiratory bronchioles.

Figure 2 shows that, for penetration volumes larger than the conducting airways (V > 130 mL), not only aerosols behave very differently from gases, but the differences between gases of different diffusivities become apparent as well. This can be explained based on the concepts of diffusion front and interdependence of transport by diffusion and convection in an asymmetrical structure (29).

1. The Diffusion Front

In Figure 3, simulations of He, SF_6, and aerosol single-breath inspirations are combined. These curves are solutions of Equation 8 for appropriate initial and boundary conditions, corresponding to the simulation of a given experiment.

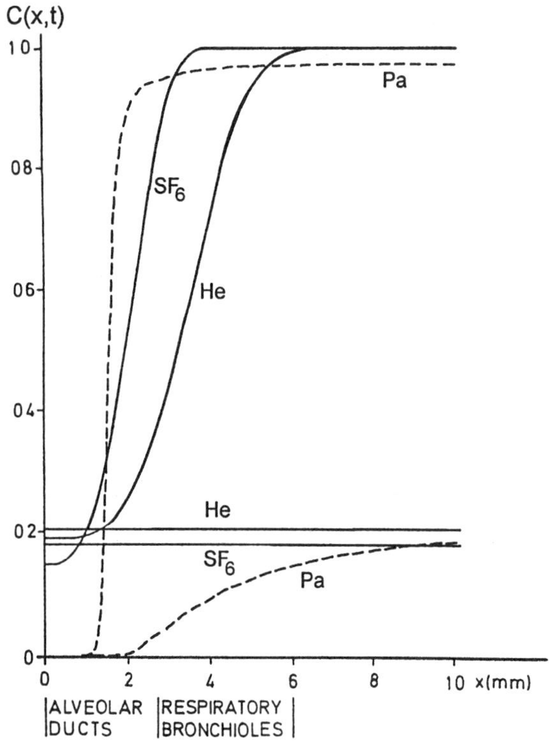

Figure 3 Representation of a 1-L inspiration of a He-SF_6-aerosol tracer mixture in O_2, followed by a 1-L expiration, both at a constant flow of 1L/s. The ordinate is the He, SF_6, and particle (Pa) concentration relative to the inspired concentration, and the abscissa is the distance to the alveolar end of a symmetrical model of the lung. Only the end inspiratory and end expiratory concentration profiles are shown. (Adapted from Ref. 34.)

The continuous lines represent the end inspiration and the end expiration He and SF_6 concentration profiles for a 1-L inspiration of an He-SF_6 tracer mixture, followed by a 1-L expiration, both at a constant flow of 1 L/s. The ordinate is the He and SF_6 concentration relative to the inspired concentration and the abscissa is the distance to the alveolar end of a symmetrical lung model. The acinar entry corresponds to $x = 6$ mm. At the end of the expiration, both the He and SF_6 concentration curves are constant. The He and SF_6 concentration profiles at the end of inspiration correspond to the so-called diffusion front, or, more appropriately, the quasistationary diffusion front. Indeed, the gas concentrations continue to increase at the alveolar end during the inspiration, but most of the concentration profile stays stationary. The diffusion front has been extensively described (29–35).

The particle concentration profile (Pa) was obtained for particles with a diameter of 1 μm and for the same breathing protocol as the He and SF_6 single-breath inspirations. Both the end inspiration and end expiration profiles are represented by dashed lines in the figure. For 1-μm particles, deposition is small, particularly in the conducting airways. Consequently, for $x = 10$ mm, the concentration at the end of inspiration is close to 1. We have already stressed that Equation 8, which assumes instantaneous radial diffusion, is only a crude approximation to describe the location of the deposition of aerosol particles within the acinus (24). Indeed, the one-dimensional approach implies a constant aerosol concentration over the cross section of the ducts. As is shown in Section III C, most of the convective displacement in the respiration zone takes place in the central channels of the alveolar ducts. Therefore, not only very large particle concentration differences are expected for the same axial position within the acini (i.e., between the airway lumen and the nearest alveoli), but also the particles should penetrate very deeply. Finally, another major difference between inspiratory gas and particle concentration profiles is that, for particles, concentration stationarity is never reached, with the dashed curve continuing to penetrate further into the acinus as inspiration proceeds.

The computation of mean particle concentration profiles along the airways, based on more realistic models, will be a major challenge during the next years. The factors that have to be incorporated in the models are not only related to the radial inhomogeneities of transport but also the influence of the gravitational field, which will depend on the duct axis orientation. These factors depend on the particle diameter.

2. The Interdependence Concept

Although the diffusion front theory is generally accepted, the interdependence concept is still considered by many scientists as a speculative exercise. Yet, both concepts come from purely theoretical approaches. However, the diffusion front has an experimental basis, owing to the technique of intrapulmonary gas sampling developed by Ludwig Engel (36,37). Furthermore, some model predictions were confirmed by experiments (38). Even so, the concept of interdependence of gas transport (by convection and diffusion in a branching structure) needs to overcome two additional obstacles: it is a more difficult concept and no direct experimental observation have been done to test model predictions.

The mammalian lung presents a unique characteristic, which, to our knowledge, is not found in any other natural or artificial structure: a to-and-fro convective movement in a multibranch cul-de-sac structure. A direct consequence is a decreasing convective velocity toward the periphery. Somewhere within the lung, the relative contribution of axial convective transport and radial diffusive transport are of the same order of magnitude that is expressed by a Peclet number close to 1. The normal asymmetrical structure of the acinus may then result in differences in inhaled gas concentrations as a consequence of the interaction between convection and diffusion. These differences persist throughout the respiratory cycle, although back-diffusion reduces them during expiration. This concept is discussed in detail elsewhere by Paiva (35).

It can be shown from simulations of aerosol transport (24) that particle expiratory concentration profiles are insensitive to acinar asymmetry. The reason for this difference with gas transport is that, for particles, Pe becomes equal to 1 only within the alveoli. Regional ventilation inhomogeneities are discussed in Chapters 12 and 18. Rosenthal (39) suggested that such inhomogeneities may interfere with the interpretation of bolus experiments. Although this effect may be relevant in disease, it is probably negligible in healthy subjects.

C. Transport in the Alveoli

The characteristic time for gas equilibration by molecular diffusion within the alveoli is of the order of microseconds, and the assumption of instantaneous intra-alveolar gas equilibration is a safe hypothesis. The simulation of intra-alveolar particle transport is a much more complex problem, and this section deals mainly with aerosols. It is therefore surprising that the first attempts to describe flow pattern with the alveolar zone of the lung were aimed at studying gas transport. Davidson and Fitz-Gerald (40) first published a detailed analysis of flow in alveolar models. Even though the equations of motion were solved analytically, several models of alveoli were considered. We show in Figure 4*A*, the streamlines in a spherical model of an alveolus with expanding walls both in an alveolar duct (*left*) and an alveolar sac (*right*). The development of digital computers and numerical techniques enabled the simulation of more realistic structures.

Two other models of alveolar ducts (also aimed at studying gas mixing) have been used in simulations of intra-acinar aerosol transport. Federspiel and

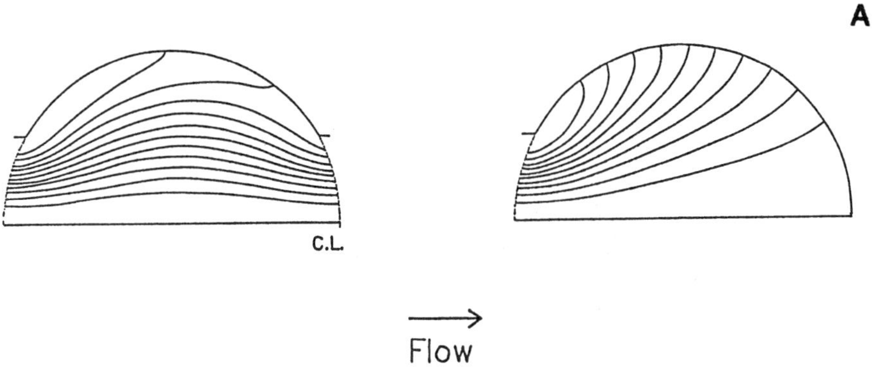

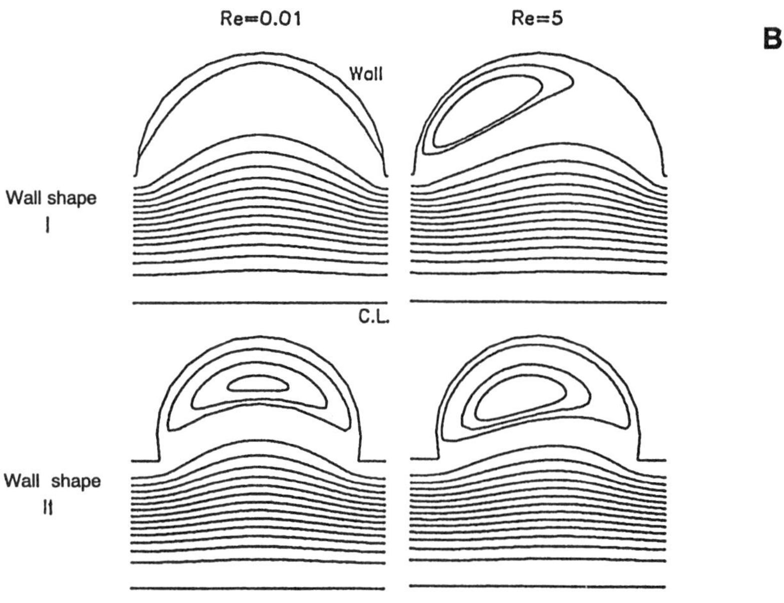

Figure 4 Flow patterns in alveolar models. **A**, streamlines in the spherical model of Davidson and Fitz-Gerald of an alveolus with expanding walls in an alveolar duct (*left*) and an alveolar sac (*right*). (Adapted from Ref. 40.) **B**, Streamlines in the model of Tsuda et al. for different Reynolds numbers and wall shapes. (From Ref. 44.) **C**, Velocity vectors in the model of Darquenne and Paiva for Re = 0.057. A different scale is used in the velocity vectors in the central channel (upper panel C) and the alveoli (lower panel C). (From Ref. 46.)

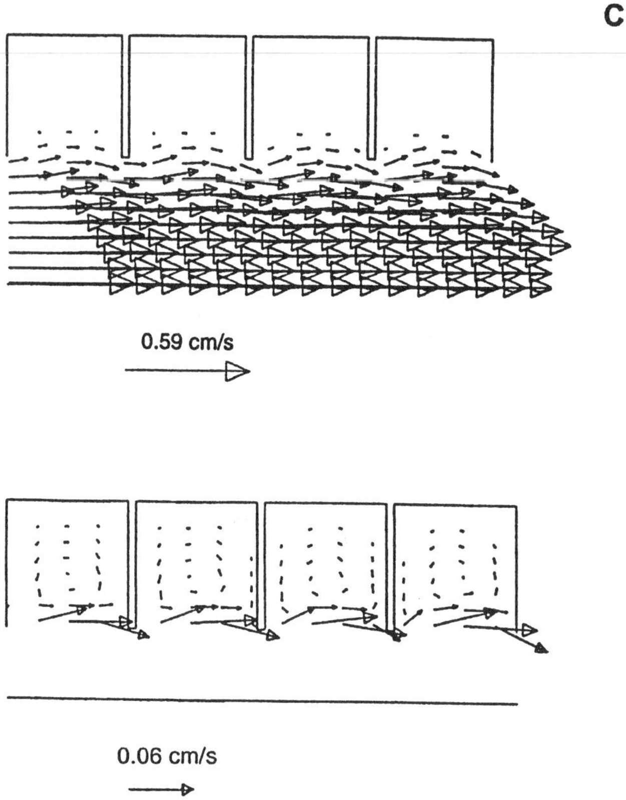

Figure 4 Continued

Fredberg (41) used a technique developed to study dispersion in porous media to evaluate the decrease in molecular axial dispersion caused by the alveolar walls. These authors also used spherical alveoli but with different apertures or mouth openings (see Figure 4*B*). They confirmed the results obtained by Paiva (42) in a model with a different geometry: cylinder with alveoli as radial slices of annular rings (represented in cross section in Figure 4*C*). Both works have shown that, in an alveolar duct, the molecular diffusion coefficient should be multiplied by s/S (Equation 8) to correct for the delay in axial molecular dispersion caused by the alveolar septa. Federspiel and Fredberg (41) and Verbanck and Paiva (43) have studied the effect of alveoli mouth opening and have shown that its effect on mixing should occur only for extreme values of the alveolar apertures.

Tsuda et al. (44,45) were the first to perform detailed computations of intra-acinar aerosol transport by solving numerically the Navier-Stokes equations for Reynolds numbers (Re) smaller than 10. Figure 4*B* shows such simulations for Re = 0.01 and Re = 5 for two different alveolar apertures. Several interesting observations were described by Tsuda et al. (44), particularly in relation to the streamlines shown in Figure 4*B*, in which recirculations were observed inside the alveoli, even for Re as small as 0.01. Furthermore, the streamline pattern is very sensitive to alveolar duct geometry, in particular at the level of the alveolar aperture. It is interesting to compare these results with those obtained by Darquenne and Paiva (46) in a different structure. Although Figure 4*C* results from a two-dimensional simulation, the vector representation shows that the intra-acinar velocities are much smaller than the velocities in the central part of the duct (lumen). A similar result is obtained from three-dimensional simulations. The two parts of Figure 4*C* represent the same simulation but with different scales for Re = 0.057. Tsuda et al. (44) have also shown that the streamlines are very sensitive to the alveolar duct geometry. Intra-acinar recirculations were found in very different geometries, and the velocity profile in the central part of the duct (Figure 4*C*) is almost identical to the parabolic profile in a cylindrical duct with a diameter equal to the airway lumen. In the Weibel model of the lung (11), the lumen represents approximately only one-fourth of the acinar volume. This shows that the presence of the alveolar septa is a major factor in the penetration of particles in the very periphery of the lung. Furthermore, very large (particle) concentration inhomogeneities are expected within any acinar duct and at any moment of the respiratory cycle. The very different convective velocities in the center of the duct in respect to the adjacent alveoli is the main reason why Equation 8 should not be used to evaluate the location of particles, and therefore particle deposition (24).

Recently, Tsuda et al. (47) have extended their previous work and have explored the possibility of chaotic behavior of fluids inside the acinus, which could be an important factor in aerosol dispersion and deposition in the lung periphery. In past analyses, it has been often assumed that acinar flow is largely viscous (Reynolds number much smaller than unity) and that it can be treated as a simple Poiseuille flow. Such a flow ought to be reversible if the alveolar motion is kinematically reversible. This simplification suits well gas transport analysis because it is primarily governed by molecular diffusion in the acinar region with minor effects of convection. Because of the typically small intrinsic motions of particles, aerosol transport and deposition are largely influenced by convection even in the lung periphery. Recent studies in fluid mechanics (48,49) showed that viscous flow can be irreversible if the flow exhibits chaotic structure. Tsuda et al. (47) tested this possibility by solving numerically the velocity field within a realistic geometrical model of an alveolated duct that expanded and contracted in a geometrically similar fashion to simulate tidal breathing. They showed that the flow pattern in the rythmically expanding alveolar duct differed from that in the rigid-walled model and exhibited a typical chaotic flow structure. They suggested that this unique flow pattern has a substantial effect on alveolar flow irreversibility that they called chaotic mixing. Chaotic mixing could be one process contributing to convective mixing in the periphery of the lung. Although the idea is attractive, the chaotic behavior is very sensitive to the geometrical boundaries and further studies are necessary to evaluate the relevance of this mechanism for the lung.

One aspect of aerosol transport related to particle deposition is the technique of evaluation of airway diameter. The possibility of computing airway dimension in vivo, both in health and disease, has been one of the most interesting applications of aerosol research in respiratory physiology. Landahl (50) gave a quantitative evaluation of airway diameter from aerosol retention in infinite tubes. This technique was applied by Palmes et al. (51), but for bolus experiments with different inhaled volumes and breathholding times. These authors compared the computed airway diameter with the diameter of the Weibel model (11) and they have found a reasonable agreement. Heyder (52) extended Landahl's analysis to a system of randomly oriented tubes. Lapp et al. (53) performed a detailed study on the variability in the size of airspaces in normal human lungs. The physical link between airway dimensions and aerosol deposition is the sedimentation velocity caused by the gravity field, the deposition being a function of end-inspiratory breathhold time. The advantage of using the bolus technique instead of aerosol breath inspirations to evaluate airway diameter is that (for monodisperse aerosol) the particles reach approximately the same zone of the lung. Gebhart et al. (54) and Heyder (55) published detailed studies on the use of aerosols to estimate pulmonary air space dimensions. However, a critical approximation in previous analysis is the assumption, as initial condition, of a uniform distribution of particles in the airways. Surprisingly, the consideration by Yu and Thiagarajan (56) of parabolic initial conditions led to minor corrections. It may be that the initial conditions are even more inhomogeneous than those considered by these authors. Finally, it is possible that realistic computations require the consideration of the complex structure of the alveolar ducts, including the alveoli.

IV. Gas and Particle Transport in Disease

The forced expiration test, in which flow is measured from total lung capacity to residual volume, is probably the most common test in pulmonology.

Phase III slope of the single breath N_2 test is the classical index of ventilation inhomogeneity. However, several factors influence this index simultaneously, which made its standardization difficult. In normal subjects, the interdependence mechanism previously described diffusion-convection-dependent inhomogeneity (DCDI) is probably the main factor influencing the slope of phase III, which would depend primarily on intra-acinar inhomogeneities, too peripheral to influence indices specific to the forced expiration curve. This is confirmed by the fact that, in asymptomatic asthmatics, the slope is frequently abnormal in the presence of otherwise normal pulmonary function (57).

In patients with emphysema, both the magnitude of He and SF_6 slopes and the differences between them are substantially greater than in healthy subjects (58). These observations could be interpreted to reflect increased diffusive impairment of gas mixing owing to enlarged peripheral air spaces. However, similar observations have been reported in asymptomatic smokers (59). The latter observation could be explained by an increased inhomogeneity of airway narrowing, resulting in increases in DCDI. The relationship between expired SF_6 and He gas concentrations during multiple breath wash-out in healthy and asthmatic subjects is distinctly different from that seen in patients with emphysema (60). These observations suggest that increased ventilation inequality in asthma occurs by convective-dependent mechanisms, whereas, in emphysema, there is an additional diffusive impairment to gas mixing among small units in the lung periphery. Single breath wash-outs performed in rats with elastase-induced emphysema suggests that the slope modifications relate mainly to elastic and not structure alterations (61).

Recently, a new index was derived from He and SF_6 slopes and a highly significant correlation was found with the degree of inflammatory and fibrotic changes of the respiratory bronchioles (62). This may open the way to finding a test for early peripheral (intra-acinar) airway dysfunction. The recent observation that in heart-lung transplant recipients who developed irreversible airflow obstruction, the SF_6-He slope difference invariably decreased and became negative (He slope larger than SF_6 slope) in four of five patients (63).

The use of aerosols in disease has been mainly in relation to measurements of deposition. In this section, we only refer to monodisperse nonradioactive aerosols used to measure dispersion and airway dimensions. A detailed account of the potential of aerosols as a diagnostic tool including other techniques has been given recently by Anderson and Dolovich (64).

A. Aerosol Bolus Dispersion

The effect of cystic fibrosis on 70 mL (1 μm) inhaled aerosol boluses was studied by Anderson et al. (65) in 11 patients. The bolus penetration volumes ranged from 100 to 700 mL and the expired bolus dispersion was characterized by the volumetric width at one-half aerosol concentration peak height and the modal shift (displacement of the maximum of the concentration curve). Patients with cystic fibrosis exhaled boluses that were broader than those exhaled by normal subjects at all penetrations. At a volume penetration of 600 mL, patients had a mean bolus half-width that was 68% greater than that of healthy subjects, and they exhaled the bolus mode 20% earlier. A very clear correlation was found between bolus spreading and the forced expiration index FEV_1 (volume expired in the first second of a forced expiration), which is a classical pulmonary functional parameter to evaluate obstruction. This indicates that bolus spreading increases in proportion to the severity of an obstructive lung disease such as cystic fibrosis.

Of particular interest was the finding of McCawley and Lippmann (66) who measured the dispersion of 0.5-μm bolus in a group of healthy nonsmoking subjects and a group of asymptomatic smokers. Although the latter presented normal lung function, the bolus dispersion was increased, suggesting early small airway abnormalities. Keefe et al. (67) examined the potential effects of ozone on 22 healthy nonsmoking male volunteers by performing 0.5-μm aerosol bolus inhalations at functional residual capacity and penetration volumes of 1.2 and 1.6 L, respectively. The principal finding of this investigation is that exposure to ozone resulted in significant widening of the expired bolus, particularly for deeper volumetric penetrations. However, the expired half-width was only weakly correlated with spirometric measures. These observations suggest that aerosol dispersion after ozone exposure reflects a different functional response than the one measured by spirometry, probably because ozone-related modifications occur in more peripheral airways than those sensitive to spirometry.

An interesting study was published by Anderson et al. (68), in which 20 asymptomatic smokers were compared with 20 age- and sex-matched nonsmokers for comparison with single-breath nitrogen test, taken as reference for small airway dysfunction. The larger difference in bolus dispersion between the groups occurred for the larger penetration volume, consistent with the results of Keefe et al. (67). For this penetration volume, a highly significant correlation was found between the dispersion and the forced expiratory volume in 1 second divided by the forced vital capacity. Smokers with abnormal spirometry (four subjects) or an abnormal single-breath nitrogen test (seven subjects) had significant increased dispersion compared with smokers with normal pulmonary function tests. A crude sensitivity-specificity analysis was performed, considering the single-breath nitrogen wash-out as the "golden standard" and the calculation led to a sensitivity of 82% and a specificity of 67%. Brand et al. (69) performed a very detailed analysis of the sensitivity-specificity test based on the receiver operating characteristics (ROC) curves for 216 randomly selected subjects (126 smokers and 90 nonsmokers). For the classical spirometric indices considered (single-breath tests were not performed), bolus dispersion showed a higher sensitivity and specificity. The same group of researchers (70) gave reference values on bolus dispersion parameters based on tests performed on 79 healthy subjects. However, dispersion measurements performed in mildly asthmatic children, also by the same group of researchers (71), did not provide benefit for clinical diagnosis.

B. Aerosol-Derived Airway Dimensions

Bronchial radioaerosol deposition and mucociliary clearance has been one of the main application of aerosols, and detailed literature can be found on the subject. Here we discuss aerosol deposition in the perspective of obtaining an evaluation of airway dimensions, the so-called effective airway diameter. As structural dimensions are already difficult to assess in normal subjects, one may expect some difficulties when this technique is extended to disease. Indeed, any model of particle deposition used for the computation of airway diameter considers implicitly that all the other parameters remain unchanged. This is always the price to be paid in any fitting procedure and probably introduces larger errors in disease. All pathological modifications, like convection-dependent inhomogeneities (CDI), are inevitably incorporated in the airway diameter, which necessarily are biased by the best ventilated zones, where the aerosols penetrate preferentially. If this limitation is kept in mind, some interesting information can nevertheless be obtained.

Hankinson et al. (72) evaluated airway dimensions in coal miners, suggesting narrower small conducting airways and abnormally large peripheral air space in these subjects. A more quantitative study was presented by Bennett and Smaldone (73). These authors estimated the mean diameter in eight subjects with chronic obstructive pulmonary disease and found it to be 0.70 ± 0.18 mm. The same technique was used in 10 subjects with normal pulmonary function and the estimated diameter was 0.36 ± 0.05 mm. In normal subjects, the computed diameter did not correlate significantly with any measure of pulmonary function, whereas, in patients, a significant correlation was only found with diffusing capacity. However, when all the data (normal and pathological) are plotted (diffusing capacity versus diameter), a curve can be drawn through all the points. The authors suggest that the decrease in diffusing capacity in disease reflects both a decrease in the alveolar surface area as well as a decrease in pulmonary blood volume, the loss in blood volume being a direct result of the loss in alveolar surface area.

Determination of air space dimensions in isolated dog lungs (74) enabled comparisons with morphometric measurements in the same lungs. Of particular interest were the results in lungs with papain-induced lung injury (75), where air space dimensions increased in some lungs and decreased in others. Some of the lungs showed gross damage yet insignificant or even negative changes in the computed dimensions. The authors suggest that these inconsistencies are related to modifications of the regional distribution of the aerosols resulting from the induced lung damage. More recently, Rosenthal (76) performed measurements of effective air space diameter in three dogs before and after papain-induced emphysema. Mean chord length measurements were performed postmortem. The average increase of effective air space computed from aerosol deposition was of 89%, but a significant correlation with the morphometric measurements was found only for the deeply penetrating boluses. Probably, the aerosol computed air space increase caused by emphysema is due only in part to real increase in the airways.

Blanchard et al. (77) applied the bolus recovery technique described by Palmes et al. (51) but in a larger number of subjects (17 males) and for different lung volumes. The comparison between effective airway diameters and Weibel's symmetric lung model (11) gives a good agreement for generation peripheral to generation 13. Furthermore, the authors tested the hypothesis that the bolus recovery technique can detect changes in air space diameter associated with a change in lung volumes by performing the tests at 57% and 87% of the total lung capacity, respectively. Assuming that the lung expands isotropically, the expected increase in the air space diameter was 15%. The observed increase ranged between 41% and 70%. The authors explain this larger than expected change in dimensions because, for the same penetration volume, the bolus travels a shorter distance into the lungs (because of the larger volume of the airways) and therefore the particles settle in larger airways. This explanation can only account for part of the observation, which may again reflect the limitations of the method of computing dimensions in vivo. The comparisons of aerosol-derived lung morphometry with lung function indices are also of interest, particularly in connection with the plethysmographical measure of airway resistance. The only significant, although weak, correlation was found between airway resistance and the computed airway diameter for a 160-mL penetration volume at 57% of the total lung capacity. This may be due to the fact that the penetration volume of 160 mL is peripheral to the airways responsible for most of the resistance.

Three recent studies from the same laboratory are also of interest. In 25 patients with chronic obstructive pulmonary disease, Beinert et al. (78) found that, for a penetration volume of 800 mL, air space dimensions were equal to 0.82 ± 0.33 mm (mean ± standard deviation) in comparison with 0.39 ± 0.05 mm in 36 healthy subjects. Furthermore, in nine patients with severe emphysema, the computed diameter was of 1.14 ± 0.31 mm. In a study on 47 children with asthma, no difference in the effective airway diameter was found with a group of normal subjects. As for the dispersion experiments, the authors suggest that aerosol measurements do not provide an obvious benefit for the clinical diagnosis of mild pediatric asthma. Finally, very detailed reference values of aerosol-derived airway morphometry were given from 79 healthy subjects (79).

Some of the difficulties described in this section are probably related to the impossibility in controlling all the other variables. It is possible that the use of more realistic models in the computation of effective air spaces will make this approach more attractive.

V. Summary

The complexity of lung structure and function and the difficulty of performing direct measurements attracted a large number of engineers and physicists into the field. Indeed, the relevant parameters are often obtained through model computations. Whatever the fascination by the modeling approach in physiology, a field finds a large interest if clinical applications are found. This is critically dependent not only on the sensitivity and specificity of the tests used but also on its simplicity. It is not yet clear whether the aerosol bolus test fulfills these conditions and whether its predictions are different from the classical lung function tests. They probably provide information not available from the classical function tests.

An intrinsic difficulty in the interpretation of gas or particle expirograms is that the interpretation depends on dispersion in the conducting airways. We have seen that, in the anatomical dead space, this dispersion is almost identical for particles and gases. This may help in the establishment of more accurate empirical formulas of axial dispersion.

Information on intra-acinar transport may come largely from single-breath tests with gases of different diffusivities. These tests have been limited to vital capacity or tidal inspirations, and the more informative gas bolus tests have only been used sporadically.

The dimensions of the alveoli are such that any direct measurement of gas concentration may be impossible. In combination with multidimensional computer simulations, the detailed postmortem localization of particle deposition may provide the basis for more realistic intra-acinar flow patterns. This will lead to a better understanding of intra-acinar transport and a better prediction of the location of particle deposition within the alveoli.

Acknowledgments

This work was supported by NASA grant NAGW 4372 and program PRODEX (Belgium).

References

1. Altshuler B, Palmes ED, Yarmus L, Nelson N. Intrapulmonary mixing of gases studied with aerosols. J Appl Physiol 1959; 14:321–327.
2. Fowler WS. Lung functions. II. The respiratory dead space. Am J Physiol 1948; 154:405–416.

3. Dollfuss RE, Milic-Emili J, Bates DV. Regional ventilation of the lung, studied with boluses of 133-xenon. Respir Physiol 1967; 2:234–246.
4. Cumming G, Jones JG, Horsfield K. Inhaled argon boluses in man. J Appl Physiol 1969; 27:447–451.
5. Heyder J, Davies CN. The breathing of half micron aerosols III. Dispersion of particles in the respiratory tract. J Aerosol Sci 1971; 2:437–452.
6. Muir DCF, Sweetland K, Love RG. Inhaled aerosol blouses in man. In: Walton WH, ed. Inhaled Particles III. Old Woking, England: Unwin Brothers, 1971:81–90.
7. Taylor GI. Dispersion of soluble matter in solvent flowing slowly through a tube. Proc R Soc Lond Ser A 1953; 219:186–203.
8. Aris R. On the dispersion of a solute in a fluid flowing through a tube (abstr). Proc R Soc Lond 1956; 235A:66–77.
9. Taylor GI. Conditions under which dispersion of a solute in a stream of solvent can be used to measure molecular diffusion. Proc R Soc Lond Ser A 1954; 225: 473–477.
10. Davies CN. Definite equations for fluid resistance spheres. Proc R Soc Lond Ser A 1945; 57:259–270.
11. Weibel ER. Morphometry of the Human Lung. New York: Academic Press, 1963.
12. Ultman J. Gas transport in the conducting airways. In: Engel LA, Paiva M, eds. Gas Mixing and Distribution in the Lung. New York: Marcel Dekker, 1985:63–136.
13. Scherer PW, Shendalman LH, Greene NM, Bouhuys A. Measurement of axial diffusivities in a model of the bronchial airways. J Appl Physiol 1975; 38:719–723.
14. Haselton FR, Scherer PW. Bronchial bifurcation and respiratory mass transport. Science 1980; 208:69–71.
15. Schroter RC, Sudlow MF. Flow patterns in models of the human bronchial airways. Respir Physiol 1969; 7:341–355.
16. Ultman JS, Doll BE, Spiegel R, Thomas MW. Longitudinal mixing in pulmonary airways—normal subjects respiring at a constant flow. J Appl Physiol 1978; 44: 297–303.
17. Lacquet LM, Van Der Linden LP, Paiva M. Transport of H_2 and SF_6 in the lungs. Respir Physiol 1975; 25:157–173.
18. Worth H, Adaro F, Piiper J. Penetration of inhaled He and SF_6 into alveolar space at low tidal volumes. J Appl Physiol 1977; 43:403–408.
19. Schulz H, Heilmann P, Hillebrecht A, Gebhart J, Meyer M, Piiper J, Heyder J. Convective and diffusive gas transport in canine intrapulmonary airways. J Appl Physiol 1992; 72:1557–1562.
20. Paiva M. Computation of the boundary conditions for diffusion in the human lung. Comput Biomed Res 1972; 5:585–595.
21. Scherer PW, Shendalman LH, Greene NM. Simultaneous diffusion and convection in single breath lung washout. Bull Math Biophys 1972; 34:393–412.
22. Taulbee DB, Yu CP. A theory of aerosol deposition in human respiratory tract. J Appl Physiol 1975; 38:77–85.
23. Taulbee DB, Yu CP, Heyder J. Aerosol transport in the human lung from analysis of single breaths. J Appl Physiol 1978; 44:803–812.
24. Darquenne C, Paiva M. One-dimensional simulation of aerosol transport and deposition in the human lung. J Appl Physiol 1994; 77:2889–2898.

25. Simone AF, Ultman JS. Longitudinal mixing by the human larynx. Respir Physiol 1982; 49:187–203.
26. Darquenne C, Brand P, Heyder J, Paiva M. Aerosol dispersion in the human lung: comparison between numerical simulations and experiments for bolus tests. J Appl Physiol 1997; 83:966–974.
27. Haefeli-Bleuer B, Weibel ER. Morphometry of the human pulmonary acinus. Anat Record 1988; 220:401–414.
28. Batycky RP, Edwards DA. Microscopic and macroscopic descriptions of gas and aerosol transport in the human lung. Chem Eng Commun 1996; Vol 148–150: 23–39.
29. Paiva M, Engel LA. Theoretical studies of gas mixing and ventilation distribution on the lung. Physiol Rev 1987; 67:750–796.
30. Engel LA. Dynamic distribution of gas flow. In: Anonymous Handbook of Physiology. The Respiratory System. 3rd ed. Bethesda, MD: American Physiological Society, 1986:575–593.
31. Paiva M, Engel LA. Gas mixing in the lung periphery. In: Chang HK, Paiva M, eds. Respiratory Physiology (Lung Biol in Health Dis) Vol. 40. New York: Marcel Dekker, 1989:245–276.
32. Engel LA. Gas mixing within the acinus of the lung. J Appl Physiol 1983; 54: 609–618.
33. Paiva M. Gas transport in the human lung. J Appl Physiol 1973; 35:401–410.
34. Paiva M, Engel LA. Pulmonary interdependence of gas transport. J Appl Physiol 1979; 47:296–305.
35. Paiva M. Theoretical studies of gas mixing in the lung. In: Engel LA, Paiva M, eds. Gas Mixing and Distribution in the Lung. New York: Marcel Dekker, 1985: 221–285.
36. Engel LA, Wood LDH, Utz G, Macklem PT. Gas mixing during inspiration. J Appl Physiol 1973; 35:18–24.
37. Engel LA, Menkes H, Wood LDH, Utz G, Joubert J, Macklem PT. Gas mixing during breath holding studied by intrapulmonary gas sampling. J Appl Physiol 1973; 35:9–17.
38. Fukuchi Y, Roussos CS, Macklem PT, Engel LA. Convection, diffusion and cardiogenic mixing: an experimental approach. Respir Physiol 1976; 26:77–90.
39. Rosenthal FS. The effect of nonuniform ventilation on the dispersion of inspired aerosol boluses: a modeling study. J Aerosol Med 1993; 6:177–197.
40. Davidson MR, Fitz-Gerald JM. Flow patterns in models of small airway units of the lung. J Fluid Mech 1972; 52:161–177.
41. Federspiel WJ, Fredberg JJ. Axial dispersion in respiratory bronchioles and alveolar ducts. J Appl Physiol 1988; 64:2614–2621.
42. Paiva M. Gaseous diffusion in an alveolar duct simulated by a digital computer. Comput Biomed Res 1974; 7:533–543.
43. Verbanck S, Paiva M. Effective axial diffusion in an expansile alveolar duct model. Respir Physiol 1988; 73:273–278.
44. Tsuda A, Butler JP, Fredberg JJ. Effects of alveolated duct structure on aerosol deposition in the pulmonary acinus. Part I: Diffusion in the absence of gravity. J Appl Physiol 1994; 76:2497–2509.

45. Tsuda A, Butler JP, Fredberg JJ. Effects of alveolated duct structure on aerosol deposition in the pulmonary acinus. Part II: Gravitational sedimentation and inertial impaction in the absence of diffusion. J Appl Physiol 1994; 76:2510–2516.
46. Darquenne C, Paiva M. Two- and three-dimensional simulations of aerosol transport and deposition in alveolar zone of human lung. J Appl Physiol 1996; 80: 1401–1414.
47. Tsuda A, Henry FS, Butler JP. Chaotic mixing of alveolated duct flow in rhythmically expanding pulmonary acinus. J Appl Physiol 1995; 79:1055–1063.
48. Aref H, Balachander S. Chaotic advection in a Stokes flow. Phys Fluids 1986; 29: 3515–3521.
49. Ottino JM, Leong CW, Rising H, Swanson PD. Morphological structures produced by mixing in chaotic flows. Nature (London) 1988; 333 (6172):419–425.
50. Landahl HD. On the removal of airborne droplets by the human respiratory tract. I: The lung. Bull Math Biophys 1950; 12:43–56.
51. Palmes ED, Wang C, Goldring RM, Altshuler B. Effect of depth of inhalation on aerosol persistence during breath holding. J Appl Physiol 1973; 34:356–360.
52. Heyder J. Gravitational deposition of aerosol particles within a system of randomly oriented tubes. J Aerosol Sci 1975; 6:133–137.
53. Lapp NL, Hankinson JL, Amandus H, Palmes ED. Variability in the size of airspaces in normal human lungs as estimated by aerosols. Thorax 1975; 30:293–299.
54. Gebhart J, Heyder J. Stahlhofen W. Use of aerosols to estimate pulmonary airspace dimensions. J Appl Physiol 1981; 51:465–476.
55. Heyder J. Charting human thoracic airways by aerosols. Clin Phys Physiol Meas 1983; 4:29–37.
56. Yu CP, Thiagarajan V. Sedimentation of aerosols in closed finite tubes in random orientation. J Aerosol Sci 1978; 9:315–320.
57. Siegler DIM, Fukuchi Y, Engel LA. Influence of bronchomotor tone on ventilation distribution in man. Am Rev Respir Dis 1976; 114:123–130.
58. Georg J, Lassen NA, Mellemgaard K, Vinther A. Diffusion in the gas phase of the lungs in normal and emphysematous subjects. Clin Sci (London) 1965; 29: 525–532.
59. Engel LA. Intraregional gas mixing and distribution. In: Engel LA, Paiva M, eds. Gas Mixing and Distribution in the Lung. New York: Marcel Dekker, 1985:287–358.
60. VonNieding G, Löllgen H, Smidt U, Lind H. Simultaneous washout of helium and sulphur hexafluoride in healthy subjects and patients with chronic bronchitis, bronchial asthma and emphysema. Am Rev Respir Dis 1977; 116:649–660.
61. González Mangado N, Peces-Barba G, Cabanillas GR, Verbanck S, Paiva M. Effect on single-breath washout and lung function of elastase-induced emphysema in rats. Am Rev Respir Dis 1993; 148:735–743.
62. Van Muylem A, DeVuyst P, Yernault J, Paiva M. Inert gas single-breath washout and structural alteration of respiratory bronchioles. Am Rev Respir Dis 1992; 146: 1167–1172.
63. Van Muylem A, Antoine M, Yernault J-C, Paiva M, Estenne M. Inert gas single-breath washout after heart-lung transplantation. Am J Crit Care Med 1995; 152: 947–952.

64. Anderson PJ, Dolovich MB. Aerosols as diagnostic tools. J Aerosol Med 1994; 7: 77–88.
65. Anderson PJ, Blanchard JD, Brain JD, Feldman HA, McNamara JJ, Heyder J. Effect of cystic fibrosis on inhaled aerosol boluses[1-3]. Am Rev Respir Dis 1989; 140: 1317–1324.
66. McCawley M, Lippmann M. Development of an aerosol dispersion test to detect early changes in lung function. Am Ind Hyg Assoc J 1988; 49:357–366.
67. Keefe MJ, Bennett PD, DeWitt P, Seal E, Strong AA, Gerrity TR. The effect of ozone exposure on the dispersion of inhaled aerosol boluses in healthy human subjects. Am Rev Respir Dis 1991; 144:23–30.
68. Anderson PJ, Hardy KG, Gann LP, Cole R, Hiller FC. Detection of small airway dysfunction in asymptomatic smokers using aerosol bolus behavior. Am J Respir Crit Care Med 1994; 150:995–1001.
69. Brand P, Tuch T, Manuwald O, Bischof W, Heinrich J, Wichmann HE, Beinert T, Heyder J. Detection of early lung impairment with aerosol bolus dispersion. Eur Respir J 1994; 7:1830–1838.
70. Brand P, Rieger C, Schulz H, Beinert T, Heyder J. Aerosol bolus dispersion in healthy subjects. Eur Respir J 1997; 10:460–467.
71. Schulz H, Schulz A, Brand P, Tuch T. Von Mutius E, Erdl R, Reinhardt D, Heyder J. Aerosol bolus dispersion and effective airway diameters in mildly asthmatic children. Eur Respir J 1995; 8:566–573.
72. Hankinson JL, Palmes ED, Lapp NL. Pulmonary air space size in coal miners. Am Rev Respir Dis 1979; 119:391–397.
73. Bennett WD, Smaldone GC. Use of aerosols to estimate mean air-space size in chronic obstructive pulmonary disease. J Appl Physiol 1988; 64:1554–1560.
74. Rosenthal FS. Lung structure parameters estimated from modeling aerosol deposition in isolated dog lungs. J Appl Physiol 1989; 67:2014–2025.
75. Rosenthal FS, Wright S. Assessment of papain-induced lung injury in isolated lungs by measurements of aerosol deposition and mixing. J Appl Physiol 1992; 72:459–467.
76. Rosenthal FS. Aerosol deposition and dispersion characterize lung injury in a canine model of emphysema. J Appl Physiol 1995; 78:1585–1595.
77. Blanchard JD, Heyder J, O'Donnell CR, Brain JD. Aerosol-derived lung morphometry: comparisons with a lung model and lung function indexes. J Appl Physiol 1991; 71:1216–1224.
78. Beinert T, Brand P, Behr J, Vogelmeier C, Heyder J. Peripheral airspace dimensions in patients with COPD. Chest 1995; 108:998–1003.
79. Brand P, Rieger C, Beinert T, Heyder J. Aerosol derived airway morphometry in healthy subjects. Eur Respir J 1995; 8:1639–1646.

Part Three

PULMONARY VENTILATION HETEROGENEITY

11

Characteristics of Respiratory System Complexity Captured via X-Ray Computed Tomography

Image Acquisition, Display, and Analysis

ERIC A. HOFFMAN

University of Iowa College of Medicine
Iowa City, Iowa

LYNNE E. OLSON

Ohio State University
Columbus, Ohio

> Of the self-organizing behaviors, two are of particular interest to the study of evolution. One is adaptation. We see it everywhere. Corporations adapt to the marketplace, brain cells adapt to signal traffic, the immune system adapts to infection, animals adapt to their food supply. We have come to think that the ability to adapt is characteristic of complex systems—and may be one reason why evolution seems to lead toward more complex organisms.
>
> *The Lost World*, Michael Crichton

I. Introduction

The primary role of the lung is gas exchange, requiring that ambient air and mixed venous blood be delivered to the alveoli so that carbon dioxide and oxygen can diffuse across the alveolar-capillary membrane. Exchange efficiency requires that ventilation be matched to perfusion within the functional unit to optimize the conditions for diffusion. The respiratory system has both active and passive mechanisms to effectively match the regional flow of fresh gas to the regional flow of mixed venous blood in normal, healthy individuals. These mechanisms result in a complex system, involving interactions between the inherent structural heterogeneity of the bronchial and vascular trees, and feedback systems designed to impose functional homeostasis by optimizing the regional exchange of respiratory gases to match the global metabolic demands of the body. A basic premise of this chapter is that the true complexity of an organ system lies in the system's functional integration within the milieu of the whole organism and the organism's drive for maximal efficiency and continued existence through compensation and adaptation. To understand such complexity, we must examine the system in the intact, dynamic state. Such an examination requires that the methodology provide the spatial and temporal resolution necessary to evaluate detail of both anatomy (airways, blood vessels, and lung parenchyma) and function (regional measures of airway reactivity, ventilation, and perfusion). X-ray computed tomography (CT) is emerging as the single modality that offers the means whereby such complexity of the respiratory components can be explored. Recent work suggests that, with the aid of computer-based image processing, it may be possible to assess temporal detail down to the level of pulmonary microvascular mean transit times and parenchymal detail allowing for a sensitive and specific quantitation of early lung disease beyond the visual resolution of the image. In this chapter we will discuss the recent advances in this modality that offer the tools for exploration of the intact lung.

Appreciating the inherent structural heterogeneity of the pulmonary tree structures (1) and understanding the complex mechanisms matching regional blood and gas flows are not merely exercises in curiosity. Applications of the knowledge gained through research in this area are expected to include improved ability to, for example: optimize arterial blood gases during anesthesia; select the best body orientation for patients requiring positive end expiratory pressure (PEEP) ventilation; detect the onset, progression, extent, and location of ventilation or perfusion disorders, such as emphysema, pulmonary fibrosis, and pulmonary emboli; cope with the altered $\dot{V}/\dot{Q}$ matching induced by exposure to abnormally high or abnormally low G forces experienced during flight within or above the earth's atmosphere; and develop specific and sensitive techniques for assessing an individual's response to therapy over time. This latter application is paramount. As we enter an era where the mapping of the human genome is nearing completion and we find the ability to modify the very genetic nature of disease and disease susceptibility, we must have sensitive, quantitative methodologies that can rapidly assess outcomes. This becomes a particularly difficult challenge when pathological changes are slow to develop, are heterogeneous, and when, as is commonly the case, multiple pathological processes, such as emphysema and fibrosis, intermingle. To achieve the needed sensitivity, not only must our measures be quantitative and obtained in vivo, but the measures must be specific to alterations of the complex pattern of structure and function at the most peripheral interfaces of such relationships (2).

With the recognition that, by design, the respiratory system is both anatomically and functionally complex and that disease processes likely interfere with the physiological mechanisms maintaining appropriately matched functional relationships within this seemingly heterogeneous system, numerous methodologies have been developed to assess ventilation, perfusion, or their functional outcome—gas exchange. While clearly useful, pulmonary function tests frequently rely on single measurements of airflows, pressures and partial pressures, and global measurements of lung volume to infer structural and functional alterations. Techniques such as single photon emission computed tomography (SPECT) imaging, positron emission tomography (PET), and the multiple inert gas technique (3) are limited by their spatial and temporal resolution and associated modeling assumptions. This chapter will explore the use of dynamic, volumetric, CT imaging, to assess lung, heart, and chest wall shapes and volumes, the structure of the bronchial and vascular trees, the textural patterns of lung parenchyma in health and disease, regional airflow and blood flow, and deviations in all of these from expected patterns of structural and functional complexity. We will discuss the advantages and disadvantages of CT. We will show examples of the use of CT imaging technology to probe normal and abnormal cardiopulmonary structure and function, and we will argue that CT technology offers a unique and comprehensive approach to evaluating the structural and functional complexity of the respiratory system in a manner that raises the standards for noninvasiveness, sensitivity, and specificity, and challenges our ability to comprehend and understand the integrative biology of the cardiopulmonary systems. It will be proposed that present-day image analysis techniques fail to adequately depict and quantify the complexity of the respiratory system and that a thorough understanding of the integrated nature of the system will require the development of new analytical techniques and scientific thought processes.

II. High-Speed X-Ray CT: Overview

Discovery of X-rays in 1895 by Roentgen, who received the Nobel Prize for his work in 1901, rapidly changed Victorian-era views of privacy, opened the door to the noninvasive exploration of the body's innermost realms, and found use in select clinical applications related to surgery, dentistry, and battlefield medicine. Through the process of learning to read X-ray images, a major paradigm shift occurred whereby pathology began to be viewed as having characteristic patterns across patients rather than presenting as unique to each person. Furthermore, principles of scientific investigation were adopted to aid clinical investigation (4). With the development of X-ray contrast agents and heart catheterization in the early 1950s, imaging began to reveal the inner dynamics of the living breathing being. When EMI Corporation released their first X-ray CT scanners in the mid-1970s, again medicine was catapulted into a new era long before the imaging method began to change our understanding of the integrated functioning of the human form with its vast number of simultaneous dynamic processes.

Image resolution has improved significantly over the past two decades to the point where so-called high-resolution CT (HRCT) (5) provides detail of lung anatomy at submillimeter resolution. HRCT generally utilizes 1–1.5-mm-thick slices and a high-frequency reconstruction algorithm that serves to enhance edges. However, there is growing appreciation regarding the need for volumetric imaging to evaluate anatomical information, and the need for very high-speed scanning if one is to evaluate the heart and lungs in motion. The image of the canine thorax from a one-of-a-kind CT scanner built at the Mayo Clinic (see below) is shown on the upper right of Figure 1 in juxtaposition with a scan obtained from a commercially available electron beam CT (EBCT) scanner. In the lower portion of the image is displayed all of the sections gathered via the dynamic spatial reconstructor (DSR) in less scanning time than was used to image a single slice by conventional X-ray CT. Placed in juxtaposition to the conventional scan, the apparently lower-resolution DSR-based image demonstrates a powerful lesson: that is, image information can be much more than what is perceived at first glance. Because the single slice shown from the DSR is one of a stack of up to 240 contiguous 1-mm-thick slices scanned simultaneously with 0.01-sec temporal resolution, images can be rearranged as shown in Figure 2 to demonstrate dynamic three-dimensional anatomy, which remains unobtainable by any other scanning system. In Figure 2, one sees the contrast agent, stop action imaged and outlining the right heart chambers, vena cavae, and the pulmonary trunk along with the right and left branches of the pulmonary artery. By reslicing the volumetric image data set in planes more appropriate to the anatomy of interest, information unmeasurable from the single thin, HRCT image can be extracted (6). Furthermore, the stack of slices can be gathered every 1/60 sec, allowing for a four-dimensional (three spatial plus time) evaluation of the heart and lungs. Professor Paul Heintzen once commented in an editorial regarding DSR images: "I am convinced that 3-D will not replace 2-D radiographic methods. They can complement each other and will coexist, as in art, where the Mona Lisa and the Venus de Milo both have their admirers. I like both, but the latter without a blurring veil" (7). What was not understood then, and is only now becoming broadly appreciated, is the notion that complex interrelationships between the multiple components of an organ system can only be understood in context, and dynamic volumetric imaging gives that important contextual information.

The techniques and clinical usefulness of conventional CT are well established for head and body imaging. Early on, Kreel (8) and later Robinson and Kreel (9) noted the change in regional lung density with varying levels of breath hold and noted that the change in attenuation coefficients (voxel gray scale) related to lung volume. They also noted that the variation in reconstructed CT

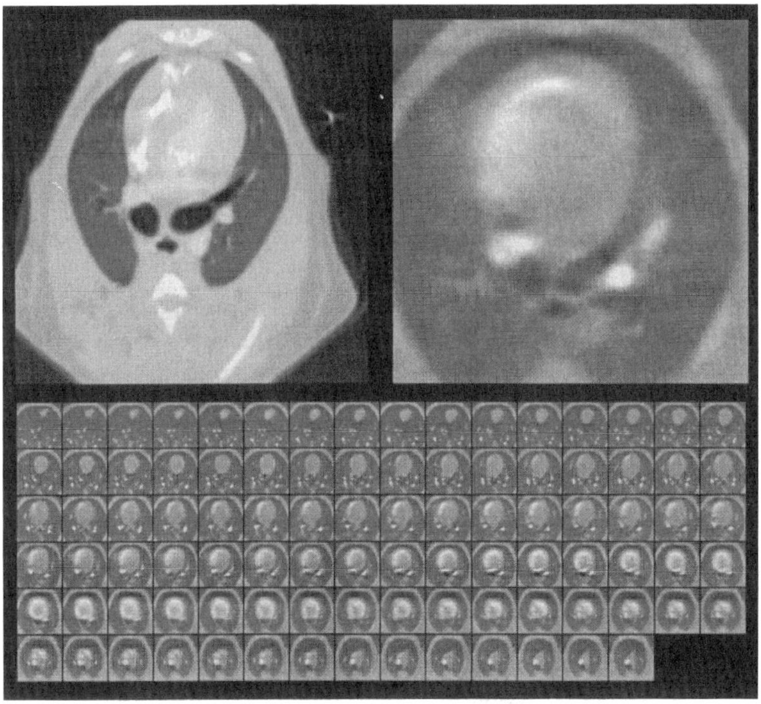

Figure 1 (Upper left) Thorax of a dog with contrast injected into the right atrium. Section is 1 mm thick and scan aperture is 0.1 sec. Imaging was via an electron beam CT scanner. (Upper right) Dog thorax at approximately the same level as depicted in the EBCT section. The section is 0.9 mm thick and the scan aperture is 0.067 sec. Imaging was via the dynamic spatial reconstructor (DSR). Because of the DSR design, at the same time that the projection data was gathered to produce the image in the upper right, all of the projections used to produce the sections in the lower panel were also gathered. Even though the EBCT image is clearly superior to the DSR for a single section, because the DSR is a true volumetric scanner, the information available by virtue of the ability to stop action image the entire heart and most of the lung provided information unachievable by any other modality. An example of such information is shown in Figure 2.

coefficients of lung tissue was much larger at functional residual capacity than at total lung capacity (TLC), an observation that correlates well with the finding that the lung is nearly uniformly expanded at TLC (10). CT is ideally suited for the evaluation of lung function and anatomy, because in-plane resolution can be brought down to well under a millimeter, with image gray scale (Hounsfield units, HU) being essentially linearly related to tissue density. Whereas the air-water interface in the lung introduces artifacts in MR images, it provides for enhanced contrast in CT scanning.

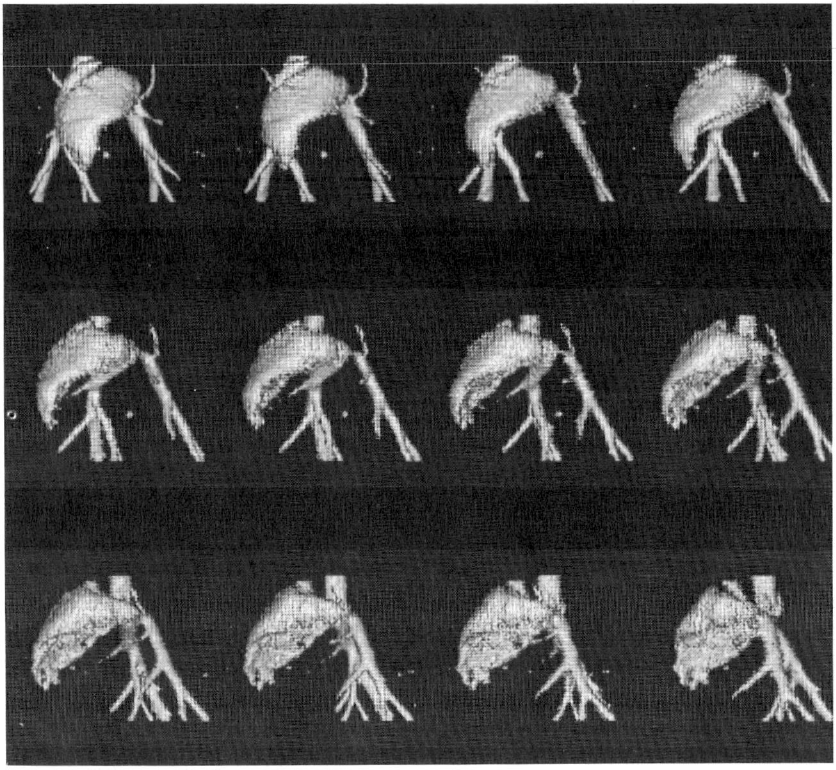

Figure 2 Multiple angles of view of a shaded surface display are shown depicting the geometry of the right heart chambers, superior and inferior vena cava, pulmonary trunk, and right and left pulmonary arteries stop-action imaged at end diastole via DSR scanning. These images of the contrast enhanced blood detected from the stack of images shown in the lower panel of Figure 1 were one of 16 such volumetric data sets available for a single heart beat, allowing investigators to evaluate cardiopulmonary mechanics in a way unachievable by any other imaging modality.

By considering the lung to be composed of structures equal in density to either air or water (lung tissue and blood density of 1.05 is very close to the density of water), it is possible to calibrate the lung density values internally for accurate assessment of regional lung air content (11). This calibration is shown in Eq. (1):

$$\text{Voxel \% air content} = [1 - (CT_x - CT_{air}/CT_{water} - CT_{air})] \times 100 \tag{1}$$

where CT_x is the original gray scale of the lung voxel (volumetric picture element) to be converted; CT_{air} is the gray scale value of voxels within a region of known 100% air content (lumen of the mainstem bronchus); and CT_{water} is a region of known 100% "water" (chamber of heart, lumen of descending aorta, lumen of pulmonary trunk, etc.). Such a correction to percent air content is demonstrated in Figure 3.

Williams et al. (12) have outlined the potential sources for measurement artifacts associated with reconstructed X-ray CT attenuation values. These include partial volume effects, beam hardening, incorrect assumptions made in reconstruction algorithms (such as ray paths and path lengths), nonlinearity of detectors, and limited-angle-of-view artifacts. Beam-hardening artifacts are induced by the polychromatic X-ray sources used in all commercial, clinical scanners. The "soft" X-ray is removed preferentially when it passes through dense structures. This artificially darkens voxels representing tissues between or near

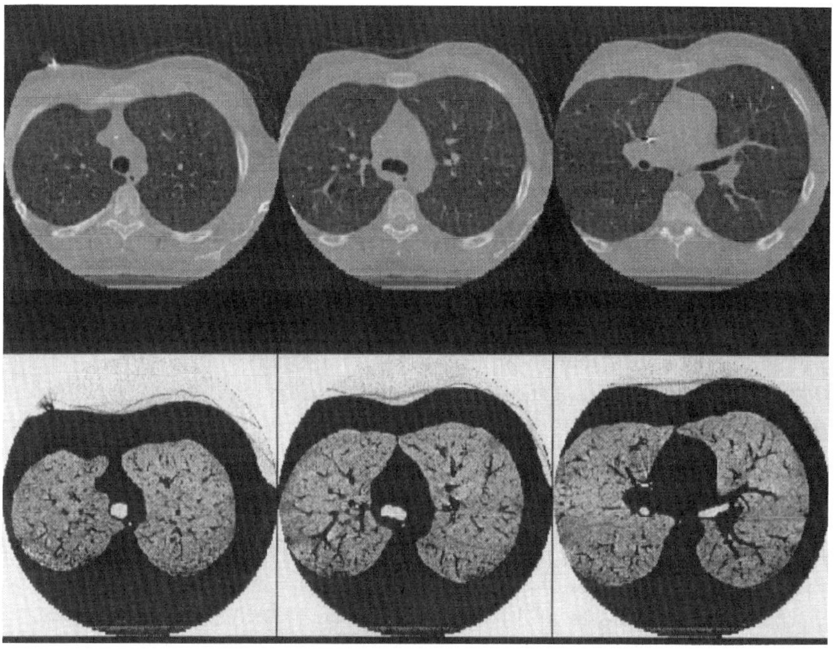

Figure 3 Three sample sections of the thorax of a normal human volunteer scanned via an EBCT scanner are depicted in the upper panel. By sampling regions of known 100% air and known 100% blood, the reconstructed voxel values for all lung regions can be converted to a value representing the percent air contained within that region of lung as depicted in the lower panel. If one images the lung at multiple inflation steps, the change in regional air content serves as an index of regional ventilation. To follow the lung during an inflation maneuver, one must image the lung volumetrically.

structures of high density, such as voxels representing lung regions near the heart or ribs. Thus, in the reconstructed image the gray scale of air inside the body differs from that of air outside the body. Corrections for this artifact have been developed (13) and correction algorithms are now incorporated into commercial reconstruction software. However, full correction can not be assumed. Calibrating the acquired images against an internal standard, such as described by Eq. (1), further reduces artifacts due to beam hardening and accounts for partial volume effects.

Early users of conventional X-ray CT examined the relationship between the acquired images and the underlying cardiopulmonary physiology. Sanders et al. (14) compared CT images with pulmonary function tests and chest radiographs with the goal of using CT to detect emphysema in patients with normal pulmonary function test results. They found that CT was as sensitive as pulmonary function tests in determining the presence of emphysema and both were more sensitive than conventional chest radiographs. Wollmer et al. (15) compared reconstructed lung density with the static lung elastic recoil pressure of smokers and nonsmokers and concluded that increased pulmonary density was a sensitive indicator of smoking-related lung pathophysiology. Vock and Salzmann (16) found lung density to be related to mean pulmonary artery pressure, pulmonary vascular resistance, and pulmonary artery wedge pressure. However, cardiopulmonary function is inherently four-dimensional, including three spatial dimensions plus time. A fundamental problem associated with conventional CT when used to image the beating heart, bellowing lung, or flowing blood is that the length of time required to complete a scan is large in comparison to the duration of the physiological event of interest.

Methodologies that have been used to quantitate parenchymal disease through CT methods have shown a high degree of correlation with even moderate disease in isolated, static lung specimens (17). Yet, these same methods have not proven to be as sensitive to early disease in vivo (18). This is most likely due to cardiogenic motion of the lung. Through the use of percutaneously implanted parenchymal markers and biplane video fluoroscopy, Wei et al. demonstrated that portions of the lung show volume changes (using four markers to form tetrahedra) during apnea that are equal to or greater than the volume change caused by a tidal breath (19). To demonstrate the effect that this has on CT studies of the lung, Reinhardt and Hoffman (20) have scanned a pig in two scanners with contrasting capabilities in regard to temporal and spatial resolution. The results are demonstrated in Figure 4. One scanner, Imatron's electron beam CT (EBCT), discussed below, has lower spatial resolution but higher temporal resolution; the other, the helical or spiral CT scanner, also discussed below, has a lower temporal resolution but higher spatial resolution. Metallic markers (1.5-mm diameter) were placed bronchoscopically into the left and right

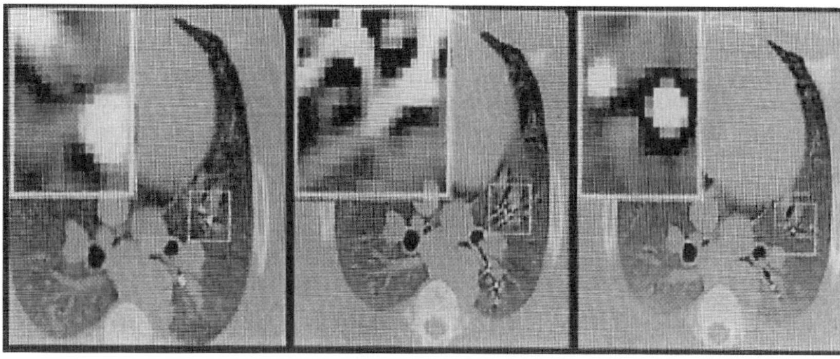

Figure 4 Three sections of the same anesthetized pig. Small metalic markers were wedged in the peripheral airways via bronchoscopy. The image in the left panel was obtained by scanning the pig alive in the EBCT scanner. Here the scan aperture was 100 msec. In the middle panel, the same lung level was scanned with the pig in a conventional helical CT scanner (Toshiba X-press). Here the pig was again alive as the scan aperture was 700 msec. (Left) The same pig in the helical scanner post mortem. Note that while the helical scanner resolution is better than the EBCT scanner, when a live subject is scanned, motion must be taken into account in assessing effective resolution. The effect of motion on the reconstruction of the markers shown in the middle panel is obvious.

lung periphery of a 100-lb anesthetized pig. The pig was scanned supine at FRC using the highest speed scanning possible (0.7 sec in Toshiba's helical scanner and 0.1 sec in the single slice mode of Imatron's EBCT scanner). As can be seen in Figure 4, with the pig alive and apneic, the markers, both close to the heart as well as at a distance, were found to be distinct and round in the reconstructed images derived from EBCT, whereas the markers were significantly distorted and nondistinct in the helical-derived images until after the pig was overdosed and rescanned both apneic and asystolic. While many physicists and radiologists, basing their views upon scans of inanimate phantoms, would argue that the helical scanner would have distinct advantages in evaluating detail of lung parenchyma, the physiologist might argue differently.

Although the most serious problem with the use of conventional CT to study the heart and lungs is motion-blurring artifact due to the length of the scan duration, there is also the problem that a single-slice image of the heart, lungs, or thoracic cavity (even if scanned at very high speed) generally cannot adequately convey the underlying volumetric, dynamic physiology. Optimizing CT technology for studying the cardiopulmonary system required the development of new CT machines, with enhanced imaging and computational hardware, and the parallel development of more robust analytical techniques.

III. State of the Art: Where Have We Been?

The prototype of dynamic volumetric X-ray CT imaging is the DSR (Fig. 5) which was designed during the mid-1970s and installed at the Mayo Clinic in 1979 (21). The DSR has a continuously rotating gantry equipped with 14 X-ray

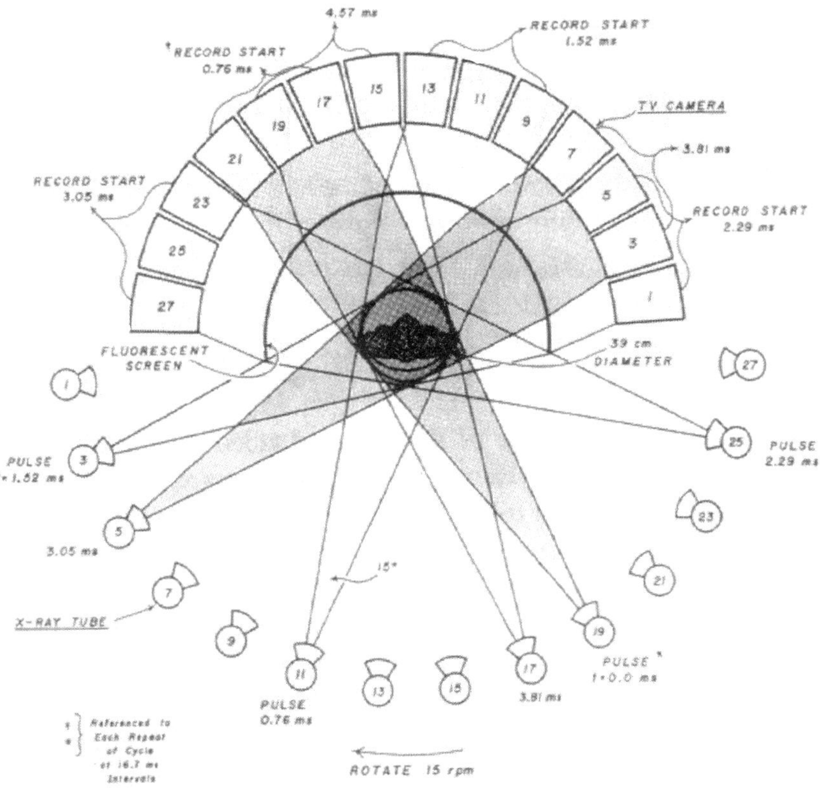

Figure 5 Schematic of the dynamic spatial reconstructor. Shown are the 14 television cameras and the justaposed 14 X-ray tubes. The 14 X-ray tubes fire synchronously with an individual X-ray pulse duration of between 100 and 700 μsec. The gantry rotates at 15 rpm such that, with the full complement of X-ray guns firing each 1/60 sec, the new 1/60-sec set of images produced on a hemicylindrical fluorescent screen represents 1.5 degrees of separation from the previous set of images. The images recorded by the television cameras were digitized either on- or off-line and a cross-sectional image of the body could be reconstructed from the multiple angles of view for each television line (or field). In this sketch, the artist is depicting that in one configuration of the scanner operation, images from flanking cameras could be used to allow for a larger field of view. (From Ref. 21, with permission.)

guns and 14 image detection systems gathering data from a hemicylindrical fluorescent screen. Up to 240 contiguous 0.9-mm-thick sections can be obtained in a period as short as 1/60 sec and the acquisition can be repeated 60 times per second. To achieve these data acquisition times, compromises were made in image detection and gray scale resolution was sacrificed. Although the DSR has remained a one-of-a-kind system, it is a true tour-de-force. The image manipulation and display techniques developed for handling the massive data sets generated by the DSR were the vanguard for techniques currently used to process and manipulate images obtained from the now commercially available volumetric scanners. In addition, as discussed below, much of the work establishing the accuracy and precision of volumetric imaging was performed on the DSR (21, 22). The primary lesson learned from the DSR was that organ systems in general, and the heart and lungs in particular, must be studied dynamically and volumetrically if one is to gain insights into the true nature of their physiology.

IV. State of the Art: Where Are We Now?

A. The Scanners

1. EBCT

One solution to the problem of collecting many angles of view, and scanning a number of contiguous slices in a short time, is provided by the EBCT (Fig. 6) produced at present by the Imatron Corporation of South San Francisco (23). In this system, the X-ray source and detection devices are stationary. The X-ray generator consists of four, fixed, parallel, pairs of semicircular tungsten target rings spanning 210 degrees about the patient, which are electromagnetically swept by a high-intensity electron beam. This creates a rotating fan beam of X-ray. Opposite each X-ray source target, multiple side-by-side scintillation crystal detectors record incident X-ray intensity. Eight transaxial slices (7-mm-thick pairs with 4-mm gaps between pairs) are scanned by sweeping the beam sequentially over the target rings and recording X-ray intensity via two fixed solid-state detector rings after the beam passes through the body. Scan speeds of 50 msec per slice pair (plus an 8-msec reset interval) are achieved; hence, eight parallel slices (scanned two per sweep) require approximately 224 msec to complete. Dynamic physiological events such as the heart beat, pulmonary blood flow, or respiratory gas turnover can be followed by gating the 50 msec/sweep of the four target rings appropriately. A single target ring can be swept repeatedly to capture one cycle of the event of interest, such as the heart beat, and then the next ring can be similarly swept, timed to the same physiological event such as the QRS complex of the electrocardiogram (ECG). In this manor, one would, for example, be able to acquire a set of slices through the heart with each heart level scanned at multiple points through a single cardiac cycle. Such

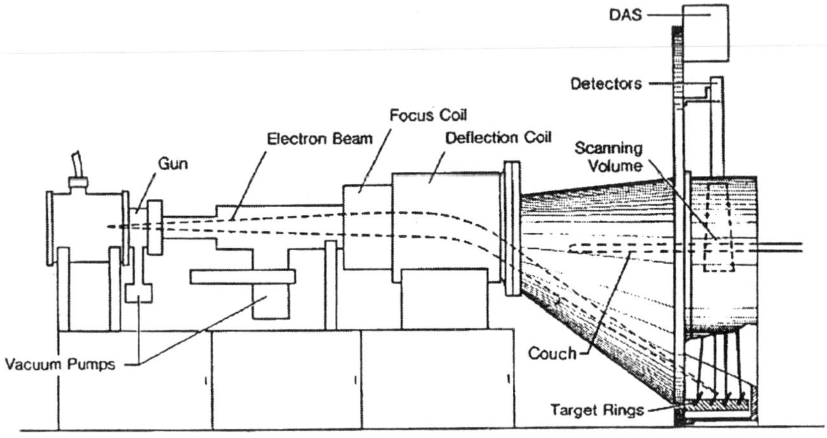

Figure 6 Schematic of the EBCT scanner. See text for full description. (Reproduced with permission from Stanford W, Rumberger J. *Ultrafast Computed Tomography in Cardiac Imaging: Principles and Practice.* Mount Kisco, NY: Futura Publishing Company, 1992.

a scanning algorithm requires that sequential cycles of a physiological event be repeatable so that when a dynamic volumetric data set is compiled from the multiple scanning sequences, the data set represents a reasonably accurate sampling of the true 4-D physiological process. To reduce the complexity of the system such that one can hope to match the limits of the scanning modality, one must, at times, resort to holding portions of the system constant such as scanning during a breath hold while watching blood flowing or the heart beating. It is possible, however, to increase the complexity of the interactions by appropriately timing the cardiac and respiratory cycles to each other to allow for scanning algorithms to be developed that evaluate cross-system interactions such as the effect of the heart on the lung or lung on the heart. This will be discussed in greater detail under the section specifically describing physiologically important observations to date via CT imaging.

Imatron has added several additional modes of scanning that allow scanning of single thin slices (as thin as 1.5 mm) in 100 msec with table motion occurring either continuously or stepwise between slice acquisitions. Here, an additional collimator is moved into place under computer control to appropriately narrow the beam emanating from the central target ring. One of the two detector rings is double-populated such that the single thin slice can be reconstructed with high spatial resolution. To date the scanner has allowed for up to 40 contiguous slices to be scanned in as little as 18 sec. The next generation of the scanner just released allows for the acquisition of up to 140 slices of the body in as little as 12 sec. One can gate each slice acquisition to the ECG, slowing total scanning time to a multiple of the time for completion of an R-R interval of the ECG. Gating minimizes the slice-to-slice variability caused by heart motion–derived variability of parenchymal spatial location. In the "continuous volume" mode of scanning the table motion is continuous as the beam is repeatedly swept along the central target ring. The beam sweep is so rapid relative to the motion occurring during the beam sweep that the result is only a slight image blurring, while allowing for very rapid acquisition of volumetric, anatomically aligned image information. In this mode, ECG gating is not possible. These rapid volumetric image acquisition modes allow for very flexible scanning algorithm development tailored to physiologically meaningful respiratory interventions, such as repeated volumetric scanning with intervening breaths to watch washout of a radiodense gas for the assessment of regional ventilation, scanning at multiple volumes of a static inflation or deflation maneuver, or scanning the lung gated to multiple points within a cardiac cycle, to name just a few examples. The primary limitations to scanning are eventually the total radiation exposure and the amount of contrast agent that is considered safe relative to the benefits to be gained by the individual and/or the scientific investigation.

When CT methodology is applied to the study of human physiology, the fact that ionizing radiation is involved places limitations on the protocol design. The EBCT scanner generates approximately the same per second dose of radiation as a conventional CT scanner. Thus, because of the shorter scan apertures, the radiation exposure is reduced. With the ability to alter the killovoltage and milliamperage of the electron beam, it would be possible to provide for lower doses of radiation. Additionally, the radiation risk is not simply proportional to the total number of slices scanned, but is more closely related to the total number of slices scanned at a fixed level of the body (per cell exposure).

Early use of X-ray occurred with extreme disregard for the dangers of radiation. Exposure levels that go far beyond radiation therapy doses used today in cancer therapy brought about skin burns, hair loss, and even death. Thomas Edison abandoned his development of X-ray technology when he recognized the risks involved (8). The radiation doses used today for volumetric scanning with EBCT are on the order of a few months of background radiation and are of no measurable risk, but concerns for the unknown have intensified.

B. Helical CT

With the growing understanding of the value of volumetric visualization, a new generation of CT machines has emerged, known as helical (or spiral) CT scanners (24). These scanners are similar to conventional CT scanners in that they most often have a single X-ray source, detector pair. However, helical CT has adopted a slip ring assembly that allows the X-ray gun and detectors to continually rotate without having to stop to unwind cabling. During this continuous revolution, the patient table is also continuously moved through the imaging field such that a helical set of X-ray-based projection images is obtained. To reconstruct individual cross-sectional images, the helical projection data are interpolated to obtain a consistent, coplanar set of projections that can be used in the reconstruction process. With greater table motion speeds, relative to the rotation speed of the X-ray gun/detector pair, the gaps in the helix widen and thus the interpolation process introduces greater image blurring. The tradeoff is body coverage in a single scan versus spatial resolution. Currently, the highest speeds achieved for X-ray gun/detector rotation are on the order of 600–700 msec. This mode of scanning provides an opportunity to obtain volumetric images of the lung within a single breath hold. However, although the rotation speed is high, 600–700 msec is nearly the full time for a cardiac cycle and thus it is not possible to eliminate cardiogenic-based image blurring and spatial uncertainty. The helical approach to CT scanning used to study respiratory system complexity will have greater limitations than are involved with the more dynamic scanning modalities such as the DSR or EBCT devices.

C. Image Acquisition Considerations

In addition to scanner resolution and speed, to aid the interpretation of the resultant images, it is important to know the physiological state of the individual at the time of scanning. This includes the need to follow both the cardiac cycle and respiratory cycle in relationship to image acquisition. Since, except under highly controlled experimental protocols commonly carried out in animal studies, it is nearly impossible to find the heart cycle and respiratory cycle events in synchrony, it is best to hold one or the other constant during scanning. Clearly it is less practical to hold the heart constant. To aid in the acquisition of images forming a consistent volumetric representation of the full apical-to-basal expanse of the lung and/or to aid in the acquisition of image data that can be compared in a meaningful way, several laboratories (25–27) have built lung volume controllers, making it possible to "encourage" the subject to hold the lung volume at a fixed and predetermined value during scanning and to keep track of all air flow in and out of the lung during interscanning periods. One such device has been discussed by Tran et al. (28). The subject is fitted with a nose plug and asked to breathe through a pneumotachometer, while the pneumotachometer signal is computer-monitored. Lung volume is calibrated by having the subject take a breath up to total lung capacity and out to residual volume defining vital capacity. Once these values are recorded, the computer then logs all airflow. A decision is made to scan at a fixed percentage of the vital capacity (difference between total lung capacity and residual volume), and the subject is instructed to take a deep breath and expire slowly. A high-frequency response balloon valve is closed at the mouth when the lung volume reaches the desired value. The subject relaxes against the closed valve and scanning commences. If the subject cannot hold his/her breath for as long as the technologist set breath hold, the subject can press a button to pause the scanner, open the valve, and alert the computer to start keeping track of airflow at the mouth. As a first application of such technology, it is imperative that radiologists begin to rigorously standardize the lung volume and body posture at which a patient is scanned. By scanning the lung at multiple volumes through use of the volume controller, a stacked image data set is acquired, which begins to allow for the study of the complex interrelationships between regional lung expansion, chest wall configuration, lobar rotation, and airway and vascular tree geometry. Figure 7 shows shaded surface displays and maximum-intensity projections of the lung of a normal human volunteer scanned at 25, 65, and 95% vital capacity using

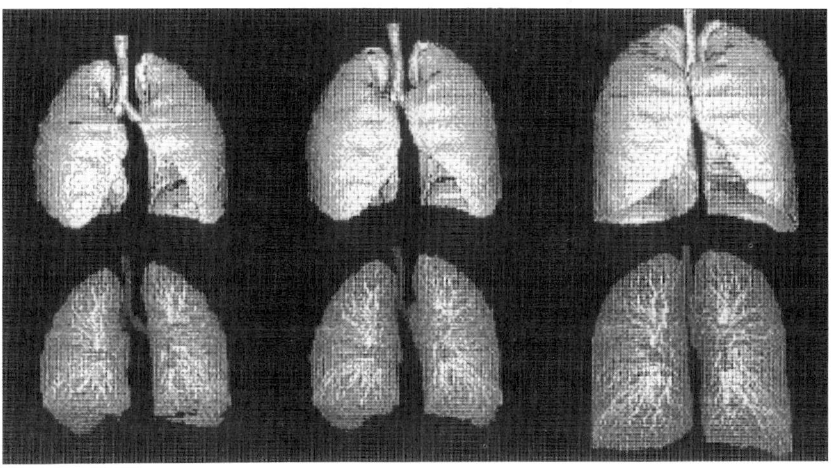

Figure 7 (Top) Shaded surface depiction and (bottom) maximum intensity projection depiction of in vivo human lungs scanned with the subject holding his breath at 40%VC, FRC, and 90%VC. The scanning time required to gather all of the slices for lung volume was long enough that the subject had to be allowed to take a number of breaths during scanning pauses. Each lung volume was scanned in three sections. The subject was brought back to the same lung volume after a period of respiration by use of a lung volume controller described in the text. If one is to use CT scanning as a quantitative tool and if the quantitation is to be used for the purposes of interpreting physiologic status of the lung, scanning must be accomplished with tight control over the lung volume and lung volumes must be standardized. (From Ref. 2, with permission.)

the volume controller. To gather data over the full extent of the lung, three acquisitions of 40 slices each were required with breathing allowed between each 40-slice run. Note the close matching of the slices and the alignment of vascular and airway markings.

V. Dynamic Measurements

A. Blood Flow and Associated Values

Regional blood flow is evaluated in either the eight-slice 8-mm or one-slice 3-mm mode of the EBCT scanner by injecting a bolus of X-ray contrast agent and following it through the myocardium or lung parenchyma at a gated time point in each of 10–12 cardiac cycles during which time respiration is suspended. Using changes in regional lung density from statically built-up pressure-volume maneuvers or xenon washout and blood flow estimated by contrast dilution methods, regional pulmonary $\dot{V}/\dot{Q}$ matching can be assessed and evaluated relative to parenchymal and vascular anatomy, chest wall configuration, cardiac position, and diaphragm geometry.

The left panel of Figure 8 shows a dye curve obtained from small regions of interest (2–3 mm on a side) placed in the main pulmonary artery and from a set of similar regions placed at varying heights within the lung "parenchyma." Intensity changes occurred in response to a 2-sec bolus injection of contrast agent within the right ventricular outflow tract. Numerous methods have been derived to evaluate regional blood flow via use of these two curves. Almost all methods apply some fit to the data, evaluate the total amount of contrast passing through the region of the main feeding artery, and the peak enhancement in the tissue region. Early assessment of the parameters involved was discussed by Axel (5), and validation studies using the Imatron scanner have been carried out for the myocardium (30). Wong et al. (31) have shown that regional tissue blood volume changes with altered regional blood flow, and when expressing blood flow as a function of regional tissue volume, one must account for the regional volume of blood.

Figure 8 Time intensity curves reflecting the passage of contrast agent through the specific regions of interest in the CT image. The highest peak was obtained from a region of interest positioned in the left pulmonary artery at a slice level not depicted here. The regional time intensity curves show a progressive diminution as one samples from dependent to nondependent lung regions, reflecting a reduction in absolute flow to those lung regions. Note that one must correct these data for the amount of lung tissue in these regions, which is also changing as a function of height in the lung. Such a correction has been carried out to obtain the data graphed in Figure 18. While the regions of interest

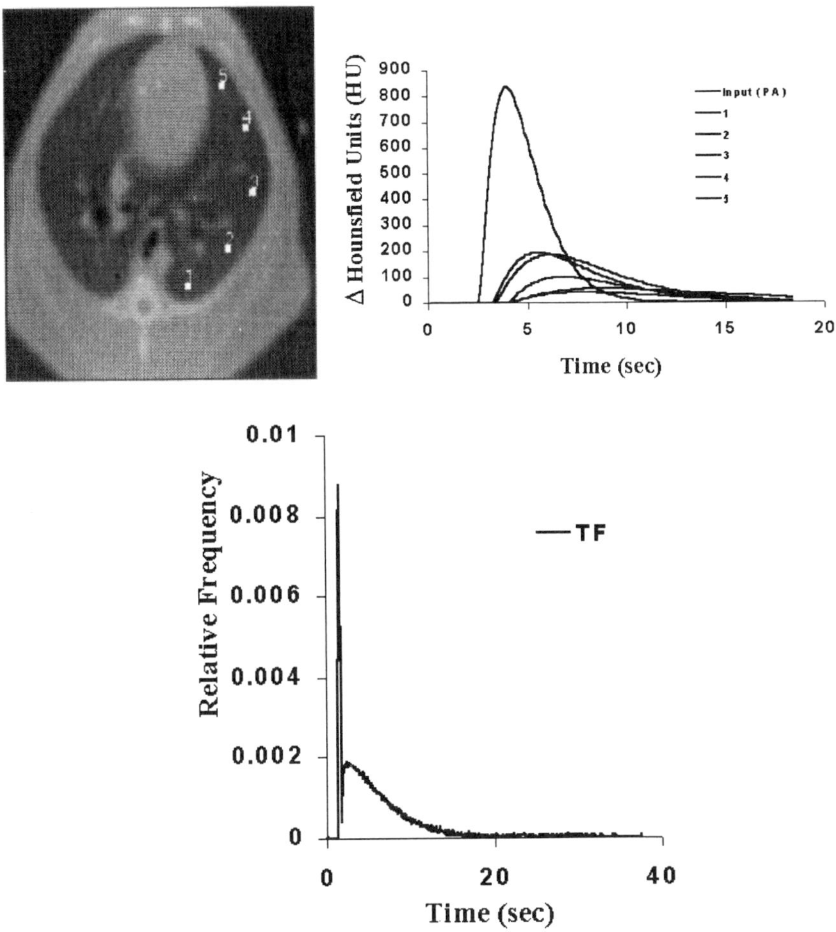

depicted are small (on the order of $1.5 \times 1.5 \times 7.0$ mm), they are not small relative to the size of the microvascular bed and most certainly there are some larger arterioles contributing to the time intensity curves. The graph in the lower panel depicts the transfer function calculated using a Fourier deconvolution approach. This transfer function, if convolved with the input curve obtained from the feeding branch of the pulmonary artery, will yield the curve sampled in the "parenchymal" region of interest. Note that this curve is bimodal. It is believed that the first sharp peak represents that portion of the function contributed by the larger arterioles. Thus if this is stripped off, and the remaining curve is convolved with the input curve, one should be able to obtain a time intensity curve representative of the microvascular bed. This curve in turn can be used to estimate regional parenchymal blood flow and microvascular mean transit times. (Work was presented in abstract form in Ref. 34.)

Blood flow and its parameters can be calculated by applying an appropriate blood flow model to samples of regional lung density changes and changes in the feeding vessel caused by contrast passage. Assuming a sharp enough bolus, such that the amount of contrast-enhanced blood leaving a region is minimal prior to the full bolus arrival, blood flow can be calculated using equations derived from a conventional microsphere approach to blood flow analysis, as described by Wolfkeil et al. (32).

$$FiCi(t) = \frac{dA}{dt} + FoCo(t) \tag{2}$$

where:

Fi = flow to the tissue from main feeding vessel
Ci = incoming concentration of indicator
Fo = flow away from tissue
Co = outgoing concentration of indicator
A = accumulated amount of indicator in tissue

By definition, the accumulated amount of indicator in a sample is simply the volume of the sample multiplied by the concentration of indicator in the feeding vessel ($A = Ci * V$). Since CT scans exhibit a linear relationship between image brightness and amount of contrast material, the amount of contrast present in a region can simply be found from the magnitude of the regional "time-intensity" curve. Thus, in terms of CT scanning:

$$\frac{Fi}{Vp} = \frac{\mathrm{CT_{peak}} - \mathrm{CT_{base}}}{\int_0^\infty \mathrm{CT_{pa}}(t)dt} \tag{3}$$

where

$\mathrm{CT_{peak}}$ = HU measured at the peak of the parenchymal dilution curve
$\mathrm{CT_{base}}$ = HU measured prior to the arrival of contrast into the region of interest
$\mathrm{CT_{pa}}$ = HU of contrast agent in the feeding pulmonary artery
Vp = the volume of parenchyma present in the region of interest

Blood flow measurements from dynamic CT images can, therefore, be calculated by relating a regional "time-intensity" curve to the curve found in the artery supplying the tissue (i.e., pulmonary artery).

As discussed earlier [Eq. (1)], to express blood flow per gram of parenchyma (V_p), we assume the region of interest (ROI) to be composed of air and "water" (i.e., blood + parenchyma) (11,33). Because of the disparate densities of these two components, we can use the CT gray scale values (Hounsfield number) of the images to calculate the fraction of each component in the ROI.

The amount of blood present within the ROI can be computed by comparing the "time-intensity" curve of the ROI to the curve in the feeding vessel.

$$\text{Blood} = \frac{\int_0^\infty \text{CT}_{\text{roi}}(t)dt}{\int_0^\infty \text{CT}_{\text{pa}}(t)dt} \tag{4}$$

Subtracting this result from the water fraction leaves the percentage of the ROI that is lung parenchyma. Multiplying the percentage of parenchyma, the number of voxels in the ROI, and the voxel dimension finally yields the volume of parenchyma (V_p) in mm^3 (g).

In Eq. (1) we have shown that, without the introduction of contrast, a voxel in the lung periphery can be assigned a percent air content value. The remainder of the voxel is composed of lung parenchyma and blood. By determining the total enhancement achieved in a region known to be 100% blood (pulmonary artery lumen) by integrating the change in HU over time and then comparing this with the integrated enhancement achieved by the blood-tissue component of the voxel of interest, one can calculate the percentage of that blood-tissue component that is blood. It is thus possible to quantitatively evaluate regional pulmonary blood flow in ml/min/g lung parenchyma throughout the lung parenchyma in a field of view that spans 8 cm cephalocaudally and up to 46 cm transaxially via the EBCT scanner.

B. Microvascular Flow Characteristics

With the concern that voxels in the lung periphery do not truly represent flow at the air/blood interface, but also represent flow in small arteries (partial volume effect), Tajik et al. (34) have sought to separate the arterial from the capillary bed curves on a voxel-by-voxel basis. Early efforts have utilized a fast Fourier transform (FFT) to take the time-intensity curve from the a feeding artery time-intensity curve (TIC) and regional parenchymal TICs into the frequency domain where the transfer function (TF) linking the two can be calculated. Image data was gathered from supine dogs imaged at FRC. The feeding pulmonary artery and regional parenchymal time-intensity data were fit to gamma variate functions, which were then used in a deconvolution-based assessment of regional pulmonary transit times and flow. A filtered FFT deconvolution scheme has been found to recover satisfactory transfer functions (TFs), which were verified by reconvolution with the input TIC to obtain curves that matched the original output TIC.

As demonstrated in the right panel of Figure 8, it has been found that such an assessment consistently yields bimodal regional TFs in the time domain consisting of an overlapping sharp, narrow peak and a second, more dispersed peak. The sharp, narrow peak is likely due to partial volume sampling of small arteries since regional TFs of samples containing a visually apparent arterial vessel contain virtually only the prominent sharp, narrow peak. Moreover, the putative arterial TF component approximates a delta function, as would be expected from a sharp bolus injection into the central circulation (RVOT).

Findings to date that support the notion that it is possible to recover the parenchymal and arterial curves for a peripheral ROI include the following observations:

The second, "parenchymal," curve disappears or is significantly reduced when an ROI is placed in a region of an apparent artery.

The height of the arterial TF component in "parenchymal" ROIs falls with lung height. This can be explained by the greater lung density in the dependent lung regions and thus a higher concentration of partial-volumed arteries and arterioles.

The mean transit time of the reconvolved parenchymal portion of the curve, when corrected for the difference in plasma versus red cell transit times to reflect the red cell rather than plasma transit (our contrast agent tags plasma), matches very closely red cell transit times reported from direct microscopic visualizations (35) through chest wall windows in dogs. Variations in "red cell mean transit time" measured via this method are (shown) in Figure 9.

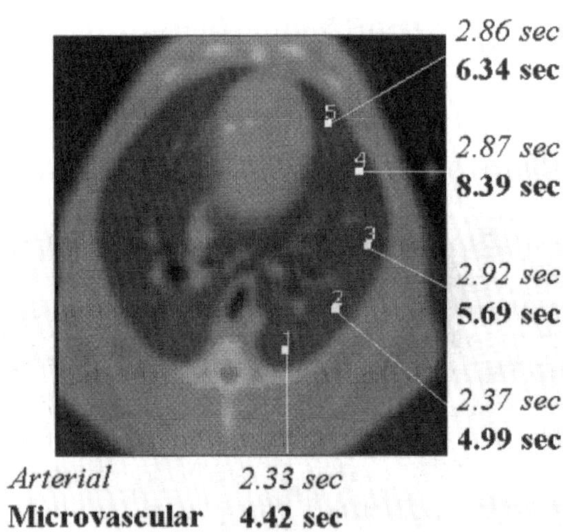

Figure 9 Methods discussed in the text and in association with Figure 8 were used to estimate arterial and microvascular mean transit times. (Data presented in abstract form in Ref. 34.)

These regional mean transit times vary as would be expected with lung height and location relative to the hilum.

The reconvolved arterial portion of the curve is a near-identical, scaled, time-shifted replicate of the TIF sampled in the main pulmonary artery.

C. Regional Ventilation

Earlier studies (11,33) using X-ray CT to evaluate regional differences in ventilation associated with body posture utilized regional density changes in the lung itself as an index of regional "ventilation." Such density changes represent changes in regional air content of the lung but do not necessarily represent fresh gas delivery. Nevertheless, important lessons were learned regarding supine/prone differences in lung function, and it was made evident that gravity alone could not account for changes in regional differences in lung function. This will be discussed in greater detail below.

To directly evaluate ventilation parameters within the reconstructed CT sections, investigators have attempted to use wash-in and wash-out of nonradioactive (stable) xenon gas. Local ventilation rate constants based on a monoexponential approach (36,37) were used to estimate regional ventilation. With 80% xenon, an enhancement of approximately 80–100 HU was achieved, and with the 30–40% xenon mixture, an enhancement of approximately 40 HU was reached. These early studies showed preliminary intriguingly good correlation with expected regional ventilation deficits predicted from visually apparent regional pulmonary pathology. A cautionary note was reported by Winkler et al. (38), who found that xenon can generate a characteristic respiratory depression. In goats, 70% equilibrated xenon decreased minute ventilation associated with a decreased respiratory rate. With closer scrutiny, one notices that lung volume was poorly controlled in these early studies, and that, because of misalignment, brightness in the subtraction images (before and after equilibration with xenon) was due more to edge artifacts than to physiologically significant ventilatory patterns.

Tajik et al. (39) have obtained preliminary data on the use of stable xenon gas as a pulmonary ventilation tracer during EBCT imaging in four pigs. Imaging protocols under development include a single-breath technique and a dynamic, multibreath wash-out technique.

As a basis for providing quantitative measures, Tajik and colleagues first assessed the Xe-concentration-X-ray attenuation relationship for the EBCT scanner. CT X-ray attenuation was found to be linearly related to xenon concentration over the entire range of xenon concentration. Linear regression analysis shows a slope of 1.55 HU enhancement per percentage increase in xenon concentration when calibrated using the EBCT scanner.

In this imaging protocol, the thorax is scanned preceding and subsequent to a single breath of 100% xenon gas. The xenon-enhanced and unenhanced

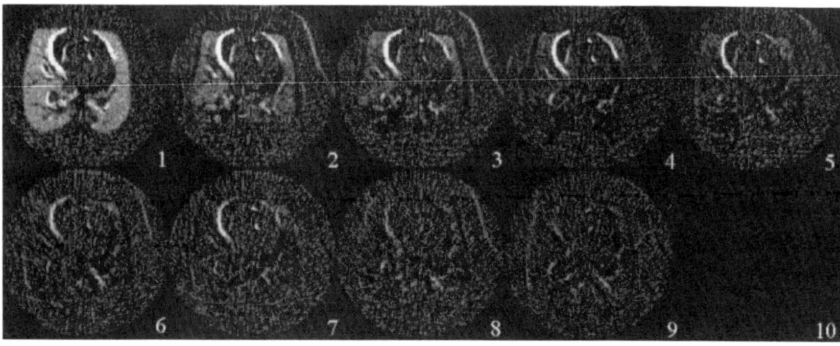

Figure 10 Images obtained via EBCT scanning. Depicted is the same level of the thorax scanned at the end of sequential breaths as equilibrated xenon gas is washed out of the lungs. The slice from the last time point (when the xenon is fully washed out) is subtracted from each of the other slices. Thus, the brighter the image, the greater is the amount of xenon gas present in that region of the lung. Note the more rapid disappearance of xenon from the dependent versus the nondependent lung regions. (Reproduced with permission from Ref. 39.)

image data sets are then digitally subtracted to represent the distribution of inhaled tracer. If the two data sets have been correctly registered (i.e., gathered at identical lung volumes), the regional image gray scale value should be directly proportional to the relative distribution of inhaled tracer gas. The subtraction images (Fig. 10) showed minimal or no edge effects, indicating that the enhanced and unenhanced scans were correctly registered. The resulting subtraction image, therefore, should depict the distribution of change in HU through the lung field due to a single deep breath of 100% xenon gas and therefore regional ventilation. The mean enhancement from the single deep breath of 100% xenon gas is 32 ± 1.85 (SE) HU in the lung parenchyma, indicating that adequate signal can be achieved with this technique.

However, when the same lung slice was scanned repeatedly during a breath hold after Xe inhalation, lung density in the dependent region began to immediately increase, and over a 10-sec apneic period the density change is on the same order of magnitude as the Xe-based enhancement. Thus, for anything other than a single-level study, conventional CT will be inadequate for evaluating regional distribution of ventilation.

1. *Validation of Regional Xenon Density Data*

As an initial validation of the equilibrium and washout data obtained from the multibreath imaging protocol, we used the equation $HU_{eq} = (\text{air fraction}*C*\text{xenon}) + HU_{baseline}$ to predict the equilibrium HU value of each sampled lung region based on regional lung air content, xenon gas concentration used during a given equilibration study, and the linear relationship between xenon concentration and HU. Use of 33 and 66% xenon gas mixtures demonstrated matches within 2 HU of that predicted.

Using the multibreath wash-out method, the following represent some of the more significant findings that serve to demonstrate the accuracy of the measures. Conclusions regarding the accuracy of the methodology came from the fact that the predicted HU changes matched those measured, and differences in wash-out between regions and various interventions matched well-understood physiological principles:

Repeating an identical multibreath imaging study three consecutive times to test the repeatability of the regional measurements indicates that respiratory and cardiac gated image acquisition during a wash-out study allows reproducible detailed regional ventilation measurements throughout the lungs.

Dependent lung regions demonstrate a significantly faster dilution of xenon relative to the nondependent region, suggesting greater ventilation in the dependent lung (Fig. 11).

As shown in Figure 12, inspiratory flow rate variations used in preliminary studies had no effect on the distribution of air flow (as indicated by xenon wash-out rates) to nondependent lung regions in the supine pig. In the dependent regions, however, wash-out is enhanced at 25 L/min inspiratory flow rate. Since at high flow rates, inertial factors and hence pathway geometry become more important in the distribution of air

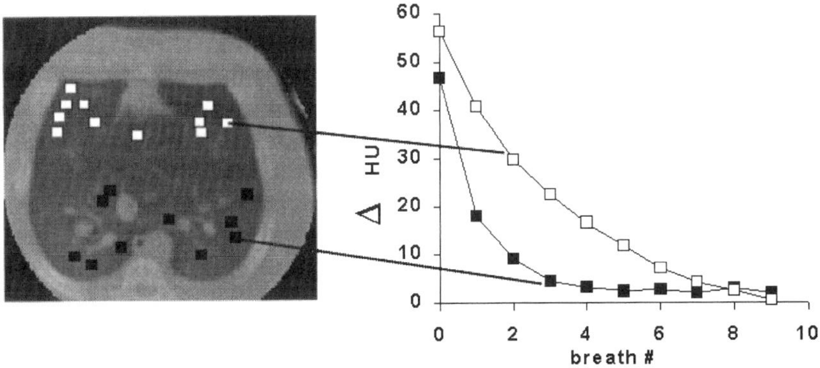

Figure 11 The same xenon washout as in Figure 10, except here a number of regions from the dependent and nondependent lung have been grouped together to depict graphically the differences in wash-out rate. (Data presented in abstract form in Ref. 39.)

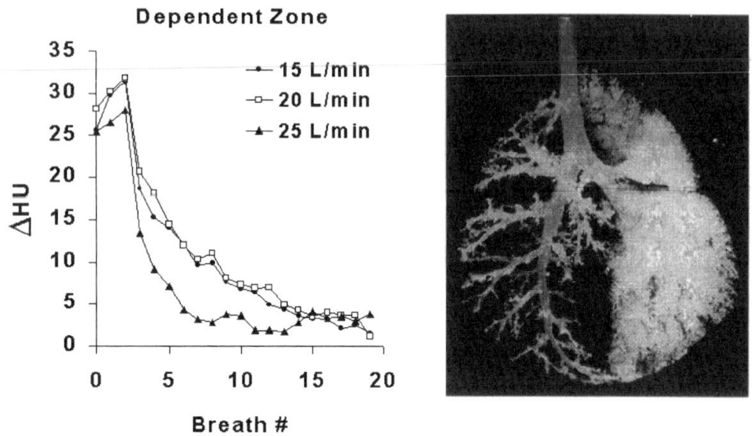

Figure 12 (Right) Airway cast of a pig lung; (left) data graphed from a pig scanned supine, anesthetized in an EBCT scanner during xenon wash-out maneuvers. As the inspiratory flow rate was increased without changing tidal volume or breaths per minute, note that the wash-out rate increases in the dependent lung region. This change was not observed in the nondependent lung regions. We believe that this preferential increase in ventilation to the dependent lung regions is reflective of the anatomy of the airway tree. The major conducting airway in a pig goes to the dependent lung region. As flow rate increases, presumably conductance plays a greater role in ventilation distribution. High-speed volumetric imaging such as is made possible by the EBCT scanner allows us for the first time to link in vivo structure to function. (Data presented in abstract form in Ref. 39. Cast of pig airway reprinted with permission from Ref. 41.)

flow (ventilation), our data indicate that the dorsal, diaphragmatic region of the pig lung (dependent lung region in a supine pig) receives an enhanced air flow distribution at higher flow rates perhaps owing to favorable airway geometry to these lung zones. Functional X-ray CT imaging may, therefore, allow us, for the first time, to explore pulmonary structure-function relationships in vivo.

D. Airway and Vascular Tree Structures

Evaluation of the airway or arterial tree has been limited, in large part, to indirect methods that detect the integrated responses of the whole system. Such measures have included pulmonary arterial blood flow assessment by contrast dilution, vascular and airway resistance calculations from measures of flows and pressures, and measurement of forced expiratory flows and volumes. More direct measurements have been achieved by visualizing surface capillaries and alveoli through pleural windows (40).

CT can assess vessel area and wall thickness in vivo, depending upon their size and orientation. When a vessel or airway crosses a slice obliquely, smaller luminal diameter structures cannot be visualized due to partial volume effects. The gray scale of an image voxel is determined by the multiple structures of varying densities within the spatial location represented. When a vessel lies oblique to the scanning plane, a voxel (considering slice thickness) is more likely to contain structures of multiple densities. Accurate evaluation of area and wall thickness requires not only adequate visualization of the structure, but also that the local long axis of the vessel or airway of interest lie perpendicular to the scanning plane. This restricts the analysis to a fraction of the tree structures. Increased sensitivity of such measures is achieved through the use of very thin slice scanning (as thin as 1–1.5 mm) and the use of high spatial frequency reconstruction algorithms to sharpen edges (HRCT). Function of smaller structures is assessed from regional in vivo–based measures of blood and air flow by contrast dilution techniques discussed above. The signal-to-noise ratio is enhanced by longer scanning times, which improve the photon statistics of the projections used to generate the reconstructed cross-sections. An additional complication when measuring structures as small as 1 or 2 mm diameter in the intact lung is caused by the effects of cardiogenic motions on image sharpness and data interpretation. Even with such limitations, new insights have been gained and we now appreciate that the response of the system is considerably heterogeneous (41,42). Specific physiological insights are discussed in greater detail in other chapters. Full exploitation of the potential for assessment of the complexity of airway physiology lies in the development of objective methods for airway detection.

A variety of different techniques have been used for airway border detection, including the adjustment of display window and level settings to rescale the image intensity values prior to measurement (43,44), methods based on manual or semiautomatic border tracing (42,45,46), and more objective, quantitative approaches such as the use of the "half-max" criteria (41,47–50). The half-max criterion is based on the assumption that the image gray level at the true airway wall will be halfway between the minimum and maximum gray levels along a ray crossing the edge. However, because of scanner blur and partial-volume effects, the half-max approach is not uniformly accurate across structures of different sizes (51); the half-max measuring technique suffers from a size-dependent measurement bias—smaller and thinner-walled airways suffer more measurement bias than the larger airways.

To address these shortcomings of the half-max approach, Reinhardt et al. (52) have developed a model-based approach for airway measurement. They explicitly model the scanning process of an ideal airway and use the model to predict the shape of the gray-level profiles of rays crossing the airway wall. Using an optimization technique, the model parameters are adjusted to minimize the difference between the predicted profile and the actual profiles observed in the data. The set of parameters that minimize the difference between the model and the data yields an estimate of the airway geometry. This approach can be accurately applied to airways of different sizes. The method is based on a two-dimensional model of an ideal airway cut perpendicular to the long axis. The centroid of the model airway is located at the origin, and the airway has inner radius l_i and outer radius l_o ($l_i < l_o$). The density of the model airway wall is unity and the density of the model airway lumen (air) is zero. The model airway is surrounded by tissue of constant density α (typically, $0 \le \alpha < 1$), which represents the lung parenchyma. Let $g(x,y)$ be the two-dimensional density profile of the ideal airway model. The scanner response to the airway is the two-dimensional convolution of the density function $g(x,y)$ and the scanner point spread function $h(x,y)$:

$$f(x,y) = A + K\int_{-\infty}^{\infty} g(x',y')h(x-x',y-y')dx'dy', \tag{5}$$

where K is a constant scale factor and A is a constant representing the background gray-level output of the scanner. Typically, $h(x,y)$ can be modeled as a symmetrical two-dimensional Gaussian curve with standard deviation sigma: $h(x,y) = e^{-(x^2+y^2)/2\sigma^2}$ (53). Without loss of generality, consider the single ray running from $x = 0$ along the x axis in the positive x direction. For this single ray, Eq. (1) can be written as:

$$f(x,0) = A + K\int_{l_i}^{l_0} e^{-(x^2+r^2)/2\sigma^2} I_0(rx/\sigma^2)r\, dr + K\alpha\int_{l_0}^{\infty} e^{-(x^2+r^2)/2\sigma^2} I_0(rx/\sigma^2)r\, dr, \tag{6}$$

where $I_0(x)$ is the modified Bessel function of order zero. A nonlinear optimization technique is used to minimize the difference between the observed ray profiles in the data and the predicted responses from the ideal airway model. The response function $f(x,0)$ in Eq. (6) can easily be differentiated with respect to the parameters l_i, l_0, K, and α, so we employ an efficient minimization technique based on the Levenberg-Marquardt algorithm (54). After the optimization, the model parameters l_i and l_0 that minimize the total error yield estimates of the airway inner and outer radius.

Reinhardt et al. have validated the model-based method using plexiglass airway phantoms (52) and excised lung tissue (55). In both cases, the model-based method gave more accurate results (less measurement bias) than the half-max approach. Measurements made on the excised lung tissue were compared to laboratory measurements made using a dissecting microscope. The mean error in estimating airway inner diameter was approximately 0.3 mm (one pixel) for the model-based approach and approximately 1.4 mm (five pixels) for the half-max method. There was no significant difference between the laboratory (microscope-based) measurements and the CT-based measurements made using the model-technique ($p < 0.01$, regression line $y = 1.03\ x + 0.09$ mm).

If one is to truly assess the airway and vascular tree structures as a function of generation, and take advantage of the airway and vascular tree structures as a roadmap to the parenchyma so that measurements can be made in the same location of the lung from maneuver to maneuver and across time, then one must image and evaluate the three-dimensional airway tree and thus one must scan the subject volumetrically. There has been little work in this area. In the realm of basic airway research, there have been exciting uses of two-dimensional CT methodologies to evaluate airway physiology (17,41,42,56–58). A number of groups using computer-based methodology for the assessment of the airways have employed the VIDA software package (59). To our knowledge, three-dimensional approaches have not yet been successfully applied to physiological investigations.

No, *reliable* automated or semiautomated method for 3-D airway tree detection in HRCT images of the in vivo lung has been published to date. The seeded region growing method adopted by Wood et al. (60,61) to study excised lungs is unreliable for peripheral airways and is inadequate for in vivo lungs. Several major limitations of HRCT make the extraction of the entire airway tree from CT image sets difficult (41,46,62): (1) in-plane image resolution is insufficient to visualize airways with a diameter smaller than 1 mm and to quantify changes in dimensions in airways smaller than 1.5 mm; (2) greater slice thickness dimensions relative to in-plane pixel dimension cause some discontinuity of bronchi between slices; and (3) the three-dimensional image data sets may not consist of perfectly contiguous slices if care has not been taken to assure a constant lung volume during scanning. Additionally, if image acquisition is not ECG-triggered, cardiogenic motion (19) can significantly alter position of the lung parenchyma and thus alter the position of airways throughout the cardiac cycle, as discussed earlier. Of these limitations, the first two can be resolved by progress in imaging technology. The third one may be minimized by computer-controlled image acquisition using CT scanner triggering (25–27).

Three-dimensional reconstruction of the airway tree has recently been performed from contiguous scanning of thin-section CT data obtained on air-inflated fixed-lung specimens (63,64). In Ref. 63, airway tree segmentation was achieved by thresholding the CT data. Due to partial-volume effect, only a few branches were reconstructed. Similarly, direct correspondence between the CT number of individual voxels and the voxel air/tissue content was used for three-dimensional visualization of bronchial and vascular pulmonary trees in Ref. 64. In Refs. 60 and 65 three-dimensional seeded region growing was used on data from an isolated lobe of a dog lung that was processed under seven static pressures ranging from 0.3 kPa to 2.0 kPa. Under best-care conditions, an anesthetized dog whose lung volume is carefully controlled and where CT slices are

ECG triggered, the region-growing method fails to reach beyond the second-generation airways in dogs that represent the size of the pediatric patients of interest here. Again, visual fly-throughs for "virtual bronchoscopy" have recently led to the belief that such problems are resolved. Visualization and detection are not the same.

Chiplunkar et al. (66) have developed a robust, automatic method to identify the first several generations of the human airway tree. The primary branches of the airway tree (first four to five generations) are identified using an *adaptive* 3D region-growing algorithm. The region growing begins with an automatically selected seed point lying in the trachea. The algorithm proceeds in multiple passes: a downward pass (apex to base) is used to identify a set of downward-growing branches and bifurcation points. An upward-growing pass (base to apex) is then used to find branches growing upward from the bifurcation points. A final pass is applied to find additional downward-growing branches. After the three region-growing passes have been applied, 3D connectivity analysis is applied to identify the set of 26-connected voxels that will represent the primary tree. Special care is taken to detect and follow in-plane branches, and to proceed past occluded airways.

The method has been applied to data sets from both normal and diseased human lungs. The diseased cases included tracheal stenosis and lung cancers. For a typical data set consisting of 40 512-by-512 pixel 3-mm-thick slices, the primary tree can be identified in approximately 12 min, with no human intervention. Figure 13 shows a surface-rendered display of the primary tree automatically extracted from a patient with advanced CF. Manually identified airway trees have been used to validate the automatic technique.

To extend the airway tree detection to the most peripherally visualized structures, an automated approach to intrathoracic airway tree detection in dogs has been developed to demonstrate the performance and computational feasibility of a knowledge-based approach to bronchial tree detection (67–73). This knowledge-based canine bronchial tree detection method consists of several stages. After determination of lung contours in the three-dimensional set of EBCT data, the primary airway tree consisting of major bronchi is identified using the approach of Chiplunkar et al. discussed above. Potential airways are determined in individual CT slices using a priori knowledge about pulmonary anatomy and contextual information (67,69,71). Using three-dimensional connectivity properties of the pulmonary airway tree and intelligent postprocessing tree growing, the three-dimensional tree is constructed from the set of adjacent slices (74). The approach has evolved considerably over the years starting with a rule-based approach, later introducing a manually trained fuzzy-logic approach, and most recently developing a fuzzy-logic approach in which the method is automatically trained using examples of manually identified trees. Instead of

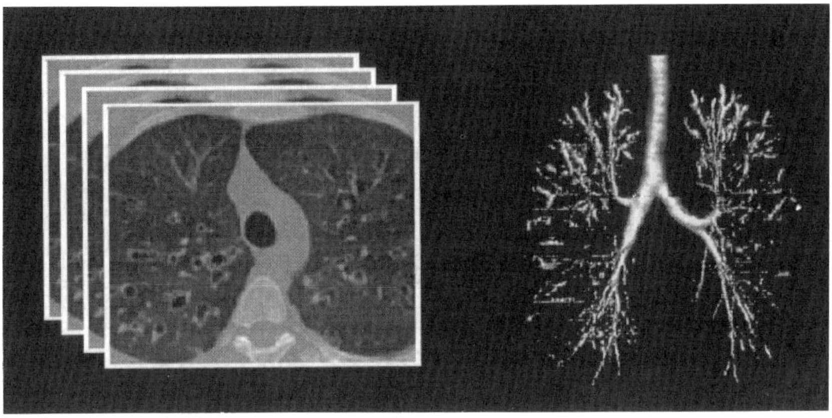

Figure 13 Noninvasive evaluation 3-D airway structure via volumetric CT scanning of a patient with cystic fibrosis, imaged via the EBCT scanner. Note the selective dilation (bronchiectasis) in the apical lung regions of this patient. (Reprinted with permission from Ref. 2.)

several man-weeks needed to manually design the fuzzy-logic parameters, the most recent implementation learns its fuzzy-logic rules and membership functions from a reasonably small number of examples and counterexamples (50 airways and 50 nonairways were used in the most recent study), and the learning stage is completely finished within about an hour of unattended computer processing. Importantly, the performance of the fuzzy-logic method that uses automated learning is virtually identical to that of the manually trained method (74). The automated training approach thus guarantees applicability of the intrathoracic airway tree detection method to a broad range of studies.

To validate all three generations of the airway tree detection method, five volumetric EBCT data sets acquired with 40 slices per set were analyzed and the computer-determined bronchial trees compared with the manually defined airway locations that served as an independent standard. Experienced observers carefully identified the independent standard following a tedious and time-consuming procedure of tracing airways on a computer screen. Manual identification of the entire airway tree required 9 hr of manual tracing and editing. In canine EBCT images, the most recent method successfully identified all airway generations determined by the experienced observer. To lay ground for future bronchial tree measurements, Ma and Sonka have developed a fully parallel method for three-dimensional thinning (75) and have shown its applicability to bronchial trees. To measure the complete geometry of the airway tree (branch lengths, cross-sectional area, rate of tapering, branch angles, etc.) it is critical to identify a highly accurate centerline of the airway tree. Others have sought to achieve such centerline finding for upper and intrathoracic airways as well as other structures including coronary arteries and the descending aorta (60,76–78). The branching structure of the lung, while fractal in nature (79) and thus exquisitely stochastically self-similar as one moves from the central to the peripheral portions of the tree, represents a highly complex network of tubing and presents greater challenges than most other vascular trees currently under investigation by use of volumetric imaging methodologies.

While studies in the mid-1980s (80,81) used more manual methodologies to demonstrate the potential accuracy of volumetric CT scanning to quantify vascular tree structures, to date the vessels have received less attention than the airways in the push for detection and quantitation. This is, in part, because of the difficulty of separating arteries from veins and the need for use of injected iodinated contrast agents to allow for the differentiation between the endoluminal blood and the vessel wall.

E. Observations

Studies of the upper airway in normal persons and patients with obstructive sleep apnea have been carried out to investigate the mechanical events governing luminal area. There is an increased active component of airway opening in inspiration in sleep apnea and a greater compliance (change in upper-airway cross-sectional area) during expiration (82–86).

Airway reactivity studies in pigs (41), designed to develop techniques for assessment of the intrathoracic airways in asthmatics, has shown that HRCT can detect changes in the peripheral (2 mm) airways before such changes are reflected in more conventional measures of pulmonary function (i.e., airway pressure and conductance) when challenged with methacholine. A recent study (87) of human asthmatic subjects has demonstrated that central airways show a greater response to methacholine than do peripheral airways whereas peripheral airways show a greater response to β-agonists. This in vivo information confirms laboratory bench observations that cholinergic receptor density is greater centrally as compared with peripheral receptor distribution while beta-receptors are more prevalent peripherally. These data were made possible through a combination of careful, objective quantification of the airways as well as through careful development of the imaging protocols. Since lung volume changes with both drugs, the lung volume controller was used to assure that the scans before and after challenge were obtained at the same lung volume. Lungs were scanned at 65% vital capacity before drug delivery and the volume below TLC was noted. After drug delivery, the lungs were scanned at the same volume below TLC rather than at a percentage of VC since RV was altered.

F. Parenchymal Characterization: An Objective Measure of Regional Pathophysiology

Computer-based methods for objective quantitation of CT data sets to compare normal and emphysematous lung are only recently gaining use in conjunction with 2D data sets. These works have largely relied on methods based upon the density histogram. These methods have ranged from the simplest form which counts the number of voxels below a cutoff density (900 HU) (5,88–98) to those that make use of measures derived from the histogram, including skewness, kurtosis, etc. (37a). We are unaware of any clinical use of 3D or 4D data sets to evaluate lung pathology, except for a few demonstration papers that have shown shaded-surface displays of the primary airway tree. Initially visual scoring systems of reduced tissue density have been used to assess emphysema (38,99–103). HRCT further enhances the resolving power of the image (102–106) allowing detection of less severe emphysema. Further studies (107) applying computerized algorithms of excised lungs showed a greater percentage of pixels with a density equivalent to that of air. This decrease in lung density compared to normal lung was thought to be caused by capillary bed destruction that was associated with emphysema. It has also been observed that 1-mm CT slices are more suitable for detecting small areas of low attenuation, and that a 5-mm collimation is more useful in detecting disruption of the vascular tree (108). Of great importance is the demonstration that HRCT performed on inflated autopsy lungs can accurately detect even mild forms of centrilobular emphysema, when compared to subsequent pathological analysis (102).

1. *Texture Analysis*

Various computer-assisted methods have successfully been used for tissue characterization using texture recognition for medical applications. Traditional methods of texture analysis can be grouped into statistical, structural, and hybrid methods (109). Methods for tissue classification typically rely on region grayscale statistical measures (i.e., mean, variance, frequency histogram) or textural measures (autocorrelation, co-occurrence matrices, un-length matrices, etc.) (5,37, 89,92,110–120). Texture analysis has been successful in detecting tumors in magnetic resonance brain imagery (116), identifying glandular tissues in mammograms (115), characterizing liver tissue (120), and analyzing cardiac echocardiograms (111,114,117). HRCT improves the ability to evaluate the lung parenchyma. Considerable recent effort has been focused on objectively measuring the density of lung tissue, either as mean lung density, or by measuring the lowest 5% of the CT scan density (5,37,89,92,110). It has been demonstrated that accurate measurements of lung tissue mean density can be an index of emphysema (5,89,92). A later study, however, showed significant lung density variation in normal individuals (110). Thus, a density-masking approach alone appears to not be sufficient to distinguish normal from diseased lung, at least in some instances, but particularly in the early stages of a disease process. More recently, the fractal concept, developed by Mandelbrot (121), has been used to characterize texture and quantify diseases. Chen et al. (120,122) devised feature vectors based on fractal Brownian motion to classify ultrasonic liver images. Various fractal models have been used for analysis of angiographic images (123), for characterization of mammographic parenchymal pattern (124), and for discrimination of chest radiographs (125). Fractal analysis of canine renal cortex has also been performed (126) to help in quantifying pathophysiological changes in renal disease. Cargill et al. (127) have estimated the surface dimension of normal lung parenchyma to be between 2.7 and 3.0. In an earlier study, we showed that the fractal dimension was a useful tool in discriminating between textures of normal and abnormal lung (119).

Significant advances in the use of tissue characterization have been made to classify parenchymal patterns in reconstructed CT data sets (128–130). Patients with emphysema, interstitial fibrosis and sarcoid were scanned to evaluate the utility of texture-based measures in classifying and quantifying the extent of lung disease.

A texture-based computer-assisted method, called the adaptive multiple-feature method (AMFM), was developed and applied (130). The AMFM method involved three steps: (1) feature extraction from the region of interest; (2) optimal feature selection based on a training set; and (3) classification of the test set. It has been shown that, by carefully controlling scanning parameters (slice thickness, reconstructed field of view, lung volume, and body posture) it is possible to have the computer characterize tissue type with a region-by-region (31×31 pixel regions throughout the lung field) match rate between human observer and computer equal to the match rate between two trained observers. The problem comes in demonstrating increased accuracy over a trained observer when the trained observer serves as the gold standard. It is of great interest that, for the match rate between observers and between computer and observers to become equal, the observers had to be given the pathological finding of the patient at the time they were assessing the image, suggesting that the observer needed to use nonimage data to support the visual assessment. Of particular note is the fact that in step 2 above (optimal feature selection), characterizing each tissue type, the features based upon the newly developed stochastic fractal measures were required to discriminate between tissue types.

Extension of this technique to cystic fibrosis has shown encouraging results. In a pilot study, one child with normal lungs was scanned for evaluation of metastatic disease and three children who demonstrated varying degrees of bronchoalveolar lavage (BAL)-based inflammation and infection were scanned. The three CF patients had the following characteristics:

1. 2% neutrophils, no bacterial growth
2. 15% neutrophils, no bacterial growth
3. 43% neutrophils, *Pseudomonas aeruginosa*, and *Staphylococcus aureus*

As shown in Figure 14, the AMFM approach to tissue characterization demonstrates a complex progression of parenchymal "texture" that is highly suggestive of increasing signs of peripheral airway disease with a progression across subjects mimicking the BAL results. The significance of this work lies in the fact that the combination of X-ray CT and computer-based image analysis provides the needed sensitivity and repeatability required for improved phenotyping of disease and outcomes analysis of pioneering new methodologies for disease intervention. It is precisely because the lung structure and physiology

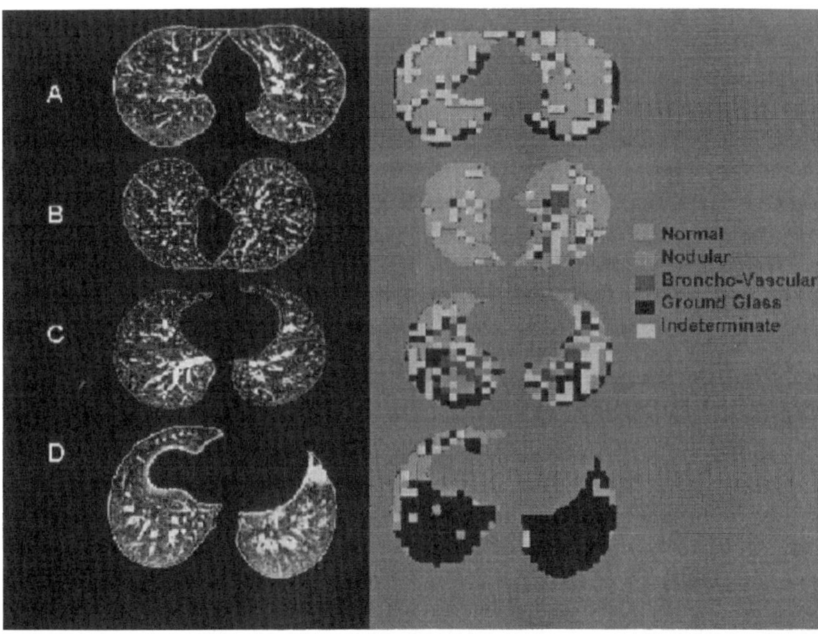

Figure 14 Lungs of four young children. (A) This child did not have cystic fibrosis, but was being scanned for possible lung metastases. (B–D) These children had cystic fibrosis but no signs of pulmonary function abnormality as judged from pulmonary function testing. Bronchoalveolar lavage revealed a neutrophil count of 2, a neutrophil count of 15, and a neutrophil count of 43 + pseudomonas in patients B, C, and D, respectively. Use of a computer-based tissue characterization method (AMFM) described in the text more fully revealed progressive patterns of tissue pathology in these otherwise asymptomatic (in regard to the PFTs) children. (Reprinted with permission from Ref. 2.)

are complex and because disease processes serve to increase the complexity that conventional methodologies of the past now fail because of their global nature.

VI. Application of the Tools in a Physiological Assessment of $\dot{V}/\dot{Q}$ Physiology

A. Heart and Lungs: Shapes and Volumes

As a first approach to evaluating the utility of these imaging tools in the study of physiology, the question was asked regarding how well the overall volume of the heart and lungs could be determined. Hoffman et al. demonstrated that the lung volumes could be detected to within 3% of excision and water displacement values (131), cardiac chamber volumes could be detected to within 5% of the water displacement measurements of radiopaque cast scanned in situ and subsequently excised (132), and ventricular muscle mass could be measured to within 5% of postmortem quantitation (133,134). The visual anatomical fidelity of the surface displays of the heart chambers and lungs correlated well with the structures apparent in the excised chamber casts and excised air-dried lungs. Subsequently, investigators have used volumetric CT imaging to evaluate dynamic heart volumes (135), diaphragm shape in the prone and supine postures (136), and lung shape following pneumonectomy and subsequent compensatory air volume replacement (137,138).

B. Regional Lung Air Content Distribution

Studies of regional lung air content distribution have led to the hypothesis that the intrathoracic position of the heart is a major determinant of the regional distribution of ventilation, and the presence of lobar fissures allows the lobes of the lungs to accommodate shape changes of the diaphragm and rib cage without altering the volumes of the alveoli (air sacs comprising the region of gas exchange with the blood). Studies of dogs on the DSR confirmed that there is a significant ventral-dorsal gradient in regional lung expansion in the supine body posture, which disappears when the dog is shifted into the prone body posture (11). Interestingly, this ventral-dorsal gradient in regional lung expansion reappeared in the nondependent lung with the dogs in the left or right lateral decubitus body postures, suggesting that gravity directly acting on the lung is not the only factor in determining regional variation in lung expansion. There are numerous factors at work including altered chest wall shape and inherent regional variations unrelated to any well-defined Cartesian coordinate system (11,33).

To reduce the analysis time in the hope of generating images offering new insights into the DSR-derived lung data sets, multinomial models were applied to the distribution of reconstructed lung air content (139). Percent air content data within the lung field is randomly sampled (usually 25% of data or 45,000 voxels) from the reconstructed lung field, which is defined as being those voxels with an air content greater than 35% and less than 90%. This image value range is selected to minimize the inclusion of lower-valued reconstruction noise and eliminate major pulmonary vessels and airways. It is important to note here that this selection criterion assures that we are not trying to fit the multinomial to "holes" such as the voxel locations representing the heart or its associated major vessels. We generally fit the data to, at most, a second-order, 10-term multinomial. Various terms can be eliminated (x,y,z or combinations thereof representing geometric orientations within the lung field). With this model, F-tests for multiple regression can be performed and assessed to indicate whether increasing or decreasing the order of the multinomial is appropriate. However, if the number of data points is very large, as in our case, all of the terms of the multinomial become significant and hence tests for "positive correlation" of the errors are used for the inclusion of additional terms instead of the F-test. Once the multinomial image is generated by identifying voxel values between 35% and 100% air content in the original image and replacing those values with values predicted by the multinomial, all voxels with an original value of less than 35 are set to zero. The original data set and the multinomial-based volume image can then be evaluated. To display function along with the complete three-dimensional geometry, air content is mapped at a fixed depth below the surface onto the lung shaded surface displays with color saturation representing air content (140). Data from the multinomial volume images for a dog studied prone and supine are depicted in Figure 15. On the left is the left lateral aspect of the lungs of the dog in the supine body posture and on the right are the same dog lungs with the dog in the prone posture. Again, note the ventral-dorsal gradient supine, which is absent prone, yet now it is apparent that in the prone posture there is a pattern to regional air content differences. However, the regional differences are not directly related to any of the major body axes. Olson and Rodarte (141) studied isolated air-filled and water-filled lung lobes suspended in water and showed that there was a considerable amount of regional inhomogeneity of lung expansion in the water-filled lung suspended in water, which was not explained by a relationship to any major axis or combination of axes. It is clear that in vivo and ex vivo, there are significant nongravitational determinants of regional ventilation differences.

With the observation that the dog manages to match ventilation and perfusion in the prone body posture without large gradients leaving the nondependent lung exposed to high, continuous strain, and with the thought that since humans in the upright posture have significant, continuous exposure of the nondependent (apical) lung region, it was hypothesized that perhaps humans have not evolved to walk upright in relationship to the cardiopulmonary system. An animal was sought that lived in the opposite body posture to the dog, and a sloth was selected. Unfortunately for the initial hypothesis, the sloth showed the same lung

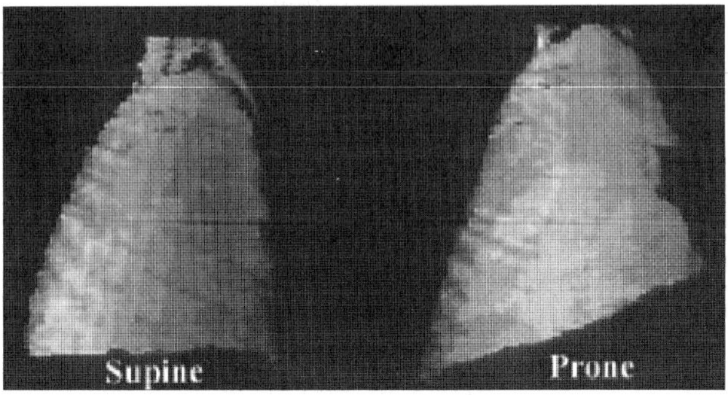

Figure 15 Shaded surface displays of the lungs of a dog scanned in the supine (left) and prone (right) body postures. The regional lung air content throughout the lung has been fitted to a polynomial function and the lung air content estimated by this polynomial function is mapped out to the surface coded in gray scale. Note the distinct ventral-to-dorsal gradient present in the supine posture, which is absent prone. While there is the absence of a ventral dorsal gradient prone, there is a distinct variation in lung air content. These data demonstrated that forces other than a direct effect of gravity play a role in determining regional lung air content. (Reproduced with permission from Ref. 139.)

density gradient supine and lack of gradient prone as was found in the dog (33). However, whereas the dog rib cage and diaphragm changed shape considerably prone versus supine, the sloth has a very rigid chest wall (22 rib pairs) and showed no significant change in chest wall geometry with change in body posture. The similarity between dog and sloth was the shift in the intrathoracic position of the heart, and we believe that it is the sternal support of the heart in the prone posture versus the lung support of the heart supine that in part alters regional lung expansion differences. Presumably, in the dog, lobar slippage is able to minimize the effects of chest wall shape changes on regional variation in lung expansion while lobar slippage may not accommodate the altered support requirements of the heart. It is interesting that the sloth is born with lobar fissures, but these fissures reportedly (142) fibrose over shortly after birth, perhaps from disuse since the rib cage does not change shape with changes in body posture. Shaded surface displays of the in vivo lungs of the dog and sloth demonstrate the altered ventral lung geometry determined by the shifts of the intrathoracic position of the heart with change in body posture.

An animal that has essentially no functional lobar fissures is the horse. Olson and Lai-Fook (143) have shown that in ponies, there is a very sharp pleural pressure gradient in the supine posture, which again is eliminated when the animal is shifted to the prone posture. The pleural pressure gradient was so steep that there is a suggestion that nearly one-third to one-half of the dorsal lung is collapsed. It is interesting to speculate that the lack of lobar fissures is in some way responsible. Miniature horses have been scanned in the DSR (144). The resulting image data, shown in Figure 16, demonstrate that there is a remarkable shape change in the diaphragm between the prone and supine body posture, with the dorsal region of the diaphragm shifting more cephalad in the supine posture, perhaps contributing to alveolar collapse in the dependent lung. As depicted in Figure 17, mechanically, the diaphragm had a piston-like motion in the supine posture while it moved in a lever arm fashion prone with the greatest motion in the dorsal region where there was the greatest amount of lung tissue. Three-dimensional images of the horse lungs demonstrated that there was not nearly as much shift of the lung geometry attributable to shift in the intrathoracic position of the heart. In the case of the horse, diaphragm shape changes appear to play an important role.

C. Blood Flow

Recent evidence suggests that blood flow may be determined in part by vascular conductance (vascular geometry) (145), and, therefore, blood flow and ventilation have nonoverlapping parameters determining their relative distribution patterns. Beck and Rehder (145) have shown that in isolated lungs, if the gravitational effect is subtracted out, the dorsal, basal region of the lower lobe receives a greater blood flow regardless of lobar posture. Looking at the geometry of the dog pulmonary arterial tree, there is a large major vessel that traverses straight toward the dorsal/basal region of the lower lobe similar to the airway anatomy depicted for the pig in Figure 12. An hypothesis might be that in the supine body posture, the gravity drives blood down and vascular conductance (vessel geometry) also drives blood down, and thus we see a ventral-to-dorsal gradient in regional perfusion. However, in the prone body posture, gravity drives blood down while perhaps vascular conductance drives blood up, and we do not see a significant ventral-dorsal pattern to regional perfusion differences. Supporting this notion, Glenny and Robertson (146) have used a fractal analysis to evaluate regional pulmonary blood flow by injecting lungs with ^{99m}Tc-labeled macroaggregated albumin and then removing the lungs after a fixation process and imaging the lung with a gamma camera. The data were found to fit a fractal model with a dimension of 1.09. The fit was greatest in the gravitational direction. However, the investigators noted that the difference between the fit in an isogravimetric plane versus the gravitational plane was small and concluded that heterogeneity of pulmonary blood flow is only secondarily influenced by gravity. Gravitationally oriented lung expansion gradients have been observed in whole-dog frozen-tissue samples (147–150). A similar gravity-dependent gradient in blood flow has been demonstrated using a variety of techniques including ^{133}Xe (151–154), radioactive microspheres (155–160), radioactive macroaggre-

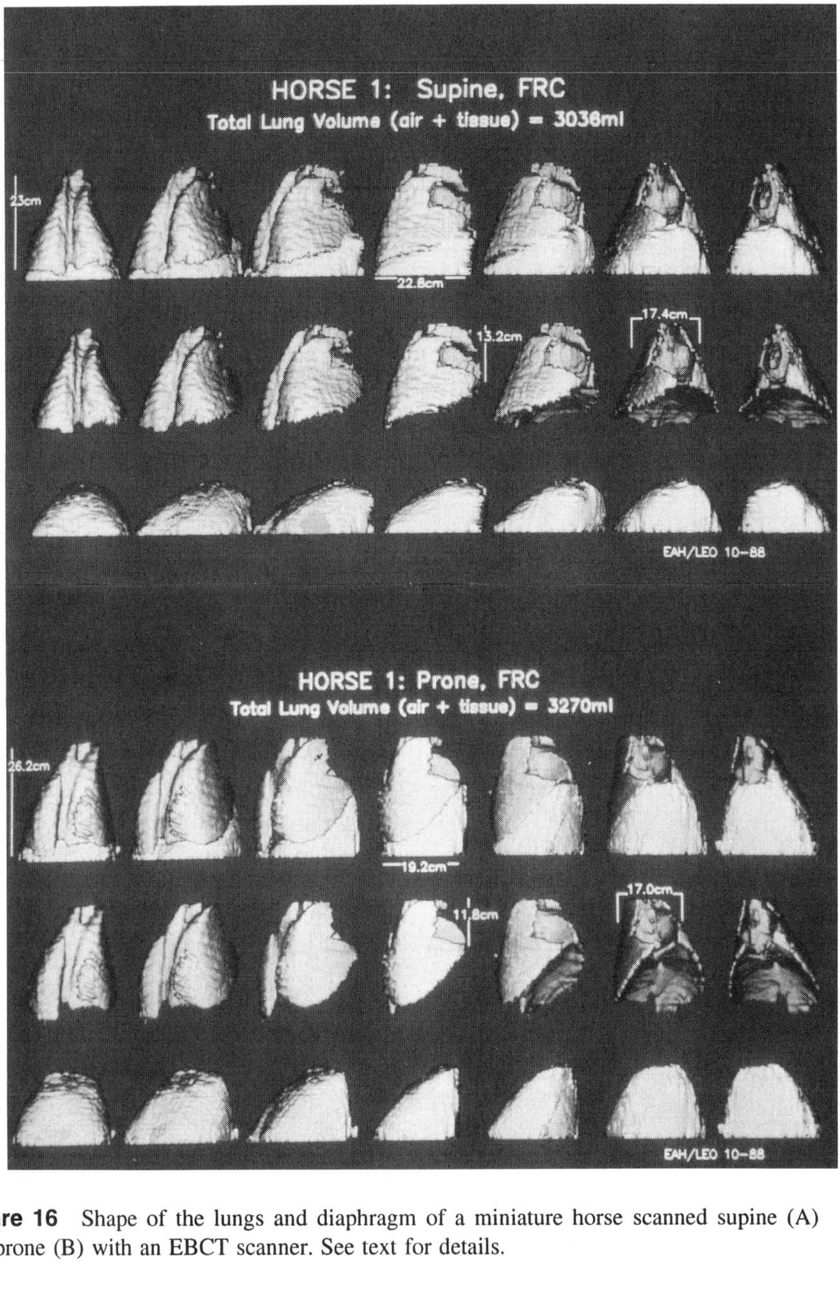

(A)

(B)

Figure 16 Shape of the lungs and diaphragm of a miniature horse scanned supine (A) and prone (B) with an EBCT scanner. See text for details.

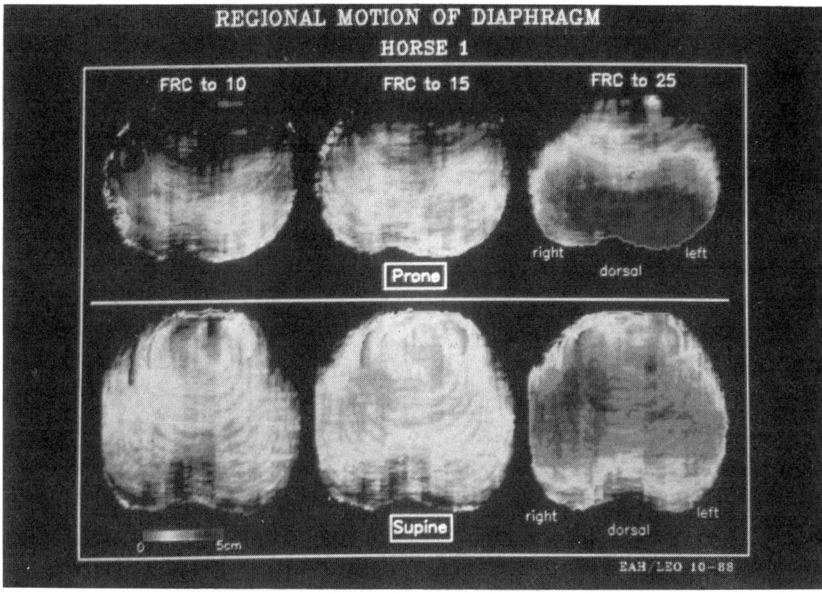

Figure 17 Projection of the diaphragm, showing the change in diaphragm position with lung inflation. Depicted are the supine (left) and prone (right) body postures. The darker the region, the greater the motion with lung inflation. These data were obtained from the same scans of a miniature horse as depicted in Figure 16.

gated albumin distribution (149,161,162), single photon emission computed tomography (163), or flow meter measurements (164). Variations in magnitude of these regional lung expansion or blood flow gradients occur by changing body positions. That is, the gradient in lung expansion and regional blood flow head-up (148,151,152,160,162,164–168) is reduced or abolished head-down (148,149, 166). An observed apex-to-base gradient in lung expansion in the supine position (169) is correlated with a supine apex-to-base gradient in blood flow (149, 160). This supine apex-to-base blood flow and lung expansion gradient is abolished or diminished in the prone body position flow (149,160,169). Similarly, Hummayr and colleagues (169) suggest the presence of a supine apex-to-base gradient in regional lung expansion. Hogg et al. (149), however, were unable to demonstrate evidence for such a gradient in frozen dogs. Recently described gradients in regional lung expansion supine that disappear prone (152,169) correlate with gradients in regional blood flow in the same body postures (162). EBCT-based measures of pulmonary blood flow in the prone versus supine body postures are shown in Figure 18. Taken in comparison to the distribution of regional lung air content and air content changes in similar body postures de-

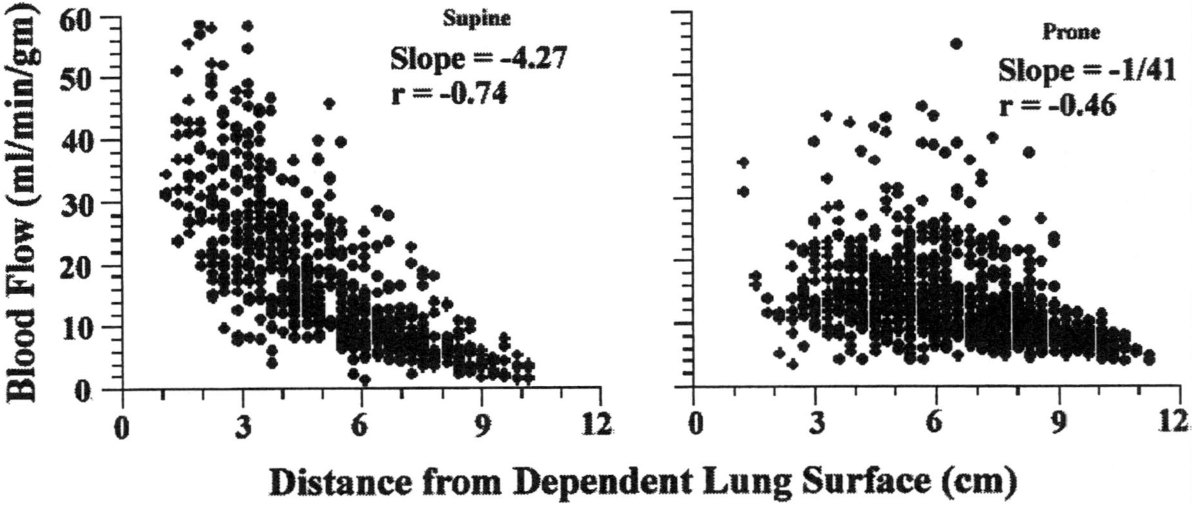

Figure 18 Regional distribution of pulmonary perfusion as detected via EBCT scanning of an anesthetized dog scanned in the supine (left) and prone (right) body postures. Note that while there is a vertical gradient in flow that is eliminated in the prone posture, there is also considerable heterogeneity of flow that is independent of lung height. Data are corrected to ml/min/g lung tissue.

picted in Figure 19, derived from DSR image data, it appears that there are factors that serve to maintain a match between regional lung expansion and regional blood flow. However, evidence demonstrating the importance of the intrathoracic location of the heart in determining regional lung expansion and the importance of vascular geometry in determining regional pulmonary blood flow suggests that these factors can contribute to the development of mismatches in ventilation-perfusion relationships.

D. Lung Growth

Conventional wisdom holds that the compensatory increase in lung air volume following pneumonectomy in rabbits can be prevented by restricting the volume of the space into which the remaining lung can expand. We applied this conventional wisdom when designing studies to investigate heart-lung interactions in rabbits. Indirect evidence from these studies suggests that the data supporting this notion may be correct only within a limited postpneumonectomy recovery

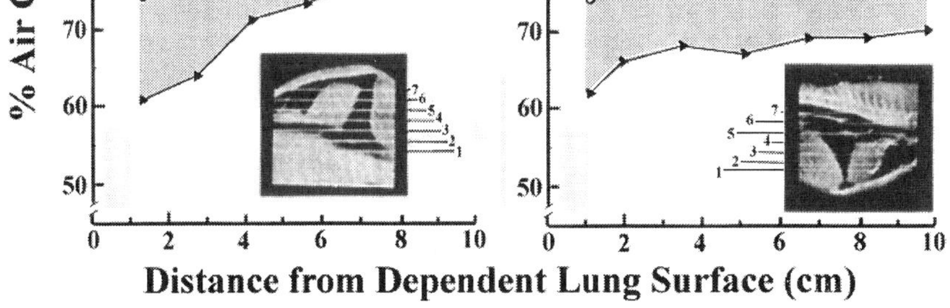

Figure 19 Regional lung air content at various lung heights with a dog scanned at three lung volumes ranging from FRC to TLC with the dog in the supine (left) and prone (right) body postures. Data were gathered via use of the dynamic spatial reconstructor. The change in regional lung air content with lung inflation is an index of regional ventilation. Thus, it is noted that there is a gradient in regional ventilation in the supine posture, which is eliminated in the prone posture. This is similar to the differences in blood flow with posture changes depicted in Figure 18. These data provided an early demonstration of the importance of mechanisms other than a direct effect of gravity on the lung being responsible for heterogeneity of lung function. (Modified with permission from Ref. 11.)

time window. Extending the recovery time appeared to permit complete restoration of lung air volume, even when the intrathoracic volume was restricted following pneumonectomy. Regional lung air content was evaluated by EBCT in sham-operated and pneumonectomized rabbits, with or without volume reduction of the left thorax following left pneumonectomy. Techniques for organizing the vast amount of information available from dynamic, volumetric CT are continually being improved and remain a challenging aspect of this technology. For this study, we elected to average data to investigate gradients in regional air content in the gravitational, cranial-caudal, and lateral directions (138). Comparing the air content gradients in the gravitational plane in the right lung in rabbits in right and left lateral recumbency indicated that interactions between the heart and the lung beneath the heart were matched by similar interactions between the abdominal contents and the lung beneath the abdominal contents (137). From this we hypothesize that the lung, chest wall, mediastinal, and abdominal contents articulate in a way that minimizes regional differences in lung air content. An additional unexpected finding was that the gravitational gradient in regional air content in rabbits in the prone position was equivalent in magnitude and direction to the gradient in rabbits in the supine position. These results differed from the results found in dogs and sloths studied in the prone and supine positions using the DSR (11,33). They serve to reinforce the lesson that the mechanical relationships between the lung and the remainder of the body are complex and likely differ among quadrupeds. Probing these species differences allows us to take advantage of the experiments of nature, and EBCT, within the current size limitations, provides a powerful technique with which to investigate these species differences.

The feasibility of using EBCT to follow the time course of the pulmonary responses to pneumonectomy was evaluated by dye-contrast studies in a subgroup of the rabbits discussed above (170). Eight rabbits, including normal, sham-operated, and pneumonectomized with and without wax-ball plombage, were studied. Both high-spatial resolution scanning of the entire lung and high-temporal resolution scanning of approximately 22% of the lung during injection of radiopaque contrast agent at FRC were performed with an EBCT scanner. As discussed above, the magnitude and distribution of pulmonary blood flow and pulmonary blood volume were estimated from the contrast injection studies. When averaged across all body positions studied, the magnitude of the differences in the volumes of the lung air, blood, and tissue between groups of rabbits was surprisingly small, given that the entire left lung (about 50% of the total lung mass) had been removed from the pneumonectomized rabbits at least 8 weeks prior to study. Although these results were consistent with conclusions reached using conventional, invasive techniques in pneumonectomized rats (171), they were unexpected for pneumonectomized rabbits with wax-ball plombage.

Consistent with findings in other animal species studied with invasive techniques, statistically significant relationships were found between regional air content, regional blood content, and regional blood flow as functions of vertical lung height, regardless of body orientation. These preliminary studies supported our inferences, from lung volume, shape, and average radiodensity data obtained by EBCT, and from direct measurements of pleural pressure, that the compensatory increase in lung air volume observed in the pneumonectomized rabbits (with and without wax-ball plombage) was due to growth of new lung tissue, rather than merely hyperexpansion of the lung tissue remaining after pneumonectomy. These results demonstrate the power of CT technology to evaluate a wide variety of lung parameters efficiently, relatively noninvasively, and therefore, in the same subject over time. Furthermore, they provide tantalizing clues that the conventional wisdom regarding the compensatory volume increase in rabbit lungs following pneumonectomy needs reevaluation. It has long been recognized that the response to pneumonectomy is complicated, in that it is known to be influenced by a variety of factors ranging from hormonal to mechanical. EBCT may provide the means to examine multiple parameters of the integrated responses, which no doubt involve multiple signaling cascades from the chest wall, to the pulmonary parenchyma, to the nuclei of the pulmonary cells, where genetic control of cell division and tissue growth resides. This may provide a means to recognize the complexity of self-reorganization associated with lung growth.

E. State of the Art: Where Are We Going?

Commercially available, clinically applicable scanning systems, including helical and electron beam CT, are capable of volumetric data acquisition in a breath hold. EBCT is capable of stop action imaging the heart and lungs simultaneously in a single or a few slices. The one-of-a-kind DSR has provided a futuristic view of the insights obtainable through dynamic volumetric data acquisition. The combined experience with these modalities has allowed for understanding of the exciting potential such modalities can play in providing the needed new insights into the complexity of basic pulmonary physiology, pathophysiology, and outcomes measures. Image display methodologies are allowing for virtual endoscopic voyages through the airways and vessels, enabling assessment of regional drug and pathogen responses, in vivo assessment of regional differences in tissue sensitivity, and geometric quantification for custom-designed laser interventions to relieve airway obstruction and the design of lifesaving new custom-built stents (2). New knowledge-based segmentation methodology is allowing for the automatic detection of the airway and vascular trees out to the limits of resolution of the scanner technologies. Tissue characterization methodology is allowing for computer-based determination and quantitation of regional pathology with a reliability unachievable by human readers. Inhaled radiodense xenon gas is providing detailed information relating to regional ventilation and lung mechanics. Use of iodinated contrast agents into the pulmonary artery is allowing us to quantitate regional blood flow normalized to regional tissue mass and to identify the presence of pulmonary emboli before a life-threatening clot is deployed, and methodology is emerging to allow us to estimate the speed of a red cell through the microvascular bed. X-ray CT has reached a state of the art where we will be able to measure lung function at the very interfaces of gas exchange. Given our state of understanding of molecular and genetic mechanisms in health and disease, it is timely that the applications of these clinically available X-ray CT scanners have moved from pure visualization tasks to accurate quantification of pulmonary structure and function.

What is quite clear now is that such quantitative measures must be tied to the three-dimensional, dynamic anatomy of the lung if one is to understand the lung in its complexity. For one to provide a sensitive measure of the onset of bronchiectasis or airway wall thickening, one must know which generation of airway is being measured. To determine change over time and/or with therapeutic interventions, one must be able to find the same airway locations. To assess the lung parenchyma over time or throughout a breath, one must be able to use the airway tree and arterial tree as a roadmap and thus one must image the lung in three dimensions. If one is to image the lung in three dimensions while the patient is breathing a radiodense gas, one must obtain the three-dimensional image in a time frame on the order of 100 msec. Much of lung pathology is a dynamic phenomenon and thus is only detectable if one is imaging the lung as air and blood are flowing. By computer detection of the lungs, lobes, airways, and airway tree and through use of morphological warping of the data to a standardized map of the standardized sublobar regions, one can begin to build a data base of normality against which to compare disease onset and progression by mapping all quantitative measures to the sublobar segments.

To achieve such a goal, we need an X-ray CT scanner that allows for the acquisition of at least 100–300 contiguous 1–1.5-mm-thick sections of the lung in 100 msec and the ability to repeat this acquisition with no more than a 10–20-msec delay. In-plane image resolution should be at least 10 and ideally 15 line pairs per centimeter (equal to or better than currently marketed scanners). Ideally, the scanner should be built to allow for scanning of human subjects in the upright or recumbent body postures. Advances in image display and analysis methodologies are critical. With such tools, it is highly likely that we will see a reclassification of lung diseases, which are currently lumped together in large part because of the global nature of the pulmonary function tests currently in practice. Advances in molecular biology, in particular, are generating new knowledge, which is allowing us to devise interventions likely to halt the onset and progression of debilitating lung diseases such as pulmonary fibrosis and emphysema, and advances in our understanding of genetically based disease puts us at the threshold of, for instance, being able to repair the cells' inability to manufacture chloride channels in cystic fibrosis. With a new-found understanding of, and the means of measure, in vivo lung complexity, we can begin to more rapidly assess the efficacy of such interventions and to better tailor the intervention to the particular lung pathology.

References

1. West GB, Brown JH, Enquist BJ. A general model for the origin of allometric scaling laws in biology. Science 1997; 276:122–126.
2. Hoffman EA, McLennan G. Assessment of pulmonary structure/function relationships and clinical outcomes measures: quantitative volumetric CT of the lung. Acad Radiol 1997; 4(11):758–776.
3. Wagner PD, Saltzman HA, West JB. Measurement of continuous distributions of ventilation-perfusion ratios: theory. J Appl Physiol 1974; 36:588–599.
4. Kevles B. Naked to the Bones. New Brunswick, NJ: Rutgers University, 1997.
5. Muller NL, Staples CA, Miller RR, Abboud RT. An objective method to quantitate emphysema using computed tomography. Chest 1988; 94:782–787.
6. Hoffman EA. An Historic Perspective of Heart and Lung Imaging. In 3-D Imaging in Medicine. Chelsea, MI: Lewis Publishers, CRC Press, 1990.
7. Heintzen PH. An appraisal of the dynamic spatial reconstructor: Investigating congenital heart disease in four dimensions. Cardiovasc Intervent Radiol 1984; 7: 138–139.
8. Kreel L. Preliminary evaluation of the EMI whole body scanner. J Belg Radiol 1976; 59:267–280.
9. Robinson PJ, Kreel L. Pulmonary tissue attenuation with computed tomography: comparison of inspiration and expiration scans. J Comput Assist Tomogr 1979; 3: 740–748.
10. Chevalier PA, Rodarte JR, Harris LD. Regional lung expansion at total lung capacity in intact vs. excised canine lungs. J Appl Physiol 1978; 45:363–369.
11. Hoffman EA. Effect of body orientation on regional lung expansion: a computed tomographic approach. J Appl Physiol 1985; 59:468–480.
12. Williams G, Bydder GM, Kreel J. The validity and use of computed tomography attenuation values. Br Med Bull 1980; 36:279–287.
13. Joseph PM, Spital RD. A method for correcting bone induced artifacts in computed tomography scanners. J Comput Assist Tomogr 1978; 2:100–108.
14. Sanders C, Nath PH, Bailey WC. Detection of emphysema with computed tomography correlation with pulmonary function tests and chest radiography. Invest Radiol 1988; 23:262–266.
15. Wollmer PU, Albrechtsson, Brauer K, Eriksson L, Jonson B, Tylen U. Measurement of pulmonary density by means of X-ray computerized tomography. Chest 1986; 90:387–391.
16. Vock P, Salzmann C. Comparison of computed tomographic lung density with

haemodynamic data of the pulmonary circulation. Clin Radiol 1986; 37:459–464.
17. Zerhouni EA, Herold CJ, Brown RH, Wetzel RC, Hirshman CA, Robotham JL, Mitzner W. High-resolution computed tomography-physiologic correlation. J Thorac Imag 1993; 8:265–272.
18. Muller NL. CT diagnosis of emphysema: it may be accurate, but is it relevant? Chest 1993; 103:329–330.
19. Wei JH, Hoffman EA, Ritman EL, Wood EH. Cardiogenic motion of right lung parenchyma in anesthetized intact dogs. J Appl Physiol 1985; 58:384–391.
20. Reinhardt JM, Hoffman EA. Quantitative pulmonary imaging: spatial and temporal considerations in HRCT. Acad Radiol (submitted).
21. Ritman EL, Robb RA, Harris LD. Imaging Physiological Functions: experience with the DSR. Philadelphia: Praeger, 1985.
22. Hoffman EA, Larsen RL. Regional pulmonary blood flow via X-ray CT and biodegradable radiopaque microspheres. Circulation 1990; 4:111–124.
23. Boyd DP, Lipton MJ. Cardiac computed tomography. Proc IEEE 1983; 71:298–307.
24. Kalender WA, Fichte H, Bautz W, Skalej M. Semiautomatic evaluation procedures for quantitative CT of the lung. J Comput Assist Tomogr 1991; 15:248–255.
25. Kalender WA, Reinmuller R, Fichte H, Behr J, Beinert T, Seissler W. Spirometrically gated CT measurement of lung density and structure. Radiology 1992; 185: 354.
26. Rienmuller R, Behr J, Kalender WA. Standardized quantitative high resolution CT in lung diseases. J Comput Assist Tomogr 1991; 15:742–749.
27. Tran BQ, Tajik JK, Chiplunkar RA, Hoffman EA. Lung volume control for quantitative X-ray CT. Ann Biomed Eng 1996; 24:S-66.
28. Tran BQ, Tajik JK, Chiplunkar RA, Hoffman EA. Dynamic lung volume tracker and controller. http://everest.radiology.uiowa.edu/nlm/volcon/volctrl.html 1996.
29. Axel L. Cerebral blood flow determination by rapid-sequence computed tomography: a theoretical analysis. Radiology 1980; 137:679–686.
30. Weiss RM, Otoadese EA, Noel MP, et al. Quantitation of absolute regional myocardial perfusion using cine computed tomography. J Am Coll Cardiol 1994; 23(5):1186–1193.
31. Wong T, Wu L, Chung N, Ritman EL. Myocardial blood flow estimated by synchronous, multislice, high speed tomography. IEEE Trans Med Imag 1989; 8:70–77.
32. Wolfkiel CJ, Ferguson JL, Chomka EV, Law WR, Labin IN, Tenzer ML, Booker M, Brundage BH. Measurement of myocardial blood flow by ultrafast computed tomography. Circulation 1987; 76:1262–1273.
33. Hoffman EA, Heffernan PB. A computer graphics-aided 3-D analysis of heart/lung interaction reconstructed via DSR scanning. Proc Comput Graph 1985; 81–92.
34. Tajik JK, Tran BQ, Hoffman EA. Assessing regional pulmonary microvascular transit times and flow using dynamic multi-slice CT. Am J Respir Crit Care Med 1996; 153:A816.
35. Presson RG, Graham JA, Hanger CC, Godbey PS, Gebb SA, Sidner RA, Glenny RW, Wagner WW. Distribution of pulmonary capillary red blood cell transit times. J Appl Physiol 1995; 79:382–388.

36. Gur D, Drayer BP, Borovetz HS, Griffith BP, Hardesty RL, Wolfson SK. Dynamic computed tomography of the lung: regional ventilation measurements. J Comp Assist Tomogr 1979; 3:749–753.
37. Gur D, Shabason L, Borovetz HS, Herbert DL, Reece GJ, Kennedy WH, Serago C. Regional pulmonary ventilation measurements by xenon enhanced dynamic computed tomography: an update. J Comp Assist Tomogr 1981; 5:678–683.
37a. Hartley PG, Galvin JR, Hunninghake GW, Merchant JW, Yagla SJ, Speakman SB, Schwartz DA. High-resolution CT-derived measures of lung density are valid indexes of interstitial lung disease. J Appl Physiol 1994; 76:271–277.
38. Winkler SS, Nielsen A, Mesina J. Respiratory depression in goats by stable xenon: implications for CT studies. J Comput Assist Tomogr 1987; 11:496–498.
39. Tajik JK, Tran BQ, Hoffman EA. Xenon enhanced CT imaging of local pulmonary ventilation. In: Proc SPIE Conf Medical Imaging. Newport Beach, CA, 1996: 40–54.
40. Wagner WWJ, Latham LP, Gillespie MN, Guenther JP, Capen RL. Direct measurement of pulmonary capillary transit times. Science 1982; 218:379–381.
41. Amirav I, Kramer SS, Grunstein MM. Hoffman EA. Assessment of methacholine-induced airway constriction by ultrafast high-resolution computed tomography. J Appl Physiol 1993; 75:2239–2250.
42. Brown RH, Herold JC, Hirshman CA, Zerhouni EA, Mitzner W. In vivo measurements of airway reactivity using high-resolution computed tomography. Am Rev Respir Dis 1991; 144:208–212.
43. Seneterre E, Paganin F, Bruel JM, Michel FB, Bousqet J. Measurement of the internal size of bronchi using high resolution computed tomography (HRCT). Eur Respir J 1994; 7:596–600.
44. Webb WR, Gamsu G, Cann CE, Proctor E. CT of a bronchial phantom: factors affecting appearance and size measurements. Invest Radiol 1984; 19:394–398.
45. Herold CJ, Brown RH, Mitzner W, Links JM, Hirshman CA, Zerhouni EA. Assessment of pulmonary airway reactivity with high-resolution CT. Radiology 1991; 181:369–374.
46. McNamara AE, Muller NL, Okazawa M, Arntorp J, Wiggs BR, Pare PD. Airway narrowing in excised canine lungs measured by high-resolution computed tomography. J Appl Physiol 1992; 73:307–316.
47. Baxter BS, Sorenson JA. Factors affecting the measurement of size and CT number in computed tomography. Invest Radiol 1981; 4:337–341.
48. D'Souza ND, Reinhardt JM, Hoffman EA. ASAP: interactive quantification of 2D airway geometry. SPIE Med Imag 1996; 2709:180–196.
49. Kramer SS, Hoffman EA, Amirav I. High resolution CT assessment of pediatric airways: structure and function. In: Proc SPIE Conf Medical Imaging, 1994.
50. Schwab RJ, Gefter WB, Kline LR, Pack AI, Hoffman EA. Dynamic imaging of the upper airway during respiration in normal subjects. J Appl Physiol 1993; 74: 1504–1514.
51. Block M, Liu YH, Harris D, Robb RA, Ritman EL. Quantitative analysis of a vascular tree model with the dynamic spatial reconstructor 1984; 8:390–400.
52. Reinhardt JM, D'Souza ND, Hoffman EA. Accurate measurement of intrathoracic airways. IEEE Trans Med Imag 1997; 16(6):820–827.

53. Assimakopoulos PA, Boyd DP, Jaschke W, Lipton MJ. Spatial resolution analysis of computed tomographic images. Invest Radiol 1986; 21:260–271.
54. Press WH, Flannery BP, Teukolsky SA, Vetterling WT. Numerical Recipes in C. Cambridge: Cambridge University Press, 1988.
55. Reinhardt JM, Raab SA, D'Souza ND, Hoffman EA. Intra-thoracic airway measurement: ex vivo validation. SPIE Med Imag 1997; 3033:69–80.
56. Brown RH, Herold C, Zerhouni EA, Mitzner W. Spontaneous airways constrict during breath holding studied by high-resolution computed tomography. Chest 1994; 106:920–924.
57. Brown RH, Herold CJ, Hirshman CA, Zerhouni EA, Mitzner W. Individual airway constrictor response heterogeneity to histamine assessed by high-resolution computed tomography. J Appl Physiol 1993; 74:2615–2620.
58. Brown RH, Mitzner W, Zerhouni E, Hirshman CA. Direct in vivo visualization of bronchodilation induced by inhalational anesthesia using high-resolution computed tomography. Anesthesiology 1993; 78:295–300.
59. Hoffman EA, Gnanaprakasam D, Gupta KB, Hoford JD, Kugelmass SD, Kulawiec RS. VIDA: an environment for multidimensional image display and analysis. SPIE Biomed Image Proc Three-Dimens Microsc 1992; 1660:694–711.
60. Wood S, Zerhouni A, Hoffman EA, Mitzner W. Measurement of three-dimensional lung tree structures using computed tomography. J Appl Physiol 1995; 79: 1687–1697.
61. Wood SA, Hoford JD, Zerhouni E, Mitzner W. A method for measurement of cross sectional area, segment length and branching angle of airway tree structures in situ. Comp Med Imag Graph 1995; 19:145–152.
62. Grenier P, Cordeau MP, Beigelman C. High-resolution computed tomography of the airways. J Thorac Imag 1993; 8:213–229.
63. Kiatoka H, Yumoto T. Three-dimensional CT of the bronchial tree. A trial using an inflated fixed lung specimen. Invest Radiol 1990; 25:813–817.
64. Ney DR, Kuhlman JE, Hruban RH, Ren H, Hutchins GM, Fishman EK. Three-dimensional CT volumetric reconstruction and display of the bronchial tree. Invest Radiol 1989; 25:736–742.
65. Wood S, Hoford J, Zerhouni E, Hoffman E, Mitzner W. Quantitative 3-D reconstruction of airway and pulmonary vascular trees using HRCT. Biomed Image Proc Biomed Visualiz 1993; 1905:316–323.
66. Chiplunkar RA, Reinhardt JM, Hoffman EA. Segmentation and quantification of the primary human airway tree from 3-D X-ray CT. Proc SPIE Conf Medical Imaging, Newport Beach, CA, 1997.
67. Park W, Hoffman EA, Sonka M. Fuzzy logic approach to extraction of intrathoracic airway trees. SPIE Med Imag 1996; 2710:210–219.
68. Park W, Hoffman EA, Sonka M. Fuzzy logic approach to extraction of intrathoracic airway trees from three-dimensional CT images. SPIE Med Imag 1996; 2710:210–219.
69. Park W, Sonka M, Hoffman EA. Segmentation of intrathoracic airway trees: a fuzzy logic approach. IEEE Trans Med Imag.
70. Sonka M, Park W, Hoffman EA. Automated detection of the intrathoracic airway

tree from volumetric X-ray CT images. Ann Biomed Eng 1995; 23(Suppl 1):S-19 (abstract).
71. Sonka M, Park W, Hoffman EA. Rule-based detection of intrathoracic airway trees. IEEE Trans Med Imag 1996; 15:314–326.
72. Sonka M, Park W, Hoffman EA. Validation of an enhanced knowledge-based method for segmentation and quantitative analysis of intrathoracic airway trees from three-dimensional CT images. SPIE Med Imag 1995; 2433:158–166.
73. Sonka M, Sundaramoorthy G, Hoffman EA. Knowledge-based segmentation of intrathoracic airways from multidimensional high resolution CT images. SPIE Med Imag 1994; 2168:73–85.
74. Park W. Automated determination of fuzzy rules and membership functions: application to analysis of pulmonary CT images. In: Electrical and Computer Engineering. Iowa City: University of Iowa, 1996:107.
75. Ma CM, Sonka M. A fully parallel 3D thinning algorithm and its applications. Computer Vision and Image Understanding 1996; 64(3):420–433.
76. Baskin K, Kusnick C, Shamsolkottabi S, Corson J, Stanford W, Thompson B, Hoffman EA. Volumetric Quantification of abdominal aortic aneurysm. SPIE Med Imag 1996; 2709:323–337.
77. Higgins M. Risk factors associated with chronic obstructive lung disease. Ann NY Acad Sci 1991; 624:7–17.
78. Story BH, Titze IR, Hoffman EA. Vocal tract area functions from magnetic resonance imaging. J Acoust Soc Am 1996; 100:537–554.
79. Weibel ER. Design of biological organisms and fractal geometry. In: Nonnenmacher TF, Losa GA, Weibel ER, eds. Fractals in Biology and Medicine. Basel, Switzerland: Birkhauser Verlag, 1994.
80. Liu YH, Hoffman EA, Hagler DJ, Seward JB, Julsrud PR, Mair DD, Ritman EL. Accuracy of pulmonary vascular dimensions estimated with the dynamic spatial reconstructor. Am J Physiol Imag 1986; 1:201–207.
81. Liu YH, Hoffman EA, Ritman EL. Measurement of three-dimensional anatomy and function of pulmonary arteries with high-speed X-ray computed tomography. Invest Radiol 1987; 22:28–36.
82. Gefter WB, Hatabu H, Hoffman EA, Ailion DC, Cutillo AG. Magnetic resonance in experimental and clinical respiratory medicine: state of the art and potential. In: Cutillo MAG, ed. Application of Magnetic Resonance to the Study of Lung. New York: Futura Publishing Company, 1996:503–537.
83. Hoffman EA, Gefter WB, Venegas J. Frontier pulmonary imaging. In: Fishman AP, ed. Update: Pulmonary Diseases and Disorders. New York: McGraw-Hill, 1992.
84. Schwab RJ, Gefter WB, Hoffman EA, Gupta KB, Pack AI. Dynamic upper airway imaging during awake respiration in normal subjects and patients with sleep disordered breathing. Am Rev Respir Dis 1993; 148:1385–400.
85. Schwab RJ, Gefter WB, Pack AI, Hoffman EA. Dynamic imaging of the upper airway during respiration in normal subjects. J Appl Physiol 1993; 74:1504–1514.
86. Schwab RJ, Gupta KB, Gefter WB, Metzger LJ, Hoffman EA, Pack AI. Upper airway and soft tissue anatomy in normal subjects and patients with sleep-disor-

dered breathing. Significance of the lateral pharyngeal walls. Am J Respir Crit Care Med 1995; 152:1673–1689.

87. Hoffman EA, Chiplunkar R, Casale TB. CT scanning confirms Beta receptor distribution is greater for smaller vs. larger airways. Respir Crit Care Med 1997; 155:A855.
88. Biernacki W, Gould GA, Whyte KF, Flenley DC. Pulmonary hemodynamics, gas exchange, and the severity of emphysema as assessed by quantitative CT scan in chronic bronchitis and emphysema. Am Rev Respir Dis 1989; 139:1509–1515.
89. Gould GA, Macnee W, McLean A, Warren PM, Redpath A, Best JJK, Lamb D, Flenley DC. CT Measurements of lung density in life can quantitate distal airspace enlargement-an essential defining feature of human emphysema. Am Rev Respir Dis 1988; 137:380–392.
90. Gould GA, Redpath AT, Ryan M, Warren PM, Best JJ, Cameron EJ, Macnee W. Parenchymal emphysema measured by CT lung density correlates with lung function in patients with bullous disease. Eur Respir J 1993; 6:698–704.
91. Gould KL. Coronary Artery Stenosis. New York: Elsevier, 1991.
92. Kinsella M, Muller NL, Abboud RT, Morrison NJ, DyBuncio A. Quantitation of Emphysema by computed tomography using a "density mask" program and correlation with pulmonary function tests. Chest 1990; 97:315–321.
93. Knudson RJ, Standen JR, Kaltenborn WT, Knudson DE, Rehm K, Habib MP, Newell JD. Expiratory computed tomography for assessment of suspected pulmonary emphysema. Chest 1991; 99:1357–1366.
94. Millar AB, Fromson B, Strickland BA, Denison DM. Computed tomography based estimates of regional gas and tissue volume of the lung in supine subjects with chronic airflow limitation or fibrosing alveolitis. Thorax 1986; 41:932–939.
95. Newman KB, Lynch DA, Newman LS, Ellegood D, Newell JD. Quantitative computed tomography detects air trapping due to asthma. Chest 1994; 106:105–109.
96. Rienmuller RK, Behr J, Kalendar WA, Schatzl M, Altmann I, Merin M, Beinert T. Standardized quantitative high resolution CT in lung diseases. J Comput Assist Tomogr 1991; 15:742–749.
97. Stern EJ, Webb WR, Gamsu G. Dynamic quantitative computed tomography: a predictor of pulmonary function in obstructive lung diseases. Invest Radiol 1994; 29:564–569.
98. Wananuki Y, Suzuki S, Nishikawa M, Miyashita A, Okubo T. Correlation of quantitative CT with selective alveolobronchogram and pulmonary function tests in emphysema. Chest 1994; 106:806–813.
99. Bergin C, Muller N, Nichols DM, Lillington G, Hogg JC, Mullen B, Grymaloski MR, Osbourne S, Pare PD. The diagnosis of emphysema. A computed tomography-pathologic correlation. Am Rev Respir Dis 1986; 133:541–546.
100. Goddard PR, Nicholson EM, Laszlo G, Watt I. Computed tomography in pulmonary emphysema. Clin Radiol 1982; 33:379–387.
101. Hayhurst MD, MacNeil W, Flenley DC, Wright D, McLean A, Lamb D, Wightman AJA, Best J. Diagnosis of pulmonary emphysema by computerized tomography. Lancet 1984; 320–322.
102. Hruban RH, Meziane MA, Zerhouni EA, Khouri NF, Fishman EK, Wheeler PS,

Dumler JS, Hutchins GM. High resolution computed tomography of inflation fixed lungs: pathologic-radiologic correlation of centrilobular emphysema. Am Rev Respir Dis 1987; 136:935–940.
103. Miller RR, Muller NL, Vedal S, Morrison NJ, Staples CA. Limitations of computed tomography in the assessment of emphysema. Am Rev Respir Dis 1989; 139:980–983.
104. Murata K, Itoh H, Senda M, Yonekura Y, Nishimura K, Izumi T, Oshima S, Torizuka K. Stratified impairment of pulmonary ventilation in diffuse panbronchiolitis. PET and CT studies. J Comput Assist Tomogr 1989; 13:48–53.
105. Sanders C. Imaging of emphysema. Semin Respir Med 1992; 13:318–330.
106. Webb WR. High-resolution computed tomography of the lung: normal and abnormal anatomy. Semin Roentgenol 1991; 26:110–117.
107. Fromson BH, Denison DM. Quantitative features in the CT of healthy lungs. Thorax 1988; 43:120–126.
108. Kuwano K, Matsuba K, Ikeda T, Murakami J, Araki A, Nishitani H, Ishida T, Yasumoto K, Shigematsu N. The diagnosis of mild emphysema. Correlation of computed tomography and pathology scores. Am Rev Respir Dis 1990; 141:169–178.
109. Sonka M, Hlavac V, Boyle R. Image Processing, Analysis and Machine Vision. London: Chapman & Hall, 1993.
110. Adams H, Bernard M, McConnochie K. An appraisal of CT pulmonary density mapping in normal subjects. Clin Radiol 1991; 43:238–242.
111. Chandrasekaran K, Aylward PE, Fleagle SR, Burns TL, Seward JB, Tajik AJ, Collins SM, Skorton DJ. Feasibility of identifying amyloid and hypertrophic cardiomyopathy with the use of computerized quantitative texture analysis of clinical echocardiographic data. J Am Coll Cardiol 1989; 13:832–840.
112. Fleagle S, Stanford W, Burns T, Skorton D. Feasibility of quantitative texture analysis of cardiac magnetic resonance imagery: preliminary results. SPIE Med Imag 1994; 2168:23–32.
113. Katsuragawa S, Kunio D, MacMahon H. Image feature analysis and computer-aided diagnosis in digital radiography: classification of normal and abnormal lungs with interstitial disease in chest images. Med Phys 1989; 16:38–44.
114. McPherson D, Aylward P, Knosp B, Bean J, Kerber R, Collins S, Skorton D. Ultrasound characterization of acute myocardial ischemia by quantitative texture analysis. Ultrason Imag 1986; 8:227–240.
115. Miller P, Astley S. Classification of breast tissue by texture analysis. Image Vision Comput 1992; 10:277–282.
116. Schad LR, Bluml S, Zuna I. MR tissue characterization of intracranial tumors by means of texture analysis. Magnet Reson Imag 1993; 11:889–896.
117. Skorton DJ, Collins SM, Nichols J, Pandian NG, Bean JA, Kerber RE. Quantitative texture analysis in two-dimensional echocardiography: application to the diagnosis of experimental myocardial contusion. Circulation 1983; 68:217–223.
118. Tully RJ, Conners RW, Harlow CA, Lodwick GS. Towards computer analysis of pulmonary infiltration. Invest Radiol 1978; 13:298–305.
119. Uppaluri R, Mitsa T, Galvin JR. Fractal analysis of high-resolution CT images as a tool for quantification of lung diseases. SPIE Med Imag 1995; 2433:133–142.

120. Wu C, Chen Y. Multi-threshold dimension vector for texture analysis and its application to liver tissue classification. Pattern Recogn 1993; 1:137–144.
121. Mandelbrot BB. The Fractal Geometry of Nature. New York: Freeman, 1983.
122. Chen D, Bovik AC. Fast image coding using simple image patterns. In: Visual Communications and Image Processing IV, Philadelphia, Pa. Bellingham, WA: SPIE, 1989:1461–1471.
123. Lundahl T, Ohley WJ, Kuklinski WS, Williams DO, Gewirtz H, Most AS. Analysis and interpolation of angiographic images by use of fractals. In: Computers in Cardiology, Linkoping, Sweden. Los Alamitos, CA: IEEE, 1985:335–358.
124. Caldwell CB, Stapleton SJ, Holdsworth DW, Jong RA, Weiser WJ, Cooke G, Yaffe MJ. Characterisation of mammographic parenchymal pattern by fractal dimension. Phys Med Biol 1990; 35:235–247.
125. Tucker DM, Correa J, Souto M, Malagari KS. A study of fractal dimension in chest images using normal and interstitial lung disease cases. SPIE Med Imag Image Proc 1993; 1898:531–539.
126. Grant PE, Lumsden CJ. Fractal analysis of renal cortical perfusion. Invest Radiol 1994; 29:16–23.
127. Cargill EB, Donohoe K, Kolodny G, Parker JA, Zimmerman RE. Analysis of lung scans using fractals. In: Proc SPIE Medical Imaging III. Bellingham, WA: SPIE, 1989:2–9.
128. Uppaluri R, Hartley PG, Hoffman EA, Sonka M, McLennan G. Validation of AMFM: a quantative regional assessment of pulmonary parenchymal pathology from HRCT. Radiology 1998 (in press).
129. Uppaluri R, Hoffman EA, Sonka M, Hunninghake GW, McLennan G. Interstitial lung disease: a quantative study using the adoptive multiple feature method. Am J Respir Crit Care Med (submitted).
130. Uppaluri R, Mitsa T, Sonka M, Hoffman EA, McLennan G. Quantification of pulmonary emphysema from lung CT images. Am J Respir Crit Care Med 1997; 156:248–254.
131. Hoffman EA, Behrenbeck T, Chevalier PA, Wood EH. Estimation of regional pleural surface expansile forces in intact dogs. J Appl Physiol 1983; 55:935–948.
132. Hoffman EA, Ritman EL. Effect of body orientation on regional lung expansion in dog and sloth. J Appl Physiol 1985; 59:481–491.
133. Iwasaki T, Sinak LJ, Hoffman EA, Robb RA, Harris LD, Bahn RC, Ritman EL. Mass of left ventricular myocardium estimated with dynamic spatial reconstructor. Am J Physiol 1984; 246:H138–142.
134. Sinak LJ, Hoffman EA, Ritman EL. Subtraction gated computed tomography with the dynamic spatial reconstructor: simultaneous evaluation of left and right heart from single right-sided bolus contrast medium injection. J Comput Assist Tomogr 1984; 8:1–9.
135. Hoffman EA, Ritman EL. Invariant total heart volume in the intact thorax. Am Physiol 1985; 249:H883–890.
136. Liu S, Margulies SS, Wilson TA. Deformation of the dog lung in the chest wall. J Appl Physiol 1990; 68:1979–1987.
137. Olson LE, Hoffman EA. Heart-lung interactions determined by electron beam X-ray CT in laterally recumbent rabbits. J Appl Physiol 1995; 78:417–427.

138. Olson LE, Hoffman EA. Lung volumes and distribution of regional air content determined by cine X-ray CT of pneumonectomized rabbits. J Appl Physiol 1994; 76:1774–1785.
139. Hoffman EA, Acharya RS, Wollins JA. Computer-aided analysis of regional lung air content using three-dimensional computed tomographic images and multinomial models. Int J Math Model 1986; 7:1099–1116.
140. Hoffman EA, Ritman EL. Shape and dimensions of cardiac chambers via computed tomography: role of imaged slice thickness and orientation. Radiology 1985; 155:739–744.
141. Olson LE, Rodarte JR. Regional differences in expansion in excised dog lung lobes. J Appl Physiol 1984; 57:1710–1714.
142. Wislocki GB. Observations on the gross and microscopic anatomy of the sloths (*Bradypus griseus griseus* Gray and *Choloepus hoffmanni* Peters). J Morphol Physiol 1928; 46:317–396.
143. Olson LE, Lai-Fook SJ. Pleural liquid pressure measured with rib capsules in anesthetized ponies. J Appl Physiol 1988; 64:102–107.
144. Hoffman EA, Ritman EL, Mason DE, Olson LE. Lung/chest wall shapes in miniature horses by X-ray CT. Physiologist 1988; 31:A222.
145. Beck KC, Rehder K. Differences in regional vascular conductance in isolated dog lungs. J Appl Physiol 1986; 61:530–538.
146. Glenny RW, Robertson HT. Fractal properties of pulmonary blood flow: characterization of spatial heterogeneity. J Appl Physiol 1990; 69:532–545.
147. Baile EM, Pare PD, Brooks LA, Hogg JC. Relationship between regional lung volume and regional pulmonary vascular resistance. J Appl Physiol 1982; 52:14–920.
148. Glazier JB, Hughes JMB, Maloney JE, West JB. Vertical gradient of alveolar size in lungs of dogs frozen intact. J Appl Physiol 1967; 23:694–705.
149. Hogg JC, Holst P, Corry P, Ruff F, Honsley E, Morris E. Effect on regional lung expansion and body position on pulmonary perfusion in dogs. J Appl Physiol 1971; 31:97–101.
150. Hogg JP, Nepszy S. Regional lung volume and pleural pressure gradient estimated from lung density in dogs. J Appl Physiol 1969; 27:198–203.
151. Anthonsien NR, Milic-Emili J. Distribution of pulmonary perfusion in erect man. J Appl Physiol 1966; 21:760–766.
152. Kaneko K, Milic-Emili J, Dolovich MB, Dawson A, Bates DV. Regional distribution of ventilation and perfusion as a function of body position. J Appl Physiol 1966; 21:767–777.
153. West JB, Dollery CT. Distribution of blood flow and the pressure-flow relations of the whole lung. J Appl Physiol 1965; 20:175–183.
154. West JB, Dollery CT, Noimark A. Distribution of blood flow in isolated lung: relation to vascular and alveolar pressures. J Appl Physiol 1964; 19:713–724.
155. Chevalier PA, Reed JHJ, Vanderberg RA, Wood EH. Effect of gravitational and intertial forces on vertical distribution of pulmonary blood flow. Aviat Space Environ Med 1978; 49:769–778.
156. Greenleaf JF, Ritman EL, Chevalier PA, Sass DJ, Wood EH. Spatial distribution of pulmonary blood flow in dogs in increased force environments. J Appl Physiol 1978; 44:384–396.

157. Greenleaf JF, Ritman EL, Sass DJ, Wood EH. Spatial distribution of pulmonary blood flow in dogs in left decubitus position. Am J Physiol 1974; 227:230–244.
158. Hedenstierna G, White FC, Mazzone R, Wagner PD. Redistribution of pulmonary blood flow in the dog with PEEP ventilation. J Appl Physiol 1979; 46:278–287.
159. Hedenstierna G, White FC, Wagner PD. Spatial distribution of pulmonary blood flow in the dog with PEEP ventilation. J Appl Physiol 1979; 47:938–946.
160. Reed JR Jr., Wood EH. Effect of body position on vertical distribution of pulmonary blood flow. J Appl Physiol 1970; 28:303–311.
161. Hoppin FG Jr., York E, Kuhl DE, Hude RW. Distribution of pulmonary blood flow as affected by transverse (+Gx) acceleration. J Appl Physiol 1967; 22:469–474.
162. Poe N. Postural influence on lobar distribution of blood flow in dogs. Proc Soc Exp Biol Med 1972; 140:118–121.
163. Maeda H, Itoh H, Ishii Y, Todo G, Mukai T, Fujita M, Kambara H, Kawai C, Toprizuka K. Pulmonary blood flow distribution measured by radionuclide-computed tomography. J Appl Physiol 1983; 54:225–233.
164. Guntheroth WG, Morgan BC, Lintermans JP. Postural effects on lobar pulmonary and systemic flow: a flowmeter study in dogs. J Appl Physiol 1967; 23:859–864.
165. Hoffman EA, Sinak LJ, Robb RA, Ritman EL. Noninvasive quantitative imaging of shape and volume of lungs. J Appl Physiol Respir Environ Exerc Physiol 1983; 54:1414–1421.
166. Hogg JP, Nepszy S. Regional lung volume and pleural pressure gradient estimated from lung density in dogs. J Appl Physiol 1969; 27:198–203.
167. Hughes JMB, Glazier JB, Maloney JE, West JB. Effect of lung volume on the distribution of pulmonary blood flow in man. Respir Physiol 1968; 4:58–72.
168. Milic-Emili J, Henderson JAM, Dolovich MB, Trop D, Kaneko K. Regional distribution of inspired gas in the lung. J Appl Physiol 1966; 21(3):749–759.
169. Hummayr R, Walters B, Chevalier PA, Rodarte JR, Olson LE. Topographical distribution of regional lung volume in anesthetized dogs. J Appl Physiol 1983; 54:1048–1056.
170. Olson LE, Wright VP, Hoffman EA. Feasibility of using high-speed electron beam X-ray CT to follow the time course of the pulmonary response to pneumonectomy in rabbits. SPIE Med Imag 1994; 2168:341–352.
171. Doerschuk CM, Sekhon HS. Pulmonary blood volume and edema in postpneumonectomy lung in rats. J Appl Physiol 1990; 69:1178–1182.

12

Measurement of Regional Ventilation by Aerosol Deposition

H. THOMAS ROBERTSON

University of Washington School of Medicine
Seattle, Washington

I. Introduction

Gas concentration measurements taken at the mouth during a single exhalation, during the course of an inert gas washout, or following administration of discrete inhaled gas boluses all have advanced our understanding of the fine-scale distribution of ventilation in the lung (1). None of the methods to analyze exhaled gas concentration profiles provide spatial information, but large-scale spatial distribution of ventilation can be determined from measurements of inhaled radionuclide tracer gases (2). A third technique utilizing measurement of intravenously infused inert gas concentrations in arterial blood, mixed venous blood, and exhaled gas, the multiple inert gas elimination technique (MIGET) (3), yields fine-scale ventilation and perfusion distributions that accurately predict respiratory gas exchange, although no spatial information is available. Given the success of these approaches, the need to further investigate the distribution of ventilation or of ventilation and perfusion in the lung could be questioned. However, the importance of some mechanisms that contribute to the matching of ventilation to perfusion remains unclear, primarily because simultaneous high-resolution spatial measurements of both ventilation and perfusion are required. Both exhaled inert gas profiles and/or MIGET can reflect interventions that alter pulmonary gas exchange, but cannot identify where the changes occur. Simultaneous spatial measurements of ventilation and perfusion represent the next step in investigation of mechanisms. Finally, modeling assumptions are incorporated into all nonspatial approaches to defining ventilation or $\dot{V}_A/\dot{Q}$ distributions. Although these models can be used to predict respiratory gas exchange, they may not accurately represent the actual distribution of ventilation and perfusion, because of assumptions made concerning the distribution of reinspired dead space gas in overall gas exchange. While it is possible that anatomically derived $\dot{V}_A/\dot{Q}$ distributions may differ from inert gas-modeled distributions, the importance of these effects are not yet defined. Again, high-resolution measurements of regional ventilation will be required to address this issue.

Interest in high-resolution measurements of regional ventilation stems from the recent appreciation of the extent of pulmonary perfusion heterogeneity (see Chapter 15). High-resolution perfusion studies reveal blood flow heterogeneity in the lung to be scale-dependent; that is, measured heterogeneity of blood flow increases with each successive improvement in resolution. The previously unanticipated extent of pulmonary blood flow heterogeneity suggests the existence of a similar scale-dependent heterogeneity of ventilation in the normal lung, as a precise match between pulmonary ventilation and blood flow is required for normal pulmonary gas exchange. This hypothesis proposes a precise match between regional ventilation and regional perfusion that mandates close integration between pulmonary parenchymal properties that determine regional ventilation and those that determine regional blood flow, and/or close coordination between local bronchiolar and arteriolar smooth muscle tone to regulate the respective flows. A second hypothesis to explain the gas exchange properties observed in normal lungs, given the high degree of spatial perfusion heterogeneity, proposes complete gas phase equilibration within gas exchange units larger than acini. The presence of larger-scale regional alveolar gas homogenization would negate effects of uneven perfusion by homogenizing end-capillary partial pressures. Gas-phase diffusion assures ventilation homogenization within alveoli, but this second hypothesis postulates sufficient convective gas mixture among acinar units to produce homogenization of gas composition at a larger scale. High-resolution measurements of ventilation and perfusion demonstrating an equal extent of heterogeneity for both measurements would support the first hypothesis, whereas the finding of a lesser degree of heterogeneity for ventilation would support the second.

High-resolution measurements of regional ventilation are technically challenging; while perfusion has been measured at an alveolar scale (see Chapter 14), current techniques for measurement of regional ventilation cannot approach that level of resolution. In this chapter limitations of resolution by established methods for measurement of regional ventilation will be discussed, with focus on the advantages and limitations of alveolar aerosol deposition to provide high-resolution estimates of regional ventilation. Results obtained from these estimates will be presented to describe the extent and spatial distribution of ventilation heterogeneity, as well as findings from simultaneously obtained spatial maps of perfusion to relate these data to overall gas exchange properties of the lung.

II. Problems with Estimation of Regional Alveolar Ventilation

When discussing the quantitation of regional alveolar ventilation, we must first acknowledge the ambiguities involved with its estimation. Regional alveolar ventilation is defined simply as the rate of delivery of fresh gas to the region of interest, but all methods developed to date to measure this quantity pose problems of interpretation. Alveolar ventilation for the entire lung has been calculated traditionally from measurements of mean arterial and mixed expired partial pressures of carbon dioxide (the Enghoff modification of the Bohr dead space). This physiological dead space includes ventilation of both conducting airways (anatomical dead space) and high $\dot{V}_A/\dot{Q}$ regions (alveolar dead space) (4). Thus, an estimate of whole-lung alveolar ventilation based on carbon dioxide exchange will be reduced by including the high $\dot{V}_A/\dot{Q}$ units with ventilation of anatomical dead space. The multiple inert gas elimination technique has been used to separate the components of anatomical and alveolar dead spaces for the entire lung, as exchange of very soluble infused inert gases reflects only "pure" inert gas dead space, without influence from high $\dot{V}_A/\dot{Q}$ regions (3). This interpretation has been clouded by recent observations that conducting airways can participate in exchange of the very soluble inert gases (5) (see also Chapter 8). This effect of inert gas exchange in the conducting airways is particularly striking when high-frequency ventilation is applied to a normal lung (6,7). Thus while gas exchange approaches can provide useful hypothetical models to describe the distribution of alveolar ventilation in the entire lung, they may either underestimate (for carbon dioxide) or overestimate (for multiple inert gases) the actual delivery of fresh gas to alveolar surfaces. Beyond limitations of gas exchange methods to define alveolar ventilation, however, these approaches cannot describe the actual spatial distribution of ventilation. Investigation of mechanisms responsible for the heterogeneity of alveolar ventilation requires different techniques.

All measurements of regional alveolar ventilation will be compromised to some extent by the tidal nature of mammalian ventilation. In gas-exchanging spaces of the lung, reinspired dead space gas precedes each arrival of fresh gas, so the volume change of an alveolar unit on inspiration overrepresents its alveolar ventilation. If each gas exchange unit reinspires its own exhaled gas, overall gas exchange is unaffected beyond the proportional reduction in alveolar ventilation (8). However, Ross and Farhi (9) postulated that if exhaled gas is completely mixed in a common dead space, that process would reduce the extent of $\dot{V}_A/\dot{Q}$ heterogeneity measured by gas exchange methods. This prediction was borne out in an experimental study by Petrini et al. (10), where the addition of common dead space reduced measured $\dot{V}_A/\dot{Q}$ heterogeneity. In adjacent regions of lung with identical perfusion but different regional ventilation, sharing a common dead space will make the alveolar gas composition of the two regions more similar. Thus, lower estimates of ventilation heterogeneity will be obtained from gas exchange measurements compared to an estimate of ventilation heterogeneity based on high-resolution measurements of regional ventilation. This difference between estimates of ventilation heterogeneity based on gas exchange or high-resolution regional measurements will be greater in lungs with high $\dot{V}_A/\dot{Q}$ heterogeneity.

An additional complication to the precise characterization of alveolar ventilation from any measurement of respiratory unit volume change was suggested from microscopic reconstructions of rat lung (11). The three-dimensional reconstructions revealed no predictable relationship between ventilatory unit size and the length of conducting airway serving that unit. Assuming ventilatory unit size would bear some relationship to its alveolar ventilation, these findings suggest that substantial heterogeneity of reinspired dead space may occur among units receiving the same fractional increase in gas volume with each breath. This presumed heterogeneity of fractional respiratory unit dead space at a microscopic level provides another interpretation of Engel's observation that over 50% of the total ventilation heterogeneity in the dog lung resided in units distal to 3-mm airways (12). The observed slope of exhaled nitrogen concentration measured at a small airway following a single breath of oxygen would be made steeper by the existence of a range of anatomical dead spaces among the contributing units to that airway. In addition, this fine-scale heterogeneity of anatomical dead space poses two problems with interpretation of any measurement of regional volume change to estimate regional alveolar ventilation. If parenchymal volume changes are used to estimate regional ventilation, neither the contributions of gas reinspired from a common dead space nor the heterogeneity of fractional dead space for different ventilatory units can be estimated.

Inhaled aerosol particles less than 2 μm in diameter deposit primarily in the alveolar spaces during resting tidal breathing (13) and appear to deposit in proportion to the volume of fresh gas entering the alveolar spaces. Zeltner et al. administered an aerosol of 0.9-μm fluorescent-labeled particles to awake hamsters and observed that nearly 95% of the aerosol particles deposited in the lungs were found in alveolar spaces (14). The overall fractional deposition of a 1-μm aerosol is approximately 30% (15); thus an estimate of alveolar ventilation will still be influenced by the reinspiration of aerosol from a common dead space. However, for aerosol sizes smaller than 1 μm, the fractional deposition increases (13). For a smaller inhaled aerosol label, such as the 0.01-μm particles of Tc-99m-labeled Technegas (16), the influence of reinspired dead space could presumably be minimized, as deposition of an inhaled bolus may exceed 80% (17,18). Thus, of all methods currently used for high-resolution measurement of regional ventilation, only aerosol deposition has the potential to minimize the influence of reinspired dead space gas on measurements of regional alveolar ventilation. The importance of reinspired dead space gas in high-resolution ventilation measurements remains problematic. High-resolution measurements of regional ventilation utilizing a range of aerosol sizes offer the best possible solution to this issue.

III. Radionuclide Images of the Intact Lung

Three different approaches with radionuclides have been used to measure regional ventilation. The first efforts described regional differences in concentrations of inhaled Xe-133 (19), soon followed by studies of regional washin and washout of the same isotope (20). Higher-resolution N-13 washout images of regional ventilation have been attained utilizing positron emission tomography (PET) (21) (see Chapter 16 for details). Administration of the very short half-life nucleotide Kr-81m in inhaled gas produces highest regional activity in the best-ventilated regions of the lung, and this activity can be related to the delivery of fresh gas by a simple mathematical model (22,23). The most popular radionuclide technique for measuring regional ventilation, however, is the inhalation of radionuclide-labeled aerosols. Radionuclide labels on inhaled aerosol particles have a long history of clinical use for investigation of regional ventilatory abnormalities (24). Aerosols permit the use of easily generated nuclides as labels instead of radioactive gases, and once the label deposits in the lung, images can be acquired over relatively long periods of time, providing higher counts and better image quality.

The in vivo radionuclide gas imaging approaches cannot appropriately represent the alveolar ventilation of regions containing a large fraction of conducting airways. Calculations made from washout images of radionuclide-labeled gases acquired over the entire ventilatory cycle will identify conducting airways as high-ventilation regions. If images gated in end-exhalation are used for calculations, conducting airways will be identified as having the same regional ventilation as the alveoli that supply them with exhaled gas. Images of the very short-life radionuclide gases acquired over the entire ventilatory cycle will register conducing airways as regions of high alveolar ventilation. Only aerosol deposition images of approximately sized radionuclide-labeled particles will identify the conducting airways as regions with no alveolar ventilation.

While convenience is an obvious advantage in obtaining in vivo radionuclide images of intact lungs, there is inevitable cost in loss of resolution. This loss of resolution is not important for many applications, but gains significance when the aim is to characterize alveolar ventilation at a resolution comparable to recent studies of perfusion heterogeneity (25–27). For in vivo images acquired on a gamma camera, a number of factors combined to cause loss of resolution. The measure of resolution commonly used for an imaging system is the full-width half-maximum. This is the width at half-height of an image profile obtained from a radiation point source. It is influenced by the gamma-camera collimator characteristics and the distance from the collimator. Additional factors that influence the accuracy of the ventilation image include scattering within tissues, loss of signal from tissue attenuation (a particular problem for radionuclides emitting low-energy photons such as Xe-133), and respiratory motion artifacts. The resolution of washout images from measurements of any gas radionuclide are limited by the rapid decrease in regional activity within a few breaths of the initiation of the washout. While Kr-81m images can be acquired over a time sufficient to produce optimal counts, these measurements are compromised in abnormal lungs by a lack of sensitivity to regions of both very high and very low specific ventilation. PET constructs images from pairs of high-energy photons produced by the annihilation reaction of a positron and an electron. It offers significant improvement in overall image resolution, although the resolution in the gas-containing lung is limited by the longer distance (roughly 10 mm) that an emitted positron has to travel before it is likely to encounter an electron. Finally, the high-resolution fidelity of all SPECT and PET radionuclide images is influenced by the reconstruction algorithm. These computational routines are designed to provide optimal resolution of boundaries between different densities. Although this goal is essential for clinical applications, it does not serve the goal of determining with-organ heterogeneity as well. Hence radionuclide image measurements taken of any organ may underrepresent the true extent of blood flow or ventilation heterogeneity. In studies of blood flow heterogeneity of the lung, we noted that even a direct image of a slice of fixed lung placed on the face of a gamma camera with an FWHM of 3 mm yields a lower measured flow heterogeneity (28) than the same slice cut into 1.9-cm^3 pieces and counted in separate vials (26). These partial-volume effects of radionuclide image acquisition and reconstruction can only be avoided by the destructive procedure of cutting the lung into small pieces and measuring activity of the individual pieces.

IV. Differences Between Aerosol Deposition and Radioactive Gas Measurements in Abnormal Lungs

Inhaled radionuclide-labeled aerosols remain the most important clinical tool to assess regional ventilation (24). Aerosol deposition on the large conducting airways can significantly impair the evaluation of the regional distribution of ventilation in patients with severe airflow obstruction (29). This deposition appears to result from the presence of flow-limiting segments within the airways during normal tidal exhalation in severely impaired patients. At those airway choke points, the lumen is so narrow that an exhaled 1-μm aerosol deposits on airway walls by inertial impaction. This artifact can be minimized with the use of Technegas as the aerosol label, as the mean particle diameter is less than 0.01 μm. The smaller aerosol diameter yields a higher fractional deposition due to enhanced movement by diffusion, and the aerosol particles remaining in the exhalate are small enough to avoid impaction at the airway walls at the flow-limiting segments. A comparison of Technegas with Xe-133 ventilation scans in patients with airflow obstruction (30) showed no airway deposition of aerosol despite the severe airflow limitation of the subjects studied.

V. CT Measurements of Regional Ventilation

The issues of radionuclide image resolution described above can be sidestepped with the higher resolution attained by rapid CT images of the washout of a high-radiodensity gas such as xenon. The same problems noted above in the discussion of the effects of reinspired dead space gas on washout images of conducting airways are present, but at least the large conducting airways can be excluded from analysis, given the high resolution of the CT images. Measurements of ventilation heterogeneity utilizing this technology are discussed in Chapter 11.

VI. Measurements of Regional Ventilation with Parenchymal Markers

Although perceptions of the extent of ventilation heterogeneity in the normal lung have been shaped by in vivo radionuclide scans, there has been a steady progression of investigations by other techniques that suggest the presence of a far greater extent of ventilation heterogeneity. Engel et al. (31) showed differences in the slope of the N_2 exhalation concentration curve among airways of different sizes following a single breath of oxygen. Engel et al. estimated that over 50% of the total ventilation heterogeneity in the lung resided in units distal to 3-mm airways. Hubmayr et al. (32) utilized radiopaque parenchymal markers in dogs to demonstrate substantial heterogeneity in regional volume changes with tidal ventilation at the 3–5-cm^3 scale, and Rodarte et al. (33) used changes in CT lung density to infer even greater ventilation heterogeneity at the (3 mm^3) scale of measurement. Wilson et al. (34) performed N_2 washouts of isolated lungs with implanted markers to further confirm these findings and to integrate them with the original observations of Engel et al. These parenchymal marker studies confirm the existence of scale-dependent heterogeneity of regional ventilation and demonstrate an overall extent of ventilation heterogeneity similar to measurements of perfusion heterogeneity made in other studies. None of the parenchymal marker studies were accompanied by simultaneous studies of regional perfusion heterogeneity, however. Nevertheless, data acquired by different parenchymal marker techniques confirm the presence of scale-dependent heterogeneity of regional ventilation present at the highest degree of resolution attained, similar in magnitude to other measurements of the heterogeneity of perfusion (25,26).

VII. Advantages of Destructive Studies of Regional Ventilation

While the in vivo radionuclide imaging methods for administered aerosols cannot yield high-resolution data, both radionuclide aerosol labels (27,35,36) and fluorescent microsphere aerosol labels (15,37) have been used to describe regional ventilation in destructive studies where the labeled lung is cut, mapped, and measured for radioactivity or fluorescence in individual pieces. Provided that an adequate radionuclide or fluorescence signal can be acquired from the cut pieces, the resolution attained depends on the size of the sampled piece. Destructive measurements on lung with deposited aerosol marker also offer the advantage of minimizing the influence of anatomical dead space on the measured regional ventilation, as insignificant amounts of aerosol deposit on all conducting airways (14,15), and the largest conducting airways can be excluded from analysis. Given the assurance that properly sized and conditioned fluorescent aerosols will label alveolar spaces, whole lung maps of regional ventilation can be constructed by systematic sectioning of the lung and measurement of fluorescent activity in each piece. Destructive sectioning studies of aerosol-labeled lung have the advantage of providing an unequivocal resolution determined by the piece size, and the potential advantage of reducing the influence of reinspired dead space gas on the estimate of alveolar ventilation. Fluorescent labels on inhaled aerosol also eliminate airborne radioactive exposure and provide several different colors for use in the course of an experiment (38).

VIII. Determinants of Aerosol Deposition in the Lung

Aerosol particles with an aerodynamic diameter greater than 2 μm have a significant fractional deposition on ciliated mucosal surfaces, and therefore do not necessarily reflect the regional distribution of ventilation. Large aerosol particles deposit primarily by inertial impaction on the conducting walls of the respiratory system. The tendency for a large aerosol particle to cross the slipstream of gas flow and stick on airways walls is proportional to the particle density, the square of its diameter, the angle of directional change of the slipstream, and velocity of the airflow (13). On the ciliated surfaces of conducting airways, the distinction between deposition and retention becomes important for sustained periods of observation, as the particles deposited on conducting airways are swept toward the larynx, and their location minutes to hours later no longer reflects the site of deposition. While the retention of large particles is an important issue for understanding the pathophysiology of environmental aerosols, the experimental methods discussed here deposit small aerosol predominantly on alveolar surface, where clearance is very slow, and measurements are taken promptly after aerosol administration. Thus for these particular applications, the distinction between deposition and retention is not important and would only become significant if aerosol were administered days prior to sacrifice.

Gravitational settling is the most important determinant of alveolar aerosol deposition for aerosols in the 1.0 μm size range. The rate of settling is a function of the square of the particle diameter and the density of the particle. A 10-μm-diameter particle of unit density settles at 2.9 mm/sec in air, whereas a 1-μm unit density particle settles at 0.033 mm/sec (13). With gravitational settling as the primary determinant of alveolar deposition in this size range, the fractional alveolar deposition of an inhaled concentration of aerosol will therefore be determined predominantly by alveolar size and alveolar residence time.

For aerosol particles smaller than 1 μm in diameter, diffusion becomes a more important force than sedimentation for alveolar deposition. For distribution by diffusion, the movement is independent of particle density and dependent on particle diameter. For a 0.1-μm-diameter particle, the mean displacement after 1 sec will be 0.064 mm, and gravitational settling 0.0008 mm (13). Modeling studies have suggested that even for the smallest aerosols, the particles will not distribute symmetrically within acini, but will be concentrated on alveolar septi intersecting the flow stream (18,39) (see also Chapter 10). Tsuda and Butler have recently proposed an additional mechanism affecting alveolar deposition of aerosol particles (40–42). They noted that minor irregularities in alveolar wall expansion produced highly irregular stream flows of aerosol particles with tidal breathing. Successively inhaled and exhaled particle streams became folded on one another, causing higher alveolar deposition than was predicted by the simple mechanism of gravitationally induced settling. The distribution of deposition had a chaotic pattern, in contrast to the random distribution produced by diffusional mechanisms. This "stretching and folding" effect on inhaled small aerosols produces convective mixing by a mechanism that is limited to the acinar regions of the lung. Since gas diffusion at that level of scale is a far faster mixing mechanism, the deposition of aerosol at the acinar level is most likely not representative of the delivery of fresh gas. This stretching and folding model was illustrated by the movement of colored silicone within silicone-ventilated rat lungs. Additional experimental support for this acinar-level convective mixing process came from a preliminary description of aerosol deposition in weightlessness (43). These authors noted that the deposition of a polystyrene 1-μm aerosol in the lungs of human subjects during transient weightlessness was significantly higher than predicted by their model, which presumed that gravitational settling was the principal mechanism of deposition for 1-μm particles (18).

IX. Ventilatory Parameters as Determinants of Deposition

Both site and extent of deposition of aerosol particles will be influenced by the ventilatory parameters chosen. Higher inspiratory flow rates will cause a greater fraction of any inspired aerosol to deposit on the conducting airways by impaction. Valberg et al. (35) showed that a 0.4-μm aerosol administered at a ventilatory frequency of <25/min demonstrated minimal large airway (>4 mm) deposition, whereas at a very high ventilatory frequency (>65/min), the large airways received a disproportionate fraction of the deposited aerosol. The other determinant of the extent of deposition is the time available within a respiratory cycle for particulate settling. As an example of this effect, we observed that the addition of a 1-sec inspiratory hold to the ventilatory pattern would increase the deposition of 1.0-μm particles from 30% to 50% (15).

X. Limitations of Aerosols for Scale of Measurement

From the preceding discussion, it is clear that within alveoli, where diffusion is the dominant mechanism for gas mixing, aerosol deposition cannot appropriately represent the distribution of ventilation. In contrast, at a subsegmental level of scale, aerosol deposition is governed by convective gas movement and appropriately represents alveolar ventilation. At the respiratory bronchiole, diffusion overcomes convection as the predominant mechanism for transport of fresh gas, while the 1-μm aerosols deposit by gravitational settling, with very little movement due to diffusion. Thus within the 40-mm^3 volume of an acinus, aerosol distribution cannot provide useful information concerning the distribution of fresh gas within that structure. However, convective mechanisms completely determine gas transport from the mouth to the final 8 mm before the alveolar surfaces are reached, and so for lung volumes that are in excess of 1.0 cm^3, uniformly sized aerosol of 1.0 μm or smaller will faithfully mark convective movement of fresh gas into the volumes at that level of scale. What remains to be better delineated is how small a lung volume can be studied by aerosol deposition with confidence that the deposition of aerosol appropriately represents the delivery of fresh gas to that volume of pulmonary parenchyma.

As the goal for high-resolution measurement of regional ventilation is to provide a more sophisticated understanding of the spatial aspects of pulmonary gas exchange, it may well be that resolution of the heterogeneity of regional ventilation is not required below an acinar level. If diffusional equilibrium within an acinus were complete in a normal tidal cycle, the perfusion heterogeneity noted within and among alveoli, described in detail in Chapter 14, may not be of functional importance, as the end-capillary gas contents will be constant for that acinus despite a considerable extent of within-acinus blood flow heterogeneity. While acinar structure may be too long and complex to constitute a single diffusion unit (44), diffusional equilibrium probably is attained within larger subdivisions of the acinus. What remains to be determined by the destructive approaches to measurement of ventilation and perfusion heterogeneity is the level of resolution needed to explain $\dot{V}_A/\dot{Q}$ heterogeneity revealed by gas exchange methods.

XI. Measurement of Fluorescent Microsphere Aerosol Deposition

Despite the importance of in vivo measurements of regional ventilation acquired with radionuclide imaging methods described above, the issues of respiratory movement, partial volume effects, the smoothing of reconstruction algorithms, and system resolution limitations all block attainment of resolution better than a few cm^3. The destructive approach of taking direct samples of fixed, labeled lung [a technique originally applied to regional blood flow measurements (45)] provides the best current solution to attaining high resolution, as the size of cut lung samples unequivocally defines the spatial resolution of the measurements. Valberg et al. (35) used both this cut-sample technique and direct radionuclide images of transverse slices of air-dried lung to investigate changes in distribution of a Tc-99m-labeled aerosol at different respiratory frequencies. Based on that aerosol study and our experience with systematic cutting and mapping of vascular-labeled inflated, dried lungs (26), we felt that the destructive approach could readily be applied to spatial mapping of inhaled aerosol distribution. The availability of several different colors of fluorescent-labeled polystyrene bead 1.0-μm aerosols (FMS) provided the opportunity to take deposition measurements in different conditions prior to sacrifice. We had previously established the accuracy of blood flow measurements with FMS in comparison to intravascularly injected radionuclide labeled microspheres (38), and believed the method could readily be applied to measurement of FMS aerosol deposition. The only difficulty with application of this fluorescence extraction method to the measurement of fluorescent aerosol deposition was the smaller FMS aerosol volume and a dye load that results in a smaller fluorescent signal.

The specifications for an aerosol generation system to produce a monodisperse aerosol of FMS were described by Zeltner et al. (14). With a similar system (described below) we demonstrated that we could generate a monodisperse aerosol of 1.0 μm FMS, and administer adequate aerosol concentrations via a ventilator to anesthetized juvenile pigs (15). The relative strength of the signal obtained in tissue cubes from the aerosol-deposited 1.0 μm FMS was weaker than that attained with the 15-μm FMS used for blood flow measurements, but the overall signal was strengthened by a 10-min aerosol administration period, a modification of the ventilator system to minimize FMS loss prior to delivery to the animal, and loading additional fluorescence into the microspheres (FMS supplied as FluoSpheres, Molecular Probes, Inc., Eugene, OR). The apparatus used to produce the FMS aerosol, the validation of aerosol composition, the methods for extraction of deposited fluorescence from lung tissue, and the data reduction procedures are described in detail in Robertson et al. (15). In summary, the protocol for ventilation labeling was a 10-min administration of FMS aerosol via a bag-in-box ventilator system. Two different color FMS labels were mixed and administered during each labeling period to provide an estimate of method error. For each aerosol-labeling experiment, 15-μm radioactive microspheres were injected intravenously during the same 10-min period to provide simultaneous measurement of regional blood blow. The animal was sacrificed, the lungs flushed free of blood, and air-dried at 25 cm H_2O inflation pressure. The dried lung was encased in a quick-setting foam, cut into 1.9-cm^3 cubes by a rectilinear coordinate system, and the cubes were weighed and mapped by their three-dimensional coordinates. Each piece had radioactivity measured, and then was soaked in a solvent to extract all fluorescent signal. We used the previously described method for measurement of total fluorescence from intravascularly injected 15-μm microspheres embedded in lung pieces (38), extracting the fluorescence by soaking the dried lung piece in solvent for 48 hr, and measuring the concentration of fluorescence in the solvent. The dried lung tissue itself has blue fluorescence, limiting the use of labels that fluoresce near that portion of the spectrum. In addition, dried lung can crumble and form fragments that float in the solvent used to leach out the fluorescent activity from the labeled lung. These pieces of lung dust in solution will scatter light and produce a significant artifact when the overall fluorescent signal is low. Again, this is predominantly a problem in the blue and blue-green regions of the spectrum. The findings described below estimated the distribution of regional ventilation in anesthetized juvenile pigs by the administration of a dry 1.0-μm aerosol of fluorescent-labeled polystyrene beads (FMS).

XII. Quantitation of Ventilation Heterogeneity

Using the system described above, the simultaneous administration of two different FMS labels to anesthetized pigs demonstrates a consistent high correlation between the two color signals, with between-color *r* values ranging between 0.98 and 0.99. The studies demonstrated that in normal animals, the extent of ventilation heterogeneity measured at the 1.9-cm^3 piece size was comparable to the extent of perfusion heterogeneity at the scale of the measurements taken. Figure 1 shows the coefficient of variation of ventilation (cross-hatched bars) and of perfusion (stippled bars) for five pigs. Similar preliminary measurements of dogs (46) have also demonstrated a comparable extent of ventilation and perfusion heterogeneity. It therefore appears that at least at the 1.9-cm^3 level of resolution, the extent of ventilation and perfusion heterogeneity in dogs and pigs is comparable. Measurements of ventilation and perfusion heterogeneity have been reported in awake goats (27) and awake sheep (37), which again demonstrated comparable degrees of ventilation and perfusion heterogeneity when measured at rest.

XIII. Temporal Heterogeneity of Ventilation

From our initial study of regional ventilation in pigs (15), measurements taken at two different times showed a good degree of correlation, with an average *r*

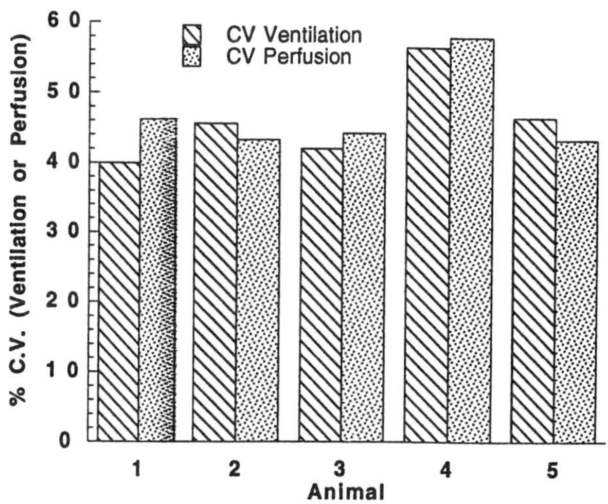

Figure 1 Comparison of the % coefficient of variation (CV) of simultaneously measured ventilation and perfusion in five juvenile pigs.

value of 0.85. For the highest correlation in that study, there was no appreciable difference between simultaneously administered microspheres and microspheres administered 30 min apart, suggesting that the variability over time can be of the same magnitude as the method error of the technique. Using only the two initial control measurements from a more current study (47), we have applied the statistical analysis from a study of temporal variation of perfusion (48) to the ventilation data. Because of the structure of this recent data set, we could divide the total variance observed among all measurements in all animals into components of structure, temporal variation, and measurement error. The factor structure, which represents the influence of anatomy on ventilation distribution, accounted for 92.9 ± 4.3% of the observed variability. Method error had a mean of 1.6% with a range of 0.6–3.3%. Temporal changes in ventilation averaged 5.6%, with a range of 0.7–9.7% among animals. The component of temporal ventilation heterogeneity is small both in normal pigs and in pigs subjected to massive pulmonary embolism (49). Presumably airway disease models will show more dramatic alterations of distribution over time.

XIV. Regional Gradients of Ventilation

In both prone pigs (15) and prone dogs (46), no significant gravitational gradients of ventilation were detected. These findings are consistent with previous studies of regional ventilation in dogs in the prone position utilizing SPECT measurements of inhaled Kr-81 activity (50) or implanted lung markers (51). Because small radial gradients of perfusion had been noted in prone dogs in a previous study, with lower flows in the most distal portions of the lobes (26), radial gradients of ventilation were sought, again using the center of each lobe as a reference point. A small radial gradient of ventilation was present, with less ventilation delivered to the most distal portion of the lobes, but this gradient accounted for less than 4% of the total variability.

A recent preliminary report by Melsom et al. of ventilation and perfusion distribution in awake sheep in rest and exercise showed a substantial redistribution of ventilation, measured by a FMS aerosol, with exercise (37). To date, this is the first report of a stimulus that substantially redistributes a FMS aerosol. Additional investigation remains to determine whether these changes result from increased deposition of aerosol on the conducting airways due to higher respiratory flow rates [as noted in the isolated lung studies of Valberg, et al. (35)], or whether they represent true changes in the distribution of ventilation during exercise.

XV. Species Differences

Comparison of the extent of ventilation heterogeneity observed in lungs of pigs compared to lungs of dogs by the aerosol deposition technique (15,46) did not show the expected differences in the extent of ventilation heterogeneity. That is, our initial hypothesis predicting a relatively lower ventilation heterogeneity in dog lungs due to increase collateral ventilation was not confirmed. An overall extent of $\dot{V}_A/\dot{Q}$ heterogeneity consistent with normal gas exchange was demonstrated in both species. Thus while the presence of extensive collateral ventilation in normal dog lungs will act to homogenize alveolar composition at an acinar scale, this effect does not appear to influence convective gas flow in the lung, nor does it influence the matching of ventilation to perfusion in normal lungs at the scale of resolution currently attained. Comparable magnitudes of ventilation and perfusion heterogeneity have been demonstrated in awake goats (27) and resting awake sheep (37) by Melsom et al.

We have failed to demonstrate any detectable differences in patterns of pulmonary aerosol deposition between dogs and pigs; however, both of these species have monopodial branching patterns, which have been demonstrated to uniformly distribute an aerosol to the smaller branching airways. Human airways, with their pattern of symmetric dichotomous branching, are more likely to demonstrate deposition of aerosol at branch points. A study comparing aerosol deposition in isolated human and dog lungs demonstrated more aerosol deposition on larger airways in the human lung (36). Thus it remains to be determined whether our approach to measurement of regional ventilation will remain valid at the high-resolution scale in primate lungs.

XVI. Validation Against Gas Exchange Methods

$\dot{V}_A/\dot{Q}$ distributions that accurately predict respiratory blood gas values are obtained from MIGET (3). The first test of the cut-piece approach was to investigate the form of the $\dot{V}_A/\dot{Q}$ distributions obtained (15). Altemeier et al. have developed a graphical presentation of the cut-piece data that permits direct comparison with the MIGET output (49). Figure 2 shows this representation from measurements of regional ventilation in a pig by FMS aerosol and regional perfusion by intravenously injected microspheres. The left panel shows a simple comparison of ventilation and perfusion for each lung piece, where the dashed line isobars describe different $\dot{V}_A/\dot{Q}$ values. The right panel shows the same data presented in the format used for MIGET (52). From these preliminary results, both approaches to quantitating $\dot{V}_A/\dot{Q}$ distributions provide comparable estimates. As another validation of our approach, simultaneous MIGET and cut-piece distributions were compared for their capacity to predict arterial blood gas values. MIGET includes a prediction of arterial respiratory blood gas measurements, based on the inert gas-derived $\dot{V}_A/\dot{Q}$ distribution and the mixed venous values for the respiratory gases. We used the $\dot{V}_A/\dot{Q}$ distribution from the cut-piece data and measurements of both mixed venous respiratory blood gases and

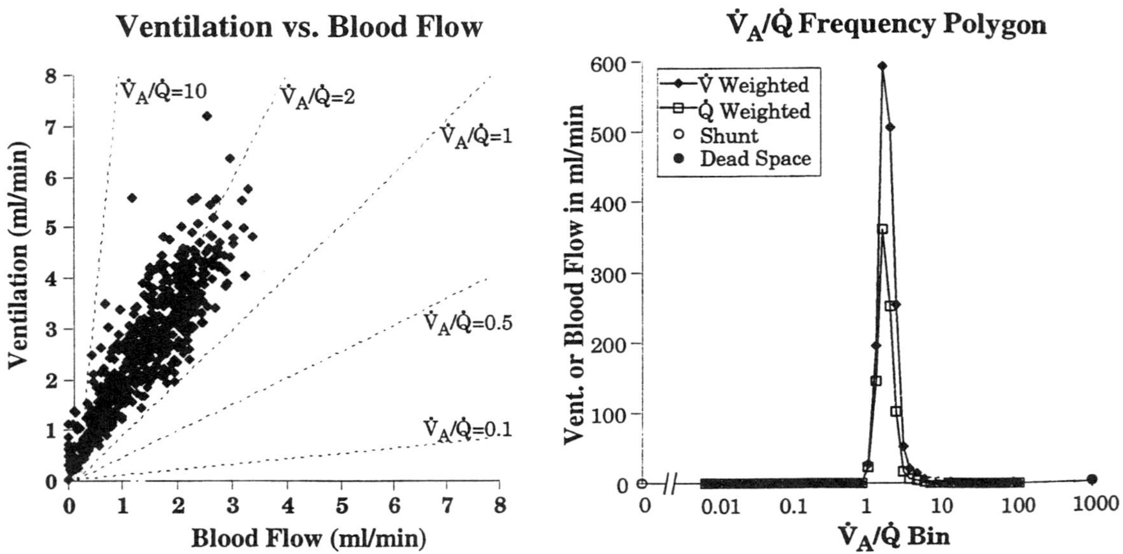

Figure 2 (Left) Plot of simultaneously measured ventilation and perfusion for each piece from a single pig lung. The diagonal dashed lines represent $\dot{V}_A/\dot{Q}$ isopleths. (Right) Same data as left panel presented as a frequency polygon, with $\dot{V}_A/\dot{Q}$ values sorted into 50 bins including shunt ($\dot{V}_A/\dot{Q} = 0$) and alveolar dead space ($\dot{V}_A/\dot{Q}$ = infinite).

mixed venous inert gases to predict the arterial respiratory gas and inert gas measurements (49). In addition to correctly predicting the arterial respiratory blood gas measurements, the arterial inert gas predictions matched the inert gas measurements as well. If borne out by further study, these results have the interesting implication that the resolution obtained with the 1.9-cm^3 cut-piece approach is sufficiently accurate to represent respiratory gas exchange, even though it appears that greater perfusion heterogeneity is present at finer scales of resolution (53).

XVII. Scale of Regional Heterogeneity of Ventilation

The extent of regional ventilation heterogeneity suggested by this aerosol deposition technique is larger than that measured by the relatively larger regional volumes demarcated by parenchymal markers (34). Wilson et al. noted, however, that their single-breath oxygen measurements suggested that there was parenchymal heterogeneity at a smaller scale than they could detect with their parenchymal marker techniques. The current FMS aerosol deposition results (15,27) are consistent with the findings from the parenchymal markers studies in that when the FMS pieces are clustered into volumes comparable to those used in the parenchymal marker studies, a similar extent of heterogeneity is noted. As noted above, the aerosol deposition approach will only be valid at the level of scale where convective transport of gas is the predominant mechanism. Additional investigation is required to define both the minimal piece size and the influence of different ventilatory parameters in obtaining physiologically meaningful FMS aerosol estimates of ventilation distribution.

XVIII. Conclusion

If an aerosol can be precisely sized, the predominant mechanism of deposition can be inferred. In the case of the 1-μm fluorescent microsphere aerosol preparation described above, deposition occurs by gravitational settling and chaotic movement within the alveolar spaces in proportion to the convective gas transport to those lung regions. At the level of scale appropriate for convective transport of gas in the lung, deposition then reflects alveolar ventilation. The extent of heterogeneity of regional ventilation suggested by aerosol deposition is large. In fact, quantitatively similar findings with lung autoradiographs following administration of a 0.4 μm technetium-labeled aerosol were reported by Valberg et al. in 1982 (35). At that time, there was no information to suggest that regional ventilation might have that extent of heterogeneity, and the authors appeared reluctant to consider regional ventilation heterogeneity as a primary explanation of their findings. Subsequent studies of heterogeneity of regional ventilation by tissue markers (32–34) demonstrated substantial degree of scale-dependent regional heterogeneity in normal lungs. Melsom et al. (27) have demonstrated a similar degree of regional heterogeneity of ventilation in goats utilizing an inhaled technetium aerosol and counting of individually cut lung pieces.

While high-resolution studies of either fluorescent or radionuclide-labeled aerosols agree on the extent and topography of the deposition of the inhaled marker, additional validation of this approach is still required. The results obtained from analysis of aerosol-labeled pieces need to be compared at comparable piece sizes to either PET or CT gas washout studies. While these results should be in agreement at an appropriate scale of resolution for the imaging studies, the direct comparison still needs to be performed. Beyond issues of validation, the fluorescent aerosol approach to the study of regional ventilation will offer a means to investigate the importance of bronchiolar tone in regional ventilation heterogeneity. Other issues for investigation include the comparison of the fractal dimension of ventilation with that of perfusion (28) and the size of the functional unit of gas exchange. While the 2-cm^3 piece-size resolution of current studies (15,27) provides an upper limit of resolution, it will be desirable to attain higher resolution, and the limits of resolution for various aerosol marker sizes need to be delineated. While smaller aerosol particles necessarily carry less fluorescent signal, they will have a higher fractional alveolar deposition and thereby provide a better index of fresh gas delivery to alveolar surface. Finally, as the principal function of the lung is as an organ of gas exchange, the gas exchange properties of the lung predicted from the simultaneous use of aerosol deposition and regional perfusion measurements need to be compared to measured exchange of respiratory gases and inert gases. The findings from simultaneous MIGET and regional measurements have shown excellent agreement in a pig model of vascular occlusion (49), but these preliminary findings need to be validated with a broad range of species and pathophysiological conditions.

References

1. Chang HK, Paiva M, eds. Respiratory Physiology: An Analytical Approach. New York: Marcel Dekker, 1989.
2. Milic-Emili J. Static distribution of lung volumes. In: Macklem PT, Mead J, eds. Mechanics of Breathing. Part 2. Bethesda: American Physiological Society, 1986: 561–574.
3. Wagner PD, Saltzman HA, West JB. Measurement of continuous distributions of ventilation-perfusion ratios: theory. J Appl Physiol 1974; 36:588–599.
4. Anthonisen NR, Fleetham JA. Ventilation: total, alveolar, and dead space. In: Farhi LE, Tenney SM, eds. Gas Exchange. Bethesda: American Physiological Society, 1987:113–130.

5. Swenson E, Robertson H, Polissar N, Middaugh M, Hlastala M. Conducting airways gas exchange: diffusion-related differences in inert gas elimination. J Appl Physiol 1992; 72:1581–1588.
6. McEvoy R, Davies N, FL M, Prutow R, Schumacker P, Wagner P, West J. Pulmonary gas exchange during high-frequency ventilation. J Appl Physiol 1982; 52: 1278–1287.
7. Robertson H, Coffey R, Standaert T, Truog W. Respiratory and inert gas exchange during high frequency ventilation. J Appl Physiol 1982; 52:683–689.
8. Fortune JB, Wagner PD. Effects of common dead space on inert gas exchange in mathematical models of the lung. J Appl Physiol 1979; 47:896–906.
9. Ross BB, Farhi LE. Dead-space ventilation as a determinant in the ventilation-perfusion concept. J Appl Physiol 1960; 15:363–371.
10. Petrini MF, Robertson HT, Hlastala MP. Interaction of series and parallel dead space in the lung. Respir Physiol 1983; 54:121–136.
11. Mercer RR, Anjilvel S, Miller FJ, Crapo JD. Inhomogeneity of ventilatory unit volume and its effect on reactive gas uptake. J Appl Physiol 1991; 70:2193–2205.
12. Engel LA, Menkes H, Wood LDH, Utz G, Joubert J, Macklem PT. Gas mixing during inspiration studied by intrapulmonary gas sampling. J Appl Physiol 1973; 35:9–17.
13. Brain JD, Valberg PA. Deposition of aerosol in the respiratory tract. Am Rev Respir Dis 1979; 120:1325–1373.
14. Zeltner TB, Sweeney TD, Skornik WA, Feldman HA, Brain JD. Retention and clearance of 0.9-μm particles inhaled by hamsters during rest or exercise. J Appl Physiol 1991; 70(3):1137–1145.
15. Robertson HT, Glenny RW, Stanford D, McInnes LM, Luchtel DL, Covert D. High-resolution maps of regional ventilation utilizing inhaled fluorescent microspheres. J Appl Physiol 1997; 82(3):943–953.
16. Burch WM, Sullivan PJ, McClaren CJ. Technegas: a new ventilation agent for lung scanning. Nucl Med Commun 1986; 7:865–871.
17. Darquenne C, Paiva M. One-dimensional simulation of aerosol transport and deposition in the human lung. J Appl Physiol 1994; 77:2889–2898.
18. Darquenne C, Paiva M. Two- and three-dimensional simulations of aerosol transport and deposition in alveolar zone of human lung. J Appl Physiol 1996; 80(4): 1401–1414.
19. Ball WC, Jr, Stewart PB, Newsham LGS, Bates DV. Regional pulmonary function studied with xenon 133. J Clin Invest 1962; 41(3):519–531.
20. Bryan AC, Bentivoglio LG, Beerel F, MacLeish H, Zidulka Z, Bates DV. Factors affecting regional distribution of ventilation and perfusion in the lung. J Appl Physiol 1964; 19:395–402.
21. Venegas JG, Yamada Y, Burnham C, Hales CA. Local gas transport in eucapnic ventilation: effects of gravity and breathing frequency. J Appl Physiol 1990; 68: 2287–2295.
22. Fazio F, Jones T. Assessment of regional ventilation by continuous inhalation of radioactive krypton-81m. Br Med J 1975; 3:673–676.
23. Amis TC, Jones T. Krypton-81m as a flow tracer in the lung: theory and quantitation. Bull Eur Physiopathol Respir 1980; 16:245–259.

24. Anderson PJ, Dolovich MB. Aerosols as diagnostic tools. J Aerosol Med 1994; 7(1):77–88.
25. Beck KC, Rehder K. Differences in regional vascular conductances in isolated dog lungs. J Appl Physiol 1986; 61(2):530–538.
26. Glenny RW, Lamm WJE, Albert RK, Robertson HT. Gravity is a minor determinant of pulmonary blood flow distribution. J Appl Physiol 1991; 71:620–629.
27. Melsom M, Kramer-Johansen J, Flatebo T, Muller C, Nicolaysen G. Distribution of pulmonary ventilation and perfusion measured simultaneously in awake goats. Acta Physiol Scand 1997; 159(3):199–208.
28. Glenny RW, Robertson HT. Fractal properties of pulmonary blood flow: characterization of spatial heterogeneity. J Appl Physiol 1990; 69:532–545.
29. Santolicandro A, Ruschi S, Fornai E, Giuntini C. Imaging of ventilation in chronic obstructive pulmonary disease. J Thorac Imag 1986; 1(2):36–53.
30. Crawford ABH, Davison A, Amis TC, Engel LA. Intrapulmonary distribution of ^{99m}Technetium labelled ultrafine carbon aerosol (Technegas) in severe airflow obstruction. Eur Respir J 1990; 3:686–692.
31. Engel LA, Utz G, Wood LDH, Macklem PT. Ventilation distribution in anatomical lung units. J Appl Physiol 1973; 37(2):194–200.
32. Hubmayr RD, Walters BJ, Chevalier PA, Rodarte JR, Olson LE. Topographical distribution of regional lung volume in anesthetized dogs. J Appl Physiol 1983; 54(4):1048–1056.
33. Rodarte JR, Chaniotakis M, Wilson TA. Variability of parenchymal expansion measured by computed tomography. J Appl Physiol 1989; 67(1):226–231.
34. Wilson TA, Olson LE, Rodarte JR. Effect of variable parenchymal expansion on gas mixing. J Appl Physiol 1987; 62(2):634–639.
35. Valberg PA, Brain JD, Sneddon SL, LeMott SR. Breathing patterns influence aerosol deposition sites in excised dog lungs. J Appl Physiol 1982; 53(4):824–837.
36. Fang C-P, Wilson JE, Spektor DM, Lippman M. Effect of lung airway branching pattern and gas composition on particle deposition in bronchial airways. III. Experimental studies with radioactively tagged aerosol in human and canine lungs. Exp Lung Res 1993; 19:377–396.
37. Melsom MN, Flatebo T, Aulie A, Sjaastad OV, Nicolaysen G. Regional pulmonary perfusion and ventilation remain well matched during exercise. Am J Respir Crit Care Med 1997; 155:A744.
38. Glenny RW, Bernard S, Brinkley M. Validation of fluorescent-labeled microspheres for measurement of regional organ perfusion. J Appl Physiol 1993; 74: 2585–2597.
39. Tsuda A, Butler JP, Fredberg JJ. Effects of alveolated duct structure on aerosol kinetics II. Gravitational sedimentation and intertial impaction. J Appl Physiol 1994; 76(6):2510–2516.
40. Tsuda A, Henry FS, Otani Y, Haber S, Butler JP. Aerosol transport and deposition in the rhythmically expanding pulmonary alveolus. J Aerosol Med 1996; 9(3):389–408.
41. Tsuda A, Otani Y, Butler JP. "Stretching and folding" convective flow mixing in a rhythmically expanding pulmonary alveolus. Am J Respir Crit Care Med 1997; 155:A744.

42. Butler JP, Tsuda A. Convective "stretching and folding", approximate entropy, and aerosol mixing in the lung. Am J Respir Crit Care Med 1977; 155:A908.
43. Darquenne C, Paiva M, West JB, Prisk GK. Deposition of aerosols in the human lung at different gravity levels. Am J Respir Crit Care Med 1997; 155:A955.
44. Weibel ER. Lung morphometry and models in respiratory physiology. In: Chang HK, Paiva M, eds. Respiratory Physiology: An Analytical Approach. New York: Marcel Dekker, 1989:1–56.
45. Hogg JC, Holst P, Corey P, Ruff F, Housley E, Morris E. Effects of regional lung expansion and body position on pulmonary perfusion in dogs. J Appl Physiol 1971; 31:97–101.
46. Robertson HT, Glenny RW. Measurement of $\dot{V}_A/\dot{Q}$ heterogeneity in anesthetized dogs utilizing deposition of inhaled and intravenously infused fluorescent-labelled microspheres. FASEB J 1996; 10:A363.
47. Robertson HT, Glenny RW. Acute occlusion of the pulmonary artery at a segmental level does not alter regional ventilation in anesthetized pigs. FASEB J 1997; 11: A2001.
48. Glenny RW, Polissar L, Robertson HT. Relative contribution of gravity to pulmonary perfusion heterogeneity. J Appl Physiol 1991; 71:2449–2452.
49. Altemeier WA, Glenny RW, Robertson HT. Flow redistribution determines change in $\dot{V}_A/\dot{Q}$ heterogeneity following vascular embolization. Am J Respir Crit Care Med 1997; 155:A117.
50. Amis TC, Jones HA, Rhodes CG, Heather JD, Hughes JMB. Regional distribution of pulmonary ventilation and perfusion in the conscious dog. Am J Vet Res 1982; 43(11):1972–1977.
51. Hubmayr RD, Rodarte JR, Walters BJ, Tonelli FM. Regional ventilation during spontaneous breathing and mechanical ventilation in dogs. J Appl Physiol 1987; 63(6):2467–2475.
52. Wagner PD, Naumann PF, Laravuso RB. Simultaneous measurement of eight foreign gases in blood by gas chromatography. J Appl Physiol 1974; 36:600–605.
53. Glenny RW, Bernard S, Ewen J, Barlow C, Kelly J, Robertson HT. Spatial distribution of pulmonary blood flow at a microscopic scale of resolution. Am J Respir Crit Care Med 1995; 151:A518.

Part Four

PULMONARY PERFUSION HETEROGENEITY

13

Complexity and Structure–Function Relationships in the Pulmonary Arterial Tree

CHRISTOPHER A. DAWSON

Medical College of Wisconsin
and Zablocki Veterans Affairs
Medical Center
Milwaukee, Wisconsin

GARY S. KRENZ and JOHN H. LINEHAN

Marquette University
Milwaukee, Wisconsin

I. Introduction

The organ source of a corrosion cast or image of an arterial tree is easily identified by its characteristic gross appearance. Both the organ and the species source can often be identified from the gross appearance of the arterial tree from a particular organ. For example, the two images in Figure 1 are recognizable as pulmonary arterial trees, but they are clearly from different species. Even though the pulmonary arterial trees from individuals of the same species may appear grossly similar and their overall function may be similar, they are not the same in detail. Thus, there are readily recognizable forms upon which certain types of variations do not alter the recognizability or, more importantly, the overall function. Because of the complexity of these structures, it is not always obvious what variations are functionally acceptable. Therefore, although it can be relatively easy to identify gross differences between arterial trees, the functionally most important details may be less obvious. For this topic, we view the pulmonary arterial tree function as distributing the blood flow appropriately among capillaries throughout the lungs while providing the appropriate impedance for the delivery of blood from the right ventricle to the pulmonary artery. Both the geometric and mechanical properties of the vessels are important, but, in this

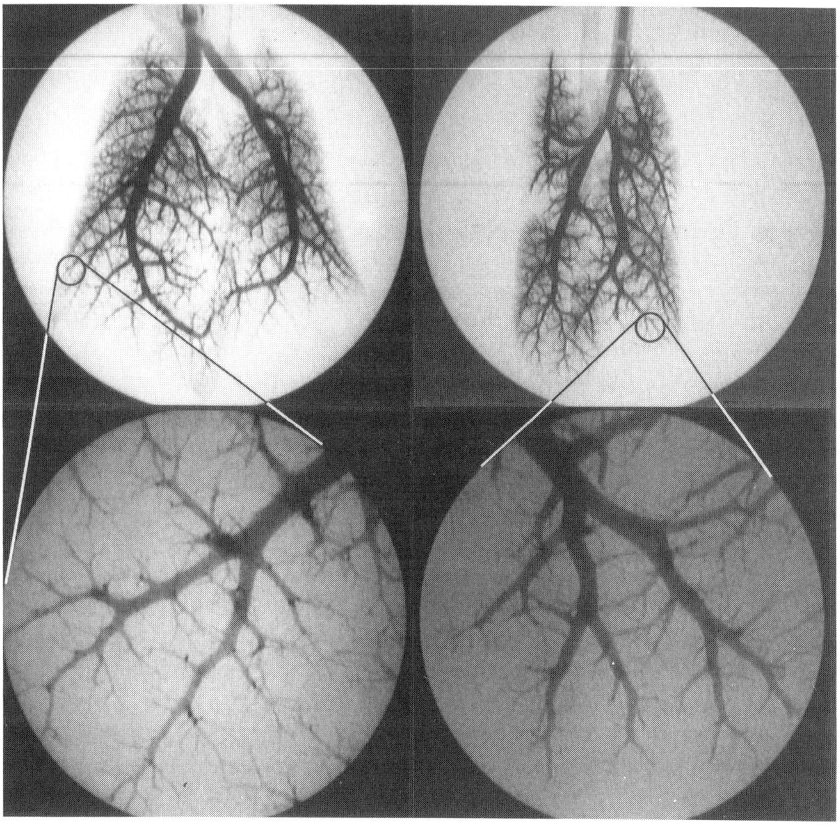

Figure 1 Images of pulmonary arterial trees from rabbit (*left*) and ferret (*right*) lungs at two levels of magnification. The two species are distinguishable at low magnification, but the differences at high magnification appear to be random variations that are not species dependent.

chapter, we concentrate on the geometry of the pulmonary arterial tree. We examine some aspects of the structure–function relationships of pulmonary arterial trees or simulated pulmonary arterial tree–like structures, looking for some unifying principles in the complex structure.

Heterogeneity is a dominant feature of the appearance of the pulmonary arterial tree, as can be appreciated from Figure 1. The routes from the main pulmonary artery to a terminal precapillary artery pass through varying numbers of vessel segments and bifurcations. The blood flow through the main pulmonary artery might be thought of as a bundle of stream tubes, each of which is the portion of the flow cross section or bundle of stream lines that will eventually pass through a terminal arteriole. The lengths of these stream tubes are quite heterogeneous. Given the complexity of the pulmonary arterial tree architecture and the sensitivity of pressure–flow relations to tree geometry (e.g., through the fourth power of vessel diameters), it is striking how consistent the pulmonary vascular pressure–flow relationship is among normal individuals. To appreciate this consistency, several points may be considered. One is that the lungs accommodate the cardiac output in a largely passive manner. Although there is a local diameter-regulating mechanism (hypoxic vasoconstriction), it does not apparently play a major role in determining the overall pulmonary pressure–flow relationship in the normal lung. This is in contrast to systemic vascular beds wherein total flow is determined by an actively controlled aortic pressure head and local active control over vessel diameters. The geometric design requirements for a passive system tend to be more stringent than for a system with active mechanisms to compensate for geometric design errors. In lieu of a major role for ongoing active compensatory mechanisms, one way to ensure the appropriate design might be to build the tree using angiogenic mechanisms that are responsive to signals related to hemodynamic function. Then, once those signals were optimized, the appropriate tree structure would be established for the future. However, the initial growth and development of the pulmonary vascular bed take place under substantially different conditions of pressure and flow than those under which it operates immediately after birth and into adult life. Thus, it is not obvious how, during fetal development, angiogenic mechanisms would be able to take advantage of signals such as local normal or shear stresses to shape the tree so that the tree structure would anticipate postnatal conditions. An alternative might be growth mechanisms that result in a structure that is robust, such that its key functions are insensitive to variations in certain geometric details. The mechanisms of pulmonary arterial tree growth and development are beyond the scope of this chapter. However, knowledge of the end result, that is, of the tree geometry, is probably an important step in the search for mechanisms controlling growth. It is certainly necessary for understanding the hemodynamic function of the tree. Our objective is to examine some design features of the pulmonary arterial tree, with particular interest in the robustness of the design with respect to hemodynamic function of the heterogeneous tree.

II. Pulmonary Arterial Tree Morphometry

The extant studies of the detailed morphometry of the entire pulmonary arterial tree have been carried out by making corrosion casts and then measuring vessel segment numbers, lengths, and diameters (1–7). Even though measurements on the more peripheral (small) vessels have generally been made on only portions of the tree, with extrapolation to the whole tree, this approach results in a large amount of data that must be summarized in some way to provide a concise quantitative description of the tree geometry. In an early (reported in 1893) attempt at quantitative pulmonary arterial tree morphometry, Miller (1) summarized the measurements on a pulmonary arterial tree cast from a dog lung by categorizing the vessel segments into nine levels: pulmonary artery, right and left branches, lobar arteries, first, second, and third order arteries, lobular arteries, atrial arteries, and sac arteries. Then, the numbers and average diameters of the vessels in each level were reported. Subsequently, consideration has been given to alternative ways of categorizing the vessels, and discussions as to the advantages of the different methods center around the kinds information retained in the morphometric summary (3,6).

These methods for summarizing the morphometric data have been categorized as centripetal and centrifugal ordering systems (8,9). The centrifugal system starts with the pulmonary artery as generation 1 (10). The right and left daughter branches are generation 2, and the generation number assigned to each vessel segment continues to increase at each bifurcation such that the generation number is equal to one plus the number of bifurcations upstream from the vessel segment in question. This system has a simple logic when applied to a symmetrical homogeneous tree, but as larger variations in the daughter diameter ratios are encountered as one moves along the actual asymmetrical heterogeneous tree, it results in grouping together of vessels of very different diameters in the same generation. Because the number of generations along each pathway can vary, the information in the number of vessels in a generation can be difficult to interpret. For example, once the terminations of short pathways are encountered, the number of vessels in a generation of an asymmetrical heterogeneous tree can decrease as the generation number increases, even though the actual number of vessel segments increases as diameters decrease.

Centripetal systems begin with the terminal (precapillary) arterioles. Horsfield (2) and Singhal et al. (4) introduced the centripetal Strahler ordering system into field of pulmonary morphometry. In the Strahler system, which was originally devised in the field of geology for analyzing river systems, the ordering begins with the terminal (precapillary) arterioles as order one. When two daughter vessel segments of the same order meet, they form a parent vessel segment of the next higher order. When two daughter vessel segments of different orders come together, the parent order number is the higher of the two daughter orders. Once the vessel segment orders have been assigned, contiguous segments of a common order are combined into vessels having the mean diameter and sum of the lengths of the combined segments. Then the number, mean diameter, and mean length of the vessels comprising each order make up the morphometric summary of the tree. For purposes of consistency within this chapter, and because other authors have found it convenient to use some of the same terms in different ways, we use the following definitions. A vessel segment is the section of vessel between two bifurcations. A vessel is comprised of the contiguous vessel segments of common Strahler order. We define the parent vessel segment at an arterial bifurcation as the upstream segment and the two daughters as the two downstream segments connected to the parent. The parent diameter is designated as D_1, the larger of the two daughters as D_2, and the smaller daughter as D_3. The largest vessel segment (i.e., the inlet vessel segment) for any tree or subtree (the portion of a tree subtended by any particular vessel segment) of interest is D_a. We define a homogeneous tree as one wherein $D_3 = D_2$ at each bifurcation, and, for a given D_1, the D_1/D_2 ratio is the same. A symmetrical tree is one in which the number of bifurcations from arterial inlet to terminal arterioles is the same for all arteriole stream tubes. In an asymmetrical tree, the number of bifurcations varies among stream tubes. When we use Strahler ordering of simulated arterial trees in what follows, the order number, j, is counted from the largest vessel to the terminal vessels. Thus, $j = n + 1 -$(Strahler order number), where n is the total number of orders. This has been referred to as the "reversed Strahler method" (8).

The Strahler system has some advantages for summarizing the morphometry of a heterogeneous asymmetrical tree. One is that the variance in dimensions in a Strahler order tends to be smaller than in a centrifugal generation. The relationship between the Strahler order number and the number of vessels in a Strahler order is also useful as is discussed below. One result of the Strahler system that has been considered a disadvantage from the hemodynamic point of view is that each order is not a full flow set (11).* However, as indicated below this may not be as important as it might first appear.

Jiang et al. (6) were concerned that the Strahler method allows overlap in the diameters of vessels in different orders. They felt that an ordering system would be more useful if each order contained an exclusive diameter range. Therefore, they introduced what they refer to as the "diameter defined" Strahler system. In this system, when two daughter vessels having diameters of D_2 and D_3 converge on parent vessel of diameter D_1, an additional criterion based on the magnitude of the differences between D_1 or D_2 and D_3 is applied in determining the parent order number. This criterion is established using an iterative

*A full flow set is, as defined by Sherman (11), comprised of any parallel set of vessel segments for which the sum of the individual flows is equal to the total flow. The two daughter vessel segments at a bifurcation are a full flow set with respect to the flow through the parent segment. The terminal vessels and the right and left branches of the main pulmonary artery are examples of full flow sets with respect to the total pulmonary blood flow. Each vessel segment may be a member of a large number of full flow sets (the smaller the vessel segment, the larger the number). Each vessel segment is also a member of a particular full flow set (a "minimum" full flow set) wherein the range of diameters is less than in any other full flow set having that vessel segment as a member. In a symmetrical homogeneous tree, an order or generation is a minimum full flow set.

method that eliminates the overlap in diameters between orders. Jiang et al. (6) also introduced the concept of the connectivity matrix to summarize the probability that a vessel from a given diameter-defined Strahler order will have a parent from any other order.

Each of these ordering systems is arbitrary in that a given vessel will end up a member of a different cohort in each system. Discussions relating to the relative merits of each system commonly state or imply that one objective is to retain functionally (hemodynamically) relevant information in the summary, but it is not always clear how well that is achieved since the functional analyses have been commonly based on homogeneous tree assumptions. In what follows, we have approached the problem of evaluating the functional consequences of the morphometry somewhat differently, partly in an attempt to avoid some aspects of the mind set that particular ordering systems may engender.

III. A Model of the Pulmonary Arterial Tree

To begin, we observe the relationships between the log N_j and log D_j obtained from number, N, and diameter, D, measurements on plastic casts of the pulmonary arterial trees of several species shown in the upper panel of Figure 2. The points represent the N and average D in the jth order or generation of vessels. In each study represented in Figure 2, the criteria used to assign a vessel to order j were different. However, the near linearity of the graphs obtained from the different species and ordering systems [including that used by Miller in 1893 (1)] suggests that linearity of this relationship is a fundamental geometric property of normal pulmonary arterial trees and that the various ordering systems used have not disrupted this relationship. This relationship can be represented by $N_j = (D_j/D_a)^{-\beta_1}$, where j increases from the inlet artery designated order 1, D_a is the order 1 artery (i.e., the largest or inlet artery), and β_1 is the magnitude of the log N_j versus log D_j slope. The consistent near linearity of these graphs is the basis of much of the following discussion.

The linearity of the mean data plotted as in Figure 2 and the recognition that the vessel segments assigned to a given order have a range of diameters and lengths have led us to consider an alternative to using an ordering system as the basis for summarizing the tree structure. Instead, we examine what might be learned from simply ranking the vessel segments comprising the tree according to their diameters. Under the assumption that no two vessel segments have exactly the same diameter, each vessel can be assigned a number, N_{cum}, which is 1 plus the number of vessel segments having diameter larger than vessel segment number N_{cum}. Assuming linearity of log N_j versus log D_j independent of ordering system down to the resolution of the morphometric measurements represented in Figure 2, the diameter of vessel number N_{cum}, namely $D(N_{cum})$, can be approximated by

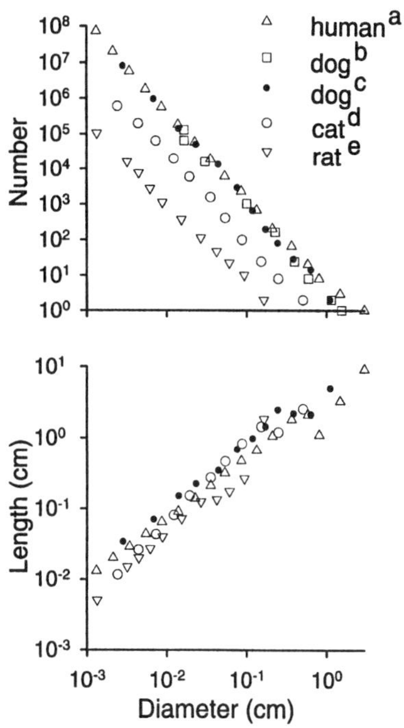

Figure 2 **Upper panel,** The relationship between vessel number, N_j, and mean diameter, D_j, from morphometric measurements on pulmonary arterial casts from human (a) (2), dog (b and c) (1,7), cat (d) (5), and rat (e) (6). **Lower panel,** The relationship between mean vessel length, L_j, and mean diameter, D_j, from the pulmonary arterial casts. (From Ref. 13. With permission from the American Physiological Society.)

$$D(N_{cum}) = D_a\left(\frac{(N_{cum}+1)}{1.5+0.5\exp(-((0.12/\beta_1)+0.44)(N_{cum}-1))}\right)^{-\frac{1}{\beta_1}} \tag{1}$$

The "approximation" has two components. One is that Equation 1 is an empirical formula for assigning vessel diameters so that for any consecutive sequence from N_{cum} to $2N_{cum} - 1$,

$$\overline{D} \sim D_a N_{cum}^{-1/\beta_1}, \text{ where } \overline{D} = \frac{1}{i} \sum_{N_{cum}=i}^{2i-1} D(N_{cum}).$$

This formula ensures that, for a symmetrical bifurcating tree constructed using a consecutive sequence of vessel segments, the log N_j versus log D_j graph is approximately linear with slope $-\beta_1$, consistent with the morphometric summary data in Figure 2.

The other component of the approximation is that, just as no two vessel segments in a tree have exactly the same diameter, no vessel segment in a real tree has exactly the same diameter as a vessel segment in another tree. On the other hand, that portion of every tree encompassing the same number of vessel segments has a vessel segment holding the same rank. Therefore, for trees with a common D_a and β_1, there is a vessel segment with rank N_{cum} and diameter roughly between $D(N_{cum} - 1)$ and $D(N_{cum} + 1)$, and, thus, with D approximately equal to $D(N_{cum})$. When N_{cum} is large, the difference between $D(N_{cum} - 1)$ and $D(N_{cum} + 1)$ must be very small, and therefore, this approximation must be quite good. Thus, even though there is no tree having vessel segments with diameters exactly corresponding to Equation 1, all trees with approximately the same β_1 and D_a must have vessel segment N_{cum} having diameter close to $D(N_{cum})$ calculated from Equation 1. Therefore, Equation 1 provides the approximate diameters of all the vessel segments comprising an arterial tree consistent with the data in Figure 2.

The lengths of the vessel segments are also quite heterogeneous, even for vessel segments in a small range in diameters. However, the morphometric data summarized in Figure 2 indicate that, for the intrapulmonary arteries, the average length, L, to D ratio is nearly independent of diameter. In other words, the graphs of the log L_j versus log D_j data are nearly linear with slopes (β_2) being close to one. Thus, in the development that follows, we make the simplifying assumption that L/D is constant. Thus, with L/D constant, Equation 1 also specifies the vessel segment lengths. The lengths of the extraparenchymal arteries are not consistent with this assumption (3), and, in what follows, we visualize the simulated arterial trees as being intrapulmonary lobar or sublobar portions of the full pulmonary arterial tree.

With respect to the objectives of this chapter, we can now examine how all the vessel segments, whose dimensions are specified by Equation 1, might be connected together to construct a simulated arterial tree, and how the ways they are connected might affect the total vascular resistance and the longitudinal distribution of resistance from a lobar artery to terminal arterioles.

There are some restrictions on how the vessel segments whose dimensions are specified by Equation 1 can be connected. These restrictions can be expressed in the following three additional assumptions: 1. the daughter diameters are always smaller than the parent diameter; 2. there are two daughters at each branch point, and 3. the terminal arterioles, those connecting to the capillaries, are the smallest vessel segments. These assumptions may not be absolutely correct, but they appear to be close enough that the exceptions are not likely to have a substantial effect on the basic conclusions that follow from their employment. Although it might occur, exceptions to the first assumption must be rare. In our experience with the dog lung, allowing that some vessel segments are very short, assumption 2 holds for about 90% of the branch points (12), and this percentage is apparently at least as high in human lungs (3). Although it is possible that there are nonterminal arteries that are smaller than the largest terminal vessel, because the arteries must connect to capillaries, which are generally the smallest vessels in the system, it does not seem likely that this is a common occurrence. Thus, assumption 3 also appears reasonable.

To construct a simulated arterial tree consistent with these three assumptions, we start with vessel segment $N_{cum} = 1$ and proceeding through $N_{cum} = (N_{tot} - 1)/2$ (where N_{tot} is the total number of segments comprising the tree), each vessel segment is randomly assigned one daughter (which will ultimately be the larger of the two daughters) from the unattached segments left in the sequence $N_{cum} - 1$ to $2N_{cum}$. After each N_{cum} through $(N_{tot} - 1)/2$ vessel has had one daughter attached, the remaining vessel segments (each of which will be the smaller of the two daughters at a bifurcation) are assigned to parents in the sequence of largest remaining daughter attached to largest remaining parent. To vary the asymmetry of the tree, limits are placed on the initial daughter assignment so that the choice of the largest daughter is limited to vessel segments having N_{cum} equal to or smaller than two times the parent N_{cum} but larger than the closest integer to x times the parent N_{cum}, where $1 < x < 2$. Thus, if x is set close to 1, the tree is more asymmetrical. Whereas, if x is set close to 2, the tree tends to be more symmetrical. Thus, this algorithm applied to vessel segments whose diameters are specified by Equation 1 provides for the construction of simulated trees consistent with the three assumptions and with varying degrees of asymmetry for a given value of β_1. For the simulations discussed below, N_{tot} was set at approximately 1 million vessel segments.

To determine the impact of asymmetry on hemodynamic function, we need a means of quantifying asymmetry. There are several possibilities. For example, the distribution of stream tube lengths might be measured. However, the Strahler ordering system provides an alternative that also provides a basis for comparison with available morphometric data. To take advantage of the Strahler system, we use the concept of branching ratio, B. Given assumption 2 above, the ratio of the number of daughter vessel segments to parent vessel segments is 2, and therefore, using this as the definition of branching ratio, B would be 2. However, for the Strahler method, the branching ratio has also been defined as the antilog of minus the slope of the graph of log N_j versus order number j (2,3). In other words, in the Strahler system, B is an average of the ratio of the number of vessels in consecutive Strahler orders. In a symmetrical tree, the Strahler B would also equal 2. However, if the number of vessel segments between pulmonary artery and terminal arterioles is distributed, the Strahler B is greater than 2. Thus, the Strahler B may be viewed as one measure of heterogeneity. In theory, the value of B could range from 2 to $(N_{tot} + 1)/2$. The latter extreme would occur if the largest $(N_{tot} - 1)/2$ vessel segments were connected together in one long trunk from which the smallest $(N_{tot} + 1)/2$ terminal vessel segments were attached. However, B has been found to be confined to a very small portion of this range (2,5–7). The reported values have ranged from 2.76 for the rat pulmonary arterial tree (6) to about 3.1 for the human (2) to 3.69 for the dog (7). In the Strahler ordered summary of the tree, the total number of Strahler vessels is less than the total number of vessel segments comprising the actual simulated tree, and the vessel length to diameter ratio is larger than the average vessel segment length to diameter ratio. Figure 3 is a diagrammatic representation of the Strahler ordering system applied to two small trees. One is symmetrical, with B = 2, and the other is constructed from the same vessel segments but is asymmetrical, with B = 2.82.

The asymmetry of the tree might also be thought of as the tree shape in the sense that, with respect to hemodynamics, the functionally important aspect of shape is the distribution of path or stream tube lengths, which is determined by the numbers and lengths of the individual vessel segments comprising a given pathway from arterial inlet to capillary inlet. In a tree constructed as indicated above, the asymmetry dominates the distribution of stream tube lengths (the shape). In a symmetrical tree, the number of vessel segments along each pathway from arterial inlet to capillary inlet is equal, and, the stream tube

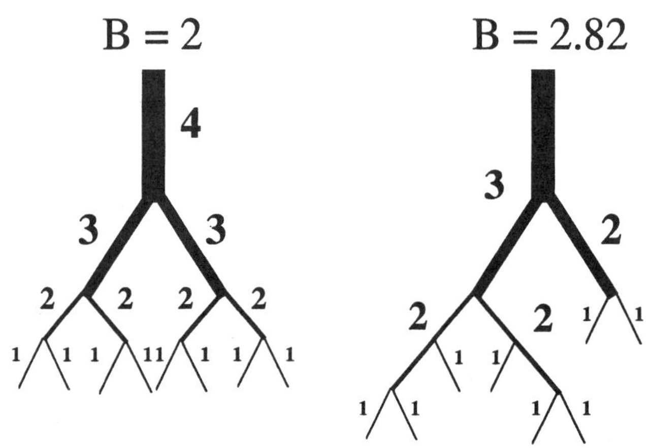

Figure 3 A diagrammatic representation of the Strahler ordering system applied to two small trees constructed with the same vessel segments but symmetrically on the left (B = 2) and asymmetrically (B = 2.82) on the right. The numbers are the Strahler orders. For the symmetrical tree on the left, the number of vessel segments, 15, equals the number of vessels, and there are four Strahler orders. For the asymmetrical tree on the right, the number of vessels, 12, is less than the number of vessel segments, and there are only three Strahler orders.

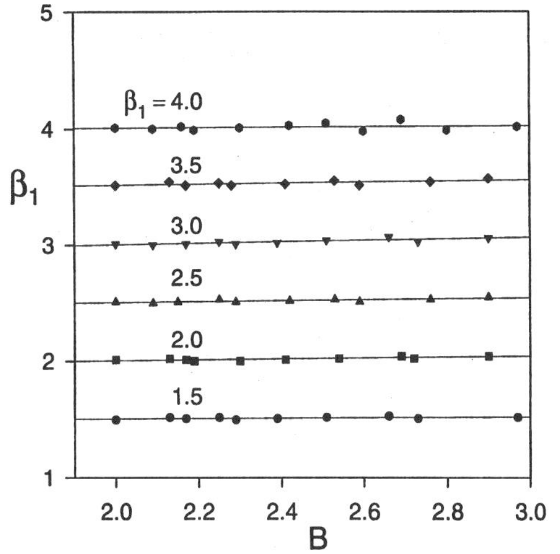

Figure 4 The impact of asymmetry, as reflected in B obtained from Strahler ordering, on the Strahler estimate of β_1 in simulated pulmonary arterial trees. The estimate of β_1 was from linear regression of log N_j versus log D_j, where j is the reversed Strahler order number. Each symbol represents one simulation. Each symbol type represents one value of β_1 used in Equation 1 in the construction of the simulated trees. The values of β_1 are indicated.

length distribution has a small coefficient of variation. This distribution widens as the tree becomes more asymmetrical.

Given B as the measure of asymmetry, we can determine the impact of asymmetry on the Strahler estimate of β_1. If one applies the Strahler method to simulated arterial trees constructed according to the above instructions, the estimate of β_1 is close to the value used to assign the vessel segment diameters in Equation 1, and is independent of B. This is shown in Figure 4, and it is the desired outcome, allowing construction of simulated trees of varying asymmetry, but which are still consistent with the morphometric data in Figure 2.

IV. Asymmetry and the Longitudinal Distribution of Pulmonary Arterial Resistance

Given the ability to construct simulated trees that are consistent with the morphometric data in Figure 2 and with assumptions 1, 2, and 3, we can investigate some functional consequences of varying the morphometric parameter β_1 and the asymmetry of the tree. One observation is that the longitudinal distribution of resistance from inlet artery to terminal arterioles is very sensitive to β_1. For this discussion, we examine the distribution of intravascular pressure (which is the inflow pressure minus the upstream resistance times the flow) as a function of cumulative intravascular volume, Q_{cum} (which is the total volume upstream from all those sites within the arterial tree where the pressure is the same). The intravascular pressure, $P(Q_{cum})$, is plotted as a function of Q_{cum} instead of diameter or distance from the arterial inlet, because in the heterogeneous tree, the pressure varies in vessel segments of a given diameter range or at given distance from the inlet. Likewise, the isobaric diameters and distances vary. Thus, Q_{cum} is a more concisely stated independent variable. Figure 5 shows examples of how, under the assumptions of Poiseuille flow in each vessel segment and common terminal arteriole outlet pressure, the pressure distribution is affected by β_1. As β_1 decreases, the intravascular pressure distribution becomes more concave with respect to the Q_{cum} axis, and the smaller vessels make a progressively larger contribution to the total resistance per unit volume. This can be appreciated by thinking of β_1 as a measure of the vessel taper along a given pathway

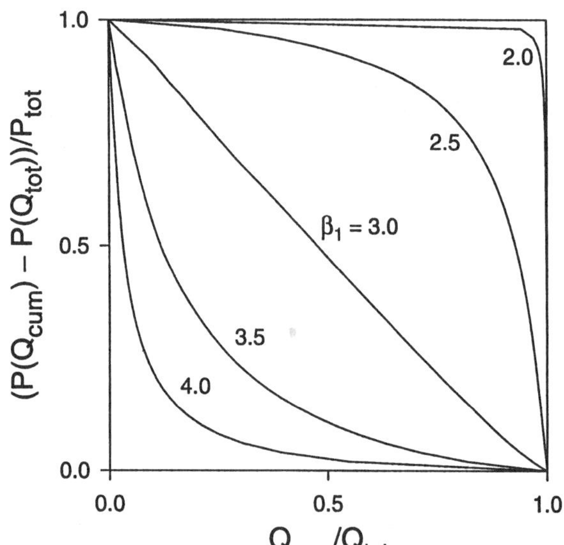

Figure 5 The effect of β_1 on the shape of the $(P(Q_{cum}) - P(Q_{tot}))/P_{tot}$ versus Q_{cum}/Q_{tot} distribution for simulated pulmonary arterial trees, where P_{tot} is the total arterial pressure decrease and Q_{tot} is the total arterial volume. $Q_{cum}/Q_{tot} = 0$ at the inlet to the simulated arterial tree and 1 at the outlet from the terminal arterioles. The simulated trees were asymmetrical with $B = 3$.

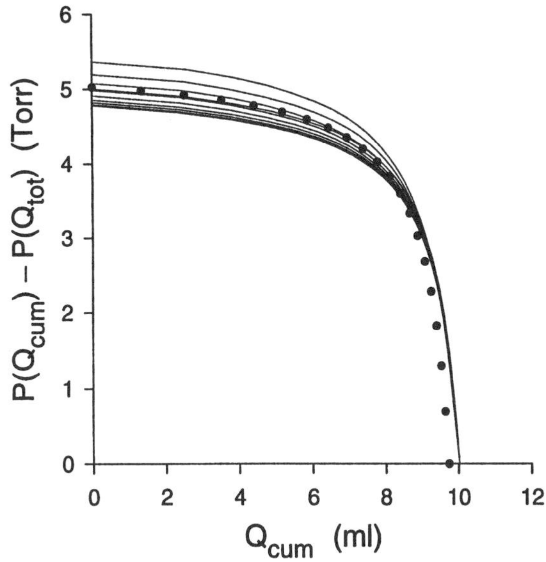

Figure 6 The impact of asymmetry on $P(Q_{cum}) - P(Q_{tot})$ versus Q_{cum} in simulated pulmonary arterial trees of about the size of the arterial tree of a dog lung lobe (39). The β_1 was set at 2.5 in these simulations and B varied from 2 to 3 (solid lines). The dotted line represents the prediction of Equation 2 given the same input parameters as used in the construction of the simulated heterogeneous trees.

or as a reflection of the trade-off between the decrease in diameters and increase in number of parallel vessels along all pathways. The total resistance can also be very sensitive to β_1, but comparisons depend on what other morphometric parameters are held constant for the comparison. For a given number of vessel segments, the total resistance is very sensitive to β_1 as is discussed below with regard to the impact of active changes in geometry as the result of vasoconstriction.

Figure 6 shows examples of $P(Q_{cum})$ graphs for simulated arterial trees having the same β_1, but different B. Both the longitudinal distribution of intravascular pressure and the total resistance are insensitive to B, that is, insensitive to the asymmetry of the tree.

Given this robustness, we examined the possibility of expressing the longitudinal distribution of intravascular pressure as a function of B, β_1, and β_2, (where β_2 is defined by $L_j = L_a(D_j/D_a)^{\beta_2}$). The following expression was derived as indicated in Reference 13.

$$P(Q_{cum}) = P_a - \frac{\dot{Q}128\mu L_a}{\pi D_a^4}\left[\frac{\left(\frac{4Q_{cum}}{\pi D_a^2 L_a}(B^{(\beta_1-\beta_2-2)/\beta_1} - 1) + 1\right)^{\frac{-\beta_1-\beta_2+4}{\beta_1-\beta_2-2}} - 1}{B^{(-\beta_1-\beta_2+4)/\beta_1} - 1}\right] \tag{2}$$

where $\dot{Q}$ is the flow, and μ is viscosity.

Equation 2 is specifically for a symmetrical homogeneous tree. However, as exemplified in Figure 6, it provides a reasonable approximation for the simulated asymmetrical heterogeneous trees when the input values of β_1, β_2, D_a, and L_a are used, and B is interpreted as the number of daughters at a bifurcation, namely 2. This is to be expected given the insensitivity to asymmetry indicated above. Equation 2 is a useful relationship for understanding the sensitivity of the resistance distribution to the morphometric parameters. For example, in Figure 4, the β_1 obtained from the Strahler ordering is virtually equal to the β_1 used in Equation 1 to construct the trees. Therefore, Equation 2 also provides a good approximation to the shape of $P(Q_{cum})$ if, instead of the input parameter values, the parameter estimates are obtained from the Strahler ordered vessels using linear regression (12). The approximation to the total pressure drop using the Strahler parameters is more variable. This is mainly because the total resistance is strongly influenced by the scaling factor D_a raised to the fourth power. Thus, the estimate of the total resistance is as sensitive to the estimate of D_a obtained from linear regression analysis of the log N_j versus log D_j of the Strahler ordered vessels as the estimate of the resistance of a single vessel segment is to the accuracy in the estimate of its diameter.

V. Arterial Tree Morphometry From Individual Bifurcations

The above observations point to β_1 as a key morphometric parameter. To exploit the central importance of β_1, it would be advantageous if there were a way to obtain the relevant morphometric information using methods that are applicable under more physiological conditions than the casting methods are. Various imaging methods provide that potential (14–18). However, in general, they have limited resolution, making centripetal ordering as a means of estimating β_1 impractical. Thus, another approach would be needed. One possibility might be as follows.

When N_{cum} is large (e.g., greater than about 20), the slope of log N_{cum} versus log $D(N_{cum})$, is virtually equal to β_1. This slope can also be expressed by Equation 3.

$$\frac{(N_{tot} - 1)\log 2}{2\left(\Sigma\ \log D_1 - \Sigma\ \log\frac{D_2 + D_3}{2}\right)} \sim \beta_1 \tag{3}$$

In Equation 3, the parent vessel segments at each bifurcation (D_1) range from D_a to $D(N_{cum} = (N_{tot} - 1)/2)$; and D_2 and D_3 (the larger and smaller daughter vessel segments, respectively, at each bifurcation) range from $D(N_{cum} = 2)$ to $D(N_{cum} = N_{tot})$. The left side of Equation 3 is also the harmonic mean of $\log 2/(\log 2D_1 - \log(D_2 + D_3))$ for each of the $(N_{tot} - 1)/2$ bifurcations of the tree. Equation 3 is not a solution to the problem because the diameters of all the vessels are not available, but it leads to a consideration of what can be learned from diameter measurements made at individual bifurcations. The relationships in Figure 2 reflect the fractal or scale-independent appearance of the pulmonary arterial tree (19). In fact, Jiang et al. (6) have referred to β_1 as a fractal dimension. (They actually obtain β_1, which they refer to as D_f, from the slope, $1 - \beta_1$, of the log of the sum of the diameters of all the vessels in an order versus the log mean diameter in that order.) Viewed as a fractal structure, the three vessel segments forming a bifurcation could be considered the repeating, scale-independent, element. Equation 3 suggests that it might be possible to use the measured parent and daughter vessel diameters from a subset of the total number of bifurcations to estimate the value of β_1. In the simulated trees, the harmonic mean of $\log 2/(\log 2D_1 - \log(D_2 + D_3))$ from sufficiently large random samples of bifurcations provides a good approximation to the value of β_1 used in their construction (which, as shown in Figure 4, is also the value obtained from the Strahler ordering).

The $\log 2/(\log 2D_1 - \log(D_2 + D_3))$ might be thought of as β_1 for a small tree consisting of only three vessel segments, and it is referred to as $\hat{\beta}_1$ in what follows. Figure 7 shows the distributions of $1/\hat{\beta}_1$ for bifurcations having D_1 in the 70 to 2900 μm diameter range obtained from measurements on microfocal x-ray angiograms from perfused dog lungs (15). The harmonic means and their distributions appear to be nearly independent of the parent diameter (D_1) range, and thus, in the range of D_1 studied, consistent with the linearity of the graphs on Figure 2.

The harmonic means of the $\hat{\beta}_1$ values estimated from the data presented in Figure 7 are lower than the values of β_1 estimated from the slopes of the data presented in Figure 2, which range from 2.15 for the rat lung (6) to 2.35 for the cat lung (5) and 2.52 (1) and 2.55 (7) for the dog lungs studied using the casting method. One difference between casting and angiographic techniques is that the longitudinal pressure distribution resulting from flow extant in the latter does not exist in the former. Because the vessels are distensible, this difference would result in a lower β_1 in the perfused arterial tree, but it is not clear that the distensibility of the vessels is sufficient to account for the entire difference.

According to Equation 2, the value of β_1 estimated from the data in Figure 7 would predict a deeply concave $P(Q_{cum})$ versus Q_{cum} relationship for the dog pulmonary arterial tree (Figure 5). When β_1 is less than 3, the graph of Equation 2 is concave downward, and most of the resistance is downstream from the

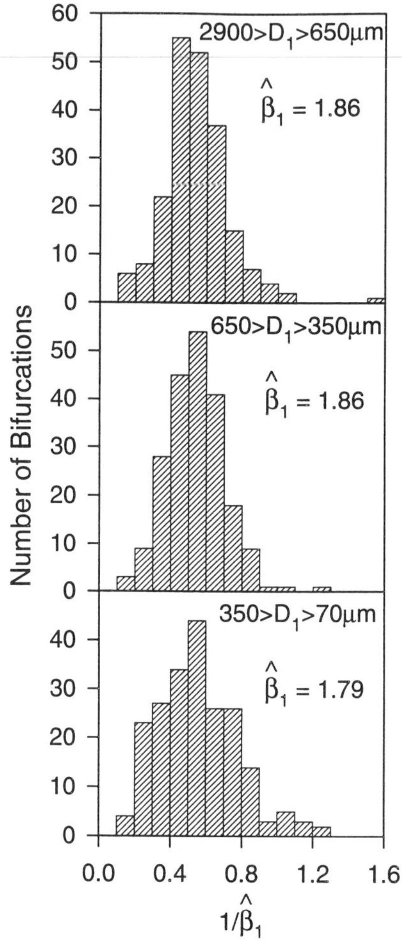

Figure 7 The distribution of $1/\hat{\beta}_l$ obtained from microfocal x-ray angiograms of dog lungs. Histograms for $1/\hat{\beta}_l$ from 630 bifurcations from the arterial tree of the dog lung left lower lobe. The parent vessel diameter range is given on each panel. The number, n, of bifurcations on each panel is 210. The harmonic mean of each $\hat{\beta}_l$ (i.e., $n/\Sigma(1/\hat{\beta}_l)$ is the estimate of β_l indicated on each panel. (From Ref. 15. With permission from the SPIE-The International Society for Optical Engineering.)

point of maximum curvature of the $P(Q_{cum})$ graph such as in Figure 5 or 6. The point of maximum curvature can serve to identify those vessels that make a substantial contribution to the total resistance (the "resistance vessels"). According to Equation 2, when $\beta_2 = 1$, and again interpreting B to be the number of daughter vessel segments at a bifurcation, namely 2, rather than the Strahler definition, then the point of maximum curvature is $(Q_{cum}/Q_{tot}, P(Q_{cum})/P_{tot}) = (c/(c+1), c/(c+1))$, where P_{tot} is $P(0) - P(Q_{tot})$, that is, the total pressure decrease across the portion of the arterial tree under consideration; $c = (2^{1/\beta_1} D_a / D_t)^{(3-\beta_1)/2}$; D_a and D_t are the inlet and terminal artery diameters, respectively, and $c/(c+1)$ is the fraction of the total pressure drop downstream from the point of maximum curvature, that is, the resistance vessel contribution to the total pressure drop. The diameter of the vessels at the point of maximum curvature would then be $(D_a D_t 2^{1/\beta_1})^{1/2}$. Given the insensitivity of the resistance distribution to the asymmetry of the simulated trees, this is probably a reasonable approximation for the asymmetrical tree as well. For vessels in the size range in Figure 7, with a $\beta_1 \sim 1.84$, if we replace D_a and D_t by the largest (2.9 mm) and smallest measured vessels (34 μm), respectively, the point of maximum curvature for that portion of the arterial tree would be estimated to be at about 380 μm diameter and more than 94% of the resistance would be in vessels smaller than that.

VI. Effects of Vasoconstriction

Changes in pulmonary arterial tree geometry can occur as the result of various phenomena such as a change in flow, lung volume, or left atrial pressure, pulmonary embolism, vascular tree remodeling associated with pulmonary vascular disease, or changes in vasomotor activity. The hypoxic vasoconstriction resulting from decreased inspired O_2 can be used to explore how the changes in pulmonary arterial tree geometry resulting from this physiologically important vasoconstrictor stimulus might be interpreted using the concepts developed above. The infusion of the pulmonary arterial constrictor agent serotonin provides another example of a change in pulmonary arterial tree geometry that is also interesting by way of contrast with hypoxic vasoconstriction. Figure 8 is an example of pulmonary arterial images obtained from perfused dog lungs under control conditions and during ventilation with low oxygen or with serotonin infusion. The relationship between the control diameter (D_c) for each vessel and its corresponding diameter during hypoxia or serotonin infusion (D_e) is shown in Figure 9. With hypoxia, it can be seen that the small vessels narrowed, but the larger vessels distended. The latter occurred because, with a constant inflow rate, the distending effect of the increase in pressure in vessels upstream from the small resistance vessels had a greater effect on their diameters than the increase in their wall tension (13). If the effect of hypoxia on the geometry of

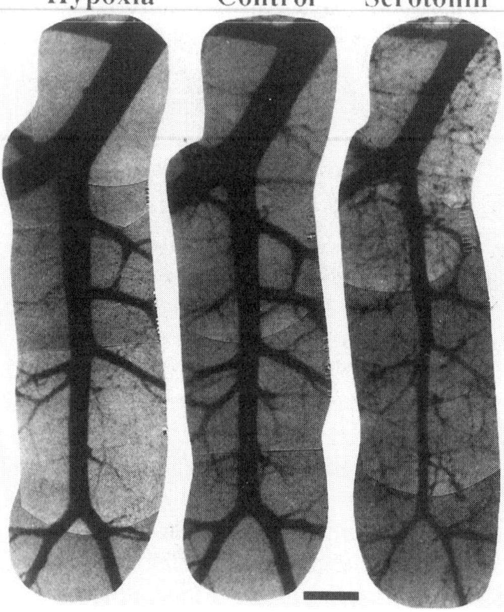

Figure 8 Images of arteries obtained from an isolated perfused dog lung during control conditions and during hypoxia or serotonin infusion. The increase in total arterial-venous pressure difference was 7.4 torr for hypoxia and 8.4 torr for serotonin. Thus, although the total increases in resistance with the two stimuli were not very different, the pattern of diameter change with respect to control diameter appears quite different. Scale bar, 2 mm. (From Ref. 14. With permission from the American Physiological Society.)

the portion of the vascular tree encompassed by vessels in the size range represented on Figure 9 had been to simply change the value of β_1, then the ratio of the hypoxic diameter to the control diameter as a function of control diameter would have been as follows:

$$D_e/D_c = \phi_1 D_c^{\phi_2} \tag{4}$$

where $\phi_1 = D_{ae}/D_{ac}^{(\beta_{1c}/\beta_{1e})}$, $\phi_2 = (\beta_{1c}/\beta_{1e}) - 1$, and the subscript "a" again identifies the largest measured vessel. This equation is the curve fit to the data on Figure 9, which appears to describe the data in the vessel size range studied reasonably well. A geometric interpretation would be that hypoxia resulted in a decrease in β_1 by about 22%. Because hypoxia did not detectably affect vessel lengths, $\beta_{2c}/\beta_{1c} = \beta_{2e}/\beta_{1e}$, which indicates that β_2 was decreased by the same fraction.

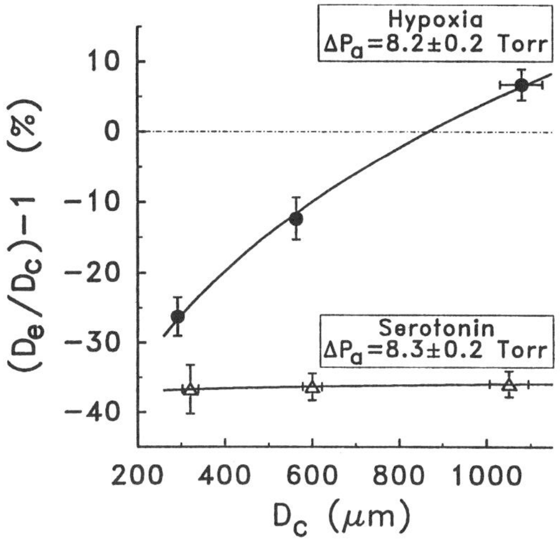

Figure 9 The relationship between the diameter during hypoxia or serotonin infusion, D_e, and the control diameter, D_c, for the pulmonary arteries in isolated perfused dog lungs. The average increase in the total arterial-venous pressure difference, ΔP_a, was about the same (8.2 torr during hypoxia and 8.3 torr during serotonin infusion, respectively), but, as in Figure 8, the pattern of the changes in arterial diameters is different. The solid lines are Equation 4 fit to the data with ϕ_1 and ϕ_2 equal to 0.145 and 0.285, respectively, for hypoxia and 0.598 and 0.010, respectively, for serotonin infusion. (From Ref. 14). With permission from the American Physiological Society.)

Thus, the average L/D increased in small vessels and decreased in large vessels. In contrast to hypoxia, when serotonin was infused, the fractional decreases in vessel diameters were essentially independent of diameter. Equation 4 applied to the serotonin data is mainly a decrease in D_a and an increase in L/D with little change in β_1 or β_2. The impact of these two stimuli on the geometry and, therefore, on the longitudinal distribution of resistance within this portion of the arterial tree was different, even though the increase in total pulmonary vascular resistance was similar. Equation 2 can be used to interpret the impact of the changes in geometry induced by the two vasoactive stimuli on the longitudinal resistance distribution within the portion of the arterial tree summarized in Figure 9 as shown in Figure 10. According to this interpretation, the total pressure drop P_{tot}, through this portion of the arterial tree during hypoxia and serotonin infusion would have been about 3.5 and 6 times, respectively, that under control conditions, P_{totc}. The volume would be significantly reduced by serotonin with little change in response to hypoxia. The differences in the shapes of the distributions of $P(Q_{cum}) - P(Q_{tot})$ reflect the differences in β_1.

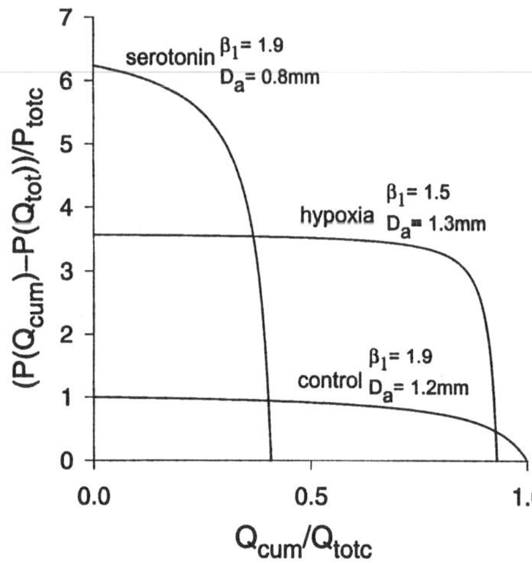

Figure 10 Comparison of $P(Q_{cum}) - P(Q_{tot})$ for control and for hypoxia- and serotonin-induced vasoconstriction predicted by Equation 2 for the vessels having control diameters in the range on Figure 9. The $P(Q_{cum}) - P(Q_{tot})$ values, normalized to the total pressure drop through the same vessels under the control conditions, P_{totc}, versus Q_{cum}, normalized to the total volume of those vessels under control conditions, Q_{totc}, were calculated using the control β_1 from Figure 7, and the changes in β_1 and β_2 obtained from Equation 4 fit to the data on Figure 9.

VII. Functional Significance of the Value of β_1

Having made the argument that β_1 is a key morphometric parameter with respect to the resistance distribution, and that it might be accessible using nondestructive methods, some consideration can be given to the significance of a given value of β_1 and the resulting concavity of $P(Q_{cum})$.

The optimization principle referred to as "Murray's Law" is one reference point that has been used to help understand how the geometry of vascular (and airway) trees relates to function. Murray (20) pointed out that, for a vascular tree with Poiseuille flow to be constructed and operated at minimum cost, where the minimum cost is defined as the minimum of the sum of the hydraulic power dissipation resulting from the flow of blood plus the metabolic power used to build and maintain the vessels (the latter being proportional to the total volume of the tree), the flow should be proportional to the third power of the diameter throughout the tree. This is a "law" in the sense that this optimality principle is mathematically demonstrable as indicated below. However, its mathematical correctness does not imply that it is the correct description of a particular vascular tree, and there has been considerable interest in determining whether vascular trees in various organs might be constructed in accordance with Murray's Law (11,17,21–25).

Murray's Law can be understood by considering the total power dissipation, W, where $W = a\dot{Q}^2L/D^4 + bD^2L/4$; $a = 128\mu/\pi$; and b = rate of work per unit volume. In other words, the flow^2 × resistance, $\dot{Q}^2 \times 128\mu L/\pi D^4$, which is the hydraulic power dissipated by flow through the system, plus the cost of construction and maintenance (e.g., metabolic work) per unit volume of the system, b, times the system volume, $D^2L/4$, is the total cost of operating the system. To minimize the total cost, this sum should be at its minimum. Because the hydraulic power term decreases with diameter and the maintenance term increases with diameter, the minimum occurs when $dW/dD = -4a\dot{Q}^2LD^{-5} + bDL/2 = 0$ or $4a\dot{Q}^2LD^{-5} = bDL/2$. Then, $\dot{Q}^2 = bD^6/8a$ and $\dot{Q} = D^3$ times the constant $(b/8a)^{1/2}$, or, if L/D were constant, times $(b/4a)^{1/2}$. In other words, assuming constant μ and b at each full flow set cross section, the sum of D^3 should be a constant. This observation is commonly stated for the three vessel segments comprising a bifurcation as $D_1^z = D_2^z + D_3^z$, where z = 3 when Murray's Law holds. The value of z for a full flow set, such as the two daughters at a bifurcation, can be estimated by the method of successive iterations. At a bifurcation where $D_2 = D_3$, $\hat{\beta}_1$ and z would be equal. It can be shown that at a bifurcation where the two daughter diameters are not equal, $z > \hat{\beta}_1$. Some implications of this inequality are discussed below.

One of the consequences of the Murray's Law optimality is that, if z = 3 at each bifurcation of the tree, the shear stress on the vessel walls, which is inversely proportional to D^3, is constant throughout the tree (21,26,27). For Poiseuille flow, shear stress $= 32\dot{Q}\mu/\pi D^3 = 8v\mu/D$. Thus, when z = 3 (i.e., $\dot{Q}$ is proportional to D^3 and mean linear velocity, v, is proportional to D), shear stress is independent of D. Because shear stress is a force that can be transduced by the endothelial lining of the blood vessels and has been shown to influence both vascular function (28,29) and growth (28,30), it is appealing to imagine that deviations from a shear stress set point might be the error signal in a feedback system controlling the architecture of the tree. However, in hetereogeneous asymmetrical vascular trees, the value of z generally varies among bifurcations. Thus, even if the average value of z were 3 (the Murray's Law value), the local shear stress would not be constant throughout the tree. To demonstrate this, simulated vascular trees were constructed as indicated above. The asymmetry of the tree was varied while the mean value of z, D_a, and the total number of vessels were held constant. Figure 11 shows how, for the same total flow, the mean of the local shear stress and the coefficient of variation in local shear stress and the coefficient of variation in z increased with increasing asymmetry, even though the mean value of z was always 3. To maintain a constant mean value of z as the tree becomes more asymmetrical and the variance in z in-

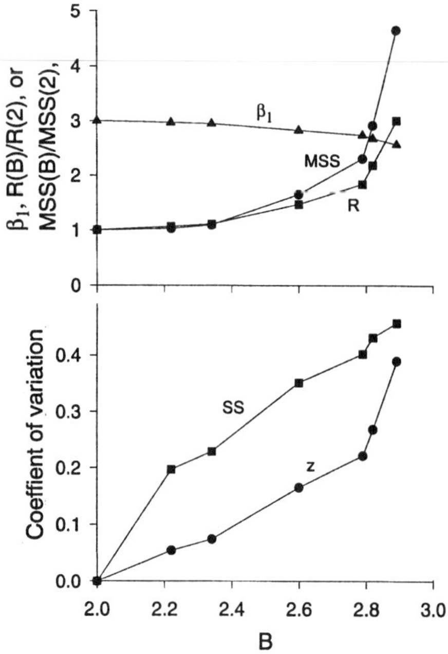

Figure 11 The impact of asymmetry, as represented by B, on simulated arterial trees all having the same mean value of $z = 3$. **Top,** The mean shear stress as a function of B, MSS(B), normalized to MSS(2); the total arterial resistance, R(B), normalized to the total resistance when $B = 2$, and β_l. Note that MSS(B) and R(B) increased with B, whereas β_l decreased. **Bottom,** The coefficient of variations in shear stress, SS, and in z increased with increasing asymmetry.

creases, β_l must decrease, and, thus, the mean shear stress and total resistance increase. This example of the impact of heterogeneity in relation to Murray's Law demonstrates that, even though we have emphasized the single parameter β_l as a key link between structure and function, there are specific functional consequences of the heterogeneity in structure that are not anticipated by averaged morphometric measurements and homogeneous assumptions.

With respect to the applicability of Murray's Law to the pulmonary arterial tree, even the average value of z appears to be significantly smaller than 3. Horsfield and Woldenberg (31) measured the diameters of the three vessel segments at nearly 2000 bifurcations of human pulmonary arterial tree casts. They found that the mean value of z was approximately 2.3, and, thus, considerably smaller than 3. The mean value of z for the same dog pulmonary arterial bifurcations as in Figure 7 is about 2.4 ± 1.2 SD and essentially independent of D_l in the range of diameters studied. At least in part because such deviations from

Murray's Law are common in vascular trees, investigations into the value of z predicted by alternative optimization principles have been carried out as well. For example, Horsfield and Woldenberg (31) point out that Uylings (32) demonstrated that the application of the general concept developed by Murray to the case of turbulent flow yields a value of $z = 2.33$. This value is close to their observed value, but the significance of this coincidence is not clear because Reynold's numbers are generally too low within the pulmonary vessels to consider this to be a fundamental optimality principle for the pulmonary arterial tree. Decreasing the power of the diameter in the maintenance cost term reduces the optimal value of z. For example, if luminal surface area rather than volume were minimized for a given hydraulic power dissipation, the optimal z would be 2.5. The inclusion of the diameter dependence of blood viscosity (the Fahraeus-Lindqvist effect) in the development of the Murray's Law optimization would also result in an optimal value of $z < 3$ in vessels smaller than about 0.3 mm in diameter, but the effect would be quite small (11).

With respect to the pulmonary arterial impedance, one might also consider the impact of the value of β_l on the longitudinal distribution of pulmonary arterial compliance as well as on resistance. The total cost of pumping the blood into the pulmonary artery includes both steady flow and oscillatory flow components. The latter depends on the pulmonary arterial input impedance, which, in turn, depends on the distributions of both compliance and resistance within the pulmonary arterial tree. Because the distensibility of the pulmonary arteries (defined as the fractional change in vessel diameter per unit change in transmural pressure) is nearly constant (independent of vessel diameter) throughout the pulmonary arterial tree (33), the vascular compliance is in nearly constant proportion to vascular volume throughout the pulmonary arterial tree (13). Thus, from Figure 5, it can be observed that if β_l were near 3, the relative longitudinal distributions of compliance (volume) and resistance would be essentially the same throughout the pulmonary arterial tree. In so far as the higher compliance per unit resistance upstream is favored for providing the appropriate pulmonary arterial input impedance, so would $\beta_l < 3$. West et al. (34) demonstrated how in large vessels with pulsitile flow the Murray's law like optimization would lead to z (or β_l in a homogeneous tree) equal to 2.

The observed deviations from $z = 3$ also serve to emphasize that optimality with respect to power dissipation is probably not the only influence of arterial diameters subject to evolutionary selection. For example, even though it is clear that the local flows can be quite heterogeneous in the lungs (35–39), there are limits on the heterogeneity in local flows consistent with optimal gas exchange efficiency. In so far as local flows may be influenced by the heterogeneity in the arterial tree structure, we can examine how the value of β_l might have an impact on the distribution of local flows. The smaller the value of β_l, the more the resistance is concentrated in the small vessels and the more the larger arteries act as a relatively constant pressure manifold through which flow can be distributed among parallel pathways with relatively small resistance over a relatively large fraction of the distance along each stream tube. This would tend to reduce the impact of the distribution of distances traveled (the shape of the tree) on the stream tube flows. To explore this effect using model simulations, one might take the point of view that the volume and shape of the lung served by the arterial tree establishes what the distribution of stream tube lengths has to be. Thus, we can examine how variations in β_l might influence the distribution of local flows if the arterial tree structure were the dominant factor controlling the flow distribution in the lungs. In the simulations, "local flows" are the flows through the terminal arterioles. Figure 12 shows an example of how the coefficient of variation in the terminal arterial flows for a simulated arterial tree of given size and shape varies with β_l. The shape of the graph on Figure 12 reflects two competing effects. One is the decrease in the contribution of the distribution in stream tube lengths to the terminal flow distribution as β_l decreases (the manifold effect). The other is the increase in total variation in diameters, and in the coefficient of variation in diameters in a minimum full flow set, as β_l decreases. If β_l is too large, the distribution of stream tube lengths dominates the terminal arterial flow distribution. If β_l is too small, the parallel variation in diameters begins to have a more dominant effect on the distribution of terminal flows. In the simulations represented in Figure 12, the minimum coefficient of variation in terminal flows occurs when β_l is near 2. The specific value of β_l at the minimum is model dependent, but this simulation reveals how the impact of geometry on the variance of the flow distribution might favor lower values of

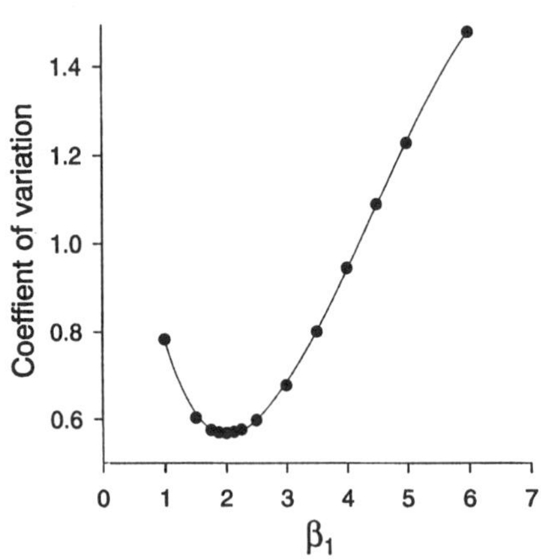

Figure 12 The impact of β_l on the coefficient of variation of the terminal flow distribution in simulated pulmonary arterial trees.

β_1 than predicted by Murray's law for a homogeneous tree. With respect to the robustness of design, the concentration of the resistance near the terminal arterioles (i.e., a small value of β_1) also means that the fine control in the biological growth algorithm can be focused near the terminal vessels where the arteriole diameters and number density have a dominant impact on total arterial tree resistance and local flows. Thus, local growth mechanisms need not include a very long memory regarding the preceding upstream growth patterns.

VIII. Summary

With respect to our objective indicated in the introduction, the simulations suggest at least two conclusions. One is that, in so far as the model tree is consistent with the actual pulmonary arterial tree morphometry, the morphometric parameter β_1 has dominant influence over the longitudinal distribution of vascular resistance, which is relatively insensitive to the asymmetry of the tree. Thus, the arterial tree design appears to be robust in this regard. Another is that the distribution of capillary perfusion, which, along with the distribution of ventilation, determines the efficiency of gas exchange in the lungs, may be one aspect of pulmonary arterial tree function that might impact on the evolutionary selection of the actual value of β_1.

The simulations used in this chapter represent some examples of ways that one might attempt to understand the complexity of the pulmonary arterial tree structure. The simulation approach has at least two potential pitfalls, one is basic to inductive reasoning, namely, that we have not tried all conceivable simulations. Thus, there may be counterexamples that we have missed. Another is that we may not have included some relevant and significant structural rule in the simulation model. One apparent limitation of the model is that the simple algorithm used to construct asymmetrical trees consistent with the morphometric data appears to be conservative in that its maximum allowable asymmetry may be somewhat less asymmetrical than in some real pulmonary arterial trees. This is reflected in the fact that the maximum value of B obtained from Strahler ordering of the simulated trees is about 3, whereas a value as high as 3.69 can be calculated for at least one pulmonary arterial tree cast (7). We suspect that the basic concepts we have discussed will prove to have validity at some level despite these limitations of the approach taken. The main objective at this point is to raise some possible ways of approaching the complexity of the pulmonary arterial structure–function relationships that might be useful to consider in future studies. At present, the data on the entire pulmonary arterial tree morphometry comes from casts from only a few lungs under a narrow range of specific conditions, which are generally not as close to those typical of the normal physiological state as one might like. Data on the morphometry of vascular trees under different physiological and pathophysiological conditions are almost nonexistent. However, modern imaging methods applied to the functioning pulmonary arterial tree (14–18) promise to provide a broader data base from which to understand pulmonary artery structure-function relationships in the future.

References

1. Miller WS. The structure of the lung. J Morphol 1893; 8:165–188.
2. Horsfield K. Morphometry of small pulmonary arteries in man. Circ Res 1978; 42: 593–597.
3. Horsfield K. Functional morphology of the pulmonary vasculature. In: Chang HK, Paiva M, eds. Respiratory Physiology: An Analytical Approach. Vol. 40. New York: Marcel Dekker, 1989:499–531.
4. Singhal S, Henderson R, Horsfield K, Harding K, Cumming G. Morphometry of the human pulmonary arterial tree. Circ Res 1973; 33:190–197.
5. Yen RT, Zhuang FY, Fung YC, Ho HH, Tremer H, Sobin SS. Morphometry of cat's pulmonary arterial tree. J Biomech Eng 1984; 106:131–136.
6. Jiang ZI, Kassab GS, Fung YC. Diameter-defined Strahler system and connectivity matrix of the pulmonary arterial tree. J Appl Physiol 1994; 76:882–892.
7. Gan RZ, Yen RT. Vascular impedance analysis in dog lung with detailed morphometric and elasticity data. J Appl Physiol 1994; 77:706–717.
8. Uylings HBM, Smit GJ, Veltman WAM. Ordering methods in quantitative analysis of branching of dendritic trees. Adv Neurol 1975; 12:247–254.
9. VanPelt J, Verwer RWH, Uylings HBM. Centrifugal-order distributions in binary topological trees. Bull Math Biol 1989; 51:511–536.
10. Weibel ER. Morphometry of the Human Lung. Berlin: Springer-Verlag, 1963.
11. Sherman TF. On connecting large vessels to small: the meaning of Murray's law. J Gen Physiol 1981; 78:431–453.
12. Krenz GS, Lin J, Dawson CA, Linehan JH. Impact of parallel heterogeneity on a continuum model of the pulmonary arterial tree. J Appl Physiol 1994; 77:660–670.
13. Krenz GS, Linehan JH, Dawson CA. A fractal continuum model of the pulmonary arterial tree. J Appl Physiol 1992; 72:2225–2237.
14. Al-Tinawi A, Krenz GS, Rickaby DA, Linehan JH, Dawson CA. Influence of hypoxia and serotonin on small pulmonary vessels. J Appl Physiol 1994; 76:56–64.
15. Dawson CA, Krenz GS, Al-Tinawi A, Linehan JH. Hemodynamic interpretation of pulmonary arterial tree images. SPIE Proceedings 1995; 2433:46–55.
16. Liu Y-H, Hoffman EA, Ritman EL. Measurement of three-dimensional anatomy and function of pulmonary arteries with high-speed x-ray computed tomography. Invest Radiol 1987; 22:28–36.
17. Liu Y-H, Ritman EL. Branching pattern of pulmonary arterial tree in anesthetized dogs. J Biomech Eng 1986; 108:289–293.
18. Wood SA, Zerhouni EA, Hoford JD, Hoffman EA, Mitzner W. Measurement of three-dimensional lung tree structures by using computed tomography. J Appl Physiol 1995; 79:1687–1697.

19. Weibel E. Fractal geometry: a design principle for living organisms. Am J Physiol 1991; 261:L361–L369.
20. Murray DC. The physiological principle of minimum work. I. The vascular system and the cost of blood volume. Proc Natl Acad Sci U S A 1926; 12:207–214.
21. Kassab GS, Fung YC. The pattern of coronary arteriolar bifurcations and the uniform shear hypothesis. Ann Biomed Eng 1995; 23:13–20.
22. LaBarbera M. Principles of Design of Fluid Transport Systems in Zoology. Science 1990; 249:992–1000.
23. Mayrovitz HN, Roy J. Microvascular blood flow: evidence indicating a cubic dependence on arteriolar diameter. Am J Physiol 1983; 245:H1031–H1038.
24. Woldenberg MJ, Horsfield K. Relation of branching angles to optimality for four cost principles. J Theor Biol 1986; 122:187–204.
25. Zamir M. Optimality principles in arterial branching. J Theor Biol 1976; 62:227–251.
26. Zamir M. Shear forces and blood vessel radii in the cardiovascular system. J Gen Physiol 1977; 69:449–461.
27. Zamir M. The role of shear forces in arterial branching. J Gen Physiol 1976; 67: 213–222.
28. Nerem RM. Hemodynamics and the vascular endothelium. J Biomech Eng 1993; 115:510–514.
29. Rubanyi GM, Freay AD, Kauser K, Johns A, Harder DR. Mechanoreception by the endothelium: mediators and mechanisms of pressure and flow-induced vascular responses. Blood Vessels 1990; 27:246–257.
30. Ohno M, Cooke JP, Dzau VJ, Gibbons GH. Fluid shear stress induces endothelial transforming growth factor beta-1 transcription and production. Modulation by potassium channel blockade. J Clin Invest 1995; 95:1363–1369.
31. Horsfield K, Woldenberg MJ. Diameters and cross-sectional areas of branches in the human pulmonary arterial tree. Anat Rec 1989; 223:245–251.
32. Uylings HBM. Optimization of diameters and bifurcation angles in lung and vascular tree structures. Bull Math Biol 1977; 39:509–520.
33. Al-Tinawi A, Madden JA, Dawson CA, Linehan JH, Harder DR, Rickaby DA. Distensibility of small arteries of the dog lung. J Appl Physiol 1991; 71:1714–1722.
34. West GB, Brown JH, Enquist BJ. A general model for the origin of allometric scaling laws in biology. Science 1977; 274:122–126.
35. Glenny RW, Polissar L, Robertson HT. Relative contribution of gravity to pulmonary perfusion heterogeneity. J Appl Physiol 1991; 71:2449–2452.
36. Glenny RW, Robertson HT. Fractal modeling of pulmonary blood flow heterogeneity. J Appl Physiol 1991; 70:1024–1030.
37. Hakim TS, Lisbona R, Dean GW. Gravity-independent inequality in pulmonary blood flow in humans. J Appl Physiol 1987; 63:1114–1121.
38. West JB, Dollery CT. Distribution of blood flow and the pressure-flow relations of the whole lung. J Appl Physiol 1965; 20:175–183.
39. Hughes JMB, Glazier JB, Maloney JE, West JB. Effect of lung volume on the distribution of pulmonary blood flow in the dog lung. J Appl Physiol 1968; 58–72.
40. Haworth ST, Linehan JH, Bronikowski TA, Dawson CA. A hemodynamic model representation of the dog lung. J Appl Physiol 1991; 70:15–26.

14

Complexity of Perfusion in the Pulmonary Gas Exchange Vessels

WILTZ W. WAGNER, JR., and ROBERT G. PRESSON, JR.

Indiana University School of Medicine
Indianapolis, Indiana

I. Introduction

Basic lung anatomy is simple: airways terminate in alveoli and the arterial and venous trees interconnect via capillaries embedded in alveolar walls. The complexity of the structure comes from its vast numbers: 300,000,000 alveoli and their accompanying 3×10^{11} capillaries (1). These numbers are so overwhelming that anatomists and, more particularly, physiologists have unabashedly simplified the lung to a one alveolus–one capillary essence (Figure 1). With time, this conceptual model has tended to become the real lung. Even some senior scientists express considerable surprise when they realize that pulmonary capillary pathways cross more than one alveolus (personal communications).

Multiple alveolar crossings by the capillaries were clearly shown by Staub and Schultz in dog, cat, and rabbit lungs (2). They perfused pulmonary arteries in isolated lungs with Sudan black-stained olive oil. Surface tension prevented the oil from penetrating further than the terminal arterioles, thereby distinguishing them from the blood-filled venules. The lungs were rapidly frozen in liquid propane, sectioned, and photomicrographed. The shortest path was measured along alveolar walls from each arteriole (<60 μm diameter) to all neighboring venules (<60 μm diameter), and the number of alveoli crossed was counted.

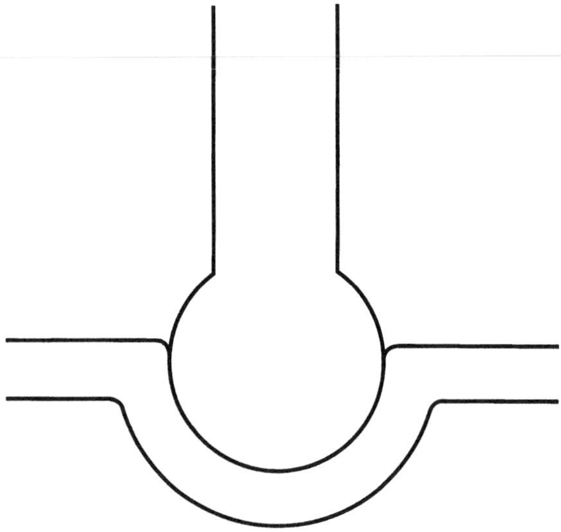

Figure 1 The essence of the lung as a gas exchanger widely used by physiologists as a model. This one alveolus–one capillary model, however, grossly oversimplifies the anatomical complexity of the lung.

These pathways crossed an average of 5–7 alveolar walls, depending on the species (Table 1). Because each alveolar wall separated two adjacent alveolar spaces, the total number of alveoli crossed was 10–14.

The measurements of Staub and Schultz were estimates of the minimum distance between arterioles and venules. Blood cells traveling through the capillaries, however, are not constrained to take the shortest pathways. Rather, the

Table 1 Multiple Alveoli Are Crossed by Pulmonary Capillaries

Species	Distance (μm)[a]	Alveoli Crossed[b]
Dog	823	7.3
Cat	850	6.1
Rabbit	603	5.4

[a]Average shortest distance from terminal arteriole to venule on the interior of the lung.
[b]Average number of alveoli crossed by a red blood cell traveling from a terminal arteriole to a venule via the shortest route.
Data from Ref. 2.

red cells traverse a range of pathways of varying distances. The scanning electron micrograph in Figure 2 illustrates some of these pathway options. Feeding and draining vessels slightly larger than capillaries are located several alveoli apart. In between lies the complex capillary bed that crosses a number of alveolar walls and provides a myriad of pathways for red cells to reach the venule. In Figure 3, an alveolar duct is cut in cross section. A small arteriole accompanies the duct. The draining venule is located several alveoli away to the right. These micrographs begin to demonstrate the complexity of the capillary network, but, because of the near two-dimensional nature of the cut tissue, the complexity is understated. To imagine the true anatomy, the sections must be rotated in three dimensions. Only then can the number of available pathways across the capillary network be appreciated. Quantification of the range of pathways in the alveolar-capillary bed is a daunting prospect. One of the few attempts to deal with the complex structure of the pulmonary microcirculation has been made by Zhuang et al. (3). These investigators identified arterioles and venules by a staining technique in vascular-injected cat lungs. The arterioles and venules were clustered in different territories giving the appearance of islands surrounded by oceans (Figure 4). Utilizing stereological analysis, they found

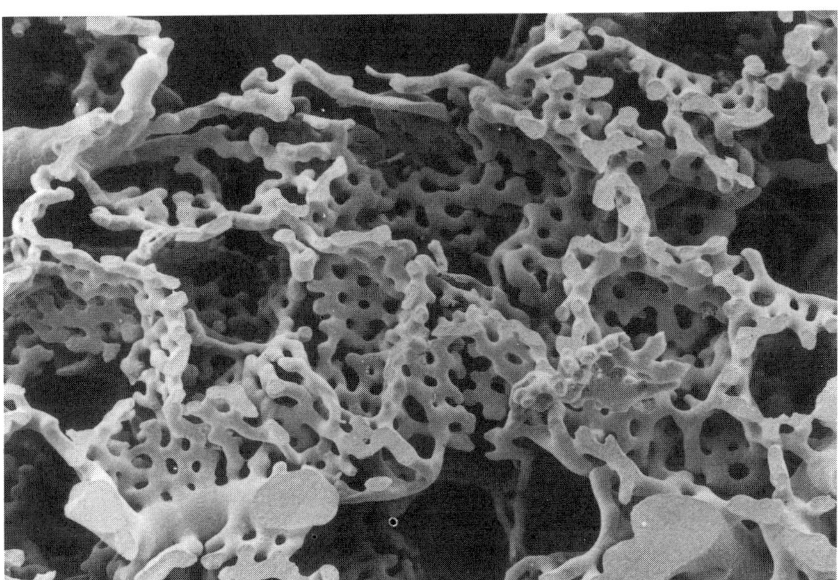

Figure 2 Scanning electron micrograph showing arterioles feeding directly into the capillary network. The capillary bed crosses several alveolar walls and provides a large number of pathway options for red cells to traverse. (Courtesy of E. R. Weibel)

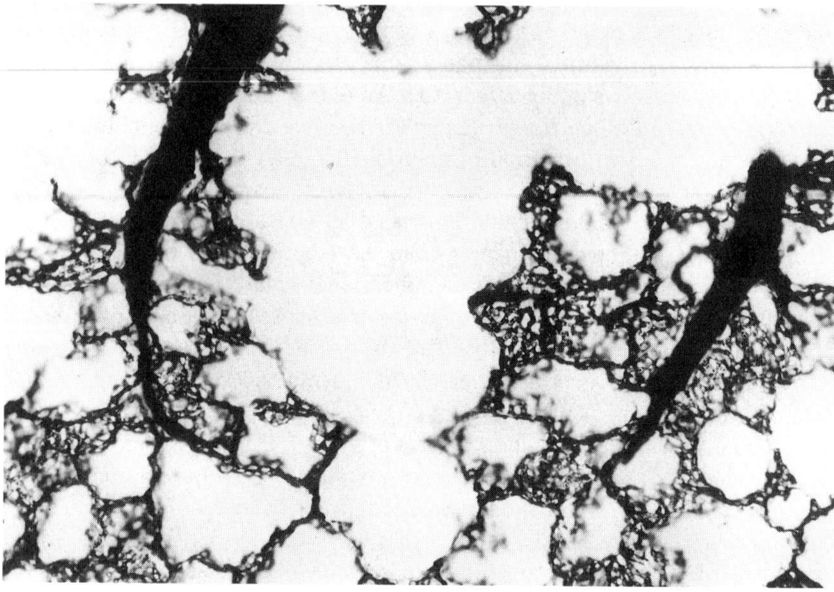

Figure 3 Cross section of an alveolar duct with accompanying arteriole. The draining venule is located several alveoli away to the right. (Courtesy of M. F. König)

that each arteriole (in the islands) was drained by an average of 1.4 venules (in the oceans). Each arteriole supplied about 25 alveoli, and each venule drained about 18 alveoli.

If the anatomical complexity was not enough to cloud the physiological understanding of the pulmonary microcirculation, additional difficulties arise from the conditions of the investigations themselves. For example, results from one species tend to be applied wholesale to all mammalian lungs. An obvious illustration of this problem comes from comparing the pulmonary physiology of quadrupeds to upright human beings. Being species chauvinists, we tend to visualize all lungs as being oriented upright, even though our pulmonary orientation is an oddity in nature. The construction and gravitational orientation is grossly different in quadrupeds, however. In the familiar canine subject, the thorax is constructed so that little of the lung lies in the most dependent part of the chest. In cross section, the internal perimeter of the thoracic cavity is heart shaped (Figure 5). The heart itself occupies much of the volume in the narrow ventral portion of the cavity, with additional volume taken up by the diaphragm (Figure 5). This arrangement leaves the large dorsal portion of the cavity available entirely for lung. If a dried specimen of dog lung is cut into isogravimetric slices

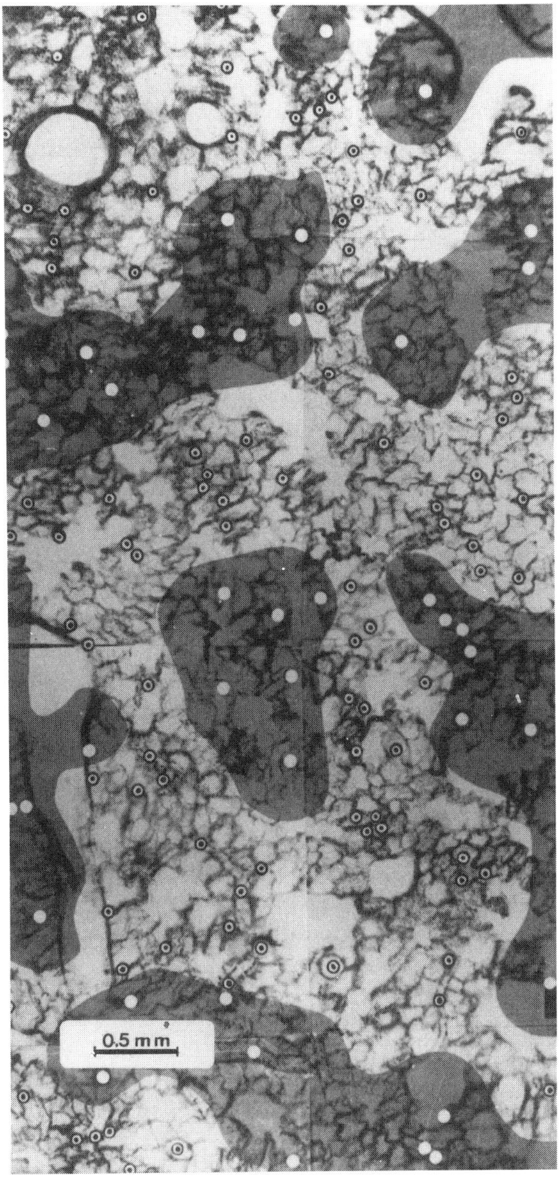

Figure 4 In vascular-injected cat lungs, arterioles and venules are clustered in different territories, giving the appearance of islands (arterioles) surrounded by oceans (venules). Stereological analysis showed that each arteriole was drained by an average of 1.4 venules. Each arteriole supplied about 25 alveoli, and each venule drained about 18 alveoli. (From Ref. 3.)

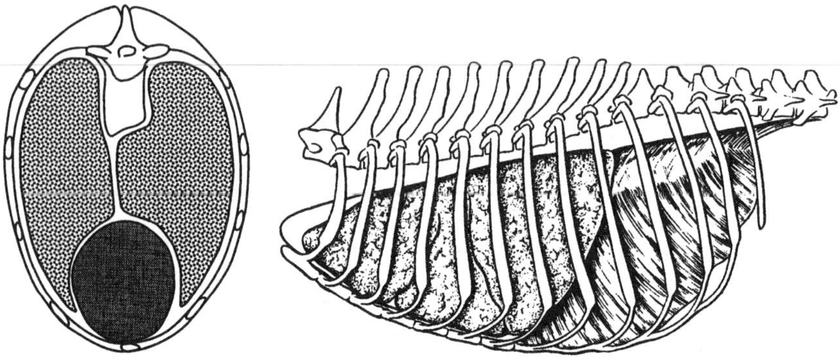

Figure 5 Transverse section of the thoracic cavity (*left*). The heart occupies much of the volume in the ventral portion of the cavity, with additional volume taken up by the diaphragm (*right*.) (Modified from Ref. 58.)

and each slice is weighed, the large majority of tissue lies in the upper half of the thorax (Figure 6). Because of this arrangement, an upward redistribution of blood flow with exercise, as has been shown in the horse (4), would recruit considerable reserves of gas exchange surface area. The relatively low vertical height of the quadruped lung compared with that of upright humans suggests that recruitment in the quadruped would require a more modest increase in pulmonary arterial pressure. Other examples of how directly comparing data from different species and different techniques leads to apparent complexity, or, more accurately, confusion, are discussed throughout this chapter.

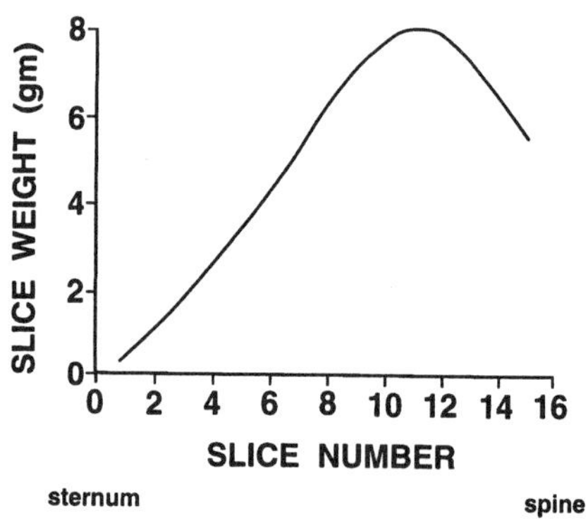

Figure 6 Coronal (isogravimetric) slices of dog lung versus weight. Unlike in the human lung, the majority of the exchange surface area lies in the upper lung.

II. The Effect of Pulmonary Microvascular Anatomy on Perfusion

Although pulmonary microvascular anatomy and its effect on perfusion is extremely complex, it is not hopelessly so. We have considerable information about the limits of complexity. During basal conditions, the vascular gas exchange reserve is not fully utilized and the blood flowing through the capillaries has a large number of pathway options. Perfusion complexity is maximal during these conditions. As is described subsequently, evidence is accumulating that, as oxygen uptake nears maximal, perfusion of the gas exchange vessels becomes simpler: nearly all of the capillaries become perfused, capillary segmental resistances likely become similar, and the transit time distribution becomes more uniform.

In trying to understand the complexities of pulmonary capillary perfusion, we consider three kinds of changes that occur in the capillary bed as cardiac output increases from rest to exercise and individual capillaries dilate in response to increasing transmural pressures. (Through common usage, opening a capillary often means opening it to red blood cell flow, whereas distention implies further enlargement after a capillary is already being perfused by red cells. Here we specify "dilate" to encompass any enlargement of a capillary diameter: from zero, to admitting plasma alone, to permitting red cell flow [recruitment], and finally to distending after red cell flow has been established.) First, as capillaries dilate sufficiently to permit the passage of red blood cells, the newly recruited capillaries add to the surface area for gas exchange. Second, as pressure continues to increase, further capillary distention occurs, which increases capillary blood volume. Third, the red blood cells flow more rapidly through the capillary bed.

Under resting conditions, it has been calculated that red blood cells become fully saturated with oxygen after crossing approximately the first one-third of the capillary bed, the remaining two-thirds serve simply as conduits. As red cell velocity increases, more and more of the total length of the capillary pathways become used for gas exchange, thereby adding to the gas exchanging portion of capillary volume and increasing the number of red blood cells that are oxygenated per unit time, that is, capillary length is recruited. In a sense, all three of these capillary changes are forms of recruitment: 1. perfusing unperfused capillaries recruits surface area directly, 2. distention recruits blood volume in gas exchange vessels as more red cells crowd into individual capillaries, and 3. as red cell velocity increases, more and more of the total length of the capillary pathways become used for gas exchange, effectively recruiting capillary length. Each change is discussed as are methods that have been used to measure the respective changes in capillary recruitment.

A. Distention

Distention of the capillaries has been studied extensively by Fung, Sobin, and Yen (5–8). Much of their work has been based on careful measurements of capillary diameters filled under various pressure conditions by a polymer, which, after having flowed into all of the vessels, formed a cast of the capillary bed (5,6). The appearance of the extraordinarily dense capillary network embedded in thin alveolar walls suggested that perfusion of the pulmonary capillaries functioned more like a sheet of flowing blood rather than flow through a network of tubes. Measurements of the polymer casts produced the relationship shown in Figure 7. In this preparation, once transmural capillary pressure ex-

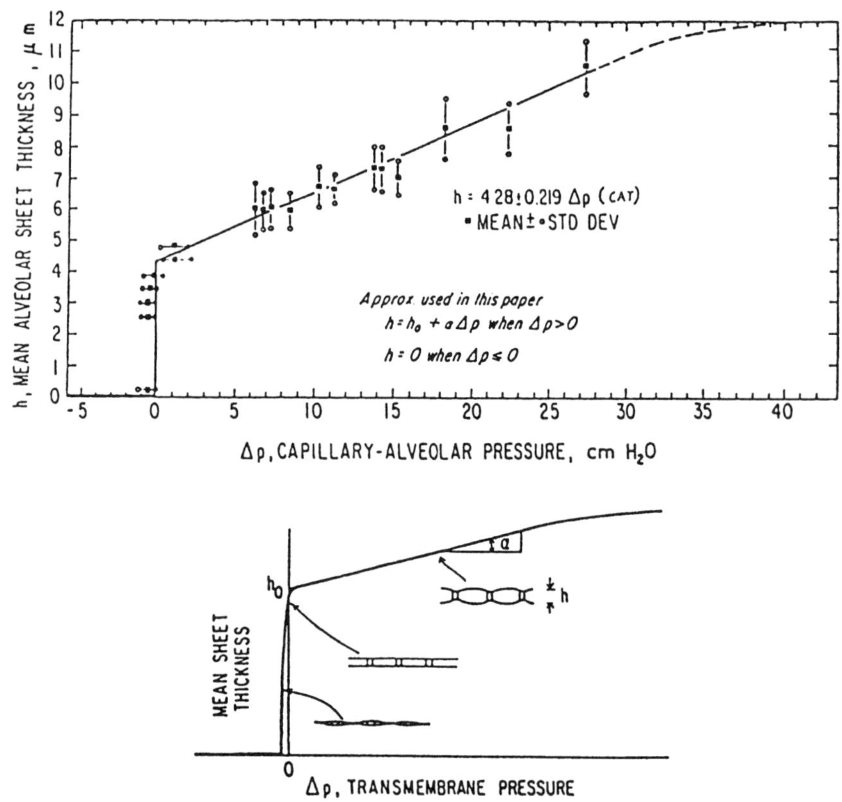

Figure 7 **Upper panel**, The nonlinear distensibility of the pulmonary capillaries in cat lungs. Transmural capillary pressure is shown on the x-axis and sheet thickness on the y-axis. The sheet remains empty until capillary pressure ≈ 0, then the sheet opens suddenly to a thickness of ~4 μm and distends linearly thereafter. **Lower panel**, Theoretical capillary shapes are shown. (From Ref. 5.)

ceeded zero, thereby exceeding alveolar pressure, the capillary bed opened suddenly to form a sheet ~4 μm thick. Additional pressure increases produced a linear increase in thickness. The sheet flow model permitted mathematical modeling of capillary hemodynamics. The complexity of other models, composed of a seemingly infinite number of tubes as wide as they were long, made it impossible to manage the mathematical analysis of flow.

Other workers have also found that the capillaries distended as pressure increased. In their classical paper, Glazier et al. (9) studied isolated perfused greyhound lungs that were rapidly frozen. The lungs were frozen under three vascular pressure conditions: 1. where alveolar pressure was greater than pulmonary arterial pressure, which, in turn, was greater than pulmonary venous pressure, and there was little or no flow ($P_A > P_{pa} > P_{pv}$ = zone 1); 2. where arterial pressure exceeded alveolar pressure but alveolar pressure was greater than venous pressure ($P_{pa} > P_A > P_{pv}$ = zone 2); and 3. where arterial pressure exceeded venous pressure and venous pressure was greater than alveolar pressure ($P_{pa} > P_{pv} > P_A$ = zone 3). In lungs frozen under zone 2 and zone 3 conditions, the capillaries distended linearly as vascular transmural pressure increased (Figure 8).

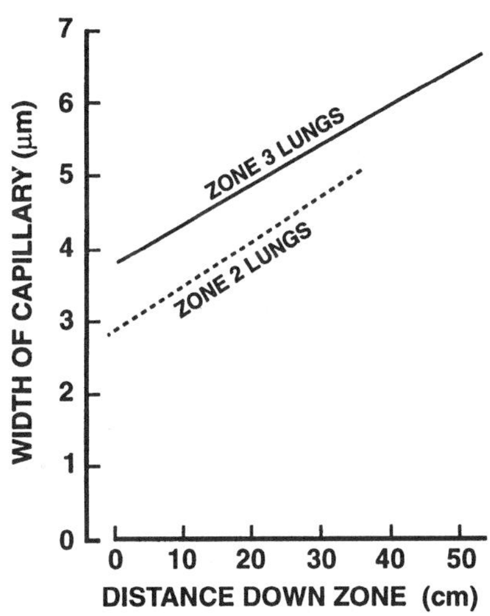

Figure 8 Capillary widths measured in dog lungs rapidly frozen under zone 2 and 3 conditions. The x-axis, distance down zone, refers to the idea that a given zone in the lung exists over a significant distance over which the transmural pressure increases. When distance down zone = 0, the width of the capillaries was measured at the uppermost level of the zone. Distension is linear under both zone 2 and 3 conditions. (Modified from Ref. 9.)

As a final note about distending capillaries, the situation becomes more complex when hematocrit is considered. In individual capillaries, hematocrit varies from moment to moment, as can readily be demonstrated by in vivo microscopy. As the capillaries distend sufficiently to admit red blood cells on edge, rouleau formations become possible. In that extreme, capillary hematocrit can reach very high values. On the other hand, large plasma gaps between red cells can reduce individual capillary segmental hematocrit to 0%. Other combinations of red cells and plasma cause the entire gamut of hematocrits to be run in a matter of seconds. These variations have not been quantitated nor have the implications for gas exchange been explored.

B. Recruitment

The model of capillary recruitment on a segment-by-segment basis has conflicted directly with the sheet flow model. This disparity between capillary recruitment models has been a difficult and important issue to resolve. The evidence supporting each idea seems solid, yet the physiological implications of each model are significantly different. Recent work by Godbey et al. (10) may have resolved the issue, because they found a way in which capillaries could be predictably recruited either segment by segment or as a sheet. The pattern of recruitment did not depend on capillary pressure or on alveolar pressure per se; rather, the recruitment pattern depended in a surprising way on the state of distention of the alveoli.

In these experiments, Godbey et al. (10) used video microscopy to quantify capillary recruitment in individual subpleural alveolar walls. Excised canine lobes were perfused with autologous blood at flow rates low enough to reduce the arteriovenous pressure gradient to <5 and often <3 mmHg. Such small gradients permitted capillary pressure to be reasonably estimated by averaging the arterial and venous pressures. In each lobe, capillary pressure was varied stepwise from airway pressure up to 30 mmHg above airway pressure by increasing the venous reservoir and adjusting the pump rate to maintain the low transcapillary pressure gradient. Capillaries began to be perfused by red blood cells at precisely the point where capillary pressure exceeded airway pressure.

At low positive airway pressures, the capillaries opened suddenly over a narrow pressure range (Figure 9*A*), exactly as predicted by the sheet flow theory (Figure 7). Even though the lobes appeared reasonably well inflated at 2 mmHg, the alveoli were unusually small in diameter (low distention) when viewed through the microscope. When airway pressure was increased to 10 mmHg, the alveoli enlarged (high distention) and the pressure–recruitment relationship became more linear (Figure 9*B*), indicating that the capillaries were being recruited segment by segment. At an inflation pressure of 15 mmHg, the pressure–recruitment relationship was essentially linear (Figure 9*C*) and alveolar size was

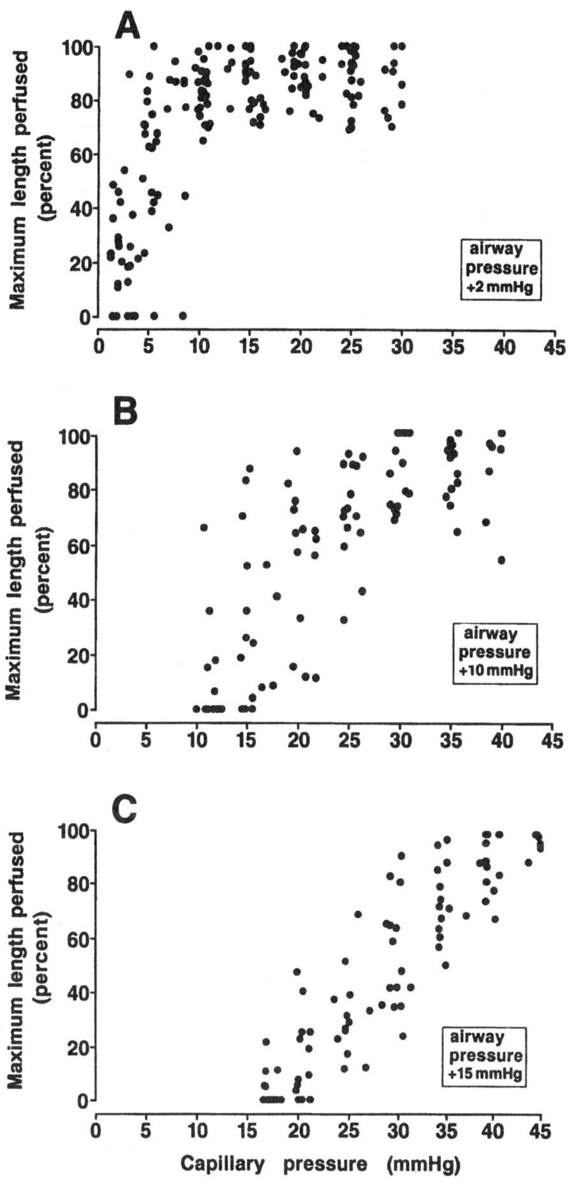

Figure 9 In excised perfused dog lung lobes, when alveolar pressure is low (**A**), the capillary bed opens suddenly and completely as alveolar pressure is exceeded by perfusion pressure; the capillaries are perfused in a sheet-like fashion. As alveolar pressure is increased (**B**) and alveoli enlarge, capillary recruitment occurs more gradually. Once the alveoli are distended (**C**), recruitment is linear. (From Ref. 10.)

similar to the size of the alveoli in the upper lung of the intact dog. The final part of the experiment was to pump perfuse canine lungs while they were sealed in the intact thorax and observe the capillaries through a window implanted in the chest wall. Lungs inflated in this more normal manner have a gradient of alveolar size, with the largest alveolar diameters (greatest distention) found in the upper lung and the smaller diameter alveoli in the lower lung (11). Because the studies were made on the uppermost surface of the lung, the observed alveoli were relatively large (comparable in size to those in the excised lobe inflated to 15 mmHg) and the recruitment relationship was linear (Figure 10), even though alveolar pressure was zero (atmospheric).

These experiments showed that each model of capillary recruitment was correct. Which model is appropriate, however, depends on the amount of alveolar distention. The sheet flow model seems more predictive for the lower lung where alveoli are small. Segment-by-segment recruitment seems more appropriate in the upper lung where alveoli are large. Although volume in the upright human lung diminishes toward the apex, the reverse is the case for quadrupeds (Figure 5). In large quadrupeds, therefore, segment-by-segment recruitment is likely to be the more accurate model for the majority of the lung.

That the state of alveolar distention could so dramatically affect capillary recruitment characteristics was unexpected and surprising. One explanation is

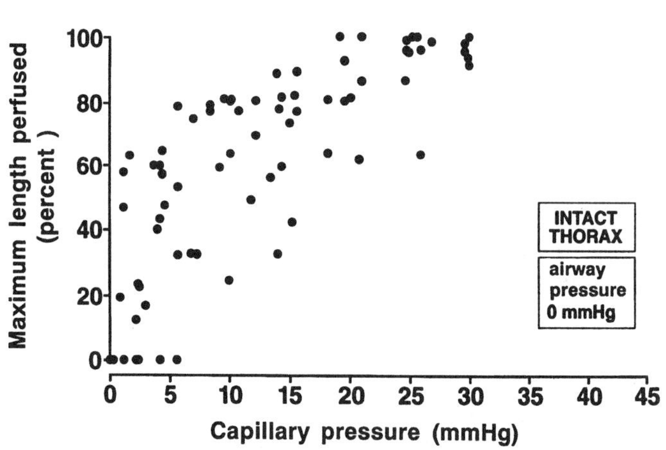

Figure 10 Recruitment pattern in lungs inflated by negative intrapleural pressure and perfused in intact canine thorax (airway pressure = 0 mmHg). Highly distended alveoli in the uppermost lung have capillary networks that are distended on a segment-by-segment basis. (Modified from Ref. 10.)

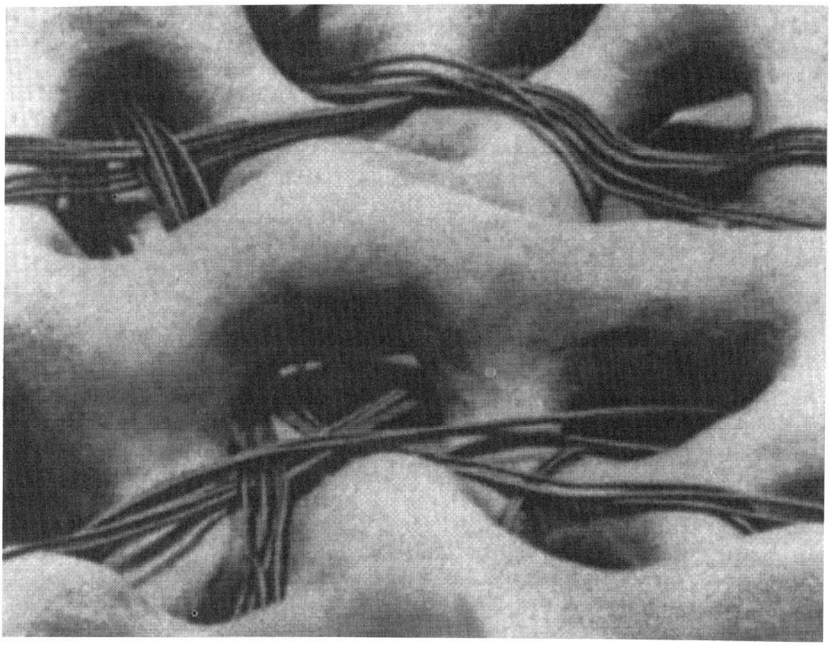

Figure 11 Model of connective tissue fibers weaving between capillary segments. When alveoli are not distended and connective tissue fibers are slack, all capillaries can be readily perfused as microvascular pressure exceeds alveolar pressure. As alveoli distend, connective tissue fibers stretch. Individual fibers become progressively taut, but not equally so. Taut fibers cross each capillary and tend to pinch the segments. The amount of pinching is thought to vary among segments, causing a range of opening pressures and therefore recruitment over a range of pressures. (Modified from Ref. 12.)

based on the anatomical observation (12) that connective tissue fibers are interlaced throughout the capillary network (Figure 11). When the lobes were inflated to low levels of distention (airway pressure = 2 mmHg), the connective fibers were slack. Under these conditions, all of the capillaries could be readily perfused as microvascular pressure exceeded alveolar pressure. As the alveoli were distended, the connective tissue fibers stretched. Individual fibers became progressively taut, but not equally so. As taut fibers crossed each capillary, they tended to pinch the segments. The amount of pinching would be likely to vary among segments and lead to a range of opening pressures and therefore recruitment over a range of pressures. Further increases in alveolar distention would make these variations more pronounced. Whether alveolar distention was caused by positive airway pressure or by the pull of gravity on a lung suspended by negative intrapleural pressure as in life (0 mmHg airway pressure), progressive capillary recruitment occurred over a wider range of capillary pressures as the alveoli enlarged. In this way, capillary recruitment on a segment-by-segment basis can be explained.

Even though these experiments seemed to resolve a long-standing conflict in interpretation, a potentially important problem remained. The assumption implicit in the observations by Godbey et al. (10) is that capillary recruitment observed on the surface of the lung accurately reflects recruitment in the interior of the lung. This assumption can be questioned because of anatomical differences between interior and subpleural capillaries. For example, the spaces between subpleural capillary segments are significantly larger than between interior segments (13–15). These larger spaces reflect the longer length of subpleural segments. The result is that subpleural networks are of a coarser mesh and occupy a smaller fraction of the alveolar wall than interior networks (15). In addition to these network density differences, subpleural canine capillaries have been shown to be about 20% larger in diameter than interior capillaries (16). The combination of these differences could potentially cause recruitment characteristics to be different between subpleural and interior locations.

To investigate whether subpleural and interior capillaries recruited similarly, Short et al. (16) studied anesthetized rats in which a wide midline thoracotomy had been performed. To obtain a large range of capillary recruitment, lungs were inflated to airway pressures of 25, 12, or 4 cmH_2O in three different groups of animals to create zones 1, 2, and 3, respectively. Liquid propane, cooled to −180°C, was poured over the inflated lungs. Pieces of frozen tissue were removed, freeze dried, sectioned 15 μm thick, and stained for histological examination. The level of capillary recruitment was measured by counting the number of red blood cells/10 μm of alveolar wall. Red blood cell counts were made in both subpleural and interior capillaries in each lung. The number of red blood cells/10 μm of alveolar wall in both interior and subpleural networks progressively decreased as higher inflation pressure was applied (Figure 12). The red blood cell counts were consistently lower in subpleural networks than in interior networks, as expected, because the capillary density was lower there. However, because subpleural counts were a constant proportion of interior counts, they correlated closely with the counts in interior networks (Figure 13). These results showed that recruitment in subpleural capillaries accurately reflected recruitment in interior capillaries.

What was unknown was whether capillaries are the only vessels that recruit in the pulmonary circulation. If arterioles or arteries can be recruited, then the recruitment of a single precapillary vessel would add significantly to capillary volume. Hanson et al. (17) investigated this issue using in vivo microscopy to study capillary segments and branches of arterioles and venules in the dog lung. With each vessel serving as its own control, observations were made dur-

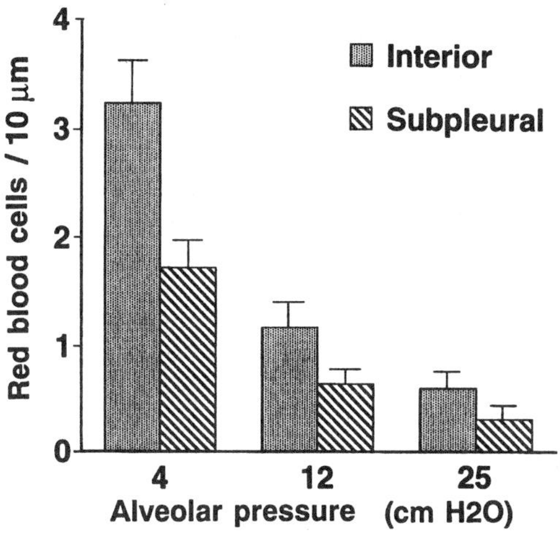

Figure 12 Number of red blood cells/10 μm length of alveolar wall for interior and subpleural capillaries in rat lungs rapidly frozen at low, medium, and high distending pressures. Both subpleural and interior measurements progressively decrease as alveolar pressure increases, showing that recruitment in subpleural capillaries accurately reflects recruitment of interior capillaries. (From Ref. 16.)

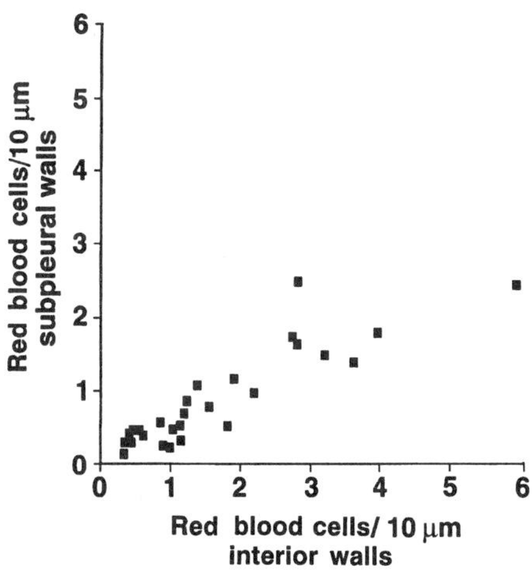

Figure 13 Correlation between red blood cell counts in subpleural and interior capillaries for 27 rats (Pearson's $r = 0.89$). As expected from embryological development of alveolar capillary networks, the interior capillary network is twice as dense as the subpleural network (From Ref. 16.)

ing low and high vascular pressures. The only vessels to recruit were capillaries, indicating that, in the dog, recruitment was exclusively a capillary event. A similar conclusion was reached in the study of Warrell et al. who studied frozen dog lungs (18).

It is not certain, however, whether the same recruitment pattern applies to all species. Godbey et al. (19), in studying supine, anesthetized, spontaneously breathing dogs, found that intravenously injected Monastral Blue dye was distributed evenly on the surface of the lung (91% ± 3% contained dye) (Figure 14). In contrast, in rabbits studied under the same conditions, there were numerous irregular unstained regions several millimeters across which resulted in an average of 77% ± 5% of the surface being perfused (Figure 14). This significant difference in surface perfusion ($p < 0.03$ by unpaired, t test) was also present in the interior of the lung (determined after the lungs were air dried and cut into gross sections). This patchy perfusion pattern has also been reported by Wang et al. (20) who used in vivo microscopy to study rabbit lungs. Because regions of this size are fed by large arterioles or small arteries, the patchy perfusion pattern suggests that recruitment of arterioles and arteries is a likely possibility in rabbits. These findings serve as an example of complexity in the pulmonary microcirculation and illustrate the kind of problem that can occur if the results from one species are applied to another.

All of the data discussed thus far have involved static or very nearly static conditions: injected vessels, frozen lungs, or vessels perfused at very low flow rates all sampled at one point in time. As valuable as those data are, they lack the dynamic quality of perfusion that exists in the living lung. It is during in vivo conditions that the complexity of the pulmonary microcirculation is most apparent. That information can only be obtained by studying the microcirculation in vivo. Data from in vivo microscopy produced the first direct evidence for a recruitable reserve of pulmonary capillaries. Those classic observations were made by Wearn et al. (21) who studied the pulmonary microcirculation on the surface of the cat lung. Not only did they demonstrate that the capillary bed was only partially perfused by red cells at any given time, but they also showed that the perfusion pattern varied with time within a single alveolar wall. Wearn et al. speculated that the changes in the capillary perfusion pattern could be explained by changes in pulmonary blood flow or pressure, but, in 1934, they lacked the techniques necessary to study these hemodynamic variables.

These important findings remained unconfirmed by direct observation for 60 years until Okada et al. (22) repeated Wearn's experiment using modern cardiovascular monitoring combined with in vivo microscopy of an intact canine preparation. During a 45-minute study period, 1-minute observations were made every 5 minutes to determine which capillaries were perfused. On average, Okada found about half of the capillaries to be perfused over the course of a total of nine observations, confirming that not all of the capillaries were per-

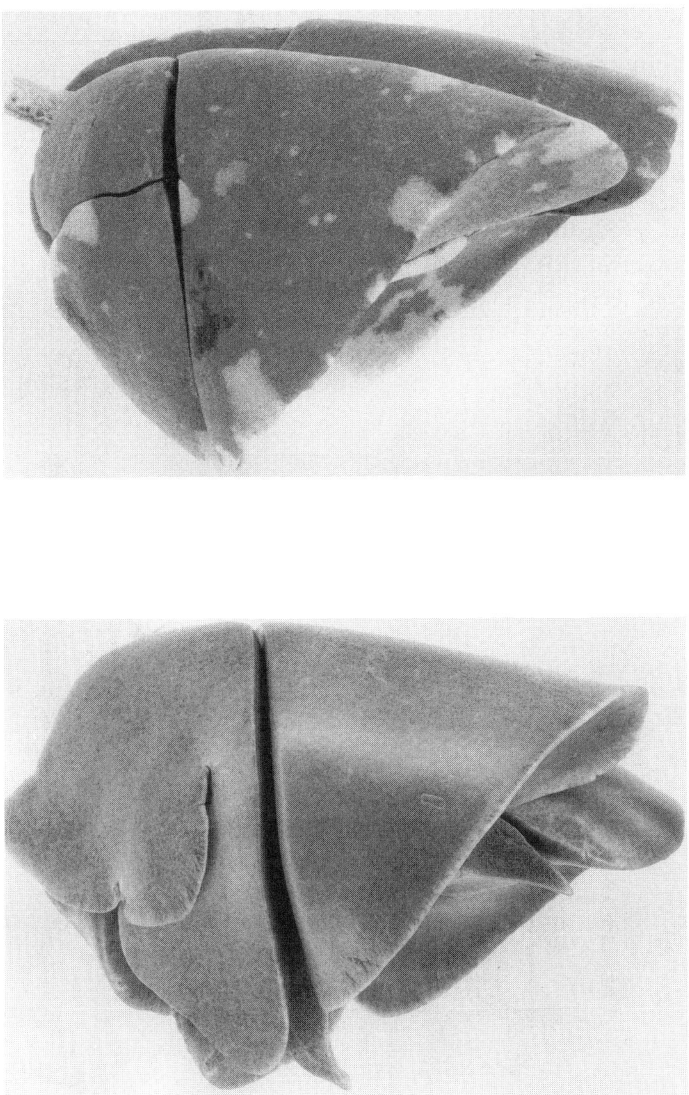

Figure 14 **Left**, Intravenously injected Monastral blue dye was distributed evenly on the surface of supine, anesthetized, spontaneously breathing dog lung (91 ± 3% of the surface contained dye). **Right**, In contrast, in rabbits studied under the same conditions, there were numerous irregular unstained regions several millimeters across, which resulted in an average of 77 ± 5% of the surface being perfused.

fused all of the time. The level of recruitment fluctuated, but the variations in perfusion did not correlate with the small fluctuations in pulmonary arterial pressure or cardiac output that occurred during the study. In most animals, the correlation was poor ($r^2 < 0.06$), which was a surprise, because previous work by this group had shown that pulmonary arterial pressure and capillary recruitment were tightly correlated (Figure 15), at least when the pressure changes were large. These findings imply that capillary perfusion alterations were being influenced by factors more subtle than small variations in pulmonary arterial pressure or cardiac output.

Two striking characteristics emerged when the perfusion of individual capillary segments was studied in detail. First, of the perfused segments, more than half were perfused by red blood cells during at least eight of the nine observations (Figure 16). This finding showed that some capillary segments had hemodynamic characteristics that were sufficiently stable to cause them to be continuously or nearly continuously perfused. These capillaries generally were interconnected to form pathways across entire alveolar walls (Figure 17). Second, the remaining half of the segments were not perfused stably. Some were perfused only once or twice during the nine 1-minute observation periods. The frequency of perfusion of the unstably perfused segments was evenly dispersed among observations (Figure 16) and resulted in considerable switching of flow among the segments within each alveolar network.

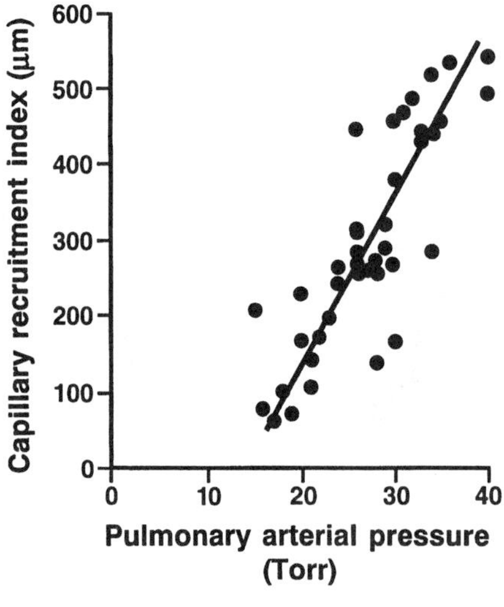

Figure 15 Capillary recruitment occurs linearly in the uppermost portion of the dog lung in vivo. Pulmonary arterial pressure was increased by airway hypoxia. (From Ref. 56.)

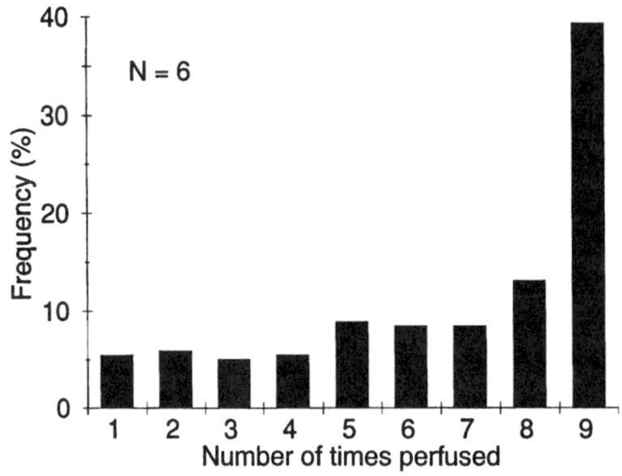

Figure 16 Fraction of total observed capillaries perfused for different numbers of observations in six dogs. A total of nine repeated observations of the same alveolar walls are shown. Half of the capillaries studied were perfused during at least eight of the nine observations. The remaining half of the segments had various degrees of intermittent perfusion and were fairly evenly distributed among different numbers of times perfused. (From Ref. 22.)

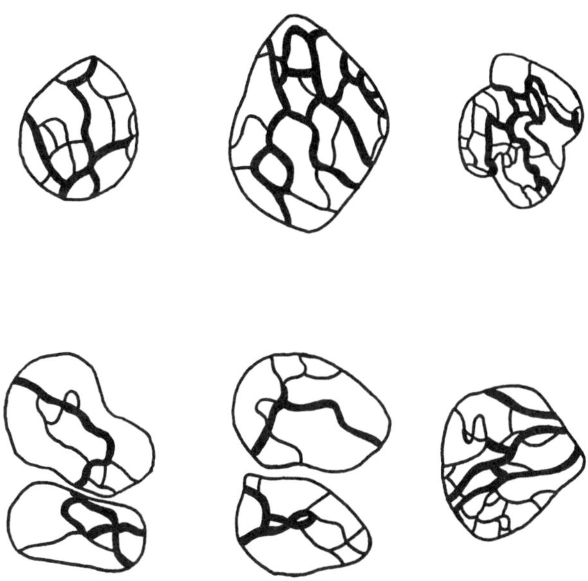

Figure 17 Frequently perfused capillary segments (thick lines) tended to form preferential pathways across alveolar walls. Six panels show one or two alveolar walls in each of six dogs. These are the same animals as in Figure 16. (From Ref. 22.)

To determine specifically whether capillary segmental resistances were stable, Okada et al. (23) again used in vivo microscopy in intact dogs. A balloon was surgically implanted in the mitral orifice. When inflated, the balloon caused left atrial pressure to increase sufficiently to recruit all of the pulmonary capillaries. Then the balloon was deflated, and pulmonary hemodynamics returned to zone 2 baseline conditions. The capillaries that remained perfused in the observed field were videotaped. The cycle of elevated pressure and baseline observation was repeated three times. Perfusion of different capillaries during each of the observations would imply that the segmental resistances within the network varied after the bed was maximally recruited. On the other hand, perfusion of a specific set of pathways each time would demonstrate that flowing blood sought a unique and repeatable combination of segments, presumably with the least total pathway resistance. During the three observations, the same capillary segments were perfused 79% of the time. An example of one experiment is shown in Figure 18. These results provided a strong indication that a reproducible combination of individual low segmental resistances determined the predominant pattern of pulmonary capillary perfusion. A number of capillaries were never perfused at baseline pressure, suggesting that even though they were opened during balloon inflation, their relatively high resistance during zone 2 perfusion kept them from being perfused.

The opening pressure of an unperfused capillary may be independent of its resistance and therefore must be studied separately. To investigate the distribution of opening pressures, an isolated, pump-perfused canine lobe combined with video microscopy was used. After pump flow was set to perfuse one-half of the capillaries in the microscopic field, the pump was turned off, and all of

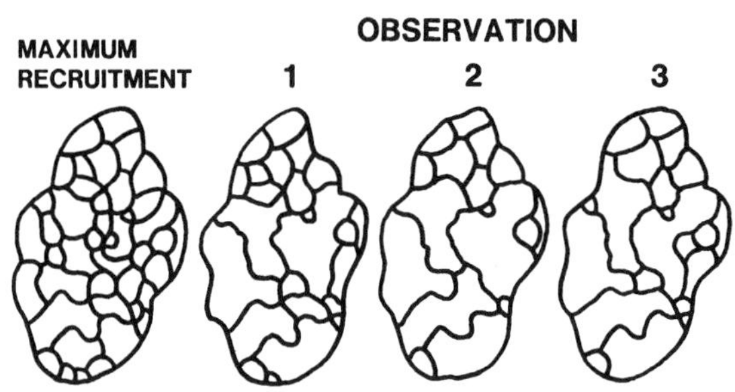

Figure 18 Typical drawing of a single alveolar wall during maximal recruitment and during each of three observation periods. In between each observation in this intact dog preparation, left atrial pressure was transiently elevated to produce maximal recruitment. The results show that some capillaries were always perfused and some were never perfused, indicating that there was a reproducible range of segmental resistances. (From Ref. 23.)

the capillaries emptied. Turning the pump back on reopened the capillaries. The on-off cycle was repeated six times with the perfusion pattern being recorded for 1 minute during each on cycle. If the same capillaries were perfused during each observation, it would demonstrate that there were stable and significant differences between individual capillary opening pressures, causing consistent recruitment of those capillaries with the lowest opening pressures. In the example shown in Figure 19, some capillary segments were perfused during each observation, some segments were never perfused, and others were intermittently perfused. To determine whether any of the capillaries were perfused more or less frequently than expected by chance, we developed a computer program to calculate all physiologically possible perfusion patterns for the observed capillary networks (24). The probability of perfusion for a segment during a single observation period was the number of possible perfusion patterns in which that segment was perfused divided by the total number of possible patterns. This single-observation probability was then used to calculate the probability of perfusion *n* out of six times for each segment. These investigators found that 40% of the capillaries in the observed networks were perfused either more or less frequently than expected by chance. They concluded that the frequently perfused segments had lower than average opening pressures, and the infrequently perfused segments had higher than average opening pressures. Overall, the implica-

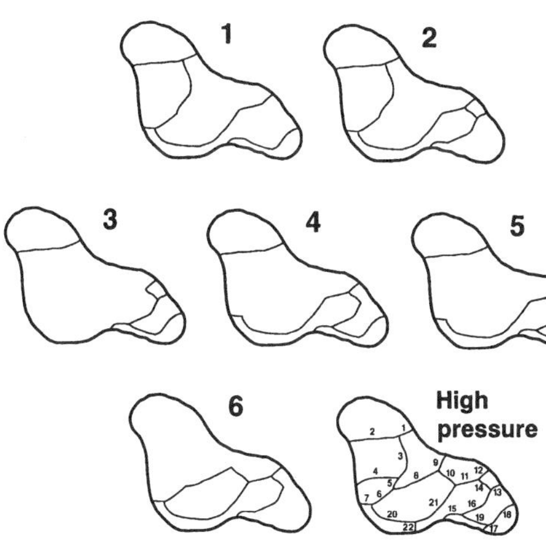

Figure 19 Typical drawing of a single alveolar wall during each of six observation periods and during high pressure, which produced maximal recruitment. In between each observation in this isolated, pump-perfused, canine lobe preparation, the pump was transiently turned off. As with capillary segmental resistances, opening pressures had a reproducible range because some segments were frequently perfused and some were never perfused. (From Ref. 60.)

tion of these experiments seems clear: there is a range of opening pressures and resistances among capillary segments which appears to be stable and exerts considerable control over the pattern of capillary perfusion.

Capillary recruitment generally refers to perfusion of new segments by a combination of red cells and plasma. However, capillaries can be perfused (recruited) by plasma alone. Recent work by Conhaim and Rodenkirch (25) has shown that capillaries in the rat lung even under zone 1 conditions have an estimated functional diameter of 1.7 μm, sufficiently large to admit plasma, but an impediment to red blood cell perfusion. König et al. (26) injected colloidal gold nanospheres (8 nm diameter) into the pulmonary circulation of rabbits. After 2 minutes, the circulation was stopped and the lungs were fixed and examined both by electron and light microscopy. They found that the entire pulmonary capillary bed was perfused by gold particles after 2 minutes, and, in later experiments, complete dispersion occurred in 10 seconds (27). This finding suggests that all of the capillaries were perfused by some of the plasma all of the time. This work suggests the following possibilities (28). The entirety of the capillary endothelium could act continuously on the plasma to perform its many metabolic functions. Red blood cell recruitment, however, would occur only when capillary pressure increased sufficiently to distend capillary segments enough for the passage of red cells. Here again, however, the caveat about interspecies comparisons must be heeded. Rabbit lungs are small and, as with other small mammals with high resting metabolic rates, rabbits are likely to have lungs that are nearly completely perfused at rest. That being the case, there would be less pulmonary reserve for exercise as exemplified by the following comparisons. The difference between oxygen uptake at rest and maximal exercise for small mammals is threefold for rats (29,30), sixfold for mice (31), sixfold for guinea pigs (32), and sixfold for hamsters (33). Larger mammals have a larger reserve: 15-fold for humans (33,34), 20-fold for horses (5,35,36), and 25-fold for dogs (37,38). Thus, it is in lungs with a large zone 2 reserve that there is a 10- to 25-fold difference in oxygen uptake between rest and maximal exercise. The small lungs, being more fully and evenly perfused at rest (39), potentially account for the widespread nanosphere distribution in rabbits.

This line of reasoning is directly supported by the experiments of Means et al. (40) who used in vivo microscopy to study the small lungs of newborn lambs. They found that all capillaries were perfused continuously during basal conditions, because there was no capillary recruitment even in the uppermost lung when pulmonary arterial pressure was doubled. By the age of 3 weeks, a particularly rapid growth period for the lamb lung (41), the older lambs had developed sufficient reserve for a 50% increase in capillary recruitment to occur when pulmonary arterial pressure was increased.

Many studies of pulmonary capillary recruitment and surface area have been published using different species, different perfusion techniques, and various perfusion media with a number of indicators that monitor endothelial uptake or metabolism in perfused regions. The results have often conflicted with one another concerning capillary recruitment and capillary volume changes. These differing conclusions add to the complexity of our understanding of pulmonary capillary function. Part of the trouble comes from comparing data that are based on plasma markers versus red blood cell markers. There is growing evidence that these markers trace different compartments, but we currently lack detailed understanding of how these compartments compare.

C. Capillary Transit Time

As red blood cells pass through the capillary network during basal conditions, oxygen and hemoglobin combine with sufficient rapidity to completely saturate hemoglobin in about the first quarter of its transit. With exercise, capillary transit times decrease as cardiac output increases. If capillary transit time becomes too rapid, red cells cross the capillaries without becoming fully saturated. A number of calculations of the length of time red cells must spend in the capillaries to become completely saturated with oxygen have been reviewed by P. D. Wagner (42). Even though a wide range of variables and assumptions were used by the investigators cited, 0.25 second consistently appeared as a reasonable bound for the minimum time required for red blood cell Po_2 to increase from 40 to 100 torr. Mixed venous Po_2 during maximal exercise can be considerably lower than 40 torr; Piiper and colleagues (43,44) have calculated that the minimum red blood cell transit time for complete saturation under these conditions is likely to exceed 0.25 second. Nevertheless, one-fourth of a second is still accepted as a reasonable estimate of the minimum time needed for complete saturation.

The predominate method for measuring pulmonary capillary transit time has been based on the diffusing capacity of the lung for carbon monoxide to compute pulmonary capillary volume. Capillary transit time can then be calculated by dividing capillary blood volume by cardiac output measured concomitantly, for example, 75 mL (capillary volume) ÷ 100 mL/s (resting cardiac output) = 0.75 second (capillary transit time). Based on this kind of calculation, it is believed that, in the resting human, red blood cells spend an average of 0.75–1.0 second in the pulmonary capillaries (42), well above the calculated 0.25-second minimum transit time. During exercise, however, hypoxemia resulting from diffusion limitation has been shown to be present in horses (45), in some elite human athletes exercising at maximal intensity at sea level (46), in exercising humans at simulated high altitude (47), and even in normal humans exercising maximally at sea level (47). Too rapid a transit time for the fastest moving red cells is implicated in these findings. Naturally, not every red cell traverses the pulmonary capillaries at the mean time. Rather, there is certain to be a range of transit times distributed about the mean with some times significantly shorter than the mean, but that important distribution has escaped measurement with nearly all methods.

During the past decade, there has been sufficient development of intensified television cameras to permit capillary transit times to be measured directly. Video fluorescence microscopy recordings of the passage of a fluorescent dye bolus through the subpleural pulmonary microcirculation have been used to obtain dye dilution curves from an arteriole and venule that shared a common capillary network. Initially, the experiments were restricted to calculation of the mean capillary transit time. At basal cardiac outputs, rabbits have a more rapid mean transit time than dogs (rabbits, 0.41–0.60 second [21,48,49] and dogs, 1.37–2.0 seconds [50–53]). There is a substantial vertical gradient of transit times in the dog lung, 10–20 seconds in the upper lung and 1.5–2.0 seconds in the lower lung (50,51,54,55). These video microscopic findings have been confirmed by Hogg and colleagues (52,53) using independent techniques. The currently available data are shown in Table 2 and reiterate the point that results from different species are likely to be significantly different.

Although the measurements of mean capillary transit time have been important, the accurate measurement of the entire distribution of transit times, including the minimum and maximum, has eluded investigators. Recently, however, Presson et al. (56) have made these measurements. These more complete measurements were possible because methods were developed to subtract the background fluorescence during passage of the dye bolus. Background fluorescence has a relatively small effect on the mean capillary transit time. However, it causes a significant distortion of the entire distribution of transit times; for example, the minimum and maximum transit times as well as variance and relative dispersion of the transit times are quite sensitive to seemingly small errors present in uncorrected curves (Figure 20). Once the arteriolar and venular dye dilution curves are corrected (Figure 20), the entire distribution of capillary transit times can be accurately computed. The wide distribution suggests a range of both path lengths and blood cell velocities, characteristics that can be qualitatively confirmed by visual observation. As blood flow was increased in this study, both the skew and kurtosis of the curves changed so that the longest times shortened and the curves approached the ideal shape, that is, a spike at 0.25 second such that all red blood cells would become saturated exactly at the downstream end of the capillaries. The more homogeneous transit time distribution (a higher, sharper peak with a narrower base) along with some capillary recruitment both acted to cause progressively more blood to transit rapidly, but not below 0.25 second, even for the most rapidly moving plasma (56).

Of course, these direct measurements of labeled plasma provide only an indirect estimate (of unknown accuracy) of the transit time of red blood cells, leaving the crucial measure of the oxygen-carrying component of blood un-

Table 2 Direct Measurements of Pulmonary Capillary Transit Times Comparing Species

Experimental Conditions	Mean Transit Time (s)	Species	Year; Reference
High zone 2, low pulmonary arterial pressure	12.3	Dog	1982; 54
High zone 2, increasing pulmonary arterial pressure	4.0		
Morphometry + radiolabeled indicator dilution		Dog	1985; 52
Upper lung	7.6		
Lower lung	0.18		
Entire lung	1.37		
Top of lung	12.3	Dog	1986; 55
Middle of lung	3.1		
Bottom of lung	1.6		
Bottom of lung (direct)	1.75	Dog	1987: 51
Concurrent transit time by diffusing capacity (whole lung)	1.85		
Morphometry + radiolabeled indicator dilution		Dog	1988; 53
Upper lung	>20		
Lower lung	0.29		
Entire lung	1.37		
Bottom of lung, cardiac output = 2.9 L/min	2.0	Dog	1990; 50
Same vessel pair, cardiac output = 9.9 L/min	0.8		
P_{AW} = 0-5 cm H_2O, Q = 80 mL/min/kg, top of lung	0.60	Rabbit	1990; 48
P_{AW} = 10 cm H_2O, Q = 60 mL/min/kg, top of lung	0.85		
P_{AW} = 15 cm H_2O, Q = 50 mL/min/kg, top of lung	1.85		
P_{AW} = 20 cm H_2O, Q = 30 mL/min/kg, top of lung	2.78		
Whole lung, pump perfused		Rabbit	1992; 20
P_{AW} = 5 cm H_2O, Q = 80, 40, 20 mL/min/kg, zone 2, top of lung	0.67, 0.89, 1.9		
P_{AW} = 5 cm H_2O, Q = 80, 40, 20 mL/min/kg, zone 3, top of lung	0.71, 1.00, 2.4		
P_{AW} = 15 cm H_2O, Q = 80, 40, 20 mL/min/kg, zone 2, top of lung	0.41, 0.63, 0.8		
P_{AW} = 15 cm H_2O, Q = 80, 40, 20 mL/min/kg, zone 3, top of lung	0.54, 0.84, 1.3		

(*continued*)

Table 2 Continued

Experimental Conditions	Mean Transit Time (s)	Species	Year; Reference
Velocity of fluorescently labeled erythrocytes from arteriole to venule during positive-pressure lung inflation	0.47	Rabbit	1993; 49
Left lower lobe, pump perfused		Dog	1994; 56
t_{mean}, Q = 400, 800, 1600 mL/min	3.3, 2.0, 1.2		
t_{min}, Q = 400, 800, 1600 mL/min	1.2, 0.93, 0.56		
t_{max}, Q = 400, 800, 1600 mL/min	10.0, 5.3, 3.0		
In tact animal, fluorescently labeled erythrocyte boluses and FITC-dextran plasma boluses		Dog	1995; 57
Red blood cells, Q = 3.9 ± 0.2 L/min	4.1		
Red blood cells, Q = 12.0 ± 0.7 L/min	1.0		
Plasma, Q = 11.9 ± 0.7 L/min	1.4		

Abbreviations: P_{AW} = airway pressure; Q = pulmonary blood flow; t = capillary transit time for average indicator (mean), fastest indicator (min), and slowest indicator (max).

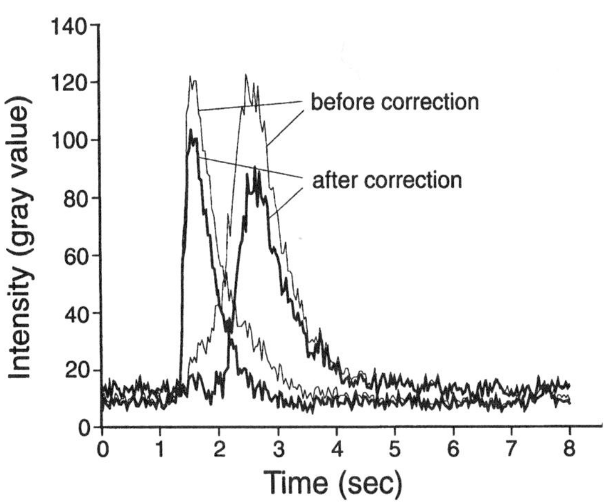

Figure 20 Dye dilution curves before and after correction for background light. Tail of uncorrected arteriolar curve is prolonged and the venular uncorrected curve takes off early, essentially at the beginning of the arteriolar curve, resulting not from the instantaneous arrival of dye but from the instantaneous arrival of background light. Heavy lines are curves after correction. (From Ref. 56.)

known. In the latest report from Presson and colleagues (57), however, the transit time distribution of fluorescently labeled red blood cells was reported. In intact dogs, they found that fluorescently labeled plasma boluses required about half again as long to traverse the capillaries as red blood cell (Figure 21), probably because of the Fahraeus effect in perfused capillaries or because of plasma alone perfusing other capillaries. This means that data obtained from the fluorescently labeled plasma dilution curves overestimated red cell transit time. Nevertheless, at the highest cardiac outputs, capillary recruitment and increasing transit time homogeneity combined, as they did for plasma capillary transit time, to prevent even the most rapidly transiting red cells from going below 0.25 second. Additionally, these measurements provided a fairly direct estimate of capillary hematocrit. That hematocrit was a mean based on the ratio of mean red blood cell transit time to mean plasma transit time through a local capillary network and provides no information about the complex variation of hematocrit that occurs moment to moment in individual capillary segments.

The fact that plasma takes ~1.4 times as long as erythrocytes to cross the capillary bed may impact on CO_2 transport, because significantly more CO_2 than

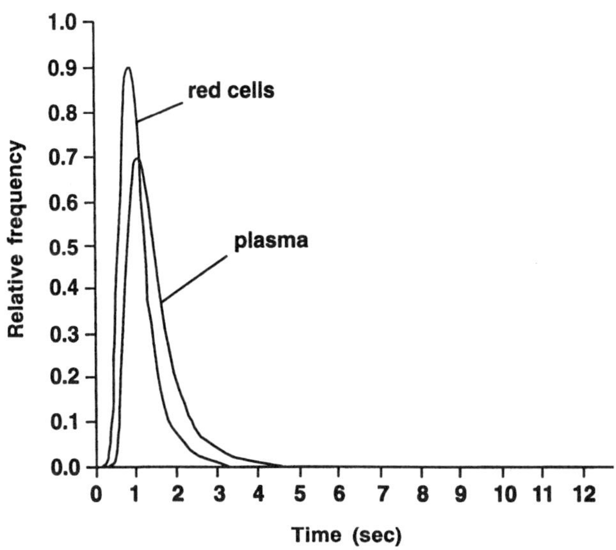

Figure 21 In intact dogs, fluorescently labeled plasma boluses require about half again as long to traverse the capillaries as red blood cells. This causes plasma dilution curves to overestimate red blood cell transit time. The mean transit times (plasma = 1.4 seconds, red blood cell = 1.0 second), the minimum transit times (plasma = 0.62 second, red blood cells = 0.40 second), and the maximum transit times (plasma = 3.5 seconds, red blood cells = 2.5 seconds) were all significantly longer for plasma. (From Ref. 57.)

O_2 is transported in plasma. However, the majority of CO_2 unloading still directly involves the erythrocyte, because of the intraerythrocytic location of carbonic anhydrase. This causes red blood cell transit time to be more important than plasma transit time per se in the transport of CO_2.

At the outset, we pointed out that the lung is conceptualized in an overly simplistic way: a single airway, single alveolus, single capillary model (Figure 1). Much evidence demonstrates that the pulmonary microcirculation behaves in an extremely complex manner with perfusion rapidly switching between capillary segments and red blood cell velocity and hematocrit continually varying. As cardiac output increases with exercise, however, a number of changes occur that cause the microcirculation to behave more homogeneously. First, as capillary pressure increases, capillary recruitment approaches 100%. Presumably, capillary resistance becomes more uniform as segments that are closed open and all segments reach the plateau of their compliance curve. Finally, the dispersion of red blood cell velocities diminishes, and the heterogeneity of capillary transit times lessens (Figure 22). The complexity of perfusion of the pulmonary microcirculation during increasing exercise, therefore, decreases and the simplistic model shown in Figure 1 becomes progressively more realistic.

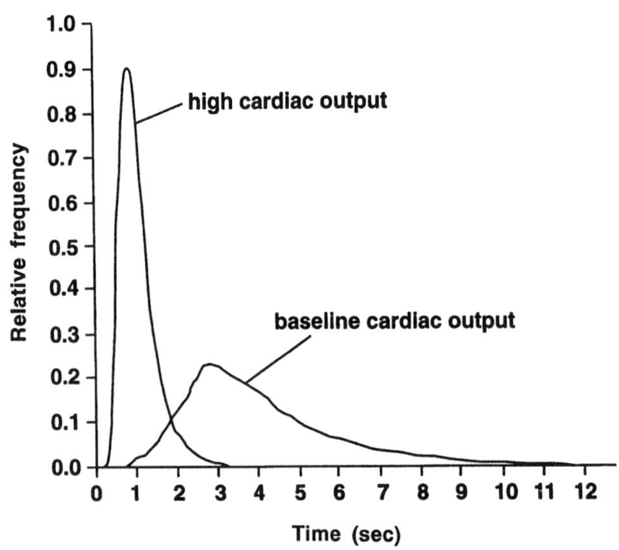

Figure 22 Even at the highest cardiac outputs (12 L/min) in this canine preparation, the minimum red blood cell transit times (0.40 second) were significantly above the calculated 0.25 second minimum for complete hemoglobin saturation. Capillary recruitment and increasing transit time homogeneity combined to prevent even the most rapidly transiting red cells from going below 0.25 second. (From Ref. 57.)

Acknowledgments

The authors thank T. M. Schmidt and T. M. Schmidt for helpful criticism of the manuscript.

References

1. Weibel ER. Morphometry of the Human Lung. New York: Academic Press, 1963.
2. Staub NC, Schultz EL. Pulmonary capillary length in dog, cat and rabbit. Respir Physiol 1968; 5:371–378.
3. Zhuang FY, Yen MRT, Fung YC, Sobin SS. How many pulmonary alveoli are supplied by a single arteriole and drained by a single venule? Microvasc Res 1985; 29:18–31.
4. Bernard SL, Glenny RW, Erickson HH, Fedde MR, Polissar N, Basaraba RJ, Hlastala MP. Minimal redistribution of pulmonary blood flow with exercise in racehorses. J Appl Physiol 1996; 81:1062–1070.
5. Fung YC, Sobin SS. Elasticity of the pulmonary alveolar sheet. Circ Res 1972; 30: 451–469.
6. Fung YC, Sobin SS. Pulmonary alveolar blood flow. Circ Res 1972; 30:470–490.
7. Fung YC, Sobin SS. Theory of sheet flow in lung alveoli. J Appl Physiol 1969; 26:472–488.
8. Fung YC, Yen RT. A new theory of pulmonary blood flow in zone 2 condition. J Appl Physiol 1986; 60:1638–1650.
9. Glazier JB, Hughes JMB, Maloney JE, West JB. Measurements of capillary dimensions and blood volume in rapidly frozen lungs. J Appl Physiol 1969; 26:65–76.
10. Godbey PS, Graham JA, Presson RG Jr, Wagner WW Jr, Lloyd TC Jr. Effect of capillary pressure and lung distention on capillary recruitment. J Appl Physiol 1995; 79:1142–1147.
11. Glazier JB, Hughes JMB, Maloney JE, West JB. Vertical gradient of alveolar size in lungs of dogs frozen intact. J Appl Physiol 1967; 23:694–705.
12. Weibel ER. The Pathway for Oxygen. Cambridge, MA: Harvard University Press, 1984.
13. Miller WS. The Lung. Springfield, IL: Charles C Thomas, 1950.
14. von Hayek H. The Human Lung. New York: Hafner, 1960.
15. Schraufnagel DE, Mehta D, Harsbarger R, Trevirnus K, Wang N. Capillary remodeling in bleomycin-induced pulmonary fibrosis. Am J Pathol 1986; 125:97–106.
16. Short AC, Montoya ML, Gebb SA, Presson RG Jr, Wagner WW Jr, Capen RL. Pulmonary capillary diameters and recruitment characteristics in subpleural and interior networks. J Appl Physiol 1996; 80:1568–1573.
17. Hanson WL, Emhardt JD, Bartek JP, Latham LP, Checkley LL, Capen RL, Wagner WW Jr. The site of recruitment in the pulmonary microcirculation. J Appl Physiol 1989; 66:2079–2083.
18. Warrell DA, Evans JW, Clarke RO, Kingaby GP, West JB. Pattern of filling in the pulmonary capillary bed. J Appl Physiol 1972; 32:346–356.

19. Godbey PS, Graham JA, Hanger CC, Presson RG Jr, Doerschuk CM, Wagner WW Jr. Microcirculatory perfusion patterns on the surface of dog and rabbit lungs. FASEB J 1992; 6:2044.
20 Wang PM, Fike CD, Kaplowitz MR, Brown LV, Ayappa I, Jahed M, Lai-Fook SJ. Effects of lung inflation and blood flow on capillary transit time in isolated rabbit lungs. J Appl Physiol 1992; 72:2420–2470.
21. Wearn JT, Ernstene AC, Bromer AW, Barr JS, German WJ, Zschiesche LJ. The normal behavior of the pulmonary blood vessels with observations on the intermittence of the flow of blood in the arterioles and capillaries. Am J Physiol 1934; 109: 236–256.
22. Okada O, Presson RG Jr, Godbey PS, Capen RL, Wagner WW Jr. Temporal capillary perfusion patterns in single alveolar walls of intact dogs. J Appl Physiol 1994; 76:380–386.
23. Okada O, Presson RG Jr, Kirk KR, Godbey PS, Capen RL, Wagner WW Jr. Capillary perfusion patterns in single alveolar walls. J Appl Physiol 1992; 72:1838–1844.
24. Hanger CC, Presson RG Jr, Okada O, Janke SJ, Watson JJ, Wagner WW Jr, Capen RL. Computer determination of perfusion patterns in pulmonary capillary networks. J Appl Physiol 1997; 82:1283–1289.
25. Conhaim RL, Rodenkirch LA. Estimated functional diameter of alveolar septal microvessels at the zone I-II border. Microcirculation 1997; 4:51–59.
26. König MF, Lucocq JM, Weibel ER. Demonstration of pulmonary vascular perfusion by electron and light microscopy. J Appl Physiol 1993; 75:1877–1883.
27. König MF, Batra S, Weibel ER. Perfusion pattern of lung microvessels after short circulation periods. Experientia 1994; 50:A4.
28. Wagner WW Jr. Pulmonary capillary perfusion by plasma (editorial). J Appl Physiol 1993; 75:1437–1438.
29. Bedford TG, Tipton CM, Wilson NC, Oppliger RA, Gisolfi CV. Maximum oxygen consumption of rats and its changes with various experimental procedures. J Appl Physiol 1979; 47:1278–1283.
30. Gonzalez NC, Sokari A, Clancy RL. Maximum oxygen uptake and arterial blood oxygenation during hypoxic exercise in rats. J Appl Physiol 1991; 71:1041–1049.
31. Chappell MA. Maximum oxygen consumption during exercise and cold exposure in deer mice, *Peromyscus maniculatus*. Respir Physiol 1984; 55:367–377.
32. Pasquis P, Lacaisse A, Dejours P. Maximum oxygen consumption in four species of small mammals. Respir Physiol 1970; 9:298–309.
33. Reeves JT, Grover RF, Cohn JE. Regulation of ventilation during exercise at 10,200 ft in athletes born at low altitude. J Appl Physiol 1967; 22:546–554.
34. Wolfel EE, Groves BM, Brooks GA, Butterfield GE, Mazzeo RS, Moore LG, Sutton JR, Vender PR, Dahms TE, McCullough RE, McCullough RG, Huang SY, Sun SF, Grover RF, Hultgren HN, Reeves JT. Oxygen transport during steady-state submaximal exercise in chronic hypoxia. J Appl Physiol 1991; 70:1129–1136.
35. Butler PJ, Woakes AJ, Smale K, Roberts CA, Hillidge CJ, Snow DH, Marlin DJ. Respiratory and cardiovascular adjustments during exercise of increasing intensity and duration and recovery in Thoroughbred racehorses. J Exp Biol 1993; 179:159–180.
36. Rose RJ, Hodgson DR, Kelso TB, McCutcheon LJ, Reid TA, Bayly WM, Gollnick

PD. Maximum O_2 uptake, O_2 debt and deficit, and muscle metabolites in thoroughbred horses. J Appl Physiol 1988; 64:781–788.

37. Musch TI, Haidet GC, Ordway GA, Longhurst JC, Mitchell JH. Dynamic exercise training in foxhounds. I. Oxygen consumption and hemodynamic responses. J Appl Physiol 1985; 59:183–189.
38. Hsia CCW, Herazo LF, Johnson RL Jr. Cardiopulmonary adaptations to pneumonectomy in dogs. I. Maximal exercise performance. J Appl Physiol 1992; 73:362–367.
39. Taylor CR, Weibel ER, Hoppeler H, Karas RH. Matching structure and function in the respiratory system: allometric and adaptive variations in energy demand. In: Wood SC, ed. Comparative Pulmonary Physiology. New York: Marcel Dekker, 1989.
40. Means LJ, Hanson WL, Mounts KO, Wagner WW Jr. Pulmonary capillary recruitment in neonatal lambs. Pediatr Res 1993; 34:596–599.
41. Davies P, Reid L, Lister G, Pitt B. Postnatal growth of the sheep lung: a morphometric study. Anat Rec 1988; 220:281–286.
42. Wagner PD. Diffusion and chemical reaction in pulmonary gas exchange. Physiol Rev 1977; 57:257–312.
43. Piiper J, Dejours P, Haab P, Rahn H. Concepts and basic equations in gas exchange physiology. Respir Physiol 1971; 13:292–304.
44. Piiper J, Scheid P. Model for capillary-alveolar equilibration with special reference to O_2 uptake in hypoxia. Respir Physiol 1981; 46:193–208.
45. Wagner PD, Gillespie JR, Landgren GL, Fedde MR, Jones BW, DeBowes RM, Pieschl RL, Erickson HH. Mechanism of exercise-induced hypoxemia in horses. J Appl Physiol 1989; 66:1227–1233.
46. Dempsey JA, Hanson PG, Henderson KS. Exercise-induced arterial hypoxaemia in healthy human subjects at sea level. J Physiol 1984; 355:61–175.
47. Wagner PD, Gale GE, Moon RE, Torre-Bueno JR, Stolp BW, Saltzman HA. Pulmonary gas exchange in humans exercising at sea level and simulated altitude. J Appl Physiol 1986; 61:260–270.
48. Wang PM, Yang QH, Lai-Fook SJ. Effect of positive airway pressure on capillary transit time in rabbit lung. J Appl Physiol 1990; 69:2262–2268.
49. Kuhnle GEH, Leipfinger FH, Goetz AE. Measurement of microhemodynamics in the ventilated rabbit lung by intravital fluorescence microscopy. J Appl Physiol 1993; 74:1462–1471.
50. Capen RL, Hanson WL, Latham LP, Dawson CA, Wagner WW Jr. Distribution of pulmonary capillary transit times in recruited networks. J Appl Physiol 1990; 69:473–478.
51. Capen RL, Latham LP, Wagner WW Jr. Comparison of direct and indirect measurements of pulmonary capillary transit time. J Appl Physiol 1987; 62:1150–1154.
52. Hogg JC, Martin BA, Lee S, McLean T. Regional differences in erythrocyte transit in normal lungs. J Appl Physiol 1985; 59:1266–1271.
53. Hogg JC, McLean T, Martin BA, Wiggs B. Erythrocyte transit and neutrophil concentration in the dog lung. J Appl Physiol 1988; 65:1217–1225.
54. Wagner WW Jr, Latham LP, Gillespie MN, Guenther J, Capen RL. Red cell transit times across pulmonary capillaries. Science 1982; 218:379–380.

55. Wagner WW Jr, Latham LP, Hanson WL, Hofmeister SE, Capen RL. Vertical gradient of pulmonary capillary transit times. J Appl Physiol 1986; 61:1270–1274.
56. Presson RG Jr, Hanger CC, Godbey PS, Graham JA, Lloyd TC Jr, Wagner WW Jr. Effect of increasing flow on the distribution of pulmonary capillary transit times. J Appl Physiol 1994; 76:1701–1711.
57. Presson RG Jr, Hanger CC, Godbey PS, Graham JA, Sidner RA, Wagner WW Jr. Distribution of pulmonary capillary red blood cell transit times. J Appl Physiol 1995; 79:382–388.
58. Miller ME, Christensen GC, Evans HE. Anatomy of the Dog. Philadelphia: WB Saunders, 1964.
59. Wagner WW Jr, Latham LP, Capen RL. Capillary recruitment during airway hypoxia: role of pulmonary arterial pressure. J Appl Physiol 1979; 47:383–387.
60. Presson RG Jr, Okada O, Hanger CC, Godbey PS, Graham JA, Glenny RW, Capen RL, Wagner WW Jr. Stability of alveolar capillary opening pressures. J Appl Physiol 1994; 77:1630–1637.

15

Regional Differences in the Lung

A Changing Perspective on Blood Flow Distribution

ROBB W. GLENNY and H. THOMAS ROBERTSON

University of Washington School of Medicine
Seattle, Washington

I. Introduction

The gravitational hypothesis explaining the distribution of both blood flow and ventilation in the lung has been a cornerstone of pulmonary physiology, influencing both the interpretation and direction of studies related to pulmonary function for the past 3 decades. The model itself has been taught to generations of students in physiology and medicine because of its reliance on simple physical principles that yield elegant explanations of lung function. However, recent studies using high-resolution methods and experiments performed in microgravity provide observations that cannot be explained by the gravitational model alone. The premise we wish to advance is that the gravitational model cannot adequately account for several experimental observations of pulmonary perfusion and that additional factors must be considered. These new proposals are based on concepts of perfusion heterogeneity and they provide new perspectives from which to explore determinants of regional blood flow.

Thomas Kuhn's seminal essay "The Structure of Scientific Revolution" describes the process by which major shifts in scientific models take place, highlighting the pace and timing of the events that are requisite to the scientific community before an established model can be replaced. It is in the context of the stages described by Kuhn that we discuss the predictions of the gravitational model and the anomalies uncovered by new high-resolution methods, and we speculate about a new model of pulmonary perfusion.

II. Kuhn's Model of Scientific Progress

Thomas Kuhn, physicist turned philosopher, formulated a view of scientific progress in which he used the term "paradigm" to be used as a set of universally recognized scientific achievements that, for a time, provide model problems and solutions to a community of scientists (1). He argues that these paradigms are woven into the fabric of every scientific group and represent the core principles that define their beliefs (1). Although the examples chosen by Kuhn represented major scientific revolutions, such as Copernican astronomy, Newtonian physics, the wave theory of light, and quantum physics, the same model of scientific progress is equally applicable to small scale paradigms, including the model we study, that of blood flow distribution in the lungs.

Scientific progress under an established paradigm, termed "normal science" is orderly and confirmatory. An established paradigm serves a number of important roles. By succinctly stating those beliefs held true by a scientific community, individuals of the group are freed from defending these facts and are able to explore more specific areas in finer detail or to concentrate efforts on solutions to other problems (1). Paradigms provide new insights by suggesting new experiments and possible outcomes. Because observations are usually analyzed in the context of the most widely accepted model, paradigms influence data interpretation by restricting the peripheral vision of researchers, making them less likely to develop conflicting theories (1).

The second form of scientific progress is revolutionary rather than evolutionary and occurs when an established paradigm is discarded. Kuhn noted that scientific progress advances in leaps or "revolutions" that are best identified by examining the paradigms of a scientific community. Kuhn postulates that the "transition from one paradigm to another via revolution is the usual developmental pattern of a mature science." This model of scientific progress is depicted in Figure 1. Initial observations are used to formulate a working model (initial paradigm). This paradigm suggests experiments, the results of which reinforce the initial paradigm. Occasionally, anomalies arise that cannot be explained. When a critical mass of inconsistencies develops, a new paradigm is proposed. This alternative model must incorporate both the anomalies and prior observations that generated the initial paradigm.

The transition from one paradigm to another does not occur through small incremental changes to the existing model. "Rather it is a reconstruction of the field from new fundamentals, a reconstruction that changes some of the field's

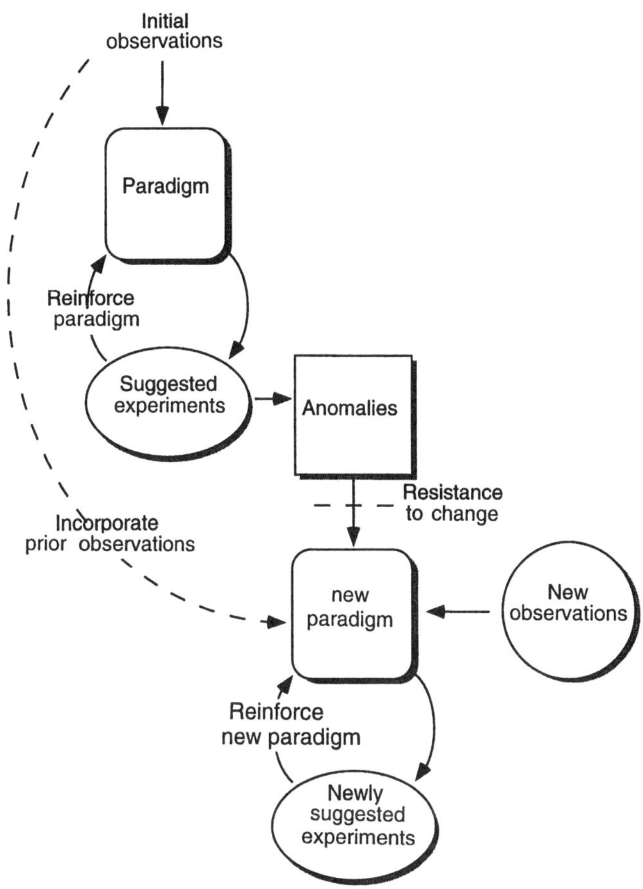

Figure 1 Kuhn's model of scientific revolutions.

most elementary theoretical generalizations . . . " (1). The fresh insights provided by a new paradigm may be the most important stimulant for scientific progress within a field because this radical reorientation provides new perspectives from which to analyze prior observations and suggests new areas of exploration.

New technologies play important roles in defining anomalies. Although the purpose of a paradigm is to explain scientific observations, it can also suggest new experiments that would not have otherwise been conceived (1). These new experiments tend to probe the boundaries of the original model, uncovering inconsistencies. New technologies reveal anomalies by providing observations not previously available. Anomalies are usually identified by investigators new to a field, because established practitioners of a community have accepted the group's paradigm and are less likely to challenge it.

Resistance to a change in paradigms is always high. Paradoxically, this resistance is crucial for scientific progress from one paradigm to another. "By ensuring that the paradigm will not too easily be surrendered, resistance guarantees that scientists will not be lightly distracted and that the anomalies that lead to the paradigm change will penetrate existing knowledge to the core" (1).

III. Initial Model and Supporting Observations

A model for the regional distribution of blood flow in the lung was first proposed by Banister and Torrance who observed that the airway pressure in excised lungs influenced pulmonary blood flow (2). They hypothesized that alveolar pressures interacted with arterial and venous pressures to act as a "sluice gate" or Starling resistor. They speculated that regional blood flow should vary with height up the lung because of changes in relative pressure differences between arterial, venous, and airway pressures. They also predicted that vertically positioned regions should exist within the lung in which blood flow was determined by either the local arterial-alveolar pressure differences or the local arterial-venous pressure differences.

The spatial distribution of pulmonary blood flow was first directly studied in elegant physiological experiments during the early 1960s. Radioactive gases were used to measure the regional distribution of blood flow by one of two methods (3–6). Either an insoluble gas was given intravenously and the radioactive counts recorded over the chest wall (Figure 2) or a soluble gas was inhaled and the clearance of the gas from the alveolar space measured in a similar fashion. In all of these studies, blood flow appeared to increase with distance down the lung. West and Dollery (7) verified the speculations of Banister and Torrance in an isolated dog lung in which arterial, venous, and alveolar pressures could be finely regulated. These observations led to the theory that gravity is an important determinant of regional pulmonary blood flow.

IV. Formulation of the Gravitational Paradigm

Hughes, West, and others synthesized the observations existing at the time into a model of pulmonary blood flow distribution (7). Briefly stated, regional blood flow is determined by the interactions between pulmonary arterial (P_a), venous (P_v), and alveolar (P_A) pressures (Figure 3). Because arterial and venous pressures increase down the lung because of increasing hydrostatic pressure, horizontal "zones" of flow are created. Within these vertically stacked zones, regional blood flow is determined by the relationship between the three pressures

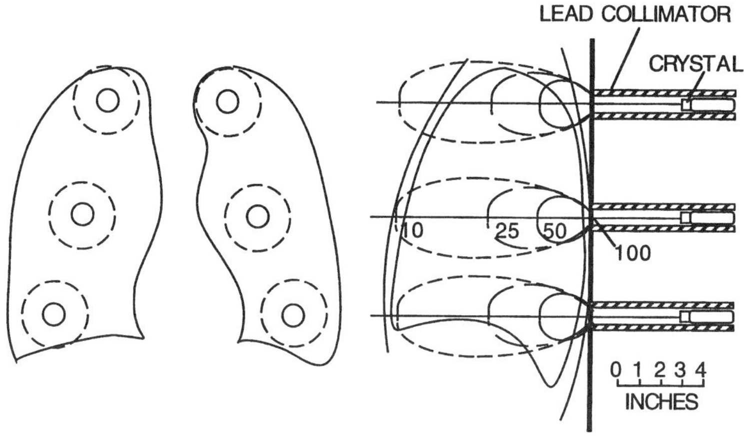

Figure 2 Placement of scintillation counters on chest wall in experiments measuring the regional distribution of blood flow. Note the relatively large regions of interest and that perfusion was measured over large horizontal planes. Numbers on the isocount curves refer to a counting rate of 100% at the end of the collimator. (Adapted from Ref. 4.)

(P_a, P_v, and P_A). In zone 1, alveolar pressure is greater than both arterial and venous pressures ($P_A > P_a > P_v$), resulting in little flow. In zone 2, flow is determined by the difference between arterial and alveolar pressures ($P_a > P_A > P_v$), producing flows that gradually increase down the lung because of arterial pressure increases while alveolar pressure remains constant. In zone 3, arterial and

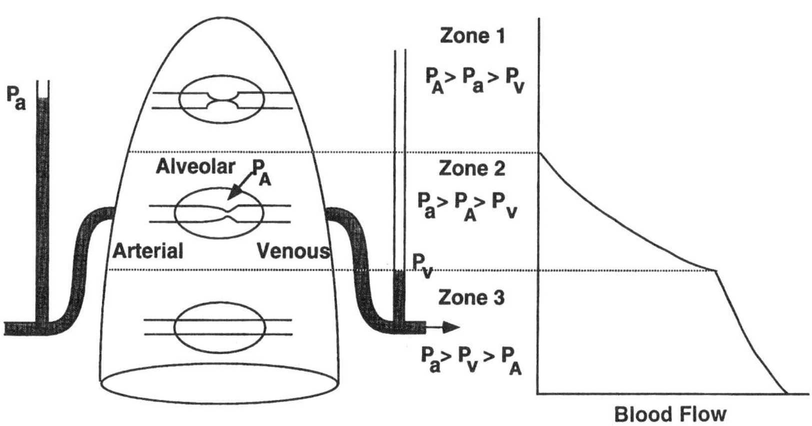

Figure 3 Gravitational model of pulmonary blood flow distribution. (Adapted from Ref. 8.)

venous pressures are greater than alveolar pressure ($P_a > P_v > P_A$), with arterial and venous pressures increasing equally down the lung. Although the driving pressure for blood flow remains constant in zone 3, flow increases down the lung because of recruitment and distention of vessels. A fourth zone of flow was subsequently added to explain the observation that blood flow decreased in the most dependent lung regions (8), although a satisfactory explanation for the fourth zone was never forthcoming.

This model of pulmonary blood flow distribution meets all of Kuhn's criteria for a paradigm. It represents generally accepted observations, provides a set of model problems to be explored, furnishes solutions to these problems, and embodies the core principles used by the scientific community interested in pulmonary physiology. Thirty years after its introduction, the gravitational model of pulmonary blood flow distribution has become the most widely accepted model and is included in every textbook of physiology. In fact, inclusion in a textbook is one of the criteria mentioned by Kuhn for a model to attain the status of a paradigm (1).

V. Model Predictions

An important function of a model is to suggest avenues of investigation and to predict the outcome of these experiments (1). Although not explicitly stated by the gravitational model, a literal interpretation predicts certain observations that were not or could not be measured until recently. A model in which regional vascular pressures are primarily determined by gravity predicts the following:

1. Regional pulmonary blood flow should be uniform within isogravitational planes where the hydrostatic and alveolar pressures are equal throughout.
2. Regional pulmonary blood flow observed in one posture (e.g., supine) should be negatively correlated with blood flow to the same regions when observed in the opposing posture (e.g., prone).
3. Most of the variability in perfusion should be explained by the height up the lung.
4. Increasing pulmonary arterial pressures during exercise should make perfusion more uniform by converting zones 1 and 2 into primarily zone 3 flow.
5. Pulmonary blood flow should become uniform under conditions of microgravity.

With the advent of high-resolution imaging methods and the space shuttle's prolonged microgravity environment, it has become possible to test these gravitational model predictions.

VI. Anomalies

The observed heterogeneity of blood flow is dependent on the spatial resolution at which it is measured (9). As the spatial resolution improves (smaller region of interest), the measured perfusion heterogeneity increases. Most of the studies reporting isogravitational heterogeneity have examined lung pieces 1–2 cm^3 in volume (10–13). At this piece size, perfusion heterogeneity is roughly 55% (coefficient of variation, 100 · SD/mean) (14). At a higher resolution, the alveolar-capillary level where gas exchange occurs, perfusion heterogeneity is even greater (15).

The discrepancies between the gravitational model predictions and these recent experimental observations have been made possible by advancing technologies that provide higher resolution data. The spatial distribution of radioactive gases was obtained using scintillation counters with poor spatial resolution relative to current standards. Figure 2 shows that the field of view of a scintillation counter was quite large. Because horizontally aligned counters measured radioactivity over large isogravitational planes, any heterogeneity within these planes could not be measured. When the spatial resolution of recently acquired data is reduced to that of older studies by averaging observations within isogravitational planes (Figure 4), height up the lung appears to be an important determinant of perfusion. However, using the higher resolution measurements, gravity is a minor determinant of pulmonary blood flow. Hence it is not the experimental results that are new but rather their resolution and interpretation.

Reed and Wood first suggested in 1970 that pulmonary blood flow may not be as homogeneous as expected from the gravitational model (16). Using methods with improved spatial resolution, they found that perfusion is not uniform within isogravitational planes and evoked regional hypoxic pulmonary vasoconstriction as a possible mechanism. They concluded that "the interrelationships of determinants of regional pulmonary blood flow in the intact animal are sufficiently complex so that achievement of an adequate description by a relatively simple model is not possible at this time" (16). Greenleaf and associates (17) confirmed the observation of heterogeneous blood flow within isogravitational planes using methods with even greater spatial resolution. Hakim and coworkers (18) used the higher resolution methods of single photon emission tomography to show considerable heterogeneity of pulmonary blood flow within isogravitational planes. A number of recent studies have confirmed the large heterogeneity of isogravitational pulmonary blood flow in a variety of laboratory animals (9,10,12,13). In all of these studies, radiolabeled blood flow markers were used and lungs of experimental animals dissected into 1 to 2 cm^3 pieces. In those studies exploring isogravitational perfusion heterogeneity, the coefficient of variation within horizontal planes was almost as large as the perfusion heterogeneity across all planes (14,19).

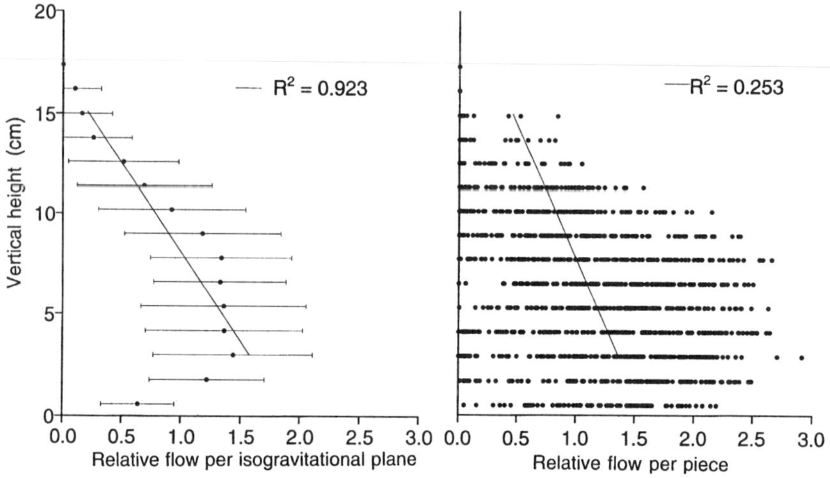

Figure 4 Effect of measurement resolution on data interpretation. Regional perfusion is plotted as a function of height up the lung. (The axes have been switched to present the data in a format consistent with Figure 3.) **Left**, When the spatial resolution of the data is reduced by averaging observations within isogravitational planes, height up the lung appears to be an important determinant of perfusion ($R^2 = 0.923$). **Right**, Using higher resolution measurements, gravity is a minor determinant of pulmonary blood flow ($R^2 = 0.253$).

Using different radiolabeled microspheres to mark perfusion, it is possible to measure blood flow to lung regions when an animal is in one posture and again when the animal is repositioned in an opposing posture. The gravitational model predicts that there should be a negative relationship between blood flow to the same piece in the two different postures (Figure 5). A dependent region should have relatively high blood flow when the animal is in one posture and, when the animal is repositioned to the opposing posture, it should become low flow because it has become nondependent. Similarly, a low-flow region that is nondependent in one posture should become a high-flow region when the animal is placed in the opposing posture. However, in anesthetized and mechanically ventilated dogs, there is a strong positive relationship between regional perfusion in the supine and prone postures (11).

If gravity is an important determinant of regional pulmonary blood flow, a strong relationship should exist between height up the lung and regional perfusion. The strength of this relationship can be gauged by the square of the linear correlation coefficient (r^2) between blood flow and vertical distance up the lung.

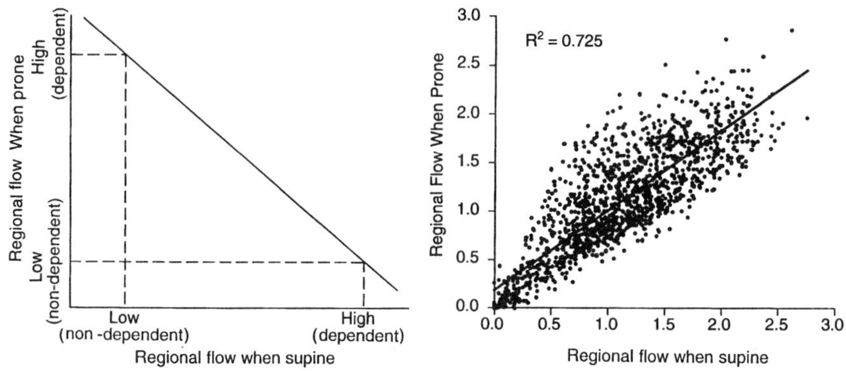

Figure 5 Relationship between regional pulmonary blood flow in opposing postures. **Left**, Theoretical relationship if gravity is the sole determinant of regional perfusion. A dependent region in the supine posture has relatively high flow, and, when the animal is turned prone, the same region becomes nondependent with relatively low flow. **Right**, Relationship between regional perfusion in supine and prone postures is positively correlated.

In anesthetized and mechanically ventilated dogs, the r^2 values for supine and prone dogs are 0.094 and 0.033, respectively (11), demonstrating that the hydrostatic pressure explains only 9.4% and 3.3% of blood flow variability in the two postures. Awake standing dogs have an average r^2 value of only 0.064 (13). In awake, standing horses with a hydrostatic gradient of nearly 60 cm, regional pulmonary blood flow was greater in the nondependent compared with the dependent regions in three of the four horses studied (Figure 6) (20).

If pulmonary perfusion heterogeneity is due primarily to the vertical stratification of zonal conditions, increasing pulmonary arterial driving pressure should recruit blood flow in the nondependent regions and make perfusion more uniform. Using high-resolution methods (1 cm^3 lung pieces), Parker and colleagues (13) studied the spatial distribution of pulmonary blood flow in standing and exercising dogs and found that perfusion heterogeneity remained constant during rest and exercise conditions. These findings have been confirmed in exercising thoroughbred horses (21).

Recent studies performed during the Spacelab Life Sciences-1 (SLS-1) mission under conditions of microgravity have shown that pulmonary perfusion remains heterogeneous in humans (22). Using hyperventilation-breath-hold, single-breath measurements, indicators of perfusion heterogeneity were reduced to approximately 60% of their preflight observations, indicating that the majority of perfusion heterogeneity persists in the absence of gravity.

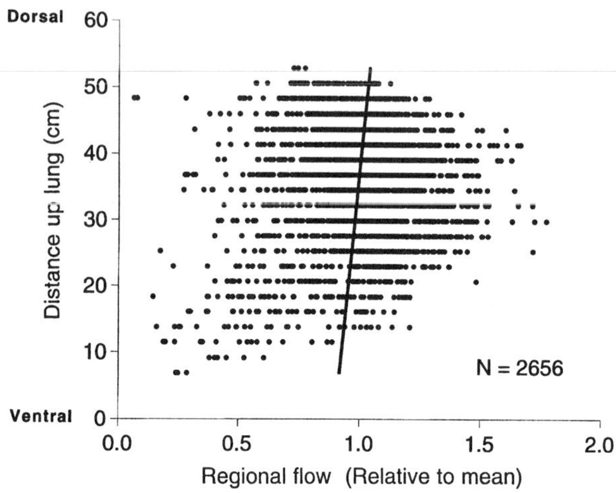

Figure 6 Regional pulmonary perfusion as a function of height up the lung in a standing horse. (The axes have been switched to present the data in a format consistent with Figure 3.) Line represents least-squares regression. Despite the large hydrostatic gradient (46 cm H_2O), blood flow tends to be slightly greater in the nondependent regions.

VII. New Observations

The high degree of perfusion heterogeneity within isogravitational planes exhibits another important property. It is not random as would be expected if it were caused by "biologic noise." When regional blood flow is determined in $\sim$2 cm^3 pieces of lung in dogs, high-flow regions are adjacent to other high-flow regions and low-flow regions are adjacent to other low-flow regions (Figure 7) (23). This relationship can be quantified using the correlation coefficient between flows to pairs of adjacent lung pieces. As the distance between regions increases, the correlation of flow decreases, eventually becoming negative at large distances. Pulmonary blood flow is therefore spatially correlated, a property that can be predicted for blood flow distributed via a progressively branching system.

Perfusion heterogeneity is less in the prone than in the supine posture in dogs (24) because of the lack of a vertical gradient of blood flow when prone. Beck and Rehder have accounted for this observation by documenting regional differences in vascular conductance in dog lungs (25). They demonstrated that, regardless of prone or supine orientation of the lung or variations in lung volume, conductance of blood flow was always greatest in the dorsal regions. They could not attribute these findings to effects of hypoxic pulmonary vasoconstriction or differences in lung expansion and concluded that regional differences in

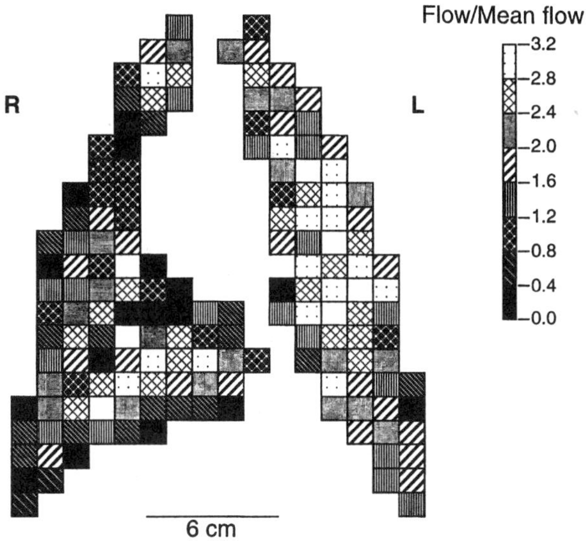

Figure 7 Distribution of regional perfusion within a coronal (isogravitational) plane at heart level: The right (R) and left (L) lungs are shown with the cardiac fossa between them. The flows have been binned into eight levels to facilitate the graphical presentation. Despite the apparent heterogeneity of flow, regional perfusion is spatially correlated with high-flow regions near other high-flow areas and low flow regions near other low flow areas. (Reproduced from Ref. 23.)

vascular anatomy have an important influence on the distribution of pulmonary blood flow (25).

A central-to-peripheral gradient in which blood flow is less peripherally has been observed (11,13,18,26). However, the magnitude of this gradient is small, roughly equivalent to the effect of gravity. The gradient has been attributed to the increased resistance in the arterial vasculature caused by the greater path lengths to the more peripheral regions.

Regional pulmonary blood flow is highly correlated over time and between rest and exercise. Using radiolabeled microspheres, regional perfusion was measured every 20 minutes in dogs over an 80- to 100-minute time interval (27). On average, the correlation coefficient of flow to the same region at different times was 0.86. In Parker's study of rest and exercising dogs (13), the correlation coefficients of flow to the same region between rest and exercise was 0.94. These high correlation coefficients indicate that, despite intervening time and dramatic changes in cardiac output, high-flow pieces remain high flow and low-flow pieces remain low flow, suggesting a structural component of the vascular system that is relatively fixed and an important determinant of regional perfusion.

Do the above observations negate the basic principles of the gravitational model? We believe they do not, but that a reorientation of perspectives is necessary with a new emphasis on the geometric structure of the pulmonary vascular tree. Variability in isogravitational pulmonary perfusion is likely caused by structural heterogeneities within the pulmonary vascular tree. In a branching vascular tree, structural heterogeneities must produce variabilities in local driving pressures and resistances. Traditionally, the gravitational model is presented with single arterial and venous hydrostatic pressures at a given vertical height (see Figure 3) (7). Whereas the hydrostatic pressure is determined by a stagnant column of blood, pressure decreases and ultimately driving pressures at the microvascular level are determined by vascular branching angles and serial resistances to flowing blood. Driving pressures within isogravitational planes should therefore be heterogeneous (28). When considering zonal conditions, the driving pressures of interest are not P_a and P_v but rather $P_{a'}$ and $P_{v'}$, where the prime indicates the local microvascular pressure.

Because of driving pressure heterogeneities at the microvascular level, more than one zonal condition can exist within an isogravitational plane. The traditional zones of blood flow described by West and colleagues are thought to be vertically stratified (see Figure 3), with a single zonal condition per horizontal plane. However, nonuniform driving pressures within an isogravitational plane can produce multiple zones within a plane. This can be demonstrated experimentally with the setup shown in Figure 8*A*. In this simple system, fluid flows from an "arterial" to a "venous" reservoir as a result of a common driving pressure of $P_a - P_v$. Flow divides into three pathways that pass through collapsible segments representing alveolar capillaries. The collapsible segments reside within a single horizontal plane and have a surrounding pressure equal to atmosphere ($P_A = 0$) (see Figure 8*B*). Because of different branching angles and resistances, pressure heterogeneities exist at the inlets and outlets of the collapsible segments. Figure 8*C* demonstrates that zones 1, 2, and 3 can exist within a single isogravitational plane.

The concept that flow is determined by the zonal conditions is commonly inferred from the diagram of the three-zone model (see Figure 3). In this diagram, blood flow increases steadily down the lung, causing zone 3 blood flow to be always greater than zone 2 flow. Zonal conditions do not determine regional flow; rather, the driving pressures and resistances within the local capillary segments determine regional flow. Consider two regions with different local pressures. In the first region, $P_{a1'} = 20$, $P_{v1'} = 1$, and $P_A = 2$ cm H_2O, and in the second region, $P_{a2'} = 4$, $P_{v2'} = 3$, and $P_A = 2$ cm H_2O. Although the first region is in zone 2 and the second region is in zone 3, the driving pressure in the first region is much greater than that in the second region, causing flow to be greater in the zone 2 region when microvascular resistances are similar.

VIII. New Model

A common framework is to compartmentalize the systemic circulation into structural segments such as arteries, arterioles, capillaries, venules, and veins. Traditionally, unique functions have been ascribed to each segment and the function of each element studied and then modeled in isolation from the other components. The problem with this approach is that the behavior of the system as a whole cannot be predicted from that of its individual elements. A shift is therefore occurring in the systemic microvascular arena away from the traditional compartmentalization of structure and function toward "networks" that integrate the macrocirculation and microcirculation (29). These networks are relatively simple models that capture the true complexity of vascular systems (30) and faithfully model the observed heterogeneity of regional perfusion (31).

We propose that an improved characterization of blood flow distribution in the lung must include the specific characteristics of the pulmonary vascular network and that the lesser effects of gravity are superimposed on these anatomical constraints. The vascular tree is an asymmetrically branching system that produces regional flows that are both heterogeneous and spatially correlated. Figure 9 is a schematic of a simple bifurcating vascular tree. Any repeating asymmetry in blood flow distribution at bifurcations cascades down the vascular tree, causing in heterogeneous regional perfusion at the terminal branches. With a sufficient number of generations in the tree, only a small amount of asymmetry is needed to produce large flow heterogeneities. We have previously shown that an asymmetry ratio as small as 53 : 47 between flows to daughter branches produces the degree of perfusion heterogeneity seen in experimental studies (32). The asymmetry of flow distribution is likely due to heterogeneities of vascular diameters, branch lengths, and branching angles. These asymmetries occur from the first bifurcation of the pulmonary arteries (33), down to the alveolar capillaries (34), and back up through the pulmonary venous system. As in an electrical circuit, flows within any portion of the network are influenced by resistances and driving pressures in every other region.

The spatial correlation of pulmonary perfusion is also likely due to the branching structure of the pulmonary vascular network (35). Figure 9 demonstrates that adjacent lung regions have similar flows caused by the shared heritage of the vascular tree. Because high-flow regions are possible only at the expense of flow to other regions, flows become dissimilar and eventually negatively correlated as the distance between regions increases. A simple network

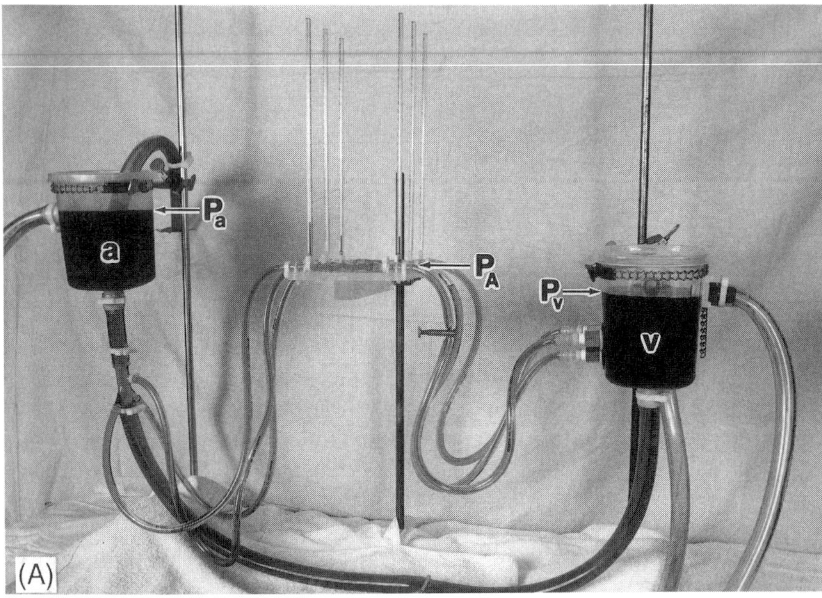

Figure 8 Simple vascular model demonstrating that all three zones can be present within an isogravitational plane. In this simple system (**A**), fluid flows from an "arterial" to a "venous" reservoir as a result of a common driving pressure of $P_a - P_v$. Flow divides into three pathways that pass through collapsible segments representing alveolar capillaries (**B**). The upright tubes are manometers reflecting the different precapillary and postcapillary pressures all within the same isogravitational plane. The collapsible segments reside within a single horizontal plane and have a surrounding pressure equal to atmosphere ($P_A = 0$). Despite a common driving pressure of $P_a - P_v$, pressure heterogeneities exist at the inlets and outlets of the collapsible (capillary) segments because of different branching angles and resistances in the vascular network. The heterogeneity of driving pressures produces multiple zonal conditions within an isogravitational plane (**C**). $P_a'2$, $P_v'2$, and $P_v'3$ are all less than alveolar pressure.

producing both heterogeneous and spatially correlated flows has been described by using a fractal model (35).

Decreased perfusion heterogeneity in prone compared with supine posture can be integrated with the regions of increased conductance in the dorsal lung regions, by means of an anatomical bias for greater flows in dorsal regions must exist. Although a structural difference between the dorsal and ventral aspects of the vascular tree has not been observed (or sought), such a difference makes teleological sense for quadrupeds. A structural bias for increased dorsal conduc-

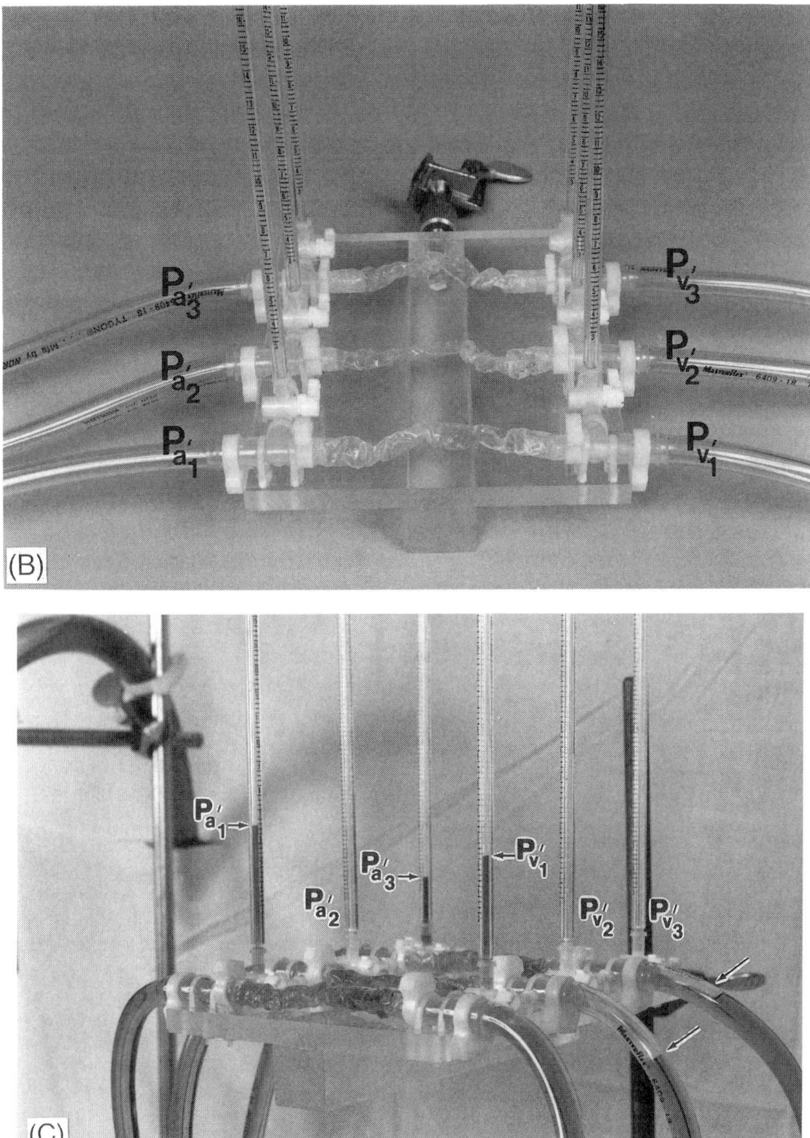

Figure 8 Continued.

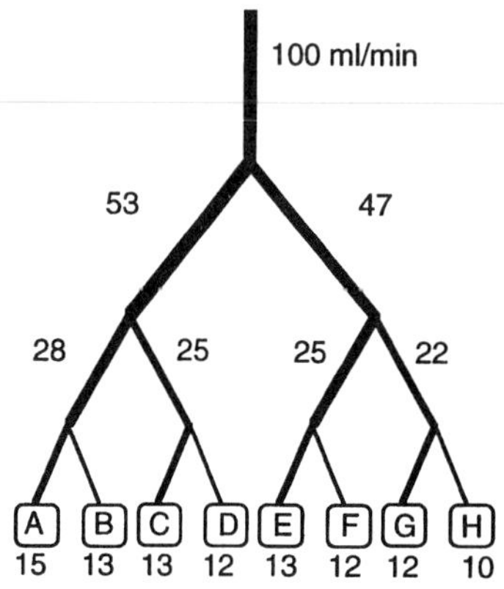

Figure 9 Simple branching vascular tree in which blood flow is distributed asymmetrically at each bifurcation. The flow asymmetry produces heterogeneous perfusion at the terminal branches, which is also spatially correlated. (Neighboring regions having similar flows: A and B have higher flows than G and H.)

tance offsets the effects of gravity and produces a more even flow distribution when prone or walking on four legs.

As a consequence of heterogeneities in the vascular network, differences in driving pressures at the capillary level must exist (28), with the potential to produce multiple zonal conditions within isogravitational planes. This concept, presented in Figure 10, focuses on microvascular pressures rather than central pulmonary arterial and venous pressures. Within each isogravitational plane, the distribution of driving pressures results in heterogeneous regional blood flow and potentially multiple zonal conditions. The heterogeneity of perfusion within isogravitational planes is depicted by the horizontal standard deviation bars shown in the graph of Figure 10.

Gravity exerts its effects on blood flow distribution by increasing the hydrostatic pressure toward dependent lung regions. Although the mean flow per isogravitational plane increases down the lung, the variability in flow within isogravitational planes produces flows that may be greater in one region than in another regardless of vertical position in the lung. Alveolar pressures influence local blood flow in the same manner described by Banister and Torrance (2) and incorporated by West (7) into the gravitational model. In contrast to the gravitational model, multiple zonal conditions may be present within a horizontal plane. Gravity alters the statistical distribution of these zones, shifting the frequency distribution toward zone 2 and 3 conditions, eventually resulting in only zone 3 conditions in the most dependent regions. The different zones within an isogravitational plane are probably not randomly distributed, but spa-

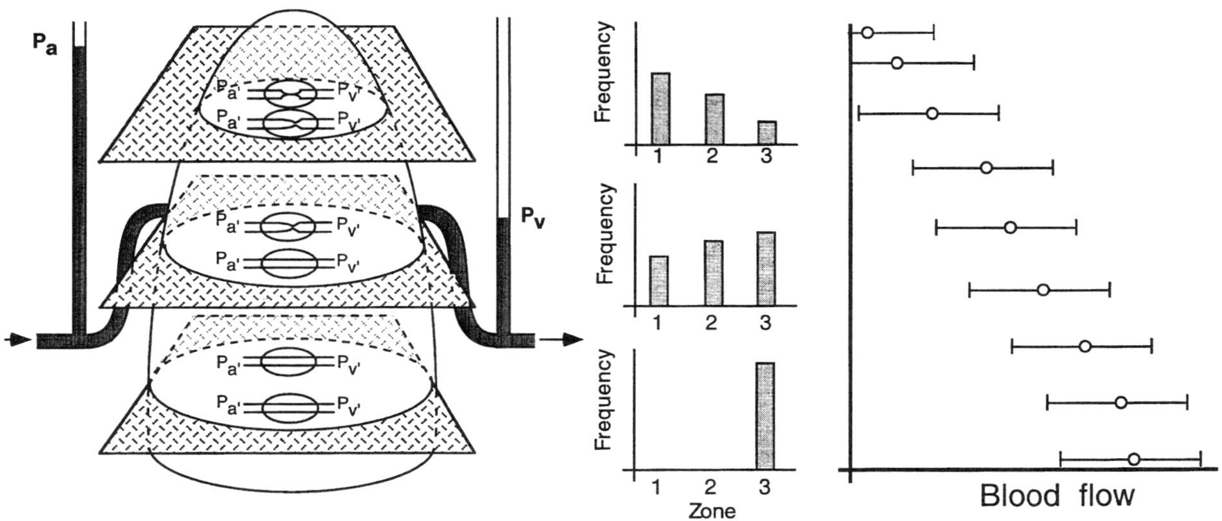

Figure 10 Model of pulmonary blood flow distribution in which regional perfusion is both heterogeneously distributed and spatially correlated within isogravitational planes. Multiple zonal conditions may exist within a horizontal plane. The mean flow per isogravitational plane increases down the lung because of the relatively smaller effect of gravity.

tially correlated, as is perfusion. The shared heritage up the vascular tree causes neighboring regions to have similar driving pressures and hence similar zonal conditions.

This representation of pulmonary blood flow is consistent with prior observations using lower resolution methods. Scintillation counters placed on the chest wall would record increasing counts down the lung bccausc of thc incrcasc in the mean flow per isogravitational plane.

IX. New Perspectives

The evidence that the gravitational paradigm of pulmonary blood flow distribution is unsatisfactory is quite strong. Historically, the effects of gravity on pulmonary blood flow distribution were noted first. However, had the technology been available to measure the spatial distribution of blood flow at the currently available level of resolution, the spatial heterogeneity of perfusion would have been noted first because of its magnitude and the relatively lesser effects of gravity noted secondarily. We believe the perspective provided by a modified model is an essential step in understanding the mechanisms responsible for efficient gas exchange in the lung. We also believe that any major changes to an established model should be aggressively challenged. If they survive the scrutiny of the scientific community, they may emerge as focal points for a renewed cycle of investigation. As with all paradigms, the model we are proposing cannot be proven. It can only be substantiated by future investigations. As stated by Kuhn, it cannot attain the status of a paradigm until it is accepted as defining the core principles belonging to a community of scientist.

We emphasize that the model we propose does not represent an incremental change to the existing gravitational model. Rather, it is a reformulation in which the heterogeneity of pulmonary blood flow is the primary focus. The reason for stating this difference is not to claim authorship of a new model but to force the reorientation that is needed to grasp the concepts of the new model. Within the context of this new perspective, old and new observation on pulmonary blood flow can be analyzed.

A new model is accompanied by new problems and new solutions. According to Kuhn, one of the most important functions of a new model is to stimulate new research. The initial direction of exploration should be to test the fidelity of this new model and to verify these new concepts. High-resolution measurements of the entire vascular network and regional perfusion are needed to relate structure to local blood flow. If the proposed model is correct, a high correlation should exist between regional blood flow and the estimated conductance of the vascular tree to a given region. Investigation of mechanisms determining pulmonary blood flow distribution should focus on the microvascular level. Pressures at multiple sites within the microvasculature of the same vascular tree are needed to confirm the heterogeneity of driving pressures within isogravitational planes. Measurements of perfusion heterogeneity at the level of gas exchange are needed to assess its true extent. With the advent of positron emission tomography (PET), the pulmonary physiology experiments of the 1960s can be repeated using higher spatial resolution methods (36).

The reorientation induced by this model also provides insights into the primary function of gas exchange in the lung. Despite the heterogeneous distribution of perfusion at the alveolar-capillary level, gases are efficiently exchanged. The traditional model of gas exchange includes a small unit of ventilation and its companion capillaries. The mechanism invoked to explain ventilation and perfusion matching has been the common effect of gravity (37). However, given the degree of isogravitational perfusion heterogeneity, gravity cannot play an important role in matching ventilation and perfusion. This prediction has recently been verified by studies done by Prisk and colleagues in SLS-1 and SIS-2 where, under conditions of microgravity, ventilation-perfusion inequalities persist (38). The authors of this study conclude that the principle determinants of ventilation-perfusion inequalities are not gravitational in origin.

These observations suggest that 1. regional ventilation is heterogeneous and intimately matched to regional perfusion or 2. the generally accepted model of gas exchange is inaccurate. In contrast to the detailed understanding of cellular function in the lung, the mechanisms responsible for the fundamental lung function of gas exchange is poorly defined (39). Studies using PET have suggested that regional ventilation and perfusion are matched via the effect of vascular blood volume on the alveolar size (40). New research should focus on the mechanisms matching regional ventilation and perfusion. This will require higher resolution measurements of ventilation and perfusion at the alveolar-capillary level.

The lung is a complex system, deriving its function from the interaction of two very complicated networks that determine regional perfusion and ventilation. The simplified models of the pulmonary vascular tree as a connection of compliant tubes, and regional ventilation as a balloon on a straw, are not adequate to characterize the variability within and the interactions between these systems. Any new model of perfusion and ventilation must incorporate the concept of heterogeneity as a principle property of the systems.

References

1. Kuhn TS. The structure of scientific revolutions. In: Neurath, ed. International Encyclopedia of Unified Science. Chicago: The University of Chicago Press, 1970.
2. Banister J, Torrance RW. The effects of tracheal pressure upon flow-pressure relations in the vascular bed of isolated lungs. Q J Exp Physiol 1960; 45:352–367.

3. Anthonisen NR, Milic-Emili J. Distribution of pulmonary perfusion in erect man. J Appl Physiol 1966; 21:760–766.
4. Ball WC, Stewart PB, Newsham, LGS, Bates DV. Regional pulmonary function studied with xenon. J Clin Invest 1962; 41:519–531.
5. Dollery CT, Gillam PMS. The distribution of blood and gas within the lungs measured by scanning after administration of 133Xe. Thorax 1963; 18:316–325.
6. Kaneko K, Milic-Emili J, Dolovich MB, Dawson A, Bates DV. Regional distribution of ventilation and perfusion as a function of body position. J Appl Physiol 1966; 21:767–777.
7. West JB, Dollery CT, Naimark A. Distribution of blood flow in isolated lung: relation to vascular and alveolar pressures. J Appl Physiol 1964; 55:1341–1348.
8. Hughes JMB, Glazier JB, Maloney JE, West JB. Effect of lung volume on the distribution of pulmonary blood flow in man. Respir Physiol 1968; 4:58–72.
9. Glenny RW, Robertson HT. Fractal properties of pulmonary blood flow: characterization of spatial heterogeneity. J Appl Physiol 1990; 69:532–545.
10. Caruthers SD, Harris TR. Effects of pulmonary blood flow on the fractal heterogeneity in sheep lungs. J Appl Physiol 1994; 77:1474–1479.
11. Glenny RW, Lamm WJ, Albert RK, Robertson HT. Gravity is a minor determinant of pulmonary blood flow distribution. J Appl Physiol 1991; 71:620–629.
12. Melsom MN, Flatebo T, Kramer-Johansen J, Aulie A, Sjaastad, OV, Iversen PO, Nicolaysen G. Both gravity and non-gravity dependent factor determine regional blood flow within the goat lung. Acta Physiol Scand 1995; 153:343–353.
13. Parker JC, Ardell JL, Hamm CR, Barman SA, Coker PJ. Regional pulmonary blood flow during rest, tilt, and exercise in unanesthetized dogs. J Appl Physiol 1995; 78: 838–846.
14. Glenny RW, Polissar L, Robertson HT. Relative contribution of gravity to pulmonary perfusion heterogeneity. J Appl Physiol 1991; 71:2449–2452.
15. Glenny RW, Bernard S, Barlow C, Kelly J, Robertson HT. Spatial distribution of pulmonary blood flow at a microscopic scale of resolution. Am J Respir Crit Care Med 1995; 151:A518.
16. Reed JH, Wood EH. Effect of body position on vertical distribution of pulmonary blood flow. J Appl Physiol 1970; 28:303–311.
17. Greenleaf JF, Ritman EL, Sass DJ, Wood EH. Spatial distribution of pulmonary blood flow in dogs in left decubitus position. Am J Physiol 1974; 227:230–244.
18. Hakim TS, Lisbona R, Dean GW. Gravity-independent inequality in pulmonary blood flow in humans. J Appl Physiol 1987; 63:1114–1121.
19. Hlastala MP, Bernard SL, Erickson HH, Fedde MR, Gaughan EM, McMurphy R, Emery MJ, Polissar N, Glenny RW. Pulmonary blood flow distribution in standing horses is not dominated by gravity. in submission (included in appendix).
20. Hlastala M, Bernard S, Erickson H, Fedde M, Emery M, Glenny R. Pulmonary perfusion heterogeneity (q) in the standing horse at rest. 1995; 151:A520.
21. Bernard S, Glenny R, Erickson H, Emery M, MP H. Pulmonary blood flow redistributes to the dorsal regions with exercise in thoroughbred racehorses. FASEB J 1995; A538.
22. Prisk GK, Guy HJB, Elliot AR, West JB. In homogeneity of pulmonary perfusion during sustained microgravity on SLS-1. J Appl Physiol 1994; 76:1730–1738.

23. Glenny RW. Spatial correlation of regional pulmonary perfusion. J Appl Physiol 1992; 72:2378–2386.
24. Beck KC, Vettermann J, Rehder K. Gas exchange in dogs in the prone and supine positions. J Appl Physiol 1992; 2292–2297.
25. Beck KC, Rehder K. Differences in regional vascular conductances in isolated dog lungs. J Appl Physiol 1986; 61:530–538.
26. Nicolaysen G, Shepard J, Onizuka M, Tanita T, Hattner RS, Staub NC. No gravity-independent gradient of blood flow distribution in dog lung. J Appl Physiol 1987; 63:540–545.
27. Glenny RW, Polissar NL, McKinney S, Robertson HT. Temporal heterogeneity of regional pulmonary perfusion is spatially clustered. J Appl Physiol 1995; 986–1001.
28. Kuhnle GE, Pries AR, Goetz AE. Distribution of microvascular pressure in arteriolar vessel trees of ventilated rabbit lungs. Am J Physiol 1993; 265:H1510–H1515.
29. Gaehtgens P. Why networks? Int J Microcirc Clin Exp 1992; 11:123–132.
30. Weibel ER. Fractal geometry: a design principle for living organisms. Am J Physiol 1991.
31. van Beek JHGM, Roger SA, Bassingthwaighte JB. Regional myocardial flow heterogeneity explained with fractal networks. Am J Physiol 1989; 257:H1670–H1680.
32. Glenny RW, Robertson HT. Fractal modeling of pulmonary blood flow heterogeneity. J Appl Physiol 1991; 70:1024–1030.
33. Horsfield K, Woldenberg MJ. Diameters and cross-sectional areas of branches in the human pulmonary arterial tree. Anat Rec 1989; 223:245–251.
34. Okada O, Presson RGJ, Kirk KR, Godbey PS, Capen RL, Wagner WWJ. Capillary perfusion patterns in single alveolar walls. J Appl Physiol 1992; 72:1838–1844.
35. Glenny RW, Robertson HT. A computer simulation of pulmonary perfusion in three dimensions. J Appl Physiol 1995; 79:357–369.
36. Rhodes CG, Hughes JMB. Pulmonary studies using positron emission tomography. Eur Respir J 1995; 8:1001–1017.
37. West JB. Regional differences in the lung. Chest 1978; 74:426–437.
38. Prisk GK, Elliot AR, Guy HJB, Kosonen JM, West JB. Pulmonary gas exchange and its determinants during sustained microgravity on Spacelabs SLS-1 and SLS-2. J Appl Physiol 1995; 79:1290–1298.
39. Marshall BE, Marshall C, Frasch F, Hanson CW. Role of hypoxic pulmonary vasoconstriction in pulmonary gas exchange and blood flow distribution: 1. Physiologic concepts. Intensive Care Med 1994; 20:291–297.
40. Brudin LH, Rhodes CG, Valind SO, Jones T, Hughes JMB. Interrelationships between regional blood flow, blood volume, and ventilation in supine humans. J Appl Physiol 1994; 76:1205–1210.

Part Five

MATCHING OF VENTILATION AND PERFUSION

16

Noninvasive Measurement of Local $\dot{V}_A$, $\dot{Q}$, and $\dot{V}_A/\dot{Q}$ Distributions by PET

JOSE G. VENEGAS

Harvard Medical School
Boston, Massachusetts

I. Introduction

Radionuclide imaging has played an important role in the evaluation of pulmonary function both clinically and in research. Early studies used inhaled ^{133}Xe gas and external radiation detectors to assess regional differences in pulmonary ventilation. Since then, imaging of radionuclides by planar gamma camera or single-photon emission computed tomography (SPECT) have become clinically established methods to assess the regional distributions of pulmonary ventilation and perfusion. Pulmonary perfusion is assessed by imaging the distribution of intravenously injected radiolabeled particles such as ^{11m}Tc-labeled macroaggregated albumin or human albumin microspheres. Pulmonary ventilation is assessed by imaging the wash-in–wash-out of ^{127}Xe or the steady-state distribution of the short lived ^{81m}Kr. Ventilation-perfusion matching is assessed from the combination of independent ventilation and perfusion scans. These scans play important roles in evaluation of patients with suspected pulmonary embolism or in estimating regional lung function before pulmonary resection is undertaken, but they suffer from quantitation errors and poor spatial resolution, which limit their research value.

Positron emission tomography (PET) is a quantitative technique with higher spatial resolution than any other nuclear medicine imaging technique. The PET imaging is based on the unique physical process that positrons undergo following their emission by beta-unstable radioisotopes. After emission, the positron follows a tortuous ionization path through the material in which it is emitted. As the positron slows down, it combines with a valence electron and undergoes the process of annihilation, emitting two high-energy (511 kvE) photons in nearly opposite directions. The high energy allows these photons to travel across body tissues and be recorded by a ring of external detectors. A coincidence event, or count, is recorded by the camera only when two opposing detectors register the arrival of photons within a very short time interval. The location of the coincident external detectors defines a line containing the origin of the radiation. Once enough counts are recorded, a tomographic image can be reconstructed using standard computed tomography (CT) algorithms. Energy attenuation by body tissues is assessed from an additional scan using an external radiation source to transmit energy across the body. Reconstruction of this "transmission" scan yields a tomographic image of tissue density, which is used to correct the emission images. These corrected images provide quantitative information of the radioactive tracer distribution within the thorax. For example, a PET image of the lungs after the gas tracer $^{13}N_2$ has been inhaled and equilibrated with the air spaces, is a direct representation of regional volume of air per unit of voxel volume. It turns out, $^{13}N_2$ is an ideal gas for imaging lung function because it is inert and has an extremely low solubility in blood and tissues, remaining mostly confined to the air spaces after inhalation.

The efficiency of the lungs as a gas exchanger is determined by the local matching of the distributions of ventilation and perfusion quantified as $\dot{V}_A/\dot{Q}$ ratio. To understand the mechanisms responsible for heterogeneity in $\dot{V}_A/\dot{Q}$, it is of vital importance to evaluate and characterize separately the contributions of $\dot{V}_A$ and $\dot{Q}$ as well as their corresponding spatial correlation. In this chapter, various PET imaging and analysis methods available to assess these variables are described, and their advantages and shortcomings are discussed.

A. General Advantages and Limitations of PET in the Lungs

The general advantages of PET for pulmonary functional imaging are its noninvasive nature and its ability to follow the kinetics and distribution of short half-life radiolabeled compounds at minimal concentrations. Depending on the nature of the labeled compound, mathematical models of tracer kinetics may need to be fitted to the imaged data to yield images of regional lung function parameters. In addition to errors caused by possible oversimplification in the formulation of such mathematical models, PET imaging has intrinsic technical limitations that need to be considered when designing experimental imaging protocols and interpreting data. These limitations include sensitivity, accuracy, and spatial and temporal resolution.

The radioactive decay events imaged by PET are a statistical process that obeys a Poisson distribution wherein the relative error of the measurement is inversely proportional to the number of events detected per voxel. Thus, to be accurate, a PET scan must include a large number of counts: this involves either high levels of radioactivity or long collection times. The levels of radioactivity used are limited by the radiation dose to the imaged subject and camera operator, and by the ability to remove or avoid false (or random) coincidences recorded by the camera from photons originating from different positron annihilations. These random coincidences are negligible in modern PET cameras even when imaging at relatively high activity levels.

The spatial resolution of PET images, defined as the width at half-height of a point source image, ranges from 4.5 to 20 mm and is determined by the geometrical design of the camera (i.e., the number and size of scintillation detecting units) and the thickness of the slice imaged. Typical slice thickness of high-resolution instruments ranges from 5 to 10 mm. Other factors can also cause additional deterioration of spatial resolution. First, positron imaging detects two photons created during the annihilation of a positron with an electron. The exact origin of the photons is, therefore, not the position of the radionuclide but some distance from it given by the finite range that the positron travels before annihilation. This range is proportional to the positron energy divided by the density of the tissue. Because the overall density of the lung is relatively lower than that of other tissues, the effect of the positron range (~3 mm) becomes a significant factor in determining resolution, particularly with a high-resolution PET camera. For a given level of activity, the count rate per voxel decreases with the cube of the voxel size; therefore, significant improvements in resolution are only feasible by increasing the sensitivity of the camera to radioactive events. A new generation of high-resolution (3 mm), high-sensitivity, three-dimensional PET cylinders has been recently developed. The Physics Research Laboratory of the Massachusetts General Hospital is testing an instrument capable of imaging at once a 10 cm long by 90 cm in diameter cylinder with a spatial resolution better than 3 mm. With this camera, it is hoped that image resolution will simply be limited by the range of the positron.

Respiratory and cardiac movement can also worsen the spatial resolution in proportion to the dimensional changes in each lung region: the radial motion of the lung during normal breathing can be as much as 1 cm in the periphery; even larger axial motions can be expected in the diaphragmatic regions. This source of error can be minimized by respiratory gated imaging. In addition to preventing capturing of lung heterogeneity of small length scales, low spatial resolution can also cause quantitative inaccuracy because of partial volume averaging of regions with a geometric scale lower than the spatial resolution of the camera. This is particularly critical in the chest wall and cardiac boundaries of the lung and in conditions of large spatial heterogeneity.

II. Imaging Techniques

A. Measurements of $\dot{Q}$

Methods for assessing regional $\dot{Q}$ with PET include direct methods, such as imaging the lung after intravenous injection of radiolabeled water $H_2{}^{15}O$ and ^{68}Ga-labeled microspheres (1) or of $^{13}N_2$ gas in saline solution (2,3) and an indirect method in which $\dot{Q}$ is derived from the ratio of independently assessed $\dot{V}_A$ and $\dot{V}_A/\dot{Q}$ images (4).

1. Intravenous Bolus Injection of ^{15}O Water

The $H_2{}^{15}O$ method (1) follows the kinetics of a bolus of tracer as it transits the lung and then equilibrates through the body. The data are then analyzed in terms of a single compartment model. Because $H_2{}^{15}O$ is freely diffused into, and out of, vascular and extravascular spaces, this method also provides information about local lung water content. A limitation to this method is imposed by the short residence time of the tracer in the lung (<10 seconds), which requires very short duration scans and results in low signal-to-noise ratio images, particularly when imaging at high spatial resolution. This limits its research use to spatial resolution scales greater than 20 mm.

2. Intravenous Injected Microspheres

The method of injecting ^{68}Ga-labeled microspheres provides a more accurate measurement of $\dot{Q}$ at high resolution. However, because the tracer has a rather long half-life (68 minutes) and remains trapped in the lungs after injection, it becomes experimentally difficult to acquire multiple measurements of $\dot{Q}$, $\dot{V}_A$ and $\dot{V}_A/\dot{Q}$ in the same subject.

3. Intravenous Bolus of $^{13}N_2$ Saline

Aside from the technical limitations, the methods described above are unable to distinguish between blood flow to gas exchanging units ($\dot{Q}_A$) from that to shunting units ($\dot{Q}_s$). At my institution, we have recently described a method to quantify $\dot{Q}_A$ and $\dot{Q}_s$ after a bolus injection of $^{13}N_2$ saline solution (5). The physical principle of the method is based on the extremely low solubility of $^{13}N_2$ gas in blood and tissues (blood gas partition coefficient $\lambda = 0.017$). Thus, after an intravenous bolus injection of $^{13}N_2$ saline during apnea, virtually all the tracer gas in the blood is transferred to gas-filled alveolar units at the first pass. In these units, the tracer content remains nearly constant during the following 30 to 60 seconds and, as ^{68}Ga-labeled microspheres, yields an accurate measurement of local $\dot{Q}$. In contrast, in nonaerated atelectatic and shunting regions, the $^{13}N_2$ tracer behaves like the tracer $H_2{}^{15}O$ and, after arrival, is removed exponentially by the continuing blood flow (Figure 1d).

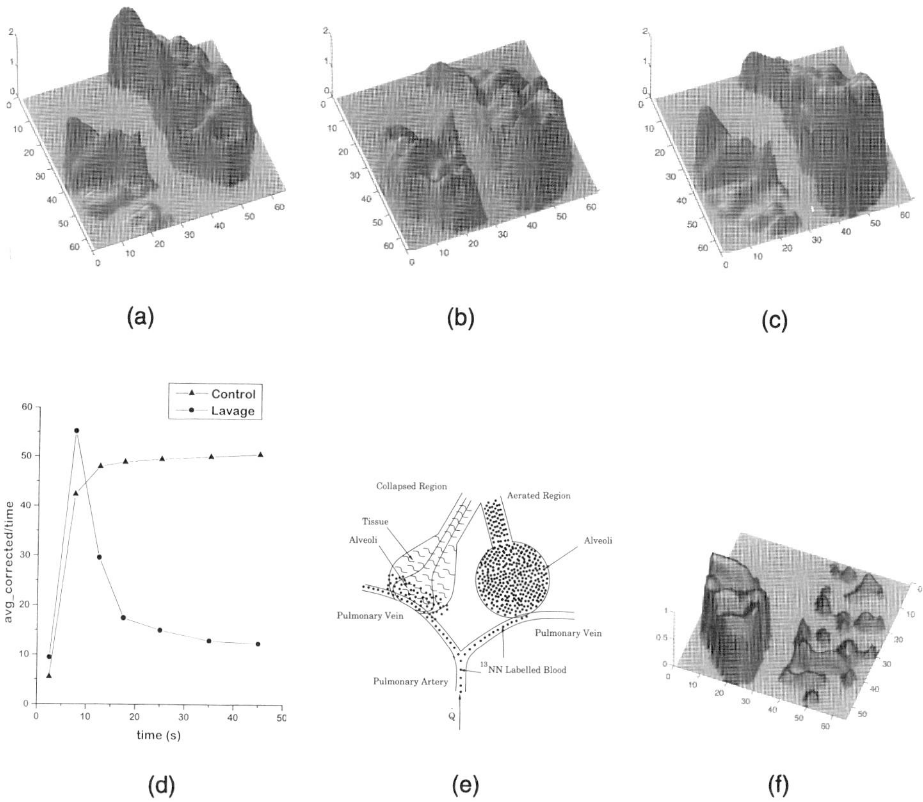

Figure 1 Cross-sectional PET images at the level of the base collected from a dog after unilateral lavage of the left lung. In the surface plots, height over the XY plane represents number of counts per voxel normalized by the mean value within the lung field. (**a**) After equilibrated inhalation of $^{13}N_2$ gas showing minimal gas content on the lavaged lung. (**b**) Image collected between 5 and 10 seconds from the $^{13}N_2$ saline bolus infusion corresponding to the peak tracer concentration in the lavaged region and thus to total $\dot{Q}$. (**c**) Image similar to (*b*), but collected after 40 seconds of bolus injection. (**d**) Plot of mean tracer concentration versus time, following a bolus injection of $^{13}N_2$ saline solution in lavaged and control regions. Note that the tracer remains in the aerated control region but falls exponentially to an asymptote in the lavaged atelectatic region. (**e**) Conceptual model of regional tracer kinetics including collapsed (or flooded) and aerated alveolar units. (**f**) Surface plot of shut fraction, Qs/Qt, derived using the model in (*e*) from the above PET data.

Experimentally, $\dot{Q}$ is measured in the following manner. Starting with a radioactive tracer–free lung, ventilation is interrupted at end exhalation and immediately a bolus of $^{13}N_2$-labeled saline is infused at a constant flow rate for 1 to 5 seconds depending on the specific activity of the infusate. At the same time as the beginning of infusion, collection of five consecutive images begins. When imaging is completed, ventilation is resumed and the tracer washed out. A sample of infusate is collected to assess its specific activity and the total activity injected.

Analysis of the images is based on a model with two parallel compartments: one for aerated alveoli and one for nonaerated atelectatic units (see Figure 1e). Application of this model to imaging data gives local indices of $\dot{Q}$ and $\dot{Q}_s/\dot{Q}$ (see Figure 1f).

Advantages of this method over other methods are that it is repeatable after a short period of tracer decay and wash-out, it has excellent signal-to-noise ratio (s/n > 100) at high resolution, and it is not affected by potential artifacts such as clustering or streaming of microspheres. More importantly, the $^{13}N_2$ method provides a way to estimate the local shunt fraction, which is not available by any other technique. This method has the limitation of requiring apnea during an imaging period of 20 to 45 seconds. This limitation, however, should not invalidate the measurement because the actual registration of $\dot{Q}$ is concluded within the first 10 seconds as the tracer is transferred to the periphery, a period too short to expect significant alterations in local perfusion. A second limitation of the method is imposed by potential interregional mixing, by diffusion and cardiogenic oscillations, of the $^{13}N_2$ gas during the apneic period of imaging, erasing heterogeneity from the PET images. However, we have found no significant differences in spatial heterogeneity of sequential images acquired during periods of apnea up to 60 seconds, suggesting that, during this period, the artifact only occurs at length scales smaller than the spatial resolution of our images (10 mm).

4. Calculated Ratio of $\dot{V}_A$ and ($\dot{V}_A/\dot{Q}$)

Regional blood flow has also been obtained indirectly (4,11) from independent measurements of $\dot{V}_A$ and $\dot{V}_A/\dot{Q}$; $\dot{V}_A$ imaged during steady-state inhalation of ^{19}Ne and $\dot{V}_A/\dot{Q}$ imaged during the steady-state intravenous infusion of $^{13}N_2$ saline solution are both described below. Although indirect, this method has the experimental advantage that is based on two measurements obtained during steady-state conditions that do not require apnea. However, because the measurements of $\dot{V}_A$ and $\dot{V}_A/\dot{Q}$ are carried out at different times, temporal fluctuation in the corresponding local distributions occurring during and between scans could affect the accuracy of the estimation of $\dot{Q}$. Furthermore, in heterogeneous diseased lungs, imaging errors intrinsic to the $\dot{V}_A$ and $\dot{V}_A/\dot{Q}$ imaging methods (see below) may combine and yield unacceptable artifacts.

B. Measurements of $\dot{V}_A$

In contrast to regional $\dot{Q}$, which can be easily defined and measured in physical units of flow rate, the concept of $\dot{V}_A$ is abstract and more difficult to quantify. The classical concept of $\dot{V}_A$ involves an idealized mechanism of convective gas transport along parallel pathways of a proximal "dead space" and a perfectly mixed alveolar compartment. Assuming that the effect of dead space is uniform, regional $\dot{V}_A$ has been estimated from local indices of lung expansion measured as changes in local lung density by CT (6), displacement of intraparenchymal markers by x-ray (7), or temporal changes in local gas content per voxel with positron imaging (8–10). However, the inference of regional gas transport from these indices of lung expansion can be misleading: 1. Dead space pathways are not strictly parallel but include common paths, making it difficult to characterize their effect on gas exchange, 2. the transition between convective, dispersive and diffusive gas transport occurs progressively and not in the sharp front assumed, and 3. mixing by diffusion and cardiogenic oscillations is not complete in the distal lung, giving rise to substantial serial and parallel gradients in respiratory gas concentrations.

Another approach to define an effective regional $\dot{V}_A$ is in terms of the rate of gas transported to or from that region. With this approach, effective $\dot{V}_A$ per unit of alveolar volume (s $\dot{V}_A$) can be estimated using PET from the steady-state distribution of a rapidly decaying inhaled isotope gas such as ^{19}Ne (11,12) or from the wash-out rate of a previously equilibrated inhaled tracer gas such as $^{13}N_2$ (13–15). Because this definition of $\dot{V}_A$ does not assume a mechanism of gas transport, it is the basis for more practical methods to quantify regional gas transport, particularly in nonconventional methods of assisted ventilation such as high frequency ventilation (13), constant flow ventilation (14) wherein the classical concept of $\dot{V}_A$ and dead space become useless.

1. Steady State Inhalation of a Short-Lived Tracer

Originally described for the tracer ^{81m}Kr and standard nuclear medicine imaging (16), this method was implemented for PET (11,17) using the gas ^{19}Ne ($T_{1/2}$ = 17.4 seconds). The method involves a continuous inhalation of the highly insoluble tracer (water–gas partition coefficient, $\lambda_{Ne} = 0.0092$) and is based on a single compartment model of the regional lung with alveolar volume V_A and tracer concentration c_A. When tracer activity in the lung has reached an equilibrium, the input activity ($\dot{V}_A$ times the inspiratory tracer concentration c_i) must be balanced by the radioactive decay within the compartment (^{19}Ne radioactive decay constant $\Lambda = 0.04$ second^{-1}) and the clearance resulting from ventilation. Using this model, specific ventilation $s\dot{V}_A = \dot{V}_A/\dot{V}_A$, can be expressed as follows:

$$s\dot{V}_A = \left(\frac{\Lambda}{\frac{c_i}{c_A} - 1}\right) \tag{1}$$

Here c_i is measured with a scintillation detector and c_A is obtained by dividing the local tracer activity, measured with PET, by the regional gas content (V_A) calculated from the transmission scan (17). The method has the advantage of allowing prolonged imaging scans, yielding images with high signal-to-noise ratios. Errors in this measurement have been estimated to be small (<10%) for normal human lungs imaged at a resolution of 17 mm, but errors could reach much higher levels when imaging at higher resolutions or in areas with low $\dot{V}_A$, where tracer concentration in conducting airways could result in more than 100% overestimation of s $\dot{V}_A$ (17).

2. *Wash-Out Rate of Equilibrated Inhaled $^{13}N_2$*

The wash-out rate from the lungs after equilibration with inhaled $^{13}N_2$ gas can also be used as an index of local specific ventilation $s\dot{V}_{A,i}$ (13,15,18,19). The method is based on the Steward-Hamilton equation, where the mean residence time of the tracer (MRT) is calculated as the integral over time of local activity during the wash-out (c[t]) divided by the initial equilibrated activity (c[0]):

$$MRT = (s\dot{V}_A)^{-1} = \frac{1}{c(0)}\int_{t=0}^{t=\infty} C(t) \cdot dt \tag{2}$$

Experimentally, c(0) is calculated from a scan collected after equilibration with the $^{13}N_2$ tracer gas, and the integral is estimated as the sum of counts collected during sequential PET imaging after correcting for radioactive decay of the tracer and truncation error caused by the finite duration of the wash-out scans. This definition is advantageous because it does not require the assumption that the local tracer wash-out follows a single exponential function (20). In diseased lungs with regions of low $s\dot{V}_{A,i}$, equilibration cannot be reached during reasonable scanning times. In those cases, however, sequential imaging collected during the wash-in and wash-out of the tracer has been used to correct for this problem (19). The $^{13}N_2$ wash-out method has also been further refined to assess s $\dot{V}_A$ from a second slower compartment (20) and to include respiratory gating (2,3). Respiratory gating is important not only to minimize spatial averaging resulting from respiratory motion but also to allow imaging of the lungs at end exhalation, a lung volume comparable to that during the apneic measurement of $\dot{Q}$. Technically, the accuracy of this method is limited in areas of high $s\dot{V}_{A,i}$ from which the tracer is rapidly removed, reducing the local count statistics. This problem is partially overcome by high initial count rates obtained with high sensitivity modern PET cameras.

Both the ^{19}Ne inhalation method and the $^{13}N_2$ wash-out method truly assess the rate at which a tracer is transported out of a resolution element. However, the measurements also include transport of tracer contained in conducting airways and unperfused alveolar units, which do not participate in the blood–air exchange of respiratory gases.

3. Wash-Out Rate After Intravenous Bolus Injection of $^{13}N_2$ Saline

At my institution, we have recently developed two PET imaging methods to assess local $\dot{V}_A$, which are not biased by the transport of tracer resident in nonperfused alveolar units and conducting airways. These methods are based on the kinetics of the tracer gas $^{13}N_2$ after it is deposited in alveolar spaces. The bolus injection method to assess $s\dot{V}_A$ ($s\dot{V}_{A,p}$ bolus) involves a rapid (2–4 seconds) intravenous bolus infusion of 5 to 10 cm^3 of $^{13}N_2$ in saline solution during apnea as in the method used to assess local $\dot{Q}$. Once the tracer is diffused into the alveoli and its concentration determined with the PET scanner, ventilation is restarted and a series of PET images are acquired as the tracer is washed out. Estimation of $s\dot{V}_{A,p}$ bolus involves the calculation of the mean residence time of the tracer during the wash-out, using a method similar to that used to calculate $s\dot{V}_{A,i}$ from the wash-out of equilibrated inhaled $^{13}N_2$ gas (see Equation 2) (10). The $^{13}N_2$ tracer is deposited in distal air spaces adjacent to the air–blood interface instead of being uniformly distributed in all air spaces. Because all perfused areas receive tracer, this method yields high signal-to-noise ratio images even in diseased lungs with areas of low $\dot{V}_A$ where tracer high concentration is maintained during the wash-out. Technically, this is a major advantage compared with the inhaled $^{13}N_2$ tracer wash-out or the steady-state ^{19}Ne inhalation method in which the corresponding tracer is diverted away from areas of low $\dot{V}_A$ yielding low signal-to-noise ratio.

4. Calculated from $\dot{Q}$ and $\dot{V}_A/\dot{Q}$

An indirect method to assess $s\dot{V}_{A,p}$ with PET ($s\dot{V}_{A,p}$ indirect) is by combining the results of a $\dot{Q}$ scan after apneic bolus injection of $^{13}N_2$ saline solution, described above, with a steady-state scan during a constant flow infusion of the same solution. As presented in more detail below, the local radioactivity per voxel recorded during steady-state constant infusion of $^{13}N_2$ saline solution is the sum of activity from alveolar and precapillary arterial blood. From a tracer mass balance, it can be shown that the alveolar content of a low solubility tracer gas is approximately proportional to the ratio of local $\dot{Q}$ to $\dot{V}_A/V_A$ or $\dot{Q}/s\dot{V}_{A,p}$. Thus, $s\dot{V}_{A,p}$ can be estimated by dividing the $\dot{Q}$ scan by the constant infusion scan after correction for precapillary blood tracer content. For this calculation to be correct, lung volumes during the apneic scan and the constant infusion steady-state scan must be comparable, thus requiring respiratory gating during the latter scans.

5. Differences Between $s\dot{V}_{A,i}$ and $s\dot{V}_{A,p}$

Because voxel ^{13}NN content after equilibration is proportional to intraregional gas volume, the measurement of local $s\dot{V}_{A,i}$ is based on tracer initially resident in all gas-filled areas including perfused and unperfused alveolar units as well as serial dead space. It can be shown that regional $s\dot{V}_{A,i}$ corresponds to a *volume-weighted* mean of local $s\dot{V}_A$ within that region. In contrast, the $^{13}N_2$ tracer after intravenous infusion is distributed in proportion to regional $\dot{Q}$ and thus is exclusively resident in perfused alveolar units. The measurement of $s\dot{V}_{A,p}$ should therefore represent a *perfusion-weighted* mean $s\dot{V}_A$ of that region.

It can be speculated that $s\dot{V}_{A,i}$ and $s\dot{V}_{A,p}$ are related but different physiological entities that are affected in different ways by heterogeneity of $\dot{V}_A$ and $\dot{Q}$ at subresolution length scales. For example, if the intraregional distribution of $\dot{V}_A$ within the resolution element was totally uniform, or was heterogeneous but spatially uncorrelated with the intraregional distribution of $\dot{Q}$, then one could expect that local $s\dot{V}_{A,i}$ and $s\dot{V}_{A,p}$ would be equal. Conversely, if the intraregional distribution of $\dot{V}_A$ was spatially correlated with the distribution of $\dot{Q}$ (intraregions of high $\dot{Q}$ having high $\dot{V}_A$), then local $s\dot{V}_{A,p}$ could be expected to exceed local $s\dot{V}_{A,i}$; subresolution regions of relative high $\dot{Q}$, weighted in the perfused tracer method, would also have high $\dot{V}_A$. This hypothesis is consistent with recent experimental data from our laboratory (2) showing that the mean values of local $s\dot{V}_{A,i}$ within the lung field $\left(\overline{s\dot{V}_{A,i}}\right)$ were correlated with, but systematically lower than, those from $s\dot{V}_{A,p}$ $\left(\overline{s\dot{V}_{A,p}}\right)$, thus suggesting the intraregional distribution of $\dot{V}_A$ at scales smaller than the resolution element in PET (1 cm^3) is spatially correlated with $\dot{Q}$.

In terms of the spatial distribution of $s\dot{V}_A$ at scales greater than the imaging resolution of PET, both methods yielded similar values of the heterogeneity index cov (defined as the mean normalized standard deviation of the regional data). Also, both methods yielded lower heterogeneity in the prone position compared with the supine (2). In the prone position, there was no significant vertical gradients in $s\dot{V}_{A,i}$ or in $s\dot{V}_{A,p}$. However, in the supine position, $s\dot{V}_{A,p}$ showed significant vertical gradients whereas $s\dot{V}_{A,i}$ did not. Also, $s\dot{V}_{A,p}$ was found to be correlated with $\dot{Q}$ in both body positions ($R_s = 0.81$ supine and 0.69 prone), whereas $s\dot{V}_{A,i}$ was not ($R_s = 0.05$ supine and 0.04 prone). The difference in results between these methods is not totally clear but it may reflect the contribution to

$s\dot{V}_{A,i}$ of tracer resident in nonperfused alveolar units (alveolar dead space) and suggest a tight spatial correlation between $\dot{V}_A$ and $\dot{Q}$ at length scales below the spatial resolution of the instrument. This interpretation would explain why local values of $s\dot{V}_{A,p}$ were greater than those of $s\dot{V}_{A,i}$ and would be compatible with significant vertical gradients in $s\dot{V}_{A,p}$ and $\dot{Q}$.

As with any method used to assess alveolar ventilation from the wash-in or wash-out of a tracer, both regional $s\dot{V}_{A,i}$ and $s\dot{V}_{A,p}0$ are affected by interregional mixing occurring in the common dead space with each breath. The physiological relevance of this effect, however, may be minimal because such a mixing must also be affecting the transport and alveolar concentrations of physiological gases. Based on these results, one could question which of these measurements of ventilation, $s\dot{V}_{A,i}$ or $s\dot{V}_{A,p}$, is more physiologically relevant. We propose that, in terms of gas exchange, $s\dot{V}_{A,p}$ ought to be more relevant than $s\dot{V}_{A,i}$ because it describes the ventilation of the most distal perfused air spaces, whereas $s\dot{V}_{A,i}$ is biased by the ventilation of regions that are not participating in the exchange of physiological gases. However, to reconcile and understand the differences between $s\dot{V}_{A,p}$ and $s\dot{V}_{A,i}$, further experimentation is needed.

C. Measurements of $\dot{V}_A/\dot{Q}$

The local matching between $\dot{V}_A$ and $\dot{Q}$ has been traditionally assessed from separate measurements of $\dot{V}_A$ and $\dot{Q}$ using conventional nuclear medicine (21,22). Aside from low resolution and the poor quantitative quality of the measurements, this approach has two fundamental problems: 1. Mismatching of $\dot{V}_A$ and $\dot{Q}$ within a resolution element yields erroneous assessment of $\dot{V}_A/\dot{Q}$ ratio and 2. because the measurements are performed at different times, dynamic changes in $\dot{Q}$ or $\dot{V}_A$, which may take place between and during measurements, result in erroneous assessments of local $\dot{V}_A/\dot{Q}$ distributions.

1. *Steady-State Infusion of $^{13}N_2$ Saline Solution*

A method of assessing $\dot{V}_A/\dot{Q}$ by imaging the lungs with PET during steady-state infusion of ^{13}N-labeled saline has obviated these problems (23,24). This method is also based on the low solubility of nitrogen (blood–gas partition coefficient $\lambda = 0.017$ at 37°C). As the tracer is infused intravenously, it reaches the pulmonary capillaries and diffuses into the alveolar air space. After equilibration across the gas–blood interface, the concentration of $^{13}N_2$ at the venous end of the capillaries should be only 1.7% of the alveolar concentration. Once a steady state is reached, the alveolar concentration of $^{13}N_2$ in aerated lung units reflects the balance between tracer delivery by the pulmonary blood flow and tracer removal by ventilation and pulmonary flow as described by the following equation:

$$c_{pa} \cdot \dot{Q} = c_A \cdot \dot{V}_A + c_A \cdot \lambda \cdot \dot{Q} \tag{3}$$

where c_{pa} and c_A are the tracer concentration of the pulmonary arterial blood and alveolar air spaces. Equation 3 can be rearranged to obtain $\dot{V}_A/\dot{Q}$ as

$$\frac{\dot{V}_A}{\dot{Q}} = \frac{c_{pa}}{c_A} - \lambda \qquad (4)$$

To derive local values of $\dot{V}_A/\dot{Q}$ during the continuous infusion of the tracer, c_A is determined from a PET scan recorded once a steady state is reached. c_{pa} may be calculated from the activity of the blood registered by the PET scan within a region of interest around the right atrium or ventricle (24) or measured directly from a pulmonary arterial blood sample using a cross-calibrated scintillation detector (3). To obtain a value of alveolar tracer content, the counts per voxel recorded in the PET scan need to be first corrected for the radioactive decay of the tracer ($T_{1/2}$ = 10 minutes). The decay-corrected tracer content ($S_{^{13}N}$) per voxel corresponds to the product of c_A times V_A plus the background activity originating from the precapillary pulmonary blood resident in pulmonary arteries and arterioles. This background activity is estimated from an additional blood volume scan recorded after labeling the erythrocytes by inhalation of ^{11}CO gas and assuming that the precapillary blood volume corresponds to 40% of the pulmonary blood volume (V_B) (24). In normal lungs, this activity does not exceed 15% of $S_{^{13}N}$. c_A can then be calculated as follows:

$$c_A = (S_{^{13}N} - 0.4 \cdot V_B \cdot c_{pa})/V_A \qquad (5)$$

where V_A can be obtained from the inhaled $^{13}N_2$ equilibrated image (2) or from a transmission san (24) as described above.

This method has been used in humans at a resolution of 17 mm (23,24) with estimated uncertainties of less than 10%. The technique has been recently refined to include respiratory gating and used to image normal dog lungs at a spatial resolution of 10 mm (2,3) and with errors of less than 5% (Figure 2). The accuracy of the constant infusion method is affected by two major assumptions: 1. that the $^{13}N_2$ alveolar concentration reaches a steady state during the scanning time and 2. that the radioactivity in nonaerated spaces within a voxel is exclusively confined to arterial blood. Although these assumptions are reasonable for normal lungs (23,24), they are not so in diseased lungs. Assumption 1 does not hold in lung regions with low $\dot{V}_A$ where reaching a steady state may take much longer than the time available for scanning.* Although the overestimation of $\dot{V}_A/\dot{Q}$ caused by a lack of steadiness on these regions can be corrected to some extent using an additional ventilation scan with ^{19}Ne (4), in areas of very low $\dot{V}_A$ or gas trapping, $^{13}N_2$ continues to accumulate throughout the infusion scan, creating "hot" spots that may saturate the PET camera and overwhelm

*Imaging time is limited by tracer decay half-life (10 minutes), the maximum level of activity allowed, or the maximal yield of the labeling process.

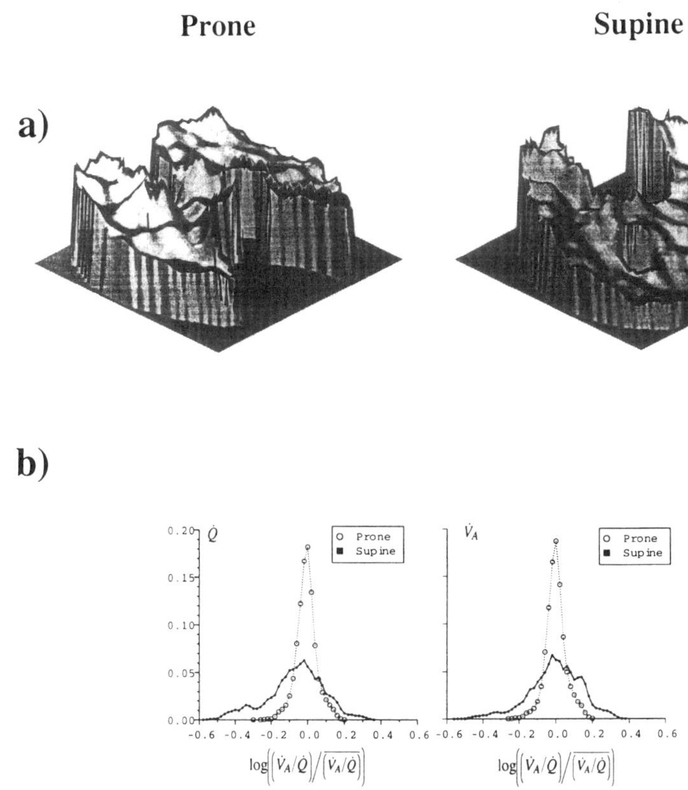

Figure 2 **a**) Images of $\dot{V}_A/\dot{Q}$ for an animal in the prone position (*left*) and for one in the supine position (*right*) in which the height of the surface over the XY plane represents the relative value of $\dot{V}_A/\dot{Q}$. **b**) Distributions of $\dot{V}_A/\dot{Q}$ as a fraction of total $\dot{Q}$ (*left*), and total $\dot{V}_A$ (*right*).

the rest of the image. Assumption 2 does not hold in lungs with atelectatic areas. Despite the low solubility of nitrogen in blood and tissues, during the constant infusion scan, $^{13}N_2$ is not exclusively confined to intravascular and air spaces, as is assumed in the calculation, but a finite amount is diffused to the extravascular lung water and tissues. In normal lungs, the amount of tracer in extravascular spaces is probably minimal, but, in areas with alveolar flooding, microatelectasis, or pulmonary edema, it can be substantially greater than the amount estimated from the assumption because the tracer labels not only the arterial side of the pulmonary vascular tree but also the venous side and the extravascular water and tissues. Another limitation of this method is the prolonged imaging time required per run because, in addition to the 15-minute constant infusion scan and the 15-minute transmission scan, each run requires an additional blood pool scan made with the longer half-life isotope ^{11}C ($T_{1/2} = 20$ minutes), limiting a feasible study to one or two experimental conditions.

2. *Wash-Out Image After Intravenous Bolus Injection of $^{13}N_2$ Saline*

At my institution, we have developed a new method to assess regional $\dot{V}_A/\dot{Q}$ that can be used in heterogeneously diseased lungs and gives simultaneous information about the distributions of $\dot{V}_A/\dot{Q}$, $s\dot{V}_{A,p}$, $\dot{Q}$, and $\dot{Q}_s$. The method is a direct consequence of the measurement of $s\dot{V}_{A,p}$ from the wash-out of an intravenously infused bolus of $^{13}N_2$ saline solution.

The image of $s\dot{V}_{A,p}$ is obtained using Equation 2; it involves dividing an image proportional to regional $\dot{Q}$ by a wash-out image (WO) made from summation of all sequential images collected during the wash-out and then corrected for truncation error, tracer radioactive decay, and missed counts resulting from respiratory gating:

$$\overline{s\dot{V}_{A,p}} \propto \dot{Q}/(\mathrm{WO})$$

It follows that the WO image is directly proportional to ($\dot{Q}/s\dot{V}_{A,p}$) (Figure 3).

This method of assessing $\dot{V}_A/\dot{Q}$, (actually $\dot{Q}/s\dot{V}_{A,p}$) has several advantages over the constant infusion method:

1. It does not require waiting for a steady state and it does not saturate the PET camera detectors in areas of low $\dot{V}_A$ because the total activity in the lung is limited to that injected in the bolus.
2. The method does not need correction for extra-alveolar tracer content because no activity remains in the pulmonary vascular tree during imaging.
3. Areas of microatelectasis can be identified from the decrease in local activity during the apneic period.
4. The method does not require a blood pool scan, thus allowing multiple serial studies.

A limitation of this method is that it requires a period of apnea for imaging $\dot{Q}$ in which local controllers of $\dot{V}_A$ and $\dot{Q}$ could be affected. This effect should be small for a short period of apnea given the similarity and correlation between images obtained with both methods in the same animal (Figure 3).

3. *Calculated Ratio of Local $s\dot{V}_A$ and Local $s\dot{Q}$*

Finally, $\dot{V}_A/\dot{Q}$ can also be indirectly calculated from the ratio of independently measured $s\dot{V}_{A,i}$ and $\dot{Q}$ normalized per unit of gas volume (s $\dot{Q}$). Aside from the discrepancies caused by differences between $s\dot{V}_{A,p}$ and $s\dot{V}_{A,i}$ discussed above, a major difference between the steady state and the wash-out methods is that one measures a distribution of $\dot{V}_A/\dot{Q}$ time averaged over the imaging period, whereas

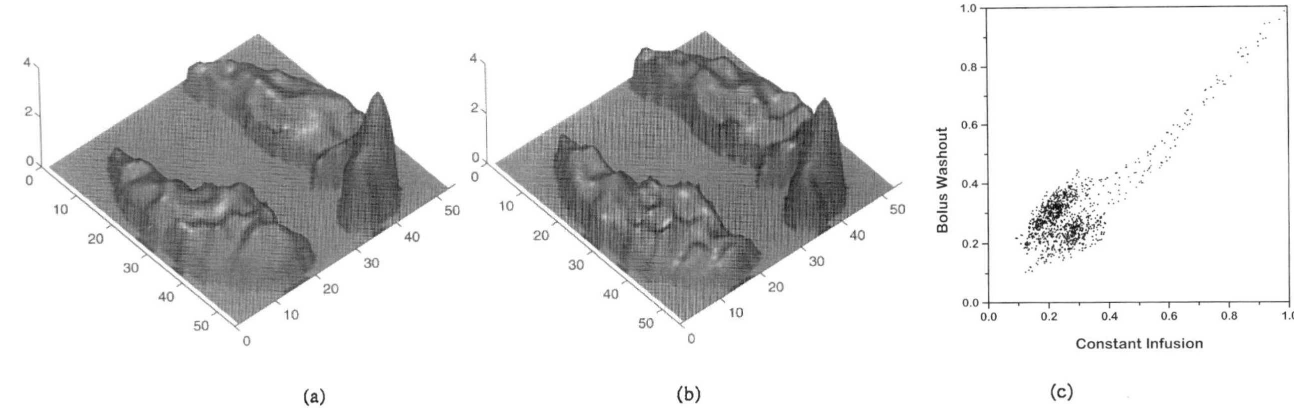

Figure 3 Illuminated surface plot of relative ($\dot{Q}/s\dot{V}_{A,p}$) for an animal with localized pneumoconstriction of a left lower lobe segment in the supine position using the constant infusion technique (**a**) and the wash-out after intravenous bolus injection of $^{13}N_2$-labeled saline (**b**). The height of the surface over the X-Y plane represents the relative value of $\dot{Q}/s\dot{V}_{A,p}$ normalized by the mean of the voxel values. (**c**) Local values of $\dot{Q}/s\dot{V}_{A,p}$ for one technique plotted against the other ($R_s = 0.82$).

the other registers the distributions of $\dot{Q}$ and $s\dot{V}_A$ during short periods separated by finite intervals ranging from a few seconds in the intravenous bolus washout method to more than 20 minutes in the indirect measurement. Thus, in otherwise physiologically stable animals, differences in heterogeneity of $\dot{V}_A/\dot{Q}$ recovered from these methods suggest the occurrence of temporal variations in the distributions of $s\dot{V}_A$ and $s\dot{Q}$. To evaluate this hypothcsis, wc measured $s\dot{V}_A/s\dot{Q}$ and $\dot{V}_A/\dot{Q}$ before and during inhalation of NO (20 ppm) in five supine and five prone anesthetized and mechanically ventilated dogs (25). We found that inhalation of NO did not significantly change the overall spatial heterogeneity ($cov^2 = (SD/mean)^2$) in $s\dot{Q}$, $s\dot{V}_A$), and $\dot{V}_A/\dot{Q}$, although it significantly ($p <$ 0.05) increased the vertical gradient in the direction of gravity of $s\dot{Q}$ from 15.1 $\pm$ 0.5 to 17.3 $\pm$ 0.6 %/cm in the supine position and from 0.9 $\pm$ 1.7 to 5.1 $\pm$ 1.3 %/cm in the prone position. By subtracting the vertical gradients by linear regression, we found that $s\dot{V}_A/s\dot{Q}$ had a residual cov^2 that was more than twice that of $\dot{V}_A/\dot{Q}$ in the prone position and more than five times that of $\dot{V}_A/\dot{Q}$ in the supine position. Inhalation of NO significantly ($p < 0.05$) reduced the residual cov^2 of $s\dot{V}_A/s\dot{Q}$ in both positions ($\Delta cov^2 = 0.023 \pm 0.01$ for prone and 0.055 $\pm$ 0.026 for supine) whereas residual cov^2 of $\dot{V}_A/\dot{Q}$ remained unchanged after NO inhalation. These findings can be explained because the images of $\dot{V}_A$ and $\dot{Q}$ register the respective distributions over relatively short periods of time ($\approx$20 seconds for $\dot{V}_A$ and <10 seconds for $\dot{Q}$), whereas the $\dot{V}_A/\dot{Q}$ image is an average more than 6 minutes of steady tracer infusion. Because $\dot{V}_A$ and $\dot{Q}$ were collected at different times, the increased heterogeneity of the $s\dot{V}_A/s\dot{Q}$ compared with that of $\dot{V}_A/\dot{Q}$ is direct evidence of a temporal variability in $\dot{V}_A$, $\dot{Q}$, or both, which would be averaged out in the constant infusion $\dot{V}_A/\dot{Q}$ image. This hypothesis is substantiated by the fact that inhaled NO, a known relaxant of bronchial and vascular smooth muscle, affects the source of temporal variability and reduces the residual heterogeneity of $s\dot{V}_A/s\dot{Q}$, making it closer to that of $\dot{V}_A/\dot{Q}$ (Figure 4).

III. Image Analysis

A. Contribution of Noise to Heterogeneity of PET Scans

To quantify regional heterogeneity in lung function from PET images, it is crucial to assess the contributions of noise to the total heterogeneity of the images. An experimental method to estimate the contributions of statistical noise to PET images (26) has been described. To a first order approximation, the contribution of noise to a PET image cov^2 is proportional to the square of the voxel size and inversely proportional to the average number of counts per voxel (n) and the effective resolution length (L) of the reconstruction filter raised to the third power (27). For an image created as a ratio of two different images of the same

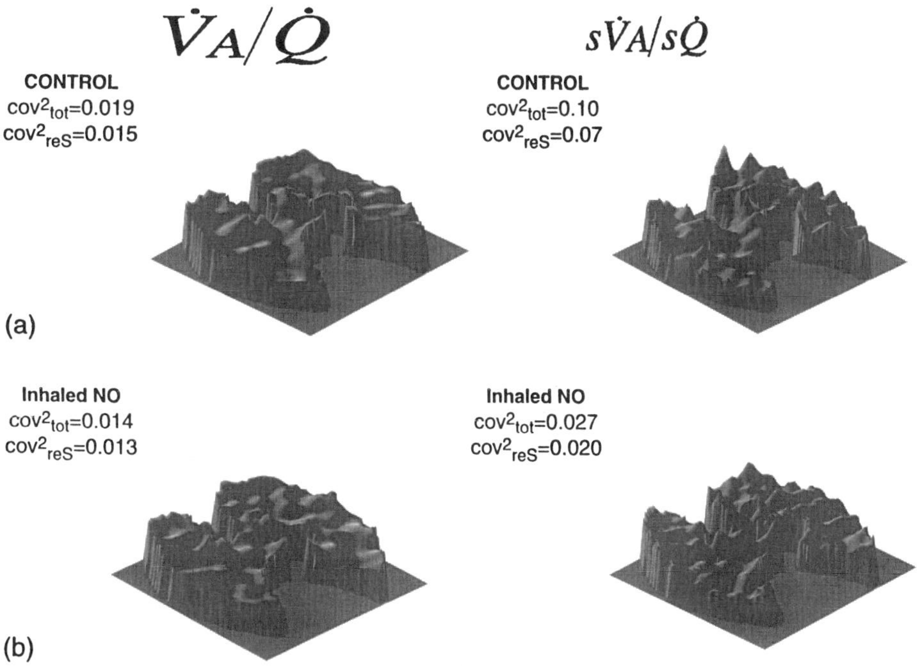

Figure 4 Surface plots from PET images of $\dot{V}_A/\dot{Q}$ (left) and $s\dot{V}_A/s\dot{Q}$ (right) of a supine animal before (a) and after (b) inhalation of NO gas at 20 ppm. Values of total and residual cov^2. The differences in heterogeneity are evidenced by the size of the ripples in these plots.

object, the contributions of the intrinsic heterogeneity of the object in each image are perfectly correlated and thus cancel out. Hence, the cov^2 of the ratio image is exclusively caused by noise and is equal to the sum of cov^2 measurements caused by noise on the respective images. Experimentally, a series of ratio images were created from different PET images of a lung phantom. For each image we obtained the proportionality factor, K, between the $cov^2_{i,j}$, measured for the ratio of images i and j and $(1/n_i + 1/n_j)/L^3$ (Figure 5b). Knowledge of the value of K allowed estimation of noise cov^2 of any image and thus estimation of their true heterogeneity. Estimates of noise from phantom and in vivo lung images using this method showed excellent agreement with estimates using the theoretical algorithm proposed by Alpert et al. (28) (see Figure 5c).

B. Characterization of the Spatial Heterogeneity

After subtracting the contribution of imaging noise, the magnitude of the spatial heterogeneity of a PET image can be characterized by the mean-normalized

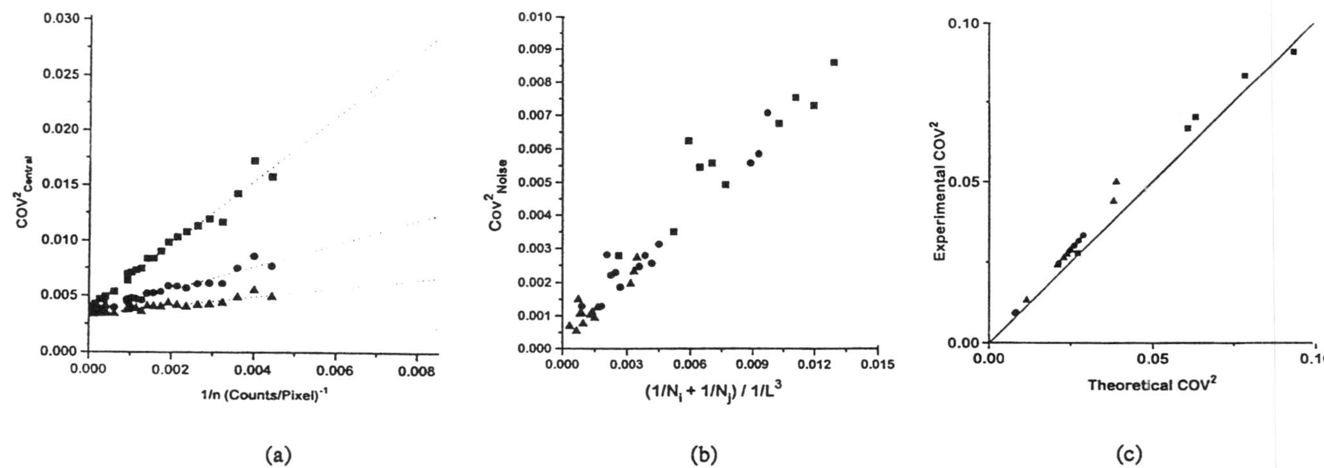

Figure 5 (**a**) Plots of cov^2 against $1/n$ for multiple images with varying number of counts per voxel (n) obtained from the center of a circular foam phantom and reconstructed at resolution lengths (L) of 0.5 (*square*), 0.71 (*circle*), and 1.0 (*triangle*) cm. The intercept of each relation corresponds to the noise-free heterogeneity of the phantom. (**b**) Plot of $cov^2_{i,j}$, against $(1/n_i + 1/n_j)L^3$ for ratio images made from pairs of multiple images with varying number of counts (n) from a lung-shaped foam phantom reconstructed at 0.5 (*square*), 0.71 (*circle*), and 1.0 (*triangle*) cm. Note that the intercept of the plot is approximately zero, which confirms the assumption that intrinsic phantom heterogeneity and inaccuracies resulting from reconstruction, attenuation correction, and edge effects are canceled out in ratio of images. (**c**) Plot of experimental estimation of PET noise cov^2 versus theoretical estimate of the same using the method described in the text. Circles and triangles are noise measured in lung phantoms; squares are noise estimated from actual lung images.

variance (cov^2) of the data within the lung field, the residual cov^2 (cov^2_{res}) remaining after removing the vertical gradient by linear regression, and the fractional contribution of such vertical gradient to the cov^2 (R^2 of the linear regression model). This analysis provides global information of the spatial heterogeneity of the image, but does not give a measure of the spatial frequency content of the heterogeneity. Intuitively, spatial frequency refers to the inverse of the length scale of the "bumps and ripples" seen in an image when presented as a surface plot (see Figures 2–4). The magnitude squared of a two-dimensional fast Fourier transform of an image yields an index of the power content (PSD) of its heterogeneity within a two-dimensional spatial frequency domain, that is, a three-dimensional plot where the X and Y axes correspond to the spatial frequency of sinusoids along vertical and horizontal directions of the image and the height of the peaks correspond to the power content of the sine waves at each spatial frequency. For a sine wave of spatial frequency, fs, along a direction (ø) the PSD has the single peak shown in Figure 6a. We found that the PSD of typical PET images, after removal any gravitational gradients by linear regression (29), included heterogeneity in all directions (see Figure 6b). Thus, to further reduce the two-dimensional PSD to a single spatial frequency axis, the data were transformed to a polar coordinate system and integrated for all angles at each radial distance from the origin. Application of this analysis to PET images showed that the total power under the PSD curve of any image, summed over all spatial frequencies, is directly proportional to the cov^2_{res} of the image (see Figure 6c). Therefore, the PSD analysis provides a quantitative way to separate the global cov^2_{res} of an image into its components of different length scales. We further developed a method to assess, and correct for, the contribution of PET-imaging noise to the PSD plot. To do this, we applied the PSD analysis to several images of noise, obtained as the ratio of multiple PET images of a lung phantom. The mean of the cov^2-normalized PSDs of these images was taken as an estimate of the characteristic PSD of PET imaging noise. This noise PSD can then be rescaled to the magnitude of the expected noise component of a PET image cov^2 and subtracted from the PSD obtained from that image. This correction yields noise-free PSDs as those illustrated in Figures 8c and 9d.

C. Contributions of $\dot{V}_A$ and $\dot{Q}$ Distributions to Heterogeneity in Local $\dot{V}_A/\dot{Q}$

The heterogeneity of functional images of $s\dot{V}_{A,p}$ or $s\dot{V}_{A,i}$, and $\dot{Q}$, can also be characterized by means of a bivariate distribution as described by Wilson and Beck (30). To obtain this bivariate distribution, the local data of $s\dot{V}_{A,p}$ and $\dot{Q}$ per voxel are first normalized by the respective means and then log-transformed. From these log-transformed data, a two-dimensional surface histogram is generated in which the vertical height of the surface above the $s\dot{V}_{A,p}$-$\dot{Q}$ plane corre-

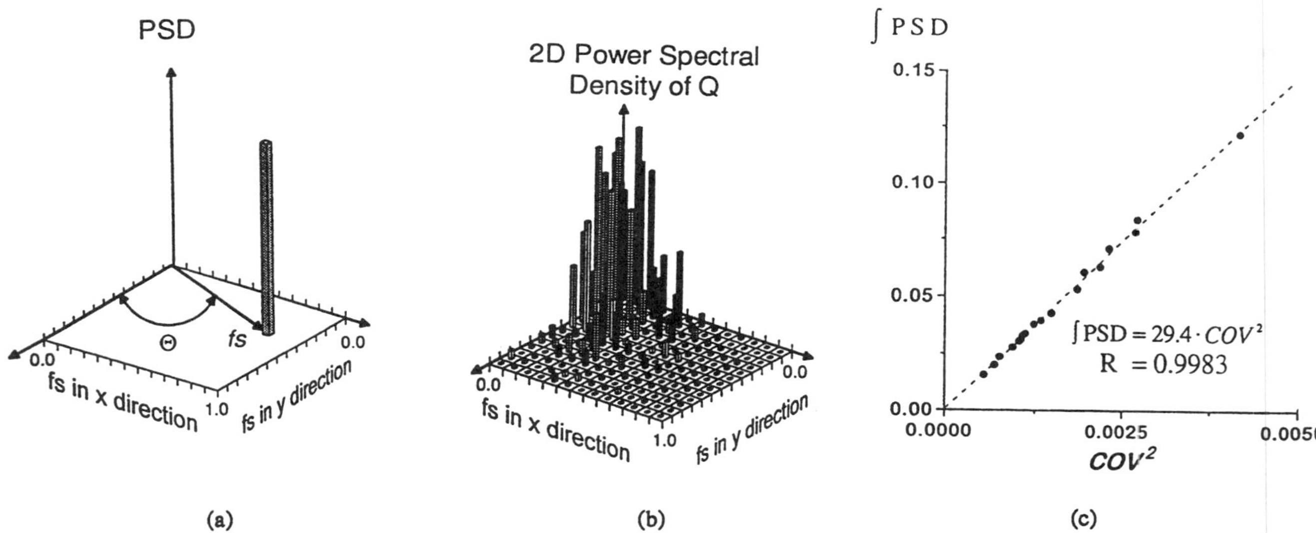

Figure 6 (**a**) Power spectral density (PSD) of a sine wave of spatial frequency, fs, along the Θ direction. (**b**) Typical two-dimensional power spectral density of a PET image of pulmonary perfusion showing heterogeneity in all directions. (**c**) Graph of the integral of (*b*) over all frequencies versus COV^2 for PET functional images of $\dot{Q}$ and $s\dot{V}_{A,p}$ showing a linear relationship between the heterogeneity estimates.

sponds to the fraction of volume of lung (or the number of voxels) that have that combination of normalized $s\dot{V}_{A,p}$ and $\dot{Q}$ values (Figure 7). As Wilson and Beck (30) noted, the integral projection of the data in the $\dot{V}_A$ or $\dot{Q}$ directions results in the logarithmic distributions of $\dot{V}_A$ and $\dot{Q}$, whereas the integral projection in a 45° direction results in a log distribution of mean-normalized $\dot{V}_A/\dot{Q}$ distribution similar to that obtained with the multiple inert gas elimination technique, MIGET. These bivariate distributions can be characterized as being unimodal or multimodal, and by their variance in the $s\dot{V}_{A,p}$, $\dot{Q}$, and 45° projections and the spatial correlation between the two variables. Note that, for the good spatial correlation of normal lungs (Figures 8a and 9a), most data lie around a

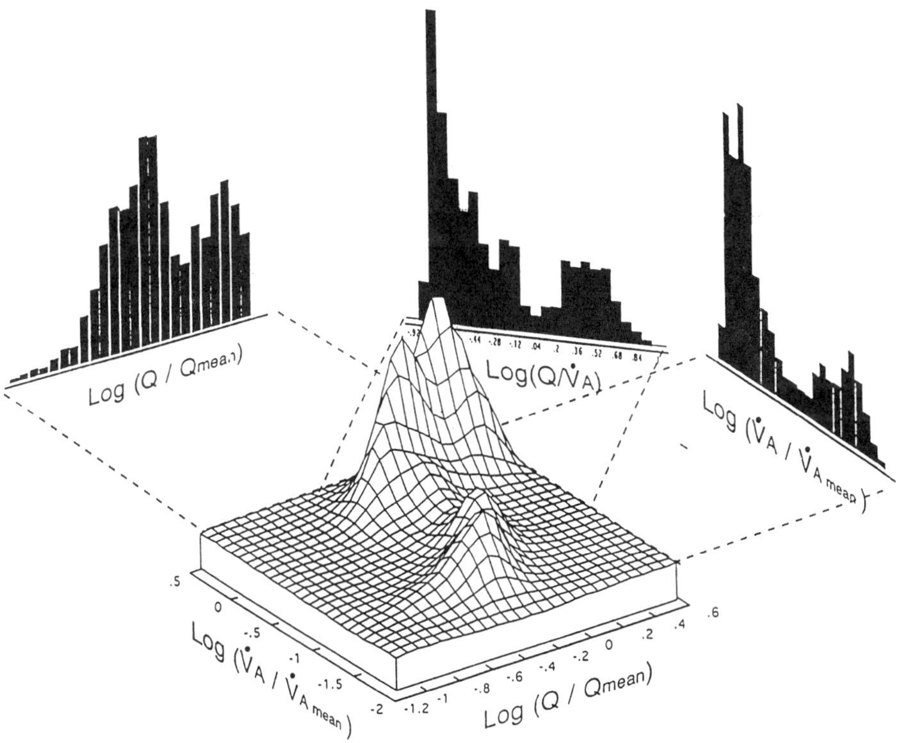

Figure 7 Bivariate distribution of log (mean-normalized $\dot{V}_A$) versus log (mean normalized $\dot{Q}$), as proposed by Wilson and Beck (30) obtained from $\dot{V}_A$ and $\dot{Q}$ scans from a unilaterally lavaged dog. The height of the surface above the $\dot{V}_A - \dot{Q}$ plane corresponds to the fraction of volume of lung (or the number of pixels) that have that combination of normalized $\dot{V}_A$ and $\dot{Q}$ values.

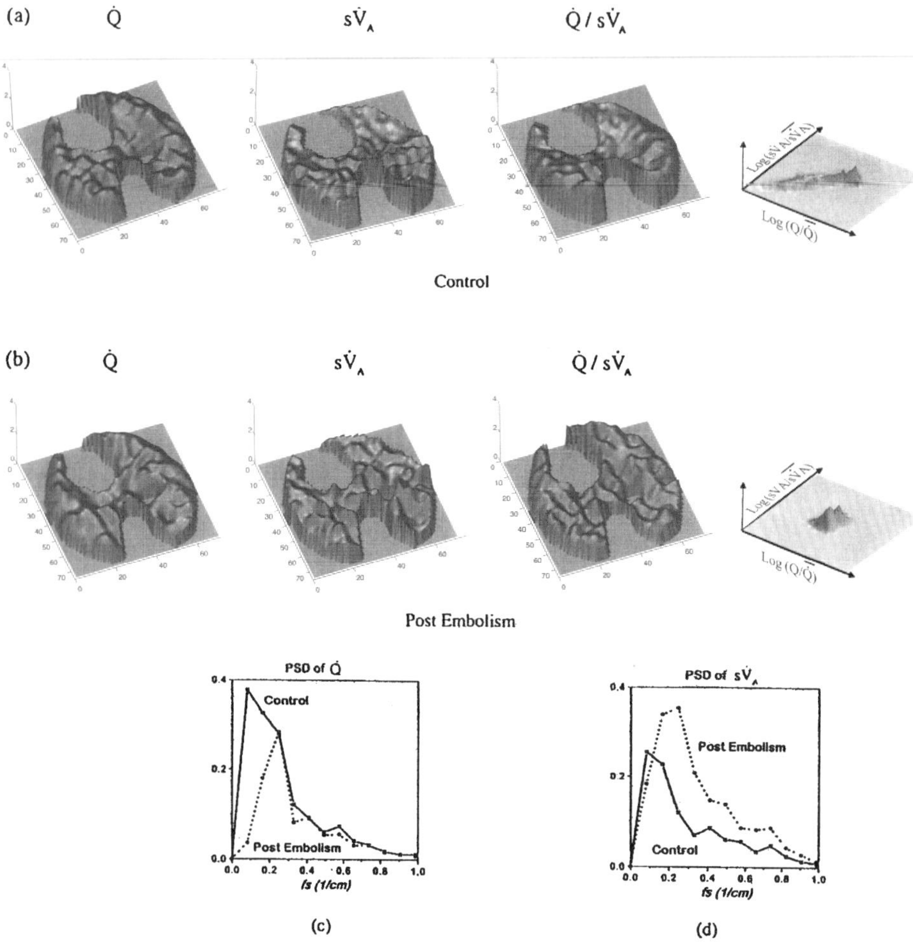

Figure 8 (**a**) From left to right, surface plots of regional perfusion ($\dot{Q}$), specific ventilation ($s\dot{V}_{A,p}$) and $\dot{Q}s\dot{V}_{A,p}$, and the bivariate distribution of $\dot{Q}$ vs $s\dot{V}_{A,p}$ from a normal supine dog. (**b**) Equivalent plots and bivariate distribution as in (*a*) after embolism with 100-μm diameter glass beads. (**c**) and (**d**) The power spectral density of $\dot{Q}$ and $s\dot{V}_{A,p}$, respectively, for both control and postembolism conditions.

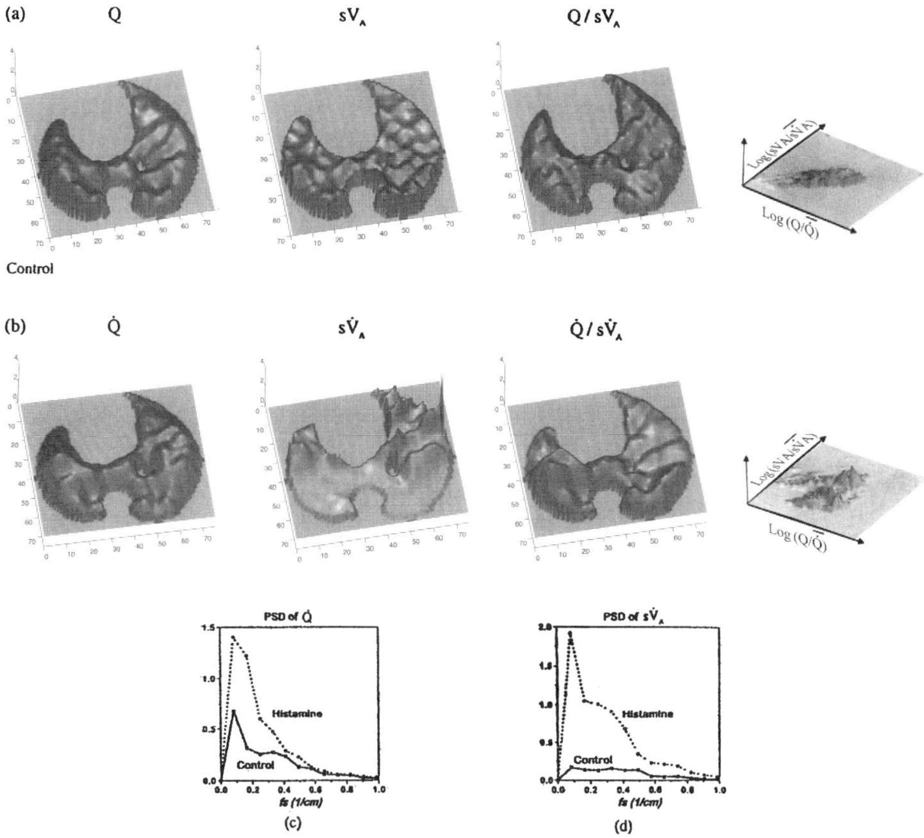

Figure 9 (**a**) From left to right, surface plots of perfusion ($\dot{Q}$), specific ventilation ($s\dot{V}_{A,p}$) and $\dot{Q}/s\dot{V}_{A,p}$, and the bivariate distribution of $\dot{Q}$ versus $s\dot{V}_{A,p}$) from a normal supine dog. (**b**) Equivalent images and bivariate distribution as in (*a*) during bronchoconstriction by steady infusion of histamine. (**c**) and (**d**) The power spectral density of $\dot{Q}$ and $s\dot{V}_{A,p}$, respectively, for both control and during histamine infusion.

45° line along a narrow band of $\dot{V}_A/\dot{Q}$s. Contrast that to the bimodal distribution from a unilaterally lavaged lung (see Figure 7) or the multimodal distribution during histamine bronchoconstriction (see Figure 9b).

IV. Regulation on $\dot{V}_A$, $\dot{Q}$, and $\dot{V}_A/\dot{Q}$ Distributions

In this section, two examples of the PET imaging methods described are given to assess the local regulation and matching of $\dot{V}_A$ and $\dot{Q}$ in heterogeneous lungs.

A. Acute Pulmonary Embolism

Using spherical beads of different dimensions, Wagner (31) defined a functional unit of gas exchange in the dog as the volume of tissue subtended by 150-μm diameter arteries (vessels associated with respiratory bronchioles). It was theorized that a local reduction in $\dot{Q}$ to areas of length scale smaller than the functional unit of gas exchange should not create areas of high $\dot{V}_A/\dot{Q}$ and, therefore, should have no direct effect on intraregional $\dot{V}_A$ distribution. Thus, we studied the effects of microembolization with 100-μm glass beads, which should only affect the distribution of $\dot{V}_A$ in response to larger scale changes in the distribution of $\dot{Q}$.

Positron emission tomography was used to measure $s\dot{V}_{A,p}$, $\dot{Q}$, and $\dot{Q}/s\dot{V}_{A,p}$ distributions before and after intravenous infusion of 100-μm glass beads and the mean P_{PA} had reached a steady value >50 cm H_2O. Ventilation with NO (80 ppm) was then carried out for 20 minutes before measuring again $s\dot{V}_{A,p}$,Q, and $\dot{Q}/s\dot{V}_{A,p}$. The spatial heterogeneity (cov^2) of the corresponding images was separated into vertical and residual components (cov^2_{res}). The PSD of the images and the spatial correlation (R_S) between $s\dot{V}_{A,p}$ and $\dot{Q}$ were also calculated.

Positron emission tomography images and summary Table 1 are presented in Figure 8. Before embolization, the distributions of $s\dot{V}_{A,p}$ and $\dot{Q}$ both had significant vertical gradients favoring the dependent regions (see Figure 8*a*) and high spatial correlation among them ($R_S = 0.92$), resulting in a rather narrow distribution of $\dot{Q}/s\dot{V}_{A,p}$ ($cov^2 = 0.057$). This is well illustrated by the narrow bivariate distribution of $s\dot{V}_{A,p}$ versus $\dot{Q}$ aligned along the line of constant $\dot{Q}/s\dot{V}_{A,p}$ (see Figure 8*a*). Embolization did not create measurable changes in peak airway pressure but dramatically *redistributed both* $\dot{Q}$ and $s\dot{V}_{A,p}$ away from dependent regions, minimizing the contribution of gravitational gradients to the cov^2 of both variables. Local changes in $s\dot{V}_{A,p}$ were highly correlated ($R_S = 0.92$) with the changes in $\dot{Q}$, but the final distributions of $\dot{Q}$ and $s\dot{V}_{A,p}$ had lowered spatial correlation ($R_S = 0.31$). Embolization decreased the cov^2_{res} of $\dot{Q}$ from 0.06 to 0.037 by reducing exclusively low spatial frequency components as demonstrated by the PSD plot. In contrast, embolisms increased the cov^2_{res} of $s\dot{V}_{A,p}$ from 0.035 to 0.056, with that increase occurring mostly at medium and high spatial frequencies. These effects changed the bivariate distribution of $s\dot{V}_{A,p}$ versus $\dot{Q}$ into a wider unimodal distribution with increased $\dot{Q}/s\dot{V}_{A,p}$ heterogeneity ($cov^2 = 0.08$). Inhalation of NO resulted in a substantial reduction in P_{PA}, a partial return of the vertical gradients, an increase in spatial correlation between $s\dot{V}_{A,p}$ and $\dot{Q}$, $R_S = 0.8$, decrease in $\dot{Q}/s\dot{V}_{A,p}$ heterogeneity to control levels.

Implications are as follows:

1. In control conditions, a high R_S between $s\dot{V}_{A,p}$ and $\dot{Q}$ explains the low cov^2 in $\dot{Q}/s\dot{V}_{A,p}$ despite highly heterogeneous distributions of $s\dot{V}_{A,p}$ and $\dot{Q}$.

2. The redistribution of $\dot{Q}$ by embolization can be explained by a greater number of beads being distributed to the areas of highest local $\dot{Q}$ and by the elevated P_{PA}.
3. The shift in $s\dot{V}_{A,p}$, however, can only be attributed to an active local controller responding to the redistribution of $\dot{Q}$ gravity, airway, and pleural pressure gradients were likely unchanged by embolization.
4. The increased cov^2 of $s\dot{V}_{A,p}$ caused by embolization occurring from medium to high spatial frequencies reflects an excellent regional adjustment of local $\dot{V}_A$ among large size regions and a less perfect adjustment at smaller length scales.
5. The remarkable redistribution in $s\dot{V}_{A,p}$ with minimal changes in airway pressures suggests that local $\dot{V}_A$ must by accurately controlled in very distal alveolar spaces with either minimal changes in local lung mechanics or with local pneumoconstriction in some areas precisely compensated by pneumorelaxation in others.
6. The vasorelaxation caused by inhalation of NO confirms previous observations of a reversible component of pulmonary hypertension during acute embolism with small glass beads (32) and suggests a potential benefit of inhaled NO in the management of acute pulmonary embolisms.

B. Bronchoconstriction

If the spatial correlation between $\dot{V}_A$ and $\dot{Q}$ is the result of the action of local active control, then intravenously infused histamine, by disturbing the local control of $\dot{V}_A$ and $\dot{Q}$, should decrease their spatial correlation. Conversely, if the spatial correlation is not a manifestation of an active local control of $\dot{V}_A$ but the result of a imaging artifacts, then correlated distributions of $s\dot{V}_{A,p}$ and $\dot{Q}$ should still be preserved after intravenous infusion of histamine.

Figure 9 summarizes the results of a study in a supine dog using the same protocol as the microembolization study except that, instead of glass beads, intravenous histamine was infused at a rate of 10 $\mu g.kg^{-1}.min^{-1}$. The effects of intravenous histamine infusion and inhaled NO on the distributions of $\dot{Q}$, $s\dot{V}_{A,p}$, $\dot{Q}/s\dot{V}_{A,p}$, blood gases, and P_{PA} were recorded. As in the microembolization experiments, the normal supine dog showed correlated ($R_S = 0.78$) distributions of $s\dot{V}_{A,p}$ and $\dot{Q}$ with vertical gradients favoring the dependent regions and resulting in a narrow and unimodal bivariate $s\dot{V}_{A,p}/\dot{Q}$ distribution ($cov^2 = 0.095$). Intravenous infusion of histamine more than doubled peak airway pressure, redistributed both $\dot{Q}$ and $s\dot{V}_{A,p}$, increasing cov^2_{res} of $\dot{Q}$ by 70% and $s\dot{V}_{A,p}$ by 700%, while totally eliminating their spatial correlation ($R_S = 0.067$). There was also a large increase in the cov^2 of $\dot{Q}/s\dot{V}_{A,p}$ with the expected decrease in oxygenation. The increases in cov^2 by histamine was mostly caused by heterogeneity of low spatial frequency for $\dot{Q}$ and of both low and medium spatial frequencies for $s\dot{V}_{A,p}$. Intravenous infusion of histamine changed the $s\dot{V}_{A,p}/\dot{Q}$ bivariate distribution from a relatively unimodal and correlated peak range along the 45° line of constant $\dot{Q}/s\dot{V}_{A,p}$ to a multimodal and uncorrelated distribution including substantial modes of low $s\dot{V}_{A,p}$ and normal and high $\dot{Q}$. Inhalation of NO resulted in a small reduction in P_{PA} and an increase in cov^2 of both $s\dot{V}_{A,p}$ and $\dot{Q}$ but also in R_S, producing a small decrease in cov^2 $\dot{Q}/s\dot{V}_{A,p}$. The increase in PA_{O_2} caused by NO was probably caused by the increased R_S and a flattening of the low $\dot{V}_A/\dot{Q}$ ridge of the bivariate distribution.

Implications are as follows. It is clear that the high degree of correlation between $\dot{Q}$ and $s\dot{V}_{A,p}$ seen in the normal lungs are not caused by imaging artifacts because infused histamine totally eliminated the spatial correlation. Instead, the data suggest that heterogeneous and uncorrelated changes in the local control of $\dot{Q}$ and $s\dot{V}_{A,p}$ were responsible for the worsening of $\dot{V}_A/\dot{Q}$ distribution during histamine infusion. The fact that the increase in cov^2 caused by histamine was more exaggerated in $s\dot{V}_{A,p}$ than in $\dot{Q}$ suggests that the primary effect of infused histamine is bronchoconstriction and pneumoconstriction. The substantial increase in the contribution of the low-to-medium range spatial frequencies to total heterogeneity suggests that the effect of airway constriction is occurring at least up to third or fourth generation airways.

V. Summary

This chapter has described the advantages and limitations of several PET imaging techniques to assess the spatial distribution of $\dot{V}_A$, $\dot{Q}$, and $\dot{V}_A/\dot{Q}$ within the lung. Although the spatial resolution of PET is limited to length scales greater than 7 mm, its ability to follow the kinetics of inert tracer gases provides a unique quantitative tool to assess in vivo and noninvasive gas transport efficiency in the lungs. Novel methods to analyze and characterize spatial heterogeneity in $\dot{V}_A$, $\dot{Q}$ and $\dot{V}_A/\dot{Q}$ in terms of the spatial correlation among them, their vertical and residual cov^2, and their power spectral density were presented. This last method provides unique information about the length scale of the heterogeneity, which is otherwise lost in a global measurement such as cov^2. Two illustrative examples of the detailed information that can be obtained from these imaging and analysis methods are presented. These studies and methods are providing new insights on exquisitely complex system behavior that originates from the ensemble of rather simple individual components.

References

1. Mintun MA, Ter-Pogossian MM, Green MA, Lich LL, Schuster DP. Quantitative measurement of regional pulmonary blood flow with positron emission tomography. J Appl Physiol 1986; 60(1):317–326.

2. Treppo S, Mijailovich SM, Venegas JG. Contributions of pulmonary perfusion ($\dot{Q}$) and ventilation ($\dot{V}_A$) to the heterogeneities in $\dot{V}_A/\dot{Q}$ measured by PET. J Appl Physiol 1997; 82(4):1163–1176.
3. Mijailovich SM, Treppo S, Venegas JG. Effects of lung motion, and tracer kinetics corrections on PET imaging of pulmonary function. J Appl Physiol 1997; 82(4): 1154–1162.
4. Brudin LH, Valind SO, Rhodes CG. Error analysis of combined measurements of regional ventilation and V/Q ratio using positron emission tomography. Phys Med Biol 1992; 37(5):1077–1093.
5. Seow D, Adrie C, Head A, Venegas JG. Assessment of intrapulmonary perfusion (Q) and shunt (Qs) with positron emission tomography (PET). Am J Respir Crit Care Med 1995; 151(4):A520.
6. Hoffman EA. Effect of body orientation on regional lung expansion: a computed tomographic approach. J Appl Physiol 1985; 59:468–480.
7. Rodarte JR, Chaniotakis M, Wilson TA. Variability of parenchymal expansion measured by computed tomography. J Appl Physiol 1989; 67(1):226–231.
8. Tsuzaki K, Hales CA, Strieder DJ, Venegas JG. Regional lung mechanics and gas transport in lungs with inhomogeneous compliance. J Appl Physiol 1993; 75(1): 206–216.
9. Venegas JG, Tsuzaki K, Fox BJ, Simon BA, Hales CA. Regional coupling between chest wall and lung expansion during HFV: a positron imaging study. J Appl Physiol 1993; 74(5):2242–2252.
10. Simon BA, Tsuzaki K, Venegas JG. Changes in regional lung mechanics and ventilation distribution after unilateral pulmonary artery occlusion. J Appl Physiol 1997; 82(3):882–891.
11. Brudin LH, Rhodes CG, Valind SO, Jones T, Jonson B, Hughes JM. Relationships between regional ventilation and vascular and extravascular volume in supine humans. J Appl Physiol 1994; 76(3):1195–1204.
12. Brudin LH, Rhodes CG, Valind SO, Jones T, Hughes JM. Interrelationships between regional blood flow, blood volume, and ventilation in supine humans. J Appl Physiol 1994; 76(3):1205–1210.
13. Yamada Y, Burnham C, Hales CA, Venegas JG. Regional mapping of gas transport during high-frequency and conventional ventilation. J Appl Physiol 1989; 66(3): 1209–1218.
14. Venegas JG, Yamada Y, Hales CA. Contributions of diffusion jet flow and cardiac activity to regional ventilation in CFV. J Appl Physiol 1991; 71(4):1540–1553.
15. Venegas JG, Yamada Y, Burnham C, Hales CA. Local gas transport in eucapnic ventilation: effects of gravity and breathing frequency. J Appl Physiol 1990; 68(6): 2287–2295.
16. Fazio F, Jones T. Assessment of regional ventilation by continuous inhalation of radioactive kripton-81m. BMJ 1975; 3:673–675.
17. Valind SO, Rhodes CG, Brudin LH, Jones T. Measurements of regional ventilation pulmonary gas volume: theory and error analysis with special reference to positron emission tomography. J Nucl Med 1991; 32(10):1037–1044.
18. Suzuki T, Iio M. [Quantitative regional alveolar volume and specific ventilation (V/VA) in healthy subjects measured with positron emission tomography] [Japanese]. Kokyu to Junkan Respir Circ 1991; 39(5):445–448.

19. Senda M, Murata K, Itoh H, Yonekura Y, Torizuka K. Quantitative evaluation of regional pulmonary ventilation using PET and nitrogen-13 gas. J Nucl Med 1986; 27(2):268–273.
20. Simon BA, Venegas JG, Analyzing 13NN lung washout curves in the presence of intraregional nonuniformities. J Appl Physiol 1994; 76(2):956–964.
21. Ross DJ, Waters PF, Waxman AD, Koerner SK, Mohsenifar Z. Regional distribution of lung perfusion and ventilation at rest and during steady-state exercise after unilateral lung transplantation. Chest 1993; 104(1):130–135.
22. Burton GH, Seed WA, Vernon P. Computer analysis of ventilation-perfusion scans for detection and assessment of lung disease. Thorax 1985; 40(7):519–525.
23. Rhodes CG, Valind SO, Brudin LH, Wollmer PE, Jones T, Hughes JMB. Quantification of regional V_A/Q ratios in humans by use of PET. I. Theory. J Appl Physiol 1989; 66:1896–1904.
24. Rhodes CG, Valind SO, Brudin LH, Wollmer PE, Jones T, Hughes JMB. Quantification of regional V_A/Q ratios in humans by use of PET. II. Procedure and normal values. J Appl Physiol 1989; 66:1905–1913.
25. Venegas JG, Treppo S, Hales CA. Inhaled NO reduces the temporal variability in regional ventilation/perfusion ratios. Am J Respir Crit Care Med 1995; 151(4): A785.
26. Venegas JG, Treppo S, Mijailovich SM. Contributions of statistical noise to spatial heterogeneity of PET images of pulmonary function. In: Medical Imaging 1994: Physiology and Function from Multidimensional Images. EA Hoffman and RS Acharya, eds. SPE-The International Society for Optical Engineering, Newport Beach, CA: 1994:361–368.
27. Brownell GL, Correia JA, Zamenhof RG. Positron instrumentation. In: Lawrence JH, Budinger TF, eds. Recent Advances in Nuclear Medicine. New York: Grune and Stratton, 1979:1–49.
28. Alpert NM, Chesler DA, Correia JA, Ackerman RH, Chang JY, Finclestein S, Davis SM, Brownell GL, Taveras JM. Estimation of the local statistical noise in emission computed tomography. IEEE Transactions on Medical Imaging 1982; MI-1(2):142–146.
29. Venegas JG, Aljuri. 2D-power spectrum analysis of spatial heterogeneity in PET images of pulmonary function N. Ann Biomed Eng 1995; 23(1):S14.
30. Wilson TA, Beck KC. Contributions of ventilation and perfusion inhomogeneities to the VA/Q distribution. J Appl Physiol 1992; 72(6):2298–2304.
31. Young I, Mazzone RW, Wagner PD. Identification of functional lung unit in the dog by graded vascular embolization. J Appl Physiol 1980; 49(1):132–141.
32. Delcroix M, Melot C, Vachiery J, Lejeune P, Leeman M, Vanderhoeft P, Naeije R. Effects of embolus size on hemodynamics and gas exchange in canine embolic pulmonary hypertension. J Appl Physiol 1990; 69(6):2251–2254.

17

Physiological Effects of Oxygen and Carbon Dioxide on $\dot{V}_A/\dot{Q}$ Heterogeneity

ERIK R. SWENSON, KAREN B. DOMINO, and MICHAEL P. HLASTALA

University of Washington School of Medicine
Seattle, Washington

I. Introduction

With development of methods that yield greater temporal and spatial resolution, there is a greater appreciation for the magnitude of regional heterogeneities in ventilation and perfusion in the normal lung. The surprising consequence of these heterogeneities is the minimal extent of equivalent inhomogeneity in regional ventilation-perfusion ($\dot{V}_A/\dot{Q}$) ratios. Such minimal mismatch rests, in part, on the fixed anatomical matching of vessels and airways as well as the dynamic mechanisms that further act to modulate and regulate regional vascular and airway conductances and regional parenchymal compliance. To a large extent, these dynamic processes are set by or are sensitive to the principal gases undergoing exchange in the lung, namely oxygen (O_2) and carbon dioxide (CO_2). This chapter describes the mechanisms, kinetics, and sites of action of O_2- and CO_2-mediated regulation of regional blood or gas flows and how these improve on the anatomical or structural meeting of blood and gas in the lung to minimize $\dot{V}_A/\dot{Q}$ mismatch in the presence of pathological changes in regional lung function. The local (intrapulmonary) influence of these gases is considered in relation to region size as is how systemic changes in O_2 and CO_2 sensed elsewhere can further influence gas exchange.

II. Oxygen

A. Pulmonary Vasculature

1. General Description

The pulmonary circulation constricts in response to alveolar hypoxia, resulting in a dual response of an increase in pulmonary artery pressure and diversion of blood flow away from the hypoxic area (1). Hypoxic pulmonary vasoconstriction (HPV) is unique to the pulmonary circulation as other circulations (coronary, cerebral, and systemic) dilate in response to hypoxia (2). HPV begins within seconds of ventilation with hypoxic gas with the speed of the pulmonary vasoconstriction related to the velocity of decline in alveolar oxygen tension (3). The HPV response is sustained for hours in the absence of respiratory alkalosis, severe systemic hypoxemia, or changes in cardiac output (4). Studies in dogs (4) and humans (5) suggested that the response to alveolar hypoxia is nearly maximal within 20 minutes, although redistribution of blood flow from atelectatic lung takes longer to be complete (6). Recent evidence that has looked at the time course of the HPV response in more detail has suggested that there are slow increases in the strength of the HPV response both in vitro (3) and in vivo (7,8,8a). Diversion of blood flow away from nonventilated liquid-filled lungs slowly intensified between 3 and 6 hours after inducing hypoxia (7). It is not clear whether this represents a characteristic of or modulation of the HPV response.

Hypoxic pulmonary vasoconstriction is the primary adaptive mechanism of the pulmonary circulation to preserve arterial blood oxygenation by increasing pulmonary vascular resistance to hypoxic alveoli, thereby diverting pulmonary blood flow away from these regions. The reduction in blood flow from poorly ventilated or hypoxic alveoli to better ventilated alveoli preserves the matching of $\dot{V}_A/\dot{Q}$ and arterial oxygenation (9).

The physiological importance of HPV is dependent upon species. Hypoxic pulmonary vasoconstriction is strongest in cows and pigs, species that lack collateral ventilation, compared with dogs, sheep, and humans, species that have well-developed collateral ventilation (10). However, consistent and strong HPV responses are obtained in these species (5,11,12), and HPV is likely to be quite significant in maintaining $\dot{V}_A/\dot{Q}$ matching in lung disease.

The success of pulmonary vasoconstriction to divert blood flow away from atelectatic or hypoxic lung regions is dependent upon the size of the hypoxic region (13,14). The smaller the hypoxic segment, the greater the blood flow reduction (e.g., flow diversion) and the smaller the increase in pulmonary arterial pressure. For instance, an 80% reduction in blood flow with a negligible increase in pulmonary artery pressure would occur when the hypoxic segment is equal to 10% of the lungs (1). A 50% diversion in blood flow would be expected with 60% of the lung as the hypoxic segment. When 100% of the lung is hypoxic, as is the case at high altitude, only pulmonary artery pressure increases and interregional flow diversion does not occur. However, with global alveolar hypoxia, the intraregional distribution of blood flow changes to a minor degree as perfusion increases to the apical portions of the lung (15,16). The increase in apical perfusion is postulated to be beneficial because it increases the vascular surface area that can participate in gas exchange.

Using fluorescent-labeled microspheres, we studied the effects of unilateral hypoxia on the distribution of pulmonary blood flow in anesthetized prone dogs (17). This technique permits detailed determination of pulmonary blood flow in small lung regions (<2 cm^3). Left lung hypoxia increases the coefficient of variation of pulmonary blood flow in the hypoxic lung, but not the hyperoxic lung. During hyperoxia, pulmonary blood flow was greatest in the hilar areas, and decreased by approximately 4%/cm with increasing linear distance from the ipsilateral hilus. This central-to-peripheral gradient has also been observed by Hakim et al. (18) using imaging methods. Left lung hypoxia decreased the hilar-to-peripheral gradient, such that hilar areas no longer had increased pulmonary blood flow compared with the peripheral areas. The HPV-flow diversion increased blood flow to the right lung but did not change the hilar-to-peripheral gradient. These results suggest that hypoxic vasoconstriction alters the regional distribution of flow in the hypoxic lung, but not in the hyperoxic lung.

2. Mechanism, Site, and Stimulus for HPV

The primary sites for constriction of the pulmonary vasculature during acute hypoxia are the small pulmonary arterioles (30–50 μm), although constriction of capillaries and pulmonary veins contributes to a small extent (19–25). Both alveolar and extra-alveolar vessels constrict in response to hypoxia (26). Intravital fluorescence microscopy has demonstrated a reduction in capillary blood flow, indicated by capillary derecruitment and a reduction in red blood cell flux and velocity in a hypoxic lung (27). Large pulmonary arterioles (>500 μm) do not participate in the usual HPV response (23) because the blood supply by the bronchial circulation increases the local vascular oxygen tension (28). However, pulmonary arteries of all sizes demonstrate HPV in vitro (28–30).

The mechanism of HPV is not definitively known. It is likely that hypoxia acts directly on the vessel wall because the vascular endothelium is not essential for the HPV response (31). The pulmonary endothelium produces prostanoid, as well as nonprostanoid, nonpeptide mediators of vascular tone. Most important are nitric oxide, the endothelium-derived relaxing factor (EDRF) (32,33), and several endothelium-derived constricting factors, including endothelin-1 and superoxide anion (34). Cultured pulmonary vascular smooth muscle cells are capable of vascular contraction (29,30). Hypoxia may cause vasoconstriction by opening calcium channels or closing potassium channels (35). A reduction in extracellular calcium markedly attenuates HPV in isolated ferret lungs (36).

Released endothelial-derived factors, such as nitric oxide, endothelin, and prostacyclin, are not mediators of the HPV response. Instead, they appear to modulate the intensity of the response. Nitric oxide is a potent pulmonary vasodilator and inhibitor of HPV (37). Endothelin-1 is a potent vasoconstrictor (34) but does not mediate HPV (38). Prostacyclin markedly attenuates HPV and reduces flow diversion away from hypoxic alveoli, resulting in reduced Pa_{O_2} (39). Endogenously produced prostacyclin appears to be responsible for the variability of HPV response in some animals, because the response is restored by administration of cyclooxygenase inhibitors (39–41).

The leukotrienes cause pulmonary vasoconstriction and increase the pulmonary pressure response to global alveolar hypoxia (42). However, their effect is due to nonspecific vasoconstriction rather than a specific potentiation of HPV, because inhibitors of leukotrienes do not attenuate HPV in regional hypoxia (43,44). Pulmonary vasoconstrictor prostaglandin $F_{2\alpha}$ also is a nonspecific vasoconstrictor that does not alter HPV-induced flow diversion (45). However, infusion of $PGF_{2\alpha}$ directly into the pulmonary artery of an atelectatic lung improved vasoconstriction in that lung and Pa_{CO_2} (46).

Autonomic innervation of the lung is not required for HPV (47), and the HPV response is present in the human transplanted lung (48). Sympathetic nerve stimulation attenuates HPV to a mild degree (49,50) and sympathetic blockade may enhance HPV (51).

The exact location and identity of the sensor for HPV are not known. The sensor is most likely in the vascular smooth muscle (29) and may involve the mitochondrial oxidative phosphorylation system and cytochrome P450 (52) or direct changes in the calcium or potassium channels in the vascular smooth muscle (53). It is also not known whether signal transduction is necessary and, if so, what is the identity of the transducer between the sensor and effector cells.

The stimulus for HPV response is a reduction in oxygen tension (P_{SO_2}) in the vicinity of the vascular smooth muscle. Although alveolar P_{O_2} is the predominant stimulus for HPV, $P_{\bar{v}O_2}$ also contributes in dogs (54) and in rats (55). $P_{\bar{v}O_2}$ is the predominant stimulus for HPV in atelectatic lung (56). $P_{\bar{v}O_2}$ may also be an important influence when it is unusually low (as with reduced cardiac output) and unusually high (as with severe stress or trauma). In isolated perfused rabbit lung, $P_{\bar{v}O_2}$ did not stimulate HPV (3).

The HPV stimulus–response curve is sigmoid in shape with a maximal HPV response observed with $P_{SO_2} < 25$ mmHg (54,57,58). A 50% HPV response is observed when P_{SO_2} is 55 mmHg. With a $P_{\bar{v}O_2}$ of 40 mmHg while breathing room air, vascular tone is increased by 15% compared to 100% O_2 and $P_{\bar{v}O_2}$ greater than 60 mmHg. With prolonged, severe global hypoxia ($P_{AO_2} = 0$ mmHg), marked pulmonary vasodilation follows a transient pulmonary vasoconstriction

(59). Because vasoconstriction to known pulmonary vasoconstrictors is absent, the pulmonary vasodilation probably represents gross metabolic failure resulting from anoxia (60).

In summary, HPV involves a direct contraction of vascular smooth muscle to hypoxia. Release of endothelial-derived factors, such as nitric oxide, endothelin, and prostacyclin do not mediate the HPV response, although they may modulate the intensity of the response. The stimulus for the HPV response (P_SO_2 is a reduction in oxygen tension in the vicinity of vascular smooth muscle (reflecting alveolar, mixed venous and bronchial arterial PO_2 in most species), with a maximal response when $P_SO_2 < 25$ mmHg. $P\bar{v}O_2$, therefore, exerts an important influence on HPV and is the stimulus for HPV in the presence of atelectasis or flooded alveoli.

3. Modifying Factors

The HPV response is influenced by multiple variables including hemodynamic variables, acid-base status, and lung disease. All these factors may profoundly influence the observed effects of anesthetic drugs and inhibitors of HPV on pulmonary hemodynamics and arterial blood oxygenation. These factors are summarized in Table 1.

a. Hemodynamic Variables

Pulmonary arterial and pulmonary venous pressures and cardiac output all affect the HPV response. Increased pulmonary arterial and venous pressures reduce the strength of HPV (61–64). In fact, the HPV response was abolished when left atrial pressure reached 25 mmHg. Increases in P_{pa} also attenuated the observed HPV response.

Cardiac output affects the observed HPV response because $P\bar{v}O_2$ and P_{pa} change with changes in cardiac output. Usually $P\bar{v}O_2$ increases when cardiac output increases and $P\bar{v}O_2$ decreases when cardiac output decreases. $P\bar{v}O_2$ and P_{pa} can act independently from each other (65). The HPV is generally reduced with increasing cardiac output. This occurs primarily because the stimulus for HPV is reduced (e.g., P_SO_2 increases) when $P\bar{v}O_2$ is increased (53). In addition, differences in pulmonary vascular recruitment and derecruitment in normoxic and hypoxic lung regions cause the curvature of the hypoxic pressure-flow curves to be increased. These differences in the pressure-flow curves cause an increase in percentage blood flown to the hypoxic lung, even with the constant $P\bar{v}O_2$ and P_SO_2. Increases in pulmonary shunt and $\dot{V}_A/\dot{Q}$ heterogeneity are observed with increases in pulmonary blood flow even in the absence of changes of $P\bar{v}O_2$ (66). As $P\bar{v}O_2$ also increases with increasing cardiac output, the resultant attenuation of HPV is marked and hypoxic lung blood flow is markedly increased with increasing cardiac output. For instance, HPV is attenuated by increased intracranial pressure because of the resultant sympathetic activation and increase in

Table 1 Factors that Attenuate HPV-Induced Flow Diversion

1. Large hypoxic lung segment
2. Increased P_{pa}
3. Increased left atrial pressure
4. Increased cardiac output
5. Increased P_vO_2
6. Severely decreased P_vO_2
7. Anemia
8. Metabolic alkalosis
9. Respiratory alkalosis
10. Acute lung injury
11. Endotoxin
12. Lung manipulation and surgery
13. Positive-end expiratory pressure (PEEP), especially normoxic lung PEEP
14. Estradiol
15. Prostacyclin (PGI_2)
16. Nitrous oxide
17. Volatile anesthetics
18. Nitric oxide
19. Sodium nitroprusside and nitroglycerin
20. Calcium-channel blockers
21. β-adrenergic receptor agonists

cardiac output (67). Although HPV is reduced, P_aO_2 may or may not decrease depending on whether the effect of the increase in shunt on P_aO_2 is greater than the influence of $P\bar{v}O_2$ on P_aO_2.

Reductions in cardiac output have an even greater influence on the HPV response and arterial blood oxygenation. In normal lung, $\dot{V}_A/\dot{Q}$ heterogeneity is also increased by reductions in pulmonary blood flow even when $P\bar{v}O_2$ is constant (68). A reduction in $P\bar{v}O_2$ may stimulate HPV in normal areas of the lung, resulting in less effective flow diversion away from the pathological lung region (14). This is especially important in regional lung disease, in which the blood flow through the hypoxic region is increased when cardiac output is low (69). Because $P\bar{v}O_2$ influences P_aO_2 even when pulmonary shunt is unchanged, P_aO_2 may be markedly reduced with low cardiac output and regional lung disease. More modest reductions in cardiac output may not affect arterial blood oxygenation but contribute to some of the observed differences in effects of drugs on HPV with in vivo versus in vitro experiments.

b. Acid-Base Status

Acid-base status profoundly influences the HPV response (12,70–73). A metabolic acidosis enhances HPV (12,72). A metabolic alkalosis inhibits HPV, with a complete reversal noted at a pH of 7.60. The HPV is blunted by a respiratory alkalosis, with an 80% inhibition observed at a pH of 7.60. However, with a chronic respiratory alkalosis, HPV is restored (71). In contrast, a respiratory acidosis does not affect HPV in dogs because of a pH-independent vasodilating effect of CO_2 (12). As HPV is significantly attenuated by a respiratory and metabolic alkalosis, $\dot{V}_A/\dot{Q}$ matching and arterial blood oxygenation in normal and abnormal lungs are impaired in the presence of a metabolic alkalosis and respiratory alkalosis (74–76).

c. Lung Injury States

HPV is attenuated by several types of acute lung injury. A diminished HPV response has been observed in a variety of lung injuries in animals as a result of hyperoxia (77), endotoxin (78–80), oleic acid (81), and *Pseudomonas* pneumonia (82,83). The HPV also appears to be blunted in humans with bacterial pneumonia (84). The HPV is also inhibited by tumor necrosis factor-alpha (TNF-α), which is released by macrophages in response to endotoxin (85). Surgical trauma and manipulation of the lungs also transiently attenuates HPV (86). Repeated intermittent exposures to hypoxia restore HPV after open-chest surgery and manipulation of pulmonary vessels (86). In contrast, repeated exposures to hypoxia do not potentiate HPV in closed-chested animals (87) and humans (11).

In many of these lung injuries, the loss of reactivity is due to the release of vasodilator prostanoids, because treatment with cyclooxygenase inhibitors restores the HPV response and oxygenation in these diseases (77,78,81,82). The variability of the HPV response with atelectasis and alveolar hypoxia in dogs is related to the release of prostacyclin (40,41,78,88). Cyclooxygenase inhibitors decrease the variability of the baseline HPV response in dogs with alveolar hypoxia (41,78) and acute atelectasis (39,40). These results suggest that attenuation of HPV in lung injury is mediated by the production of vasodilating prostanoids (such as prostacyclin) by the endothelium. Nitric oxide probably does not mediate the loss of HPV in lung injury, such as in *Pseudomonas* pneumonia (83) and TNF-α (85).

d. Other Factors

Lung inflation, as with positive end-expiratory pressure (PEEP), may attenuate HPV (89). This is likely to be encountered clinically when PEEP is administered to the ventilated lung during one-lung anesthesia and when PEEP is used to treat regional lung disease such as a pneumonia or pulmonary contusion. In these situations, PEEP may increase blood flow through the nonventilated lung, thereby increasing pulmonary shunt and decreasing P_aO_2.

Hypoxic pulmonary vasoconstriction is also attenuated by estradiol, because the HPV response is greater in males than in females (90). Cellular elements of the blood may also modulate the HPV response, because the HPV response is transient (91), not as intense (92) in the absence of a blood perfusate.

The red blood cells may prevent the accumulation of an inhibitor or release a factor that enhances vascular responsiveness. This is not related to a general decline of the preparation. Acute isovolemic anemia increases intrapulmonary shunt during atelectasis in rabbits (93).

e. Pharmacological Agents

Pharmacological agents that increase cyclic adenosine monophosphate (AMP) or cyclic guanosine monophosphate (GMP) cause pulmonary vasodilation and may attenuate hypoxic pulmonary vasoconstriction. In contrast, agents that decrease the cyclic nucleotides increase pulmonary vascular tone and may improve hypoxic pulmonary vasoconstriction, as long as pulmonary artery pressures are not elevated to levels that depress HPV. The net result of a particular drug on gas exchange is complex and depends on its hemodynamic effects and whether it dilates injured as well as noninjured vessels.

Nitric oxide decreases pulmonary vascular tone in response to alveolar hypoxia by increasing cyclic GMP. Inhaled nitric oxide selectivity decreases pulmonary artery pressure and attenuates HPV (37). Sodium nitroprusside and nitroglycerin attenuate HPV owing to release of nitric oxide (94,95). The HPV is attenuated by isoproterenol (96), whereas beta-receptor blockade may enhance HPV (50,97). The HPV response is also attenuated by calcium channel blockers (98,99).

f. Anesthetic Agents

The intravenous anesthetics, including pentobarbital, opioids, droperidol, and ketamine, have been traditionally believed to have little influence on the pulmonary vasoconstrictor response to alveolar hypoxia (100,101). However, recent studies by Wetzel and colleagues (102) have demonstrated that pentobarbital has complex and significant effects on the regulation of pulmonary vascular tone, including the response to alveolar hypoxia. The pulmonary pressor response to global hypoxia was modestly attenuated by pentobarbital when studied in isolated sheep lungs (102).

The direct pulmonary vascular effect of inhalational anesthetics is the dose-dependent inhibition of HPV (27,100,103). The mechanism of inhibition of HPV most likely involves suppression of calcium ion channels, because volatile anesthetics reduce calcium flux in other vascular beds (104). In contrast to marked inhibition of HPV in vitro, inhalational anesthetics have variable and inconclusive effects on HPV in intact animals and humans (94,105,106) because of the secondary cardiovascular and autonomic effects of the anesthetic.

B. Airways

In contrast to its marked effect on the pulmonary vasculature, oxygen has a smaller effect on the airways. Alveolar hypoxia causes bronchoconstriction in animals and humans (107–112) although dogs show large airway dilation by CT scanning with inhalation of 7% O_2 (112a). Airways resistance increased by 20% in normal humans with inhalation of 10%–12% oxygen (111). Collateral airways resistance was increased by 37% with hypoxic ventilation (113). Alveolar hypoxia also enhances nonspecific bronchial reactivity in sheep (107). Histamine and carbachol-induced increases in airways resistance were greater during alveolar hypoxia (107).

Inhalation of a hyperoxic gas mixture reduces bronchoconstriction in patients with chronic obstructive pulmonary disease (COPD) (108,114). Maximal expiratory flow rates increased in patients with severe COPD when 30% O_2 was inspired (114). Whereas the absolute increases in flow rates were small for the normal adult, the increases represented changes of 20%–25% for these patients (114). Hyperoxia also attenuates bronchial responsiveness to methacholine in asthmatic patients (115).

Multiple mechanisms may be involved in hypoxia-induced bronchoconstriction. The bronchoconstriction may be secondary to a decrease in CO_2 tension, because hypoxia decreases local perfusion. Hypocapnic bronchoconstriction may result (see Section III). Secondary changes in CO_2 may be important in bronchoconstriction and increases in collateral resistance with regional alveolar hypoxia. The effect of hypoxia on collateral resistance is abolished by administration of 5% CO_2. With global alveolar hypoxia, bronchoconstriction may be partially mediated by increased vagal tone (110,114). Nonspecific bronchial reactivity may be increased because of hypoxia-induced release of mast cell mediators (107).

C. Ventilation/Perfusion Relationships

Because HPV causes flow diversion away from hypoxic or atelectatic alveoli, it is the most important physiological adaptation of the lung to help preserve Pa_{O_2}. HPV improves oxygenation in regional lung disease, such as pneumonia or pulmonary contusion. Because of the increased ability to divert blood flow away from hypoxic lung segments with smaller segments, P_aO_2 is better maintained when small rather than large areas of the lung are rendered hypoxic. For instance, if 30% of the lung is hypoxic, while the remainder receives 100% O_2 P_aO_2 would be expected to decrease to 100 mmHg if HPV is absent (1). However, a P_aO_2 of 400 mmHg would be expected in the presence of HPV. With greater percentages of the lung being hypoxic, HPV is less effective in improving the observed P_aO_2. Blockade of HPV by administration of hyperoxic gas mixtures worsens $\dot{V}_A/\dot{Q}$ relationships in many forms of lung disease in animals (116) and humans (117,118). HPV has a smaller role in the preservation of $\dot{V}_A/\dot{Q}$ matching in the normal lung. Blockade of HPV by 100% O_2 did not affect $\dot{V}_A/\dot{Q}$ heterogeneity in humans (118) and animals (116) with normal lungs.

Alveolar hypoxia has variable effects on $\dot{V}_A/\dot{Q}$ relationships in normal lungs, ranging from no effect (119), mild deterioration in the distribution of $\dot{V}_A/\dot{Q}$ ratios (120), to slight improvement in $\dot{V}_A/\dot{Q}$ heterogeneity (76). The variable results are due to concurrent changes in cardiac output, pulmonary artery pressure, and possibly ventilation. For instance, when blood flow and ventilation were constrained to baseline values, mild improvement in $\dot{V}_A/\dot{Q}$ matching was noted (120). Administration of a hypoxic gas mixture to a region of the lung helps to preserve $\dot{V}_A/\dot{Q}$ matching in the entire lung by increasing $\dot{V}_A/\dot{Q}$ heterogeneity in the hypoxic lobe and decreasing $\dot{V}_A/\dot{Q}$ heterogeneity in the hyperoxic lobes (9).

III. Carbon Dioxide

A. Pulmonary Vasculature

Von Euler and Liljestrand (2) were the first to propose that local hypercapnia may control pulmonary blood flow in a homeostatic manner analogous to local hypoxia. However, controversy remains not only regarding the magnitude of the vasoconstrictor effect but also whether in some circumstances CO_2 is inert or may indeed be vasodilating as it is in the systemic vasculature. For these reasons and because local P_{CO_2} changes in alveolar gas are much less than the corresponding local P_{O_2} changes associated with fluctuations in regional perfusion and ventilation, it has been argued that the CO_2 effects are likely insignificant in the active regulation of $\dot{V}_A/\dot{Q}$ matching (121).

A variety of factors may account for some of the reported differences in pulmonary vascular CO_2 reactivity. These are given in Table 2, which also lists several factors known to affect HPV that have been neglected for CO_2.

1. *Effects of Inhaled CO_2 in Whole Animal Studies*

In most mammalian species, inhalation of 5%–10% CO_2 in normoxic gas mixtures is vasoconstricting (57,122,123) but not in all (124–126). With regards to species differences, it appears that CO_2 pulmonary vasoreactivity follows that for O_2 (127), with dogs, rats, and rabbits having the least responsiveness, primates having an intermediate responsiveness, and pigs, sheep, and cats having the greatest responsiveness. The best data in awake and anesthetized normoxic humans show that breathing 3%–10% CO_2 is vasoconstricting, with pulmonary artery pressure increasing 30%–50% with CO_2 inhalation, but, because cardiac output also increases, pulmonary vascular resistance increases to a lesser (25%–35%) extent (128,129).

The interpretation of the direct effects of CO_2 on the pulmonary vasculature in vivo is hampered by several possible important systemic influences. The first is whether arterial and systemic hypercapnia might limit the local vascular response to CO_2. For instance, hypoxic stimulation of the peripheral chemoreceptors blunts HPV via vagal innervation of the lung (51,130). Although it has

Table 2 Factors Affecting Pulmonary Vascular CO_2 Reactivity and Effective Responses

- A. Known factors
  1. Species differences
  2. Vessel type and caliber
  3. Lung region size
  4. Mode of CO_2 change
     - a. Inhalation
       - Change in ventilation versus F_ICO_2
     - b. Perfusion
       - Change in blood flow versus $P_{\bar{v}}CO_2$
  5. Local Po_2
- B. Undetermined but possible factors
  1. Systemic oxygenation and acid-base status
     - a. Central versus peripheral chemoreceptor response
     - b. Changes in bronchial blood flow and Po_2 and/or Pco_2
  2. Anesthetics
  3. Carbonic anhydrase inhibition
  4. Lung injury/manipulation
  5. Endogenous cytokines and vasoactive mediators
  6. Vasoactive drugs
  7. Hematocrit
  8. Lung volume/positive end-expiratory pressure
  9. Cardiac output, PA and LA pressures

not been investigated, hypercapnic and acidemic stimulation of the peripheral chemoreceptors might reduce hypercapnic pulmonary vasoconstriction in an analogous fashion. General activation of the sympathetic nervous system with hypercapnic acidosis, however, does not appear to blunt the hypercapnic pulmonary vasoconstrictor response (131). Locally, changes in bronchial arterial Pco_2 may be important in modifying the pulmonary vascular response to CO_2 although this has never been studied as it has for bronchial arterial Po_2 and HPV (28). Because the bronchial arteries are systemic blood vessels that dilate with increasing CO_2 (132), one might predict that with increasing bronchial blood flow, increased oxygen delivery to the pulmonary vascular smooth muscle, and increased wash-out of CO_2 might blunt any local downstream vasoconstrictor influence.

2. *Effects of Inhaled CO_2 in Isolated Lung and Lobe Studies*

Studies in isolated lungs or in situ lobes have the virtue of eliminating many of the systemic influences mentioned above and, in principle, should yield a more accurate picture of the direct effects of CO_2 on the pulmonary vasculature. Indeed, normoxic ventilation of isolated perfused lungs or in situ lobes with 5%–10% CO_2 in dogs (131), cats (133), monkeys (134), rabbits (135), and sheep (136) causes elevations of pulmonary artery pressure and vascular resistance. Several species, including the rat and ferret, show little to no vasoconstriction with CO_2 (137,138). Hypocapnia (usually produced by hyperventilation) causes slight vasodilation in normoxia probably because baseline resistance is already low (12,136). When equally hypercapnic loads are imposed on a lobe to yield the same alveolar P_{CO_2} either by CO_2 inhalation or perfusion of hypercapnic blood but without altering arterial P_{CO_2}, the increase in pulmonary vascular resistance is greater with precapillary hypercapnia (hypercapnic blood) than with alveolar hypercapnia (CO_2 inhalation) (139). Bergofsky et al. (122) also showed that at an equivalent lobar arterial blood pH, the increase in vascular resistance was no different between perfusates made acidic with CO_2 or fixed acids.

Several studies have suggested a possible dilating action of CO_2 in addition to its vasoconstricting effect. In studies documenting overt vasodilation (2,140), this was observed only with inhalation of >15% CO_2, which may simply represent a direct paralytic effect of very high CO_2 of no physiological relevance. Indirectly, others have deduced that CO_2 has a dilating action based upon lesser constriction with hypercapnic acidosis in normoxia than that occurring with an equal metabolic stimulus. However, in these experiments, metabolic acid was delivered by blood and CO_2 by inhalation, which may not have been strictly equivalent stimuli (141–143). Similar evidence for a competing vasodilator influence of CO_2 on hypoxic pulmonary vasoconstriction has been found (2,144), again with differences in the mode of delivery of the two acidic perturbations.

Although it is not easy to arrive at a definitive conclusion about the pulmonary vasoreactivity to CO_2, in general, acidic and hypercapnic perturbations are vasoconstricting, at least in the range of $P_{CO_2} < 80$ mmHg and $pH > 7.10$, and hypocapnia is vasodilating when there is preexisting vasoconstriction such as with hypoxia. With more acidic stress, there may be direct paralyzing effects or systemic influences that counteract local vasoconstriction. It should not be discounted that CO_2 may have a vasodilating action, which, under certain conditions, can blunt but rarely override its own acidic vasoconstricting effect.

3. Sites and Mechanisms of CO_2 Response

Carbon dioxide acts on the pulmonary vasculature at several sites. Hyde et al. (145) and Bergofsky et al (139) used isolated perfused cat lungs and various combinations of forward and retrograde perfusions with either CO_2 inhalation or hypercapnic blood perfusion combined with diffusing capacity measurements of capillary blood volume to demonstrate that both arteries and veins constrict with CO_2. Similar changes in capillary blood volume in humans breathing CO_2 were found by Rankin et al. (146), suggesting pulmonary venoconstriction. Direct measurements of vessel caliber in response to CO_2 have only been done in the cat (147) in which it was found that 10% CO_2 inhalation caused no changes in diameter of small muscular pulmonary arterioles (100–200 μm) nevertheless that were responsive to hypoxia. These findings, taken as a whole, suggest that CO_2 is vasoconstricting both to veins and arteries but that, in contrast to hypoxia, the effect is on larger vessels. With the advent of high-resolution computed tomography (HRCT), it is possible to assess vessel caliber noninvasively. This approach may yield considerable valuable data in combination with traditional hemodynamic measurements.

Very little is certain about how CO_2 acts on the vasculature. Traditionally, it has been considered that the resultant hydrogen ion concentration changes were largely responsible, with acidosis and alkalosis causing, respectively, constriction and dilation. Experiments comparing CO_2 inhalation and hyperventilation to blood perfusates of differing acid-base status largely confirm the vasoconstricting stimulus of low pH both in normoxia (12,122) and hypoxia (72,103,148). It is not known whether extracellular pH (pH_e) or intracellular pH (pH_i) is the more important stimulus in the pulmonary vasculature because CO_2 reduces very quickly both pH_e and pH_i. In brain blood vessels, pH_e is responsible for CO_2 reactivity (149), but this has not been systematically studied in the lung. Although a number of in vitro studies employing pulmonary artery strips or isolated perfused lungs have reported a controlling influence of intracellular pH (36,150–152), only stimuli other than CO_2 were used. Thus, the relevance of these sometimes very nonphysiological stimuli to in vivo conditions may be argued, because it is changes in P_{CO_2} (from changes in regional ventilation and perfusion which cause both intracellular and extracellular acidosis) and extracellular pH (from changes in systemic acid-base disturbances altering mixed venous blood pH), which are of physiological and clinical interest.

Of the many agents with vasoactivity in the pulmonary circulation, only a few have been investigated as possible mediators of the CO_2 response and no definite picture emerges. As in the systemic circulation (153), changes in P_{CO_2} and pH alter arachidonate metabolism in the lung, with extreme acidosis suppressing both thromboxane and prostacyclin synthesis in the lung (154); however, over more physiological pH values (7.2 to 7.7), the changes are slight. A mediator of recent interest is nitric oxide (NO), which plays an important part in hypercapnic vasodilation of the systemic vasculature (155,156). It has been shown in cultured systemic vascular endothelial cells that NO synthase, the rate-limiting enzyme in NO generation, is extremely pH sensitive: ~4% change in activity per 0.01 pH unit difference (157). If endogenous NO production plays a role in setting airway and vascular tone, this may be an important mechanism by which CO_2 exerts its effects. In the isolated buffer perfused rabbit lung, hypocapnic alkalosis and hypercapnic acidosis, respectively, decreased and increased pulmonary vascular NO synthesis (135). Inhibition of this CO_2-mediated production of NO by nitric oxide synthase inhibitors results in greater CO_2 vasoconstriction in the range of 5%–10% inhaled CO_2 in the dog and rabbit (135,158) but not with extremely high concentrations (15% CO_2) in the rat (159). Thus, as in the systemic blood vessels, CO_2 mediates NO release, and this may also explain partly the relatively weaker vasoconstriction of hypercapnic acidosis when compared with metabolically induced acidosis.

4. *Kinetics of the CO_2 Response*

The speed at which CO_2 constricts the vasculature and diverts blood flow in normoxia has not been studied systematically, but the data of Barer et al. (57), Viles and Shepherd (143), and Johnson et al. (160) show the response is maximal in less than 3 minutes with a half-time of roughly 90 seconds (57). In hypoxia, the data show a more complex time course. Orchard et al. (161) found an acute response with a half-time of roughly 60–90 seconds, a response equal to or slightly faster than that for acute hypoxic pulmonary vasoconstriction (162,163). However, when alveolar gas tensions are allowed to vary as a region responds to hypoxia by vasoconstriction, a progressively dampening oscillatory pattern of blood flow develops (164), reflecting the effect of varying blood flow on CO_2 delivery into a lung region, which, in turn, alters the strength of HPV. These oscillations disappear and blood flow declines monotonically when alveolar P_{CO_2} is held constant. In a model analysis, Grant and Schneider (165) found that these findings could only be explained by incorporating a vasoconstrictor response into changes in H^+ and a dilator response into molecular CO_2, interacting with a monotonic vasoconstrictor response to hypoxia. Both the CO_2 and H^+ responses had time constants of 4.8 minutes, much slower than the few direct measurements cited above. No studies have taken measurements of these kinetics beyond 5 minutes to establish whether longer time courses are present, but it is possible, as shown for HPV (7), that there might be slower responses that may take several hours to reach maximum effect.

5. *Effects of Region Size on Changes in Blood Flow in Response to CO_2*

The ability of CO_2 to constrict pulmonary vessels, divert blood flow to other portions of the vascular bed, and alter total pulmonary vascular resistance depends on the size of the region experiencing a change in its CO_2. Thus, when a hypercapnic stimulus is applied to both lungs in vivo or in vitro, there is usually vasoconstriction because all regions experience greater CO_2. However, this does not preclude a heterogeneous response such that some regions, possibly those with the lowest CO_2 (high $\dot{V}_A/\dot{Q}$ regions) may have greater vasoconstriction than areas of low $\dot{V}_A/\dot{Q}$ because the high $\dot{V}_A/\dot{Q}$ regions may experience a greater relative increase in CO_2. Although this has not been studied in a systematic manner, one study suggests that inhaled CO_2 may reduce regional perfusion heterogeneity. Using radioactive xenon and external counters on the upright (head up) dog, Dugard and Naimark (166) found that inspired CO_2 further reduced the caudal-cephalad perfusion gradient when compared to hypoxia alone. This question requires investigation with more sophisticated methods of spatial resolution such as microsphere analysis or positron emission tomography.

As definitively demonstrated for hypoxic pulmonary vasoconstriction (13), hypercapnic vasoconstriction is a more effective mechanism for redistributing blood flow the smaller the lung region involved. Twining et al. (167) found that 10% CO_2 administered to a single lung in conscious humans caused a 10% diversion of blood flow to the normocapnic lung. In a similar design, Borst et al. (168) found that unilateral administration of 5% CO_2 in cats produced a 20% shift in blood flow away from the hypercapnic lung. In the dog, using changes in mixed venous P_{CO_2} (from 45 to >90 mmHg), Hyman et al. (142) found no diversion of blood flow. In contrast, Barer et al. (57) used inspired CO_2 and showed a 20%–30% reduction of perfusion from a hypercapnic lobe with an equivalent increase in alveolar P_{CO_2}. The striking differences between these studies are not easily reconciled, but they suggest an important difference in the manner by which a lung region becomes hypercapnic, alluded to earlier, that has not been systematically studied. Sheehan and Farhi (136) noted even greater blood flow diversion (40%) in the isolated right apical lobe (RAL) of the sheep (15% of total lung volume) with elevation of the alveolar P_{CO_2} from 40 to 60 mmHg by administration of 5%–6% CO_2. Figure 1 shows the extent of perfusion shifts with both hypoxic and hypercapnic alveolar gas tensions. The only study

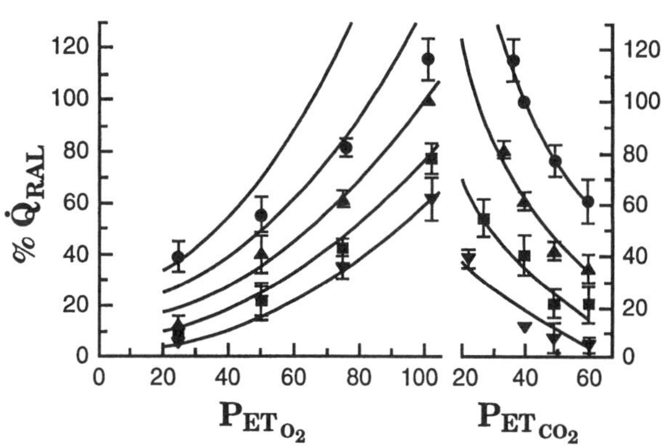

Figure 1 Extent of perfusion shifts both with hypoxic and hypercapnic alveolar gas tensions. (From Ref. 136.)

to examine this question at an even smaller region size (approximately 1%–2% of total lung volume) found no flow diversion with 8% inspired CO_2 in contrast to inspired hypoxia (169). These limited data across a variety of species suggest that hypercapnic vasoconstriction becomes more effective at blood flow diversion the smaller the involved lung region but that the site of control may not extend beyond the sublobular level.

B. Airways and Parenchyma

Venrath et al. (170) were the first to suggest that CO_2 might alter local ventilation to promote $\dot{V}_A/\dot{Q}$ matching based on observations that temporary pulmonary artery occlusion to one lung causes ventilation to decrease to that lung and increase in the contralateral lung, and that a decrease in alveolar P_{CO_2} causes bronchoconstriction in isolated cat lungs (171). Although CO_2 does not affect pulmonary vascular resistance as profoundly as does oxygen, it has significantly greater impact on the airways and parenchyma.

1. *Effects of Inhaled CO_2*

Reported effects of inhaling different concentrations of CO_2 on respiratory mechanics are conflicting, with much of the same variability noted for effects on pulmonary vascular resistance. Table 3 lists some of the factors known to affect airway CO_2 reactivity, in many cases analogous to those affecting pulmonary vascular CO_2 reactivity. Most studies in resting nonhyperventilating animals show CO_2 inhalation to be bronchoconstricting (172–174), although in some, depending on the concentration of inhaled CO_2 and type of measurement of airflow resistance, there is no effect (173,175) or dilation (176). The same tendency toward bronchoconstriction holds for studies in humans breathing low levels of CO_2 (111,177), but others have found bronchodilation (178). In contrast, all studies done in animals and humans with hyperventilation, which itself is bronchoconstricting, document that addition of inhaled CO_2 to correct hypocapnia restores normal bronchomotor tone (111,178–180). Likewise, adding CO_2 to the inspired gas of nonperfused lung regions abolishes the bronchoconstriction caused by the resultant low airway and alveolar P_{CO_2} (173,181,182).

When changes in airway and alveolar CO_2 are the result of changes in blood flow or CO_2 content, Samanek and Aviado (174) showed that increased blood flow (and thus increased CO_2 delivery) in the isolated lobe of the dog increased alveolar P_{CO_2} and caused bronchodilation. When total pulmonary blood flow or mixed venous P_{CO_2} are increased to augment pulmonary CO_2 delivery in anesthetized but spontaneously breathing dogs whose systemic and pulmonary circulations are isolated to control arterial P_{CO_2}, ventilation increases with increased pulmonary CO_2 delivery (183). Although these workers attributed the increased ventilation to stimulation of intrapulmonary CO_2 receptors, it is

Table 3 Factors Affecting Airway/Parenchymal CO_2 Reactivity and Effective Responses

A. Known factors
   1. Species differences
   2. Airway caliber
   3. Lung regions size
   4. Mode of CO_2 change
      a. Inhalation
         Change in ventilation versus F_ICO_2
      b. Perfusion
         Change in blood flow versus $P_{\bar{v}}CO_2$
   5. Carbonic anhydrase inhibition
   6. Lung volume and positive end-expiratory pressure
   7. Extent of collateral ventilation
   8. Systemic acid-base status
      a. Chemoreceptor response
      b. Central chemoreceptor stimulated bronchoconstriction
      c. Peripheral chemoreceptor stimulated bronchoconstriction

B. Undetermined but possible factors
   1. Anesthetics
   2. Lung injury/manipulation
   3. Endogenous cytokines and bronchoactive mediators
   4. Bronchoactive drugs
   5. Changes in bronchial blood flow and PO_2 and/or PCO_2

possible that the resultant increases in airway and alveolar PCO_2 may have caused bronchodilation and thus an increase in ventilation for the same neural input to the respiratory muscles.

2. Mechanisms and Sites of Pulmonary Bronchial Reactivity to CO_2

The apparent contradiction that both hypocapnia and hypercapnia are bronchoconstricting can be explained by antagonistic local and systemic effects of CO_2 on the airways. Ingram (173) explored this systemically by studying all combinations of altered airway (local) PCO_2 and arterial (systemic) PCO_2. When arterial PCO_2 was held constant, lowered airway PCO_2 caused bronchoconstriction, but elevated airway PCO_2 did not appear to produce any bronchodilation. When airway PCO_2 was held constant, increased arterial PCO_2 was bronchoconstricting but there was no bronchodilation with arterial hypocapnia. The effects of airway hypocapnia and arterial hypercapnia were additive.

The bronchoconstricting effects of systemic hypercapnia are largely mediated via efferent vagal parasympathetic nonmyelinated pathways and can be blocked by parasympatholytic interventions such as vagotomy and atropine administration (109,111,173,176,184). The larger bronchi are the site of vagally mediated reflex bronchoconstriction (173), there being little vagal innervation beyond the large conducting airways. The sensors for systemic hypercapnic bronchoconstriction are located within the brain (184). Hypercapnic stimulation of the peripheral chemoreceptors in isolation, on the other hand, induces bronchodilation (112,185) and, in vivo, this response may thus oppose the centrally mediated bronchoconstriction.

The local effects of CO_2 that cause bronchoconstriction with hypocapnia (173,178,180–182) and bronchodilation with hypercapnia (174,178) are direct actions because they are not attenuated or abolished by alterations in lung innervation (173,174) and are observed in isolated preparations of airway smooth muscle (186,187). The effects of CO_2 on bronchial smooth muscle appear to follow those expected with the change in H^+ ion concentration (187,188) but no studies have been attempted to determine whether the response is more dependent on pH_e or pH_i changes. The effects of P_{CO_2} and pH that regulate airway smooth muscle tone are mediated by changes in calcium uptake from the extracellular space. Verapamil, a Ca^{2+} channel antagonist, blocks the bronchoconstriction of voluntary hyperventilation (180) and attenuates the effects of changes in extracellular pH and P_{CO_2} in isolated airway strips constricted with cholinergic agonists (186,187).

Bronchodilating effects of CO_2 extend from the trachea and large conducting airways (186) to distal airways (189). As noted above, in vivo studies that result in systemic hypercapnia usually do not find evidence for large airway bronchodilation because any direct effect is usually overridden by reflex bronchoconstriction. When more sensitive techniques are used to separate the changes in resistance of large and small airways, small airways bronchodilation can be detected (178,189) even with central airway bronchoconstriction. The HRCT scanning of airway caliber combined with measurements of airway resistance has considerable potential to locate anatomically the sites and direction of CO_2 responsiveness.

One of the more important sites of bronchodilation with CO_2 is at the level of airways and channels that constitute pathways for collateral ventilation (189,190). There are large species differences in collateral ventilation (191) such that species with extensive collateral ventilation (dog) show greater CO_2 responsiveness than animals (sheep and pig) with little collateral ventilation. Lung volume may be an important determinant of the magnitude of collateral ventilation because large tidal volumes or positive end-expiratory pressure blunts the bronchodilating effect of CO_2 (192,193).

Changes in CO_2 may also affect total and local parenchymal compliance. In studies involving pulmonary artery occlusion and CO_2 inhalation, static compliance is reduced (pneumoconstriction) with maneuvers that generate local hypocapnia, and it can be prevented by inhalation of CO_2 (181,182). Short duration inhalation of CO_2 increases static compliance and total lung capacity (173,177). The phenomenon of hypocapnic pneumoconstriction and hypercapnic pneumodilation have not been adequately explained but may be due to distal smooth muscle relaxation with CO_2 beyond the nonrespiratory conducting airways, promoting greater collateral ventilation (190), or it may be due to pH-mediated enhancement of the surface tension–lowering properties of surfactant (194).

3. *Kinetics of the CO_2 Response*

The kinetics of CO_2-induced changes in ventilation and airway resistance are rapid, occurring within 5–10 seconds with a half-time of roughly 60–90 seconds (76,176,182). We (211) used acetazolamide, a carbonic anhydrase inhibitor in dogs, to slow the rate at which local tissue pH changed following occlusion of the pulmonary artery to that region and measured the regional ventilation and its rate of change. In the control state, the half-time of ventilation redistribution away from the nonperfused lobe was roughly 75 seconds, which increased to 160 seconds with acetazolamide (Figure 2). Equivalent slowing of the rate of return of lobar ventilation with return of blood flow was also observed, providing evidence that it is changes in pH rather than CO_2 that initiate the bronchoactive effects of CO_2. Hypocapnic bronchoconstriction at the small airways and changes in collateral ventilation exhibit tachyphylaxis when the stimulus is maintained for greater than 30 minutes (195). This is not altered by changes in cholinergic mechanisms nor by histamine or prostaglandins, but it might be explained by a return of intracellular pH toward normal by mechanisms of intracellular pH defense in smooth muscle and lung tissue.

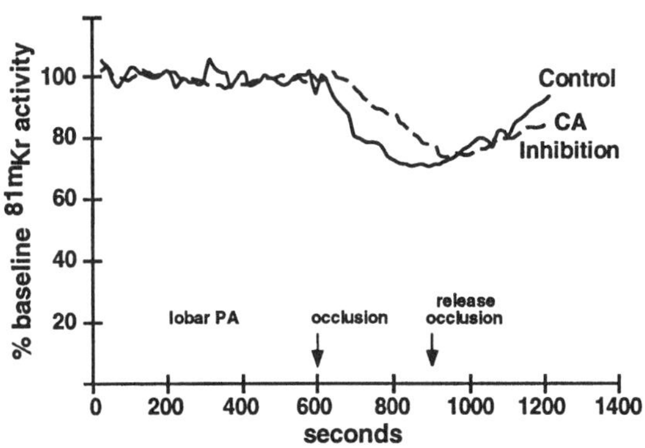

Figure 2 Kinetics of lobar ventilation changes in the dog following acute lobar vascular occlusion and release of occlusion showing the slowing of redistribution of homeostatic ventilation redistribution with inhibition of carbonic anhydrase. (From Ref. 211.)

4. Effects of Lung Region Size on Changes in Ventilation in Response to CO_2

In a similar fashion to CO_2 vasoreactivity and blood flow redistribution, the ability of regional ventilation to be diverted in response to a change in its local CO_2 is a function of region size. Near complete cessation of blood flow into a single lung of dog and human causes a 25%–35% diversion of ventilation to the perfused lung whose blood flow is correspondingly increased (181,182). At the lobar level in the dog, there is a 45% shift of ventilation with loss of blood flow (76), and this increases to almost 70% at the segmental and subsegmental level (196). With increases in blood flow at the lobar level, Samanek and Aviado (174) found that lobar ventilation increased in parallel with blood flow, although they could not quantitate the absolute magnitude. However, in contrast to these studies, Robertson and Glenny (1997) found that pigs show no ventilation redistribution following lobar pulmonary artery occlusion.

The magnitude of ventilation redistribution in the canine and human experiments was likely maximized over the natural response because, in many cases, the test region was separately ventilated, thus preventing reinspiration of CO_2 eliminated from other regions into the common dead space. In vivo, this would buffer the decrease or increase in CO_2 with changes in blood flow and thus blunt the magnitude of ventilation shift. Furthermore, airway blood flow via the bronchial circulation would also buffer any changes in local airway P_{CO_2} because the bronchial circulation is capable of significant CO_2 exchange with the airways (198). At a very peripheral level, mechanical interdependence between lung units within a lobe will also limit local ventilation redistribution in that Grant et al. (169) found subsegmental tidal volume in ferrets was not altered by large variations in inspired CO_2. It is not readily explicable but nevertheless intriguing that the ability to redistribute ventilation in response to a change in perfusion appears to be correlated with the extent of collateral ventilation, being minimal in ferrets and pigs but greater in dogs and humans.

C. Gas Exchange and $\dot{V}_A/\dot{Q}$ Relationships

The relevance of local CO_2-mediated vascular, airway, and parenchymal effects in the efficiency of gas exchange and in $\dot{V}_A/\dot{Q}$ matching has never been accorded the same attention as for oxygen, whose effects are predominantly on regional perfusion and much less on the regional distribution of ventilation. Although vascular effects of O_2 are quantitatively larger than any of the CO_2 actions described above, especially because venous blood to gas phase differences for O_2 and interregional P_{O_2} heterogeneities are much greater, changes in lung tissue and gas phase CO_2, both globally and regionally, have an important influence on gas exchange efficiency. This has been studied to a greater extent with imposed global changes in CO_2 and only more recently at the regional level, which may mimic better the physiological state of the lungs.

1. *Effects of Inspired CO_2 on Gas Exchange and $\dot{V}_A/\dot{Q}$ Heterogeneity*

Investigations in the 1960s and 1970s revealed the curious finding that addition of CO_2 to the inspired gas could increase arterial P_{O_2} even at constant ventilation (193,199). Some of the improvements observed were simply a consequence of the respiratory acidosis generating a rightward shift in the O_2-dissociation curve (Bohr effect), which has the effect of reducing the alveolar-arterial O_2 difference for any degree of venous admixture or $\dot{V}_A/\dot{Q}$ mismatch (200). However, neither changes in blood gas chemistry nor the small changes in cardiac output, metabolic rate, or pulmonary arterial pressures could explain the full effect, and it was assumed that regional $\dot{V}_A/\dot{Q}$ heterogeneity was reduced. We have shown in both normally ventilated dogs (76) and hyperventilated dogs (75) and in hyperventilated pigs (201) that $\dot{V}_A/\dot{Q}$ heterogeneity measured with the multiple inert gas elimination technique (MIGET) can be reduced 30%–50% by inhalation of 2%–4% CO_2. In the dog, Domino et al. (75) and Tsukimoto et al. (202) have shown that the effect is considerably attenuated with large tidal volumes and/or PEEP just as was reported by Ingram et al. (193) for the (A-a)P_{O_2} difference with PEEP. The reason for this may be the loss of any recruitable collateral ventilatory pathways when tidal or functional residual lung volumes are high (191).

In addition to reducing $\dot{V}_A/\dot{Q}$ heterogeneity, inspired CO_2 also improves respiratory gas exchange by its reduction in dead space ventilation, which may decrease as much as 30% (76). The exact cause of reduced dead space and therefore greater alveolar ventilation is not certain. It may reflect singly, or in combination, large central airway bronchoconstriction, reducing the volume of the non-gas–exchanging conducting airways (173), increased bronchial blood flow by inspired CO_2 (132) enhancing gas exchange by the more distal airways, especially for CO_2 whose effective solubility is about 20 times that for O_2 (203) or the slight increase in pulmonary artery pressure and cardiac output with hypercapnia (204) recruiting alveolar dead space. If CO_2 reduces the actual volume of the common dead space, then the effective improvement in $\dot{V}_A/\dot{Q}$ inequality with inspired CO_2 may be somewhat underestimated with MIGET because of the loss of gas mixing in the diminished common dead space (202). When external dead space is added, the resulting measured dead space is less than the sum of the intrapulmonary and added dead spaces (202,205). The ensuing hypercapnia may act in the same fashion as inspired CO_2, although there may be important unexplained differences between the elevated CO_2 added exogenously (with

CO_2 present in the airways in both cycles of respiration) and CO_2 retention with increases in dead space (with CO_2 absent in the inspired gas).

In normally ventilated dogs, 3%–4% inspired CO_2 reduces the calculated (A-a)P_{O_2} difference by approximately 3 mmHg in normoxia, by 19 mmHg with hyperoxic (50% O_2) inhalation, and by 1.5 mmHg with hypoxic (15% O_2) inhalation, and it reduces the normal arterial-mixed expired P_{CO_2} difference from 16 to 2 mmHg (76,193,206). In the dog, the effect of CO_2 is probably not through any enhancement of HPV (76) because similar benefits were seen in the dogs ventilated with 50% O_2 (HPV minimized). In experiments designed to test for the presence of putative intrapulmonary CO_2 receptors in the control of breathing in mammals, Shirer et al. (207) added 12% CO_2 to different portions of the inspirate in spontaneously air-breathing ponies and found that CO_2 added to the latter half of inspiration increased arterial PO_2 ($\sim$12 mmHg) almost equal to that observed with continuous 6% CO_2 inhalation but did not increase ventilation or arterial P_{CO_2}. These findings suggest that the improvements in gas exchange efficiency with inspired CO_2 in vivo are the result of local responses in the lung and are not dependent on any systemic acid-base change.

The effect of inspired CO_2 on $\dot{V}_A/\dot{Q}$ mismatch appears to be mediated largely by changes in pH because the improvements of gas exchange with CO_2 always followed the changes in pH no matter how the pH was changed (CO_2 versus metabolic acid or base) (208). However, in normocapnic nonhyperventilated dogs, metabolic acidosis itself does not improve $\dot{V}_A/\dot{Q}$ matching (209,210), suggesting some differences between respiratory and metabolic acidosis and the manner in which the acidic stimulus is delivered (blood versus inspired gas). The primacy of CO_2-mediated pH changes also is supported indirectly by the results with CA inhibition, whose main effect is to reduce the catalytic rate at which a change in CO_2 (brought about by a fluctuation in regional blood flow) generates a new H^+ concentration (210). Acetazolamide slowed the rate of ventilation redistribution following pulmonary lobar artery occlusion and worsened the degree of $\dot{V}_A/\dot{Q}$ mismatch with cyclical blood flow fluctuations (211).

Whether inspired CO_2 principally reduces the heterogeneity of regional perfusion or ventilation cannot be ascertained by MIGET because the indices of perfusion and ventilation dispersions derived from inert gas excretion data are relative to the mean or normalized $\dot{V}_A/\dot{Q}$ ratio and not to the mean of the perfusion or ventilation distributions. Thus, other methods must be used to study this question. We have assessed the heterogeneity of regional ventilation in dogs and pigs by simultaneous multiple breath wash-outs of helium and nitrogen and have shown that inspired CO_2 reduces peripheral ventilation heterogeneity in the dog (208) but not in the pig (201). Given the multiple effects of CO_2, it is not altogether surprising that the mode of improvement in $\dot{V}_A/\dot{Q}$ heterogeneity may differ between species, such as the dog and pig, which have differing pulmonary vasoreactivity and collateral ventilation (212). Studies employing inhaled and vascular microspheres should provide more definitive answers.

2. *The Role of CO_2 in $\dot{V}_A/\dot{Q}$ Matching During Spontaneous Fluctuations in Regional Ventilation and Perfusion*

Homeostasis is a central tenet of physiology and it is generally assumed that regulatory systems act to keep different variables in a near steady state. However, it is becoming increasingly clear that many physiological systems are not stable in a strict sense but show highly complex dynamic fluctuations. With regard to the lung, there are oscillations in total ventilation, functional residual capacity, cardiac output, and arterial blood gases, with differing cycles, some as short as 20–120 seconds (213–215). Recently, Glenny et al. (216) have demonstrated that there are nonrandom fluctuations in regional perfusion of the lung in otherwise unperturbed dogs in region sizes as small as 2 cc over intervals of 20 minutes, which account for approximately 18% of the total perfusion heterogeneity. Further preliminary data from out laboratory with microsphere analysis show that these fluctuations extend as far out as days and as short as minute-by-minute.

If short duration fluctuations in regional perfusion (and possibly of regional ventilation) are asynchronous, they could contribute to overall $\dot{V}_A/\dot{Q}$ mismatch if not rapidly matched by compensatory changes in their respective accompanying gas or blood flow. Although Wagner et al. (216a) have shown that $\dot{V}_A/\dot{Q}$ heterogeneity shows very little temporal variability on the time scale of hours-to-days, it has not been examined whether there are greater or lesser fluctuations in shorter time intervals. Alveolar and tissue P_{CO_2} changes resulting from spontaneous fluctuations in $\dot{V}_A$ and $\dot{Q}$ are likely to be small (2–4 mmHg), being bounded by the mixed venous P_{CO_2} and alveolar P_{CO_2} of that region. Although the changes are small, Sheehan and Farhi (136) have shown that these P_{CO_2} changes can cause up to 10%–20% blood flow diversion in lobar segments. The reason for this sensitivity to small changes in P_{CO_2} may lie in the much larger pH changes they can evoke in the more acidic and poorly buffered lung interstitium and alveolar airway fluids, where values as low as pH: 6.2, HCO_3^-: 2 mM, and protein: 0.2 g/L have been measured (217,218).

Because a number of vascular, airway, and parenchymal properties are pH sensitive in a manner that causes appropriate matching changes in ventilation in response to perfusion changes and vice versa, we inhibited lung CA activity to slow the rate at which local pH with any spontaneous $\dot{V}_A$ or $\dot{Q}$ fluctuations would change and showed greater $\dot{V}_A/\dot{Q}$ heterogeneity in the normal dog lung (Figure 3). We proposed that CA inhibition unmasks an element of $\dot{V}_A/\dot{Q}$ mismatch arising from a failure to rapidly match these spontaneous short duration fluctua-

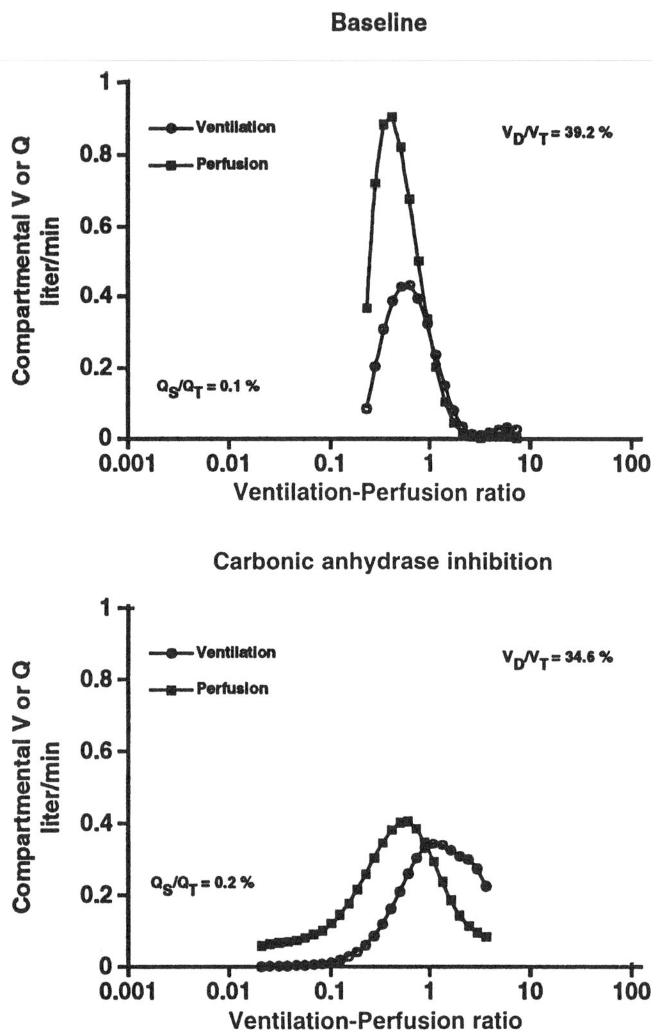

Figure 3 $\dot{V}_A/\dot{Q}$ distributions in the dog before and after inhibition of carbonic anhydrase showing increased heterogeneity with loss of rapid CA-mediated pH-sensitive mechanisms of $\dot{V}_A/\dot{Q}$ matching. (From Ref. 210.)

tions, although it could not be ruled out that new fixed regional heterogeneity had not developed. To test the concept more directly, we imposed a known regional perfusion fluctuation (cyclic lobar pulmonary artery occlusion and release) and demonstrated that there was a doubling of the measured $\dot{V}_A/\dot{Q}$ heterogeneity with lung CA inhibition (211). Similar experiments with imposed fluctuations in regional ventilation and CA inhibition to test whether the rate of blood flow diversion (more strongly dependent on HPV) is also dependent upon the kinetics of CO_2 and H^+ equilibration have not been performed, but we have recently shown that CA inhibition slows HPV (219).

The importance of CO_2-medicated responses by the vasculature and airways in $\dot{V}_A/\dot{Q}$ matching remains to be further quantified. Our studies with CA inhibition (210,211) and those of Sheehan and Farhi (136) are strongly suggestive, but studies with selective inhibitors of these processes (none are presently known) and better quantification of the magnitude of regional blood and gas flow fluctuations are needed. Such data could be useful in extending the modeling of the effect of local blood flow and ventilation control on gas exchange as already defined for O_2 regulation of local perfusion. Grant (220) has shown that HPV appears to be most homeostatic in regions of low $\dot{V}_A/\dot{Q}$. With CO_2 having much stronger effects on local ventilation than O_2, it might be predicted that CO_2 would act more powerfully in regions of higher $\dot{V}_A/\dot{Q}$ where the local P_{CO_2} is lower and the data suggest that changes in CO_2 are more potent.

IV. Summary

Local changes of both O_2 and CO_2 have significant effects on both the pulmonary vasculature and pulmonary airways and, hence, overall pulmonary gas exchange efficiency. The efficiency of the effect of both gases varies amongst the species and is influenced by regional size, anesthesia, acid-base status, and presence of lung disease. O_2 and CO_2 responses are relatively rapid (within seconds) and largely complete within several minutes. The combined influence of the two respiratory gases serves to maintain very efficient gas exchange in the normal lung and minimizes the deterioration of gas exchange in the diseased lung.

References

1. Marshall BE, Marshall C. Continuity of response to hypoxic pulmonary vasoconstriction. J Appl Physiol 1980; 49:189–196.
2. Euler UV, Liljestrand G. Observations on the pulmonary arterial blood pressure response in the cat. Acta Physiol Scand 1946; 12:301–320.
3. Weissmann N, Grimminger F, Walmrath D, Seeger W. Hypoxic vasoconstriction in buffer-perfused rabbit lungs. Respir Physiol 1995; 100:159–169.

4. Domino KB, Chen L, Alexander CM, Williams JJ, Marshall C, Marshall BE. Time course and responses of sustained hypoxic pulmonary vasoconstriction in the dog. Anesthesiol 1984; 60:562–566.
5. Carlsson AJ, Bindslev L, Santesson J, Gottlieb I, Hendenstierna G. Hypoxic pulmonary vasoconstriction in the human lung: the effect of prolonged unilateral hypoxic challenge during anaesthesia. Acta Anaesthesiol Scand 1985; 29:346–351.
6. Glasser SA, Domino KB, Lindgren L, Purcella P, Marshall C, Marshall BE. Pulmonary blood pressure and flow during atelectasis in the dog. Anesthesiology 1983; 59:225–231.
7. Vejlstrup N, Dorrington K. Intense slow hypoxic pulmonary vasoconstriction in gas-filled and liquid-filled lungs; an in vivo study in the rabbit. Acta Physiol Scand 1993; 148:305–313.
8. Vejlstrup NJ, O'Neill M, Nagyova B, Dorrington KL. Time course of hypoxic pulmonary vasoconstriction: a rabbit model of regional hypoxia. Am J Respir Crit Care Med 1997; 155:216–221.
8a. Dorrington KL, Clar C, Young JD, Jonas M, Tansley JG, Robbins PA. Time course of the human pulmonary vascular response to 8 hours of isocapnic hypoxia. Am J Physiol 1997; 273:H1126–H1134.
9. Domino KB, Hlastala MP, Eisenstein BL, Cheney FW. Effect of regional alveolar hypoxia on gas exchange in dogs. J Appl Physiol 1989; 67:730–735.
10. Kuriyama T, Wagner WW. Collateral ventilation may protect against high-altitude pulmonary hypertension. J Appl Physiol 1981; 51:1251–1256.
11. Bindslev L, Jolin A, Hedenstierna G, Baehrendtz S, Santesson J. Hypoxic pulmonary vasoconstriction in the human lung: effect of repeated hypoxic challenges during anesthesia. Anesthesiology 1985; 62:621–625.
12. Brimioulle S, Lejeune P, Vachiery J-L, Leeman M, Melot C, Naeije R. Effects of acidosis and alkalosis on hypoxic pulmonary vasoconstriction in dogs. Am J Physiol 1990; 258:H347–H353.
13. Marshall B, Marshall C. A model for hypoxic constriction of the pulmonary circulation. J Appl Physiol 1988; 64:68–77.
14. Marshall BE, Marshall C, BJ, Saidman LJ. Hypoxic pulmonary vasoconstriction in dogs: effects of lung segment size and oxygen tension. J Appl Physiol 1981; 31:1543–1551.
15. Dawson A. Regional pulmonary blood flow in sitting and supine man during and after acute hypoxia. J Clin Invest 1969; 48:301–310.
16. Neumann PH, Kivlen CM, Johnson A, Minnear FL, MAB. Effect of alveolar hypoxia on regional pulmonary perfusion. J Appl Physiol 1984; 56:338–342.
17. Mann CM, Domino KB, Walther SM, Glenny RW, Hlastala MP. Redistribution of pulmonary blood flow during unilateral hypoxia in prone and supine dogs. J Appl Physiol 1998 (in press).
19. Dawson CA, Grimm DJ, Linehan JH. Influence of hypoxia on the longitudinal distribution of pulmonary vascular resistance. J Appl Physiol 1978; 44:493–498.
20. Dawson CA, Grimm DJ, Linehan JH. Lung inflation and longitudinal distribution of pulmonary vascular resistance during hypoxia. J Appl Physiol 1979; 47:532–536.

21. Groh J, Kuhnle GEH, Kuebler WM, Goetz AE. An experimental model for simultaneous quantitative analysis of pulmonary micro- and macrocirculation during unilateral hypoxia in vivo. Res Exp Med 1992; 192:431–441.
22. Hakim TS, Michel RP, Minami H, Chang HK. Site of pulmonary hypoxic vasoconstriction studies with arterial and venous occlusion. J Appl Physiol 1983; 54: 1298–1302.
23. Madden JA, Dawson CA, Harder DR. Hypoxia-induced activation in small isolated pulmonary arteries from the cat. J Appl Physiol 1985; 59:113–118.
24. Nagasaka Y, Bhattacharya J, Nanjo S, Gropper MA, Staub NC. Micropuncture measurement of lung microvascular pressure profile during hypoxia in cats. Circ Res 1984; 54:90–95.
25. Zhao Y, Packer CS, Rhoades RA. Pulmonary vein contracts in response to hypoxia. Am J Physiol 1993; 265:L87–L92.
26. Sylvester JT, Mitzner W, Ngeow Y, Permutt S. Hypoxic constriction of alveolar and extra-alveolar vessels in isolated pig lungs. J Appl Physiol 1983; 54:1660–1666.
27. Groh J, Kuhnle GEH, Sckell A, Ney L, Goetz AE. Isoflurane inhibits hypoxic pulmonary vasoconstriction: an in vivo fluorescence microscopic study in rabbits. Anesthesiology 1994; 81:1436–1444.
28. Marshall B, Marshall C, Magno M, Lilagan P, Pietra G. Influence of bronchial arterial PO_2 on pulmonary vascular resistance. J Appl Physiol 1991; 70:405–415.
29. Madden JA, Vadula MS, Kurup VP. Effects of hypoxia and other vasoactive agents on pulmonary and cerebral artery smooth muscle cells. Am J Physiol 1992; 263:L384–L393.
30. Murray TR, Chen L, Marshall BE, Macarak EJ. Hypoxic contraction of cultured pulmonary vascular smooth muscle cells. Am J Respir Cell Mol Biol 1990; 3: 457–465.
31. Marshall C, Marshall BE. Hypoxic pulmonary vasoconstriction is not endothelium dependent. Proc Soc Exp Biol Med 1992; 201:267–270.
32. Ignarro LJ, Byrns RE, Buga GM, Wood KS. Endothelium-derived relaxing factor from pulmonary artery and vein possesses pharmacologic and chemical properties identical to those of nitric oxide radical. Circ Res 1987; 61:866–879.
33. Palmer RMJ, Ferrige AG, Moncada S. Nitric oxide release accounts for the biological activity of endothelium-derived relaxing factor. Nature 1987; 327:524–526.
34. Yanagisawa M, Kurihara H, Kimura S, Tomobe Y, Kobayashi M, Mitsue Y, Yazaki Y. A novel potent vasoconstriction peptide produced by vascular endothelial cells. Nature 1988; 332:411–415.
35. Tolins M, Weir EK, Chesler E, Nelson DP, From AHL. Pulmonary vascular tone is increased by a voltage-dependent calcium channel potentiator. J Appl Physiol 1986; 60:942–948.
36. Farrukh IS, Michael JR. Cellular mechanisms that control pulmonary vascular tone during hypoxia and normoxia. Possible role of CA^{2+} ATPases. Am Rev Respir Dis 1992; 145:1389–1397.
37. Frostell CG, Blomqvist H, Hedenstierna G, Lundberg J, Zapol WM. Inhaled nitric oxide selectively reverses human hypoxic pulmonary vasoconstriction without causing systemic vasodilation. Anesthesiology 1993; 78:427–435.

38. Wong J, Vanderford PA, Winters JW, Chang R, Soifer SJ, Fineman JR. Endothelin-1 does not mediate acute hypoxic pulmonary vasoconstriction in the intact newborn lamb. J Cardiovasc Pharmacol 1993; 22:S262–S266.
39. Sprague RS, Stephenson AH, Lonigro AJ. Prostaglandin I_2 supports blood flow to hypoxic alveoli in anesthetized dogs. J Appl Physiol 1984; 56:1246–1251.
40. Garrett RC, Thomas HMI. Relation of prostanoids to strength of hypoxic vasoconstriction in dogs with lobar atelectasis. J Appl Physiol 1985; 59:72–77.
41. Hales CA, Rouse ET, Slate JL. Influence of aspirin and indomethacin on variability of alveolar hypoxic vasoconstriction. J Appl Physiol 1978; 45:33–39.
42. Leeman M, Lejeune P, Hallemans R, Mélot CN, R. Effects of increased pulmonary vascular tone on gas exchange in canine oleic acid pulmonary edema. J Appl Physiol 1988; 65:662–668.
43. Gottlieb JE, McGeady M, Adkinson NF, Sylvester JT. Effects of cyclo- and lipoxygenase inhibitors on hypoxic vasoconstriction in isolated ferret lungs. J Appl Physiol 1988; 64:936–943.
44. Schuster DP, Dennis DR. Leukotriene inhibitors do not block hypoxic pulmonary vasoconstriction in dogs. J Appl Physiol 1987; 62:1808–1813.
45. Chen L, Miller FL, Malmkvist G, Cooley R, Marshall C, Marshall BE. Intravenous $PGF_{2\alpha}$ infusion does not enhance hypoxic pulmonary vasoconstriction during canine one-lung hypoxia. Anesthesiology 1988; 68:226–233.
46. Scherer R, Vigfusson G, Hultsch E, Van Aken H, Lawin P. Prostaglandin F_2 improves oxygen tension and reduces venous admisture during one-lung ventilation in anesthetized paralyzed dogs. Anesthesiology 1985; 62:23–26.
47. Lodato RF, MJR, Murray PA. Absence of neural modulation of hypoxic pulmonary vasoconstriction in conscious dogs. J Appl Physiol 1988; 65: – .
48. Robin ED, Theodore J, Burke CM, Oesterle SN, Fowler MB, Jamieson SW, Baldwin JC, Morris AJ, Hunt SA, Vankessel A, Stinson EB, Shumway NE. Hypoxic pulmonary vasoconstriction persists in the human transplanted lung. Clin Sci 1987; 72:283–287.
49. Kadowitz J, Hyman AL. Effect of sympathetic nerve stimulation on pulmonary vascular resistance in the dog. Circ Res 1973; 32:221–227.
50. Porcelli RJ, Viau AT, Haftchi NE, Befgofsky EH. β-receptor influence on lung vasoconstrictor responses to hypoxia and humoral agents. J Appl Physiol 1977; 43:612–616.
51. Naeije R, Lejeune P, Leeman M, Melot C, Closset J. Pulmonary vascular responses to surgical chemodenervation and chemical sympathectomy in dogs. J Appl Physiol 1989; 66:42–50.
52. Miller MA, Hales CA. Role of cytochrome P-450 in alveolar hypoxic pulmonary vasoconstriction in dogs. J Clin Invest 1979; 64:666–673.
53. Post JM, Hume JR, Archer SL, Weir EK. Direct role for potassium channel inhibition in hypoxic pulmonary vasoconstriction. Am J Physiol 1992; 262:C882–C890.
54. Marshall B, Marshall C, Frasch F, Hanson C. Role of hypoxic pulmonary vasoconstriction in pulmonary gas exchange and blood flow distribution. Intensive Care Med 1994; 20:291–297.
55. Marshall C, Marshall BE. Site and sensitivity for stimulation of hypoxic pulmonary vasoconstriction. J Appl Physiol 1983; 55:711–716.
56. Domino KB, Wetstein L, Glasser SA, Lindgren L, Marshall C, Harken AH, Mar-

shall BE. Influence of $P_{\bar{V}}O_2$ on blood flow to atelectatic lung. Anesthesiology 1983; 59:428–434.

57. Barer G, Howard P, Shaw J. Stimulus-response curves for the pulmonary vascular bed to hypoxia and hypecapnia. J Physiol 1970; 211:139–155.
58. De Cannière D, Stefanidis C, Hallemans R, Delcroix M, Brimioulle S, Naeije R. Stimulus-response curves for hypoxic pulmonary vasoconstriction in piglets. Cardiovasc Res 1992; 26:944–949.
59. Sylvester JT, Harabin AL, Peake MD, Frank RS. Vasodilator and constrictor responses to hypoxia in isolated pig lungs. J Appl Physiol 1980; 49:820–825.
60. Harabin AL, Peake MD, Sylvester JT. Effect of severe hypoxia on the pulmonary vascular response to vasoconstrictor agents. J Appl Physiol 1981; 50:561–565.
61. Benumof J, Wahrenbrock E. Blunted hypoxic pulmonary vasoconstriction by increased lung vascular pressures. J Appl Physiol 1975; 38:846–850.
62. De Cannière D, Stefanidis C, Hallemans R, Delcroix M, Lejeune P, Naeije R. Increased left atrial pressure inhibits hypoxic pulmonary vasoconstriction. J Appl Physiol 1994; 76:1502–1506.
63. Gu S, Ducas J, Schick U, Prewitt RM. Effects of left atrial pressure on the pulmonary vascular response to hypoxic ventilation. J Appl Physiol 1991; 70:1991–1995.
64. Lejeune P, De Smet J-M, De Francquen P, Leeman M, Brimioulle S, Hallemans R, Mélot C, Naeije R. Inhibition of hypoxic pulmonary vasoconstriction by increased left atrial pressure in dogs. Am J Physiol 1990; 259:H93–H100.
65. Sandavol J, Long GR, Skoog C, Wood LDH, Oppenheimer L. Independent influence of blood flow rate and mixed venous PO_2 on shunt fraction. J Appl Physiol 1983; 55:1128–1133.
66. Domino KB, Eisenstein BL, Cheney FW, Hlastala MP. Pulmonary blood flow and ventilation-perfusion heterogeneity. J Appl Physiol 1991; 71:252–258.
67. Domino KB, Hlastala MP, Cheney FW. Effect of increased intracranial pressure on regional hypoxic pulmonary vasoconstriction. Anesthesiology 1990; 72:490–495.
68. Ohlsson J, Middaugh M, Hlastala MP. Reduction of lung perfusion increases $\dot{V}_A/\dot{Q}$ heterogeneity. J Appl Physiol 1989; 66:2423–2430.
69. Colley PS, Cheney FW, Butler J. Mechanism of change in pulmonary shunt flow with hemorrhage. J Appl Physiol 1977; 42:196–201.
70. Bindslev L, Jolin-Carlsson A, Santesson J, Gottlieb I. Hypoxic pulmonary vasoconstriction in man: effects of hyperventilation. Acta Anaesthesiol Scand 1985; 29:547–551.
71. Gordon J, Martinez F, Keller P, Tod M, Madden J. Differing effects of acute and prolonged alkalosis on hypoxic pulmonary vasoconstriction. Am Rev Respir Dis 1993; 148:1651–1656.
72. Lejeune P, Brimioulle S, Leeman M, Hallemans R, Mélot C, Naeije. Enhancement of hypoxic pulmonary vasoconstriction by metabolic acidosis in dogs. Anesthesiology 1990; 73:256–264.
73. Marshall C, Lindgren L, Marshall BE. Effects of halothane, enflurane, and isoflurane on hypoxic pulmonary vasoconstriction in rat lungs in vitro. Anesthesiology 1984; 60:304–308.
74. Domino K, Swenson E, Polissar NL, Lu Y, Eisenstein B, Hlastala M. Effect of inspired CO_2 on ventilation and perfusion heterogeneity in hyperventilated dogs. J Appl Physiol 1993; 75:1309–1317.

75. Domino KB, Lu Y, Eisenstein BL, Hlastala MP. Hypocapnia worsens arterial blood oxygenation and increases $\dot{V}_A/\dot{Q}$ heterogeneity in canine pulmonary edema. Anesthesiology 1993; 78:91–97.
76. Swenson E, Robertson H, Hlastala M. Effects of inspired carbon dioxide on ventilation-perfusion matching in normoxia, hypoxia, and hyperoxia. Am J Respir Crit Care Med 1994; 149:1563–1569.
77. Newman JH, McMurtry IF, Reeves JT. Blunted pulmonary pressor responses to hypoxia in blood perfused, ventilated lungs isolated from oxygen toxic rats: Possible role of prostaglandins. Prostaglandins 1981; 22:11–20.
78. Hales CA, Sonne L, Peterson M, Kong D, Miller M, Watkins WD. Role of thromboxane and prostacyclin in pulmonary vasomotor changes after endotoxin in dogs. J Clin Invest 1981; 68:497–505.
79. Hutchison AA, Ogletree ML, Snapper JR, Brigham KL. Effect of endotoxemia on hypoxic pulmonary vasoconstriction in unanesthetized sheep. J Appl Physiol 1985; 58:1463–1468.
80. Reeves JT, Grover RF. Blockade of acute hypoxic pulmonary hypertension by endotoxin. J Appl Physiol 1974; 36:328–332.
81. Leeman M, Delcroix M, Vachiéry J-L, Mélot C, Naeije R. Blunted hypoxic vasoconstriction in oleic acid lung injury: effect of cyclooxygenase inhibitors. J Appl Physiol 1992; 72:251–258.
82. Hanly P, Sienko A, Light RB. Effect of cyclooxygenase blockade on gas exchange and hemodynamics in *Pseudomonas* pneumonia. J Appl Physiol 1987; 63:1829–1836.
83. McCormack DG, Paterson NAM. Loss of hypoxic pulmonary vasoconstriction in chronic pneumonia is not mediated by nitric oxide. Am J Physiol 1993; 265: H1523–H1528.
84. Lampron N, Lemaire F, Teisseire B, Hart A, Palot M, Matamis D, Lorino AM. Mechanical ventilation with 100% oxygen does not increase intrapulmonary shunt in patients with severe bacterial pneumonia. Am Rev Respir Dis 1985; 131:409–413.
85. Johnson D, Hurst T, Wilson T, Murphy F, Saxema A, To T, Mayers I. N^G-monomethyl-L-arginine does not restore loss of hypoxic pulmonary vasoconstriction induced by TNF-α. J Appl Physiol 1993; 75:618–625.
86. Pirlo AF, Benumof JL, Trousdale FR. Potentiation of lobar hypoxic pulmonary vasoconstriction by intermittent hypoxia in dogs. Anesthesiol. 55: – .
87. Chen L, Miller FL, Williams JJ, Alexander CM, Domino KB, Marshall C, Marshall BE. Hypoxic pulmonary vasoconstriction is not potentiated by repeated intermittent hypoxia in closed chest dogs. Anesthesiology 1985; 63: – .
88. Thomas HMI, Garrett RC. Strength of hypoxic vasoconstriction determines shunt fraction in dogs with atelectasis. J Appl Physiol 1982; 53:44–51.
89. Lejeune P, Vachiery J-L, De Smet J-M, Leeman M, Brimioulle S, Delcroix M, Mélot C, Naeije R. PEEP inhibits hypoxic pulmonary vasoconstriction in dogs. J Appl Physiol 1991; 70:1867–1873.
90. Wetzel RC, Zacur HA, Sylvester JT. Effect of puberty and estradiol on hypoxic vasomotor response in isolate sheep lungs. J Appl Physiol 1984; 56:1199–1203.
91. McMurtry IF, Hookway BW, Roos SD. Red blood cells but not platelets prolong vascular reactivity of isolated rat lungs. Am J Physiol 1978; 234:H186–191.

92. Hakim TS, Macek AS. Role of erythrocyte deformability in the acute hypoxic pressor response in the pulmonary vasculature. Respir Physiol 1988; 72:95–100.
93. Deem S, Bishop MJ, Alberts MK. Effect of anemia on intrapulmonary shunt during atelectasis in rabbits. J Appl Physiol 1995; 79:1951–1957.
94. Naeije R, Lejeune P, Leeman M, Mélot C, Deloof T. Pulmonary arterial pressure-flow plots in dogs: effects of isoflurane and nitroprusside. J Appl Physiol 1987; 63:969–977.
95. Parsons GB, Leventhal JP, Hansen MM, Goldstein JD. Effect of sodium nitroprusside on hypoxic pulmonary vasoconstriction in the dog. J Appl Physiol 1981; 51: 288–292.
96. Furman WR, Summer WR, Kennedy TP, Sylvester JT. Comparison of the effects of dobutamine, dopamine, and isoproterenol on hypoxic pulmonary vasoconstriction in the pig. Crit Care Med 1982; 10:371–374.
97. Shirai M, Shinco T, Ninomiya I. β-adrenergic mechanisms attenuate hypoxic pulmonary vasoconstriction during systemic hypoxia in cats. Am J Physiol 1994; 266:1777–1785.
98. McMurtry IF, Davidson AB, Reeves JT, Grover RF. Inhibition of hypoxic pulmonary vasoconstriction by calcium antagonists in isolated rat lungs. Circ Res 1976; 38:99–104.
99. Tucker A, McMurtry IF, Grover RF, Reeves JT. Attenuation of hypoxic pulmonary vasoconstriction by verapamil in intact dogs. Proc Soc Exp Biol Med 1976; 151:611–614.
100. Bjertnaes L-J. Hypoxia-induced vasoconstriction in isolated perfused lungs exposed to injectable or inhalation anesthetics. Acta Anaesthesiol Scand 1977; 21: 133–147.
101. Mathers J, Benumof JL, Wahrenbrock EA. General anesthetics and regional hypoxic pulmonary vasoconstriction. Anesthesiology 1977; 46:111–114.
102. Wetzel RC, Martin LD. Pentobarbital attenuates pulmonary vasoconstriction in isolated sheep lungs. Am J Physiol 1989; 257:H898–H903.
103. Marshall C, Lindgren L, Marshall B. Metabolic and respiratory hydrogen ion effects on hypoxic pulmonary vasoconstriction. J Appl Physiol 1984; 57:545–550.
104. Buljubasic N, Rusch NJ, Marijic J, Kampine JP, Bosnjak ZA. Effects of halothane and isoflurane on calcium and potassium channel currents in canine coronary arterial cells. Anesthesiology 1992; 76:990–998.
105. Carlsson AJ, Bindslev L, Hedenstierna G. Hypoxia-induced pulmonary vasoconstriction in the human lung: the effect of isoflurane anesthesia. Anesthesiology 1987; 66:312–316.
106. Domino KB, Borowec L, Alexander CM, Williams JJ, Chen L, Marshall C, Marshall BE. Influence of isoflurane of hypoxic pulmonary vasoconstriction in dogs. Anesthesiology 1986; 64:423–429.
107. Ahmed T, Marchette B. Hypoxia enhances nonspecific bronchial reactivity. Am Rev Respir Dis 1985; 132:839–844.
108. Astin TW, Penman RWB. Airway obstruction due to hypoxemia in patients with chronic lung disease. Am Rev Respir Dis 1967; 95:567–574.
109. Green M, Widdicombe J. The effects of ventilation of dogs with different gas mixtures on airway calibre and lung mechanics. J Physiol 1966; 186:363–381.

110. Nadel J, Widdicombe J. Effect of changes in blood gas tensions and carotid sinus pressure on tracheal volume and total lung volume. J Physiol 1962; 163:13–33.
111. Sterling G. The mechanism of bronchoconstriction due to hypocapnia in man. 1968; 34:277–285.
112. Widdicombe J. Chemoreceptor control of the airways. Respir Physiol 1992; 87: 373–381.
112a. Wetzel RC, Herold CJ, Zehouni EA, Robotham JL. Hypoxic bronchodilation. J Appl Physiol 1992; 73:1202–1206.
113. Traystman RJ, BGK, Menkes HA. Local regulation of collateral ventilation by oxygen and carbon dioxide. J Appl Physiol 1976; 40:819–823.
114. Libby DM, Briscoe WA, King TKC. Relief of hypoxia-related bronchoconstriction by breathing 30 percent oxygen. Am Rev Respir Dis 1981; 123:171–175.
115. Inoue H, Inoue C, Okayama M, Sekizawa K, Hida W, Takishima T. Breathing 30 percent oxygen attenuates bronchial responsiveness to methacholine in asthmatic patients. Eur Respir J 1989; 1:506–512.
116. Wagner PD, Laravuso B, Goldzimmer E, Naumann PF, West JB. Distributions of ventilation-perfusion ratios in dogs with normal and abnormal lungs. J Appl Physiol 1975; 38:1099–1109.
117. Guenard H, Verhas M, Todd-Prokopek A, Solvignon F, Crouzel C, Manigne P, Soussaline F. Effects of oxygen breathing on regional distribution of ventilation and perfusion in hypoxemic patients with chronic lung disease. Am Rev Respir Dis 1982; 125:12–17.
118. Wagner PD, Laravuso RB, Uhl RR, West JB. Continuous distributions of ventilation-perfusion ratios in normal subjects breathing air and 100% O_2. J Clin Invest 1974; 54:54–68.
119. Wagner PD, Gale GE, Moon RE, Torre-Bueno JR, Stolp BW, Saltzman HA. Pulmonary gas exchange in humans exercising at sea level and simulated altitude. J Appl Physiol 1986; 61:267–270.
120. Mélot C, Naeije R, Hallemans R, Lejeune P, Moles P. Hypoxic pulmonary vasoconstriction and pulmonary gas exchange in normal man. Respir Physiol 1987; 68:11–27.
121. Hughes J. Lung gas tensions and active regulation of ventilation/perfusion ratios in health and disease. Br J Dis Chest 1975; 69:153–170.
122. Bergofsky E, Lehr D, Fishman A. The effect of changes in hydrogen ion concentration on the pulmonary circulation. J Clin Invest 1962; 41:1492–1502.
123. Brimioulle S, Vachiery J-L, Lejeune P, Leeman M, Melot C, Naeije R. Acid-base status affects gas exchange in canine oleic acid pulmonary edema. Am J Physiol 1991; 260:H1080–1086.
124. Durand J, Leroy LM, RBB. Effects of hypoxia and hypercapnia on the repartition of pulmonary blood flow in supine subjects. Prog Respir Res 1970; 5:156–165.
125. Horwitz L, Bishop V, Stone H. Effects of hypercapnia on the cardiovascular system on conscious dogs. J Appl Physiol 1968; 25:346–348.
126. Matalon S, Nesarajah M, Krasney J, Farhi L. Effects of acute hypercapnia on the central and peripheral circulation of conscious sheep. J Appl Physiol 1983; 54: 803–808.
127. Tenney S. A phylogenetic perspective of control of the pulmonary circulation. Weir & Reeves, eds. 1989:3–31.

128. Fullerton D, Kirson L, St Cyr J, Albert J, Whitman G. The influence of respiratory acid-base status on adult pulmonary vascular resistance before and after cardiopulmonary bypass. Chest 1993; 103:1091–1095.
129. Kiely D, Cargill R, Lipworth B. Effects of hypercapnia on hemodynamic, inotropic, lusitropic, and electrophysiologic indices in humans. Chest 1996; 109:1215–1221.
130. Wilson L, Levitzky M. Chemoreflex blunting of hypoxic pulmonary vasoconstriction is vagally mediated. J Appl Physiol 1989; 66:782–791.
131. Nishikawa T, Naito H. Clonidine modulation of hemodynamic and catecholamine responses associated with hypoxia or hypercapnia in dogs. Anesthesiol 1996; 84: 672–685.
132. Baile E, Pare P. Response of the bronchial circulation to acute hypoxemia and hypercarbia in the dog. J Appl Physiol 1983; 55:1474–1479.
133. Duke H, Killick E, Marchant J. Changes in pH of the perfusate during hypoxia in isolated perfused cat lungs. J Physiol 1960; 153:413–422.
134. Hebb C, Nimmo-Smith R. Pulmonary vasoconstriction in response to inhalation of CO_2 in the isolated perfused lungs of Macacus rhesus. Q J Exp Physiol 1949; 34:159–163.
135. Yamaguchi K, Takasugi T, Fujita H, Mori M, Oyamada Y, Suzucki K, Miyata A, Suzuki Y. Endothelial modulation of pH-dependent pressor response in isolated perfused rabbit lungs. Am J Physiol 1996; 270:H252–H258.
136. Sheehan D, Farhi L. Local pulmonary blood flow: control and gas exchange. Respir Physiol 1993; 94:91–107.
137. Barer G, Shaw J. Pulmonary vasodilator and vasoconstrictor actions of carbon dioxide. J Physiol 1971; 213:633–645.
138. Emery C, Sloan P, Mohammed F, Barer G. The action of hypercapnia during hypoxia on pulmonary vessels. Bull Eur Physiolpath Respir 1977; 13:763–776.
139. Bergofsky E, Haas F, Porcelli R. Determination of the sensitive vascular sites from which hypoxia and hypercapnia elicit rises in pulmonary artery pressure. Fed Proc 1968; 27:1420–1425.
140. Peters R. Effect of unilateral carbon dioxide breathing on pulmonary blood flow. Am J Physiol 1957; 191:399–403.
141. Barer G, Howard P, McCurrie J. The effect of carbon dioxide and changes in blood pH on pulmonary vascular resistance in cats. Clin Sci 1967; 32:361–376.
142. Hyman A, Woolverton W, Guth P, Ichinose H. The pulmonary vasopressor response to decreases in blood pH in intact dogs. J Clin Invest 1971; 50:1028–1043.
143. Viles P, Shepherd J. Evidence for a dilator action of carbon dioxide on the pulmonary vessels of the cat. Circ Res 1968; 22:325–332.
144. Benumof JL, Wahrenbrock EA. Local effects of anesthetics on regional hypoxic pulmonary vasoconstriction. Anesthesiology 1975; 43:525–532.
145. Hyde R, Lawson W, Forster R. Influence of carbon dioxide on pulmonary vasculature. J Appl Physiol 1964; 19:734–744.
146. Rankin J, McNeill R, Forster R. Influence of increased alveolar CO_2 tension on pulmonary diffusing capacity for CO in man. J Appl Physiol 1960; 15:543–549.
147. Kato M, Staub N. Response of small pulmonary arteries to unilobar hypoxia and hypercapnia. Circ Res 1966; 19:426–440.
148. Malik A, Kidd B. The independent effects of changes in H^+ and CO_2 concentra-

tions on pulmonary hemodynamics of intact dogs. Can J Physiol Pharmacol 1973; 51:139–147.

149. Tian R, Vogel P, Lassen NA, Mulvany F, Andreasen F, Aalkjaer C. Role of extracellular and intracellular acidosis for hypercapnia-induced inhibition of tension of isolated rat cerebral arteries. Circ Res 1995; 76:269–275.
150. Krampetz I, Rhoades R. Intracellular pH: effect on pulmonary arterial smooth muscle. Am J Physiol 1991; 260:L516–L521.
151. Lloyd T. Influences of PO_2 and pH on resting and active tensions of pulmonary arterial strips. J Appl Physiol 1967; 22:1101–1109.
152. Raffestin B, McMurtry I. Effects of intracellular pH on hypoxic vasoconstriction in rat lungs. J Appl Physiol 1987; 63:2524–2531.
153. Parfenova H, Shibata M, Zuckerman S, Leffler CW. CO_2 and cerebral circulation in newborn pigs: cyclic nucleotides and prostanoids in vascular regulation. Am J Physiol 1994; 266:1494–1501.
154. Farrukh I, Gurtner G, Terry P, Tohidi W, Yang J, Adkinson N, Michael J. Effect of pH on pulmonary vascular tone, reactivity, and arachidonate metabolism. J Appl Physiol 1989; 67:445–452.
155. Gurevicius J, Salem M, Metwally A, Silver J, Crystal G. Contribution of nitric oxide to coronary vasodilation during hypercapnic acidosis. Am J Physiol 1995; 268:H39–H47.
156. Horvath I, Sandor N, Ruttner Z, McLaughlin A. Role of nitric oxide in regulating cerebrocortical oxygen consumption and blood flow during hypercapnia. J Cereb Blood Flow Metab 1994; 14:503–509.
157. Fleming I, Hecker M, Busse R. Intracellular alkalinization induced by bradykinin systains activation of the constitutive nitric oxide synthase in endothelial cells. Circ Res 1994; 00:00–00.
158. Brogan T, Hlastala M, Swenson E. Pulmonary nitric oxide synthase inhibition: effects on $\dot{V}_A/\dot{Q}$ matching and response to inspired CO_2 in the dog. FASEB J 1995; 9:A130.
159. Baudouin S, Evans T. Action of carbon dioxide on hypoxic vasoconstriction in the rat lung: evidence against specific endothelium derived relaxing factor-mediated vasodilation. Crit Care Med 1993; 21:740–746.
160. Johnson DH, Chang PC, Hurst TS, Reynolds FB, Lang SA, Mayers I. Changes in $P_{ET}CO_2$ and pulmonary blood flow after bronchial occlusion in dogs. Can J Anesthesiol 1992; 39:184–191.
161. Orchard C, Sanchez de Leon R, Sykes M. The relationship between hypoxic pulmonary vasoconstriction and arterial oxygen tension in the intact dog. J Physiol 1983; 338:61–74.
162. Morrell N, Nijran K, Biggs T, Seed W. Magnitude and time course of acute hypoxic pulmonary vasoconstriction in man. Respir Physiol 1995; 100:271–281.
163. Sheehan D, Klocke R, Farhi L. Pulmonary hypoxic vasoconstriction: How strong? How fast? Respir Physiol 1992; 87:357–372.
164. Benumof J, Mathers J, Wahrenbrock E. Cyclic hypoxic pulmonary vasoconstriction induced by concomitant carbon dioxide changes. J Appl Physiol 1976; 41:466–469.
165. Grant B, Schneider A. Dynamic response of local pulmonary blood flow to alveolar gas tensions: analysis. J Appl Physiol 1983; 54:445–452.

166. Dugard A, Naimark A. Effect of hypoxia on distribution of pulmonary blood flow. J Appl Physiol 1967; 23:663–671.
167. Twining R, Lopez-Majano V, Wagner H, Chernick V, Dutton R. Effect of regional hypercapnia on the distribution of pulmonary blood flow in man. Johns Hopkins Med J 1968; 123:95–103.
168. Borst H, Whittenburger J, Berglund E, McGregor M. Effects of unilateral hypoxia and hypercapnia on pulmonary blood flow distribution in the dog. Am J Physiol 1957; 191:446–452.
169. Grant B, Davies E, Jones H, Hughes J. Local regulation of pulmonary blood flow and ventilation-perfusion ratios in the coatimundi. J Appl Physiol 1976; 40:216–228.
170. Venrath H, Rotthoff R, Valentin H, Bolt W. Bronchospirographische untersuchungen bei durchblutsstorungen im kleinem kreislauf. Beitr Klin Tuberk 1952; 107:291–299.
171. Nisell O. Some aspects of the pulmonary circulation and ventilation. Int Arch Allergy 1952; 3:142–158.
172. Barer G, Astin T, Shaw J, Warren P. Bronchomotor effects of respired gases. Bull Physiopath Respir 1972; 8:459–465.
173. Ingram R. Effects of airway versus arterial CO_2 changes on lung mechanics in dogs. J Appl Physiol 1975; 38:603–607.
174. Samanek M, Aviado D. Interrelationships between pulmonary blood flow and bronchomotor tone: PO_2 and PCO_2. Anesthesiology 1967; 22:719–730.
175. Sly P, Bates J, Kochi T, Okubo S, Milic-Emili J. Frequency dependent effects of hypercapnia on respiratory mechanics of cats. J Appl Physiol 1987; 62:444–450.
176. Delpierre S, Jammes Y, Mei N, Mathiout M, Grimaud. Mise en evidence de l'origine vagale reflexe des effets bronchoconstricteurs du CO_2 chez le chat. J Physiol 1980; 76:889–891.
177. Rodarte J, Hyatt R. Effect of acute exposure to CO_2 on lung mechanics in normal man. Respir Physiol 1973; 17:135–145.
178. Elshout FVD, Herwaarden CV, Folgering H. Effects of hypercapnia and hypocapnia on respiratory resistance in normal and asthmatic subjects. Thorax 1991; 46: 28–32.
179. Monkcom W, Patterson RW. Ventilation-perfusion inequalities resulting from hypocapnic changes in lung mechanics. J Thorac Cardiovasc Surg 1972; 63:577–584.
180. Twort C, Neild J, Cameron I. The effect of verapamil and inspired CO_2 on the bronchoconstriction provoked by hyperventilation in normal humans. Clin Sci 1985; 69:361–364.
181. Severinghaus J, Swenson E, Finley T, Lategola M, Williams J. Unilateral hypoventilation produced in dogs by occluding one pulmonary artery. J Appl Physiol 1961; 16:53–60.
182. Swenson E, Finley T, Guzman S. Unilateral hypoventilation in man during temporary occlusion of one pulmonary artery. J Clin Invest 1961; 40:828–835.
183. Green J, Sheldon M. Ventilator changes associated with changes in pulmonary blood flow in dogs. J Appl Physiol 1983; 54:997–1002.
184. Daly Md, Lambertsen C, Schweitzer A. The effects upon the bronchial musculature of altering the oxygen and carbon dioxide tensions of the blood perfusing the brain. J Physiol 1953; 119:292–341.
185. Daly Md, Schweitzer A. Reflex bronchomotor responses to stimulation of recep-

tors in the regions of the carotid sinus and the arch of the aorta in the dog and cat. J Physiol 1951; 113:442–462.
186. Croxton T, Lande B, Hirschman C. Role of intracellular pH in relaxation of porcine tracheal smooth muscle by respiratory gases. Am J Physiol 1995; 268:L207–L213.
187. Twort C, Cameron I. Effects of PCO_2, pH, and extracellular calcium on contraction or airway smooth muscle from rats. Respir Physiol 1986; 66:259–267.
188. Stephens N, Mitchell R. Effect of respiratory acidosis and activity on airway smooth muscle intracellular pH. J Appl Physiol 1977; 42:408–412.
189. Kikuchi R, Kikuchi K, Hildebrandt J, Yanai M, Sekizawa K, Sasaki H. Dependence of colateral and small airway resistances of CO_2 and volume in dog lobes. Respir Physiol 1995; 100:245–252.
190. Traystman R, Terry P, Menkes H. Carbon dioxide: a major determinant of collateral ventilation. J Appl Physiol 1978; 45:69–74.
191. Delaunois L. Anatomy and physiology of collateral respiratory pathways. Eur Respir J 1992; 2:893–904.
192. Batra G, Traystman R, Rudnick H, Menkes H. Effects of body position and cholinergic blockade on mechanics of collateral ventilation. J Appl Physiol 1981; 50: 358–362.
193. Ingram R, Rinlay G, Bradford J. Relationship of $AaDO_2$ to airway PCO_2 in dog lungs. J Appl Physiol 1976; 40:720–724.
194. Wildeboer-Venema F. Influences of nitrogen, air and alveolar gas upon surface tension of lung surfactant. Respir Physiol 1984; 1–14.
195. Kolbe J, Kleeberger S, Menkes H, Spannhake E. Hypocapnia-induced constriction of the canine peripheral airways exhibit tachyphylaxis. J Appl Physiol 1987; 63: 497–504.
196. Levy S, Simmons D. Redistribution of alveolar ventilation following thromboembolism in the dog. J Appl Physiol 1974; 36:60–68.
197. Robertson HT, Glenny RW. Acute occlusion of the pulmonary artery at a segmental level does not alter regional ventilation in pigs. FASEB J. 1997; 11:A2001.
198. Hlastala M, Swenson E. Airway gas exchange. In: Lenfant C, ed. The Bronchial Circulation. New York: Marcel Dekker, 1992:417–441.
199. Haas F, Bergofsky E. Effect of pulmonary vasoconstriction on balance between ventilation and perfusion. J Appl Physiol 1968; 24:491–497.
200. Turek Z, Kreuzer F. Effects of shifts of the O_2 dissociation curve upon alveolar-arterial O_2 gradients in computer models of the lung with ventilation-perfusion mismatching. Respir Physiol 1981; 45:133–139.
201. Domino KB, Swenson ER, Emery M, Hlastala MP. Ventilation heterogeneity is increased in hypocapnic dogs but not pigs. Respir Physiol 1998; 111:89–100.
202. Tsukimoto K, Arcos J, Schaffartzik W, Wagner P. Effect of common dead space on V_A/Q distribution in the dog. J Appl Physiol 1990; 68:2488–2493.
203. Hlastala M, Berger A. Physiology of Respiration. New York: Oxford University Press, 1996.
204. Prys-Roberts C, Kelman GR, Greenbaum R, Kain ML, Bay J. Hemodynamics and alveolar-arterial PO_2 differences at varying P_aCO_2 in anesthetized man. J Appl Physiol 1968; 25:80–87.

205. Petrini M, Robertson H, Hlastala M. Interaction of series and parallel dead space in the lung. Respir Physiol 1983; 54:121–136.
206. Scheid P, Meyer M, Piiper J. Arterial-expired PCO_2 differences in the dog during acute hypercapnia. J Appl Physiol 1979; 47:1074–1078.
207. Shirer H, Orr J, Loker J. Inspiratory airway CO_2 loading in the pony. J Appl Physiol 1984; 57:1097–1103.
208. Domino KB, Swenson ER, Hlastala MP. Hypocapnia-induced ventilation-perfusion mismatch: a direct CO_2 or pH-mediated effect? Am J Respir Crit Care Med 1995; 152:1534–1539.
209. Frans A, Clerbaux T, Willems E, Kreuzer F. Effect of metabolic acidosis on pulmonary gas exchange of artificially ventilated dogs. J Appl Physiol 1993: 74: 2301–2308.
210. Swenson E, Robertson H, Hlastala M. Effects of carbonic anhydrase inhibition on ventilation-perfusion matching in the dog lung. J Clin Invest 1993; 92:702–709.
211. Swenson E, Graham M, Hlastala M. Acetazolamide slows V_A/Q matching after changes in regional blood flow. J Appl Physiol 1995; 78:1312–1318.
212. Kuriyama T, Latham LP, Horwitz LD, Reeves JT, Wagner WW. Role of collateral ventilation in ventilation-perfusion balance. J Appl Physiol 1984; 56:1500–1506.
213. Hlastala MP, Wranne B, Lenfant CJ. Cyclical variations in FRC and other respiratory variables in resting man. J Appl Physiol 1973; 34:670–676.
214. Lenfant C. Time-dependent variations of pulmonary gas exchange in normal man at rest. J Appl Physiol 1967; 22:675–684.
215. Sackner MA, Dougherty R, Atkins N, Culver D, Poole D, Stout F, Wanner A. Techniques of pulmonary capillary blood flow determination. Bull Physiol Path Respir 1973; 9:1189–1202.
216. Glenny R, Polissar NL, McKinney S, Robertson HT. Temporal heterogeneity of regional pulmonary perfusion is spatially clustered. J Appl Physiol 1995; 79:986–1001.
216a. Wagner PD, Hedenstierna G, Bylin G, Lagerstrand R. Reproducibility of the multiple inert gas elimination technique. J Appl Physiol 1987; 62:1740–1746.
217. Neilson DW, Goerke J, Clements JA. Alveolar subphase pH in the lungs of anesthetized rabbits. Proc Natl Acad Sci USA 1981; 78:7119–7123.
218. Robinson N, Kyle H, Webber S, Widdicombe JG. Electrolyte and other chemical concentrations in tracheal airway surface liquid and mucus. J Appl Physiol 1989; 66:2129–2135.
219. Swenson ER, Brogan TV, Hedges RG, Deem S. Acetazolamide slows hypoxic pulmonary vasoconstriction. Am J Respir Crit Care Med 1998 (in press).
220. Grant BJB. Effect of local pulmonary blood flow control on gas exchange: theory. J Appl Physiol 1982; 53:1100–1109.

18

Ventilation–Perfusion Heterogeneity
Insights from Comparative Physiology

SUSAN R. HOPKINS and FRANK L. POWELL

University of California, San Diego
La Jolla, California

I. Introduction

The lungs of all vertebrates evolved, in part, to solve the common problem of providing adequate oxygen to fuel the metabolic activities that are necessary for survival and propagation of a species. However, the range of O_2 demands that vertebrate lungs must meet is huge and varies within a single animal up to 1000-fold during different states such as hibernation, sleep, wakefulness, and exercise (1). Oxygen demands also vary among animals of different size, and also depending on their degree of body temperature regulation and mode of locomotion. An animal's ecological niche also creates large variations in O_2 *demand* by determining its energy budget. Finally, there are large variations in O_2 *supply* in different ecological niches, for example, at different altitudes.

Evolutionary solutions to different versions of the O_2 supply and demand problem have produced several different types of vertebrate lungs. The complexity of vertebrate lungs ranges from simple sacklike lungs in some amphibians and reptiles, to highly subdivided homogeneous branching structures such as the mammalian alveolar lung and heterogeneous respiratory systems such as the parabronchial lung and air sac system in birds (Figure 1). Therefore, comparative studies may offer valuable insights about the importance of lung complexity

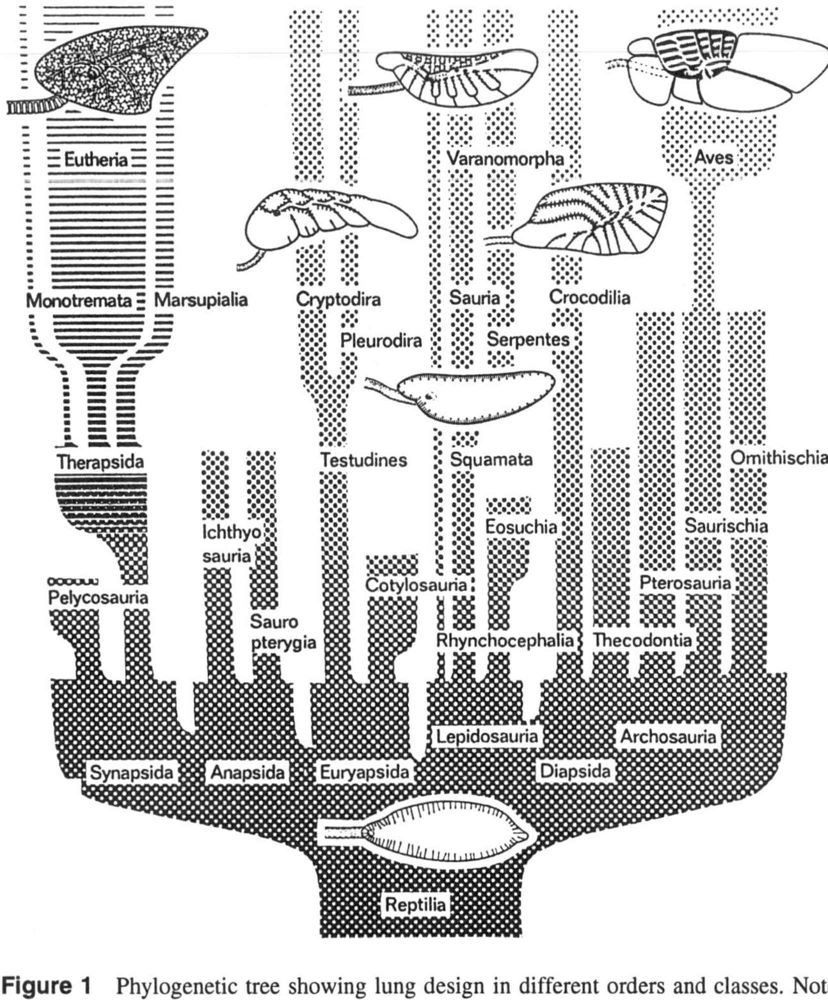

Figure 1 Phylogenetic tree showing lung design in different orders and classes. Note the structure of the homogeneously partitioned lung, which is characteristic of mammals, compared to the heterogeneous air sac parabronchial lung of the birds. The reptile lungs (although less complex) have features of both. (From Ref. 77.)

for respiratory function. For example, as lungs evolved to meet higher O_2 demands, diffusing capacity was increased by subdividing the lung into smaller gas exchange units. One could hypothesize that the "benefit" of increased diffusing capacity is greater than the potential "cost" of increased ventilation-perfusion ($\dot{V}/\dot{Q}$) heterogeneity between gas exchange units. Physiological measurements in animals with different lung designs can be used to test this hypothesis.

However, one must exercise caution in attributing "adaptive significance" to a physiological characteristic, such as lung complexity, when using a comparative approach. First, lungs have also evolved for many nonrespiratory functions, particularly in nonmammalian species. For example, aquatic reptiles must adjust lung volume to achieve neutral buoyancy during surfacing or diving when avoiding predators or pursuing prey (2). Reptilian lungs and avian air sacs serve social functions by inflating during sexual displays and acting as resonators for mating calls (3) (varanid lizards can inflate their apparent body size by 40% or more when threatened by a natural enemy [2]). Second, evolution does not operate on a "clean slate" and lung design in modern species reflects their ancestry. Many lung designs might satisfy the respiratory needs of relatively primitive organisms, which may not require the exquisite balance between O_2 supply and demand, for example, that a modern homeotherm requires. Therefore, a variety of lung structures might have satisfied the respiratory needs of primitive vertebrates, and the diversity of lung structure and complexity in modern animals may reflect aspects of evolution that have nothing to do with respiration *per se*.

In summarizing, comparative physiology has the potential to teach several lessons about general properties of complexity in the respiratory system, but it may or may not explain the reasons for differences in complexity and lung design in different species.

II. Lesson One: Although Lung Structure Differs Between Species, Spatial Ventilation–Perfusion Heterogeneity Is Similar

Increased diffusing capacity for oxygen is essential to increase metabolic rate. Mammals and birds have high metabolic rates compared to reptiles, and complex respiratory systems with very different lung structures have evolved to accommodate the need for oxygen to fuel their metabolic machinery. The mammalian lung is structurally the most uniform compared that in other vertebrates. In mammals, the function of ventilation and gas exchange is shared by the respiratory bronchioles, alveolar ducts, and alveoli. Less than 20% of the total lung volume (i.e., trachea, bronchi, bronchioles) is dedicated solely to ventilation. Consequently, the vast majority of the lung volume is composed of relatively homogeneous tissues (respiratory bronchioles, alveolar ducts, and alveolar sacs), which have the dual function of ventilation and gas exchange.

On the other hand, the bird respiratory system has complete separation of the function of ventilation and gas exchange between the air sacs and the lung (parabronchi), respectively. In the bird, nine air sacs act as bellows to ventilate the lungs and occupy approximately 90% of the total respiratory system volume. The remaining 10% is the lung. The bird lung is a small constant volume structure, consisting of open-ended parabronchi arranged in parallel and connected at both ends to secondary bronchi that act as conducting airways. The parabronchi are perfused along their entire length by pulmonary mixed venous blood, and ventilation and perfusion can be thought of as occurring at right angles to one another, so gas exchange in a bird lung is described by a cross-current model (4). The theoretical efficiency of the cross-current lung is greater than that of the alveolar lung, and, in hypoxia, the measured arterial Po_2 can exceed the expired Po_2.

It is perhaps easier to understand the large morphometric differences between two such highly evolved and metabolically active groups such as birds and mammals when the structural diversity of the reptiles is considered. Reptiles, from which both birds and mammals are derived, have the greatest structural variability in their lungs of any vertebrate class (5). As discussed previously, the need to satisfy constraints other than that of gas exchange, such as the need to vocalize or to fly away from predators, may result in selection for a different structure than would be expected from gas exchange constraints alone.

Reptiles form an interesting intermediate between birds and mammals in terms of lung structure. Reptilian lung types can be divided into single chambered (unicameral), few chambered (paucicameral), and the more complex many chambered (multicameral lung) (6). Reptiles typically have much lower metabolic rates and can be considered energy conservers compared to comparably sized birds and mammals. Even so, within reptile species, there is considerable variability in the demands for oxygen, and lung structure has evolved accordingly. For example, the varanid lizards are known for their relatively high metabolic scopes (7,8) and active behavior patterns in the wild. Larger animals may travel several kilometers in a day in search of prey. These reptiles have relatively complex multicameral lungs with a high respiratory surface area compared to other species (9). By contrast, the tegu lizard has a respiratory surface area that is approximately 50% less. In the tegu, the lung is essentially a large air sac with a tissue-free central lumen and a relatively simple parenchymal layer formed into honeycomb-like falveoli (9).

Figure 1 summarizes these structural differences with a schematic diagram of the lungs of mammals, birds, and representatives from four reptilian families: turtles, varanid lizards, crocodilians, and tegu lizard. In these animals, the gross architecture of the lung can be partitioned into air-containing spaces, which function primarily for conduction of gas, and lung parenchyma, across which gas exchange occurs. Figure 2 shows how the amount of total lung volume devoted to conduction of air and gas exchange varies substantially in reptiles between the two extremes defined by birds and mammals. However, even though the amount of partitioning between conduction/ventilation and gas exchange is similar between, for example, the tegu and the birds on a gross basis, there are marked differences on a microscopic basis in the complexity of the

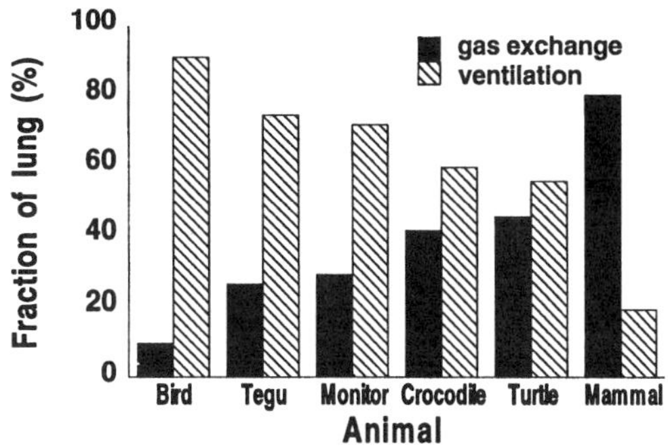

Figure 2 Fraction of the lung devoted to ventilation and gas exchange in different vertebrates. (Data from Ref. 78.)

parenchymal structure. The mass specific respiratory surface area across which gas exchange occurs is an order of magnitude higher in the birds and mammals than in the reptiles.

This diversity of lung complexity raises questions about how ventilation ($\dot{V}$) and perfusion ($\dot{Q}$) are distributed in lungs of different design. The multiple inert gas elimination technique (MIGET) can be used to measure $\dot{V}/\dot{Q}$ distributions (10,11). The physiological consequences of $\dot{V}/\dot{Q}$ heterogeneity can also be studied with MIGET. Comparing inert gas and Po_2 measurements allows one to distinguish among spatial $\dot{V}/\dot{Q}$ heterogeneity, intrapulmonary shunting, and diffusion limitation as causes of decreased O_2 transfer across the lung in a variety of experimental situations (10,11). Despite marked variations in lung structure, both with respect to gross and microscopic structure, the similarities in spatial $\dot{V}/\dot{Q}$ heterogeneity are more striking than the differences. As can be seen in Figure 3, the shape of the $\dot{V}/\dot{Q}$ distribution recovered from mammals, birds, and a variety of reptiles are smooth and unimodal, although the mean $\dot{V}/\dot{Q}$ ratio varies. Additionally, the degree of heterogeneity present in these different lung structures is remarkably similar across species, as indicated by the dispersion of the distribution about the mean (logSD$\dot{Q}$ in the case of blood flow and logSD$\dot{V}$ in the case of ventilation).

These distributions can be contrasted with one obtained from a patient with chronic obstructive pulmonary disease (COPD) (Figure 4). Here, this particular distribution is bimodal with a substantial portion of the pulmonary blood flow to areas of low $\dot{V}/\dot{Q}$ ratio. The log SD$\dot{Q}$ is 2.0, approximately double that obtained from the tegu, and almost an order of magnitude greater than resting distributions obtained from the mammals, reflecting the marked degree of $\dot{V}/\dot{Q}$ heterogeneity present. Thus, the differences in spatial ventilation-perfusion matching are less across species than between healthy and diseased lungs from the same species.

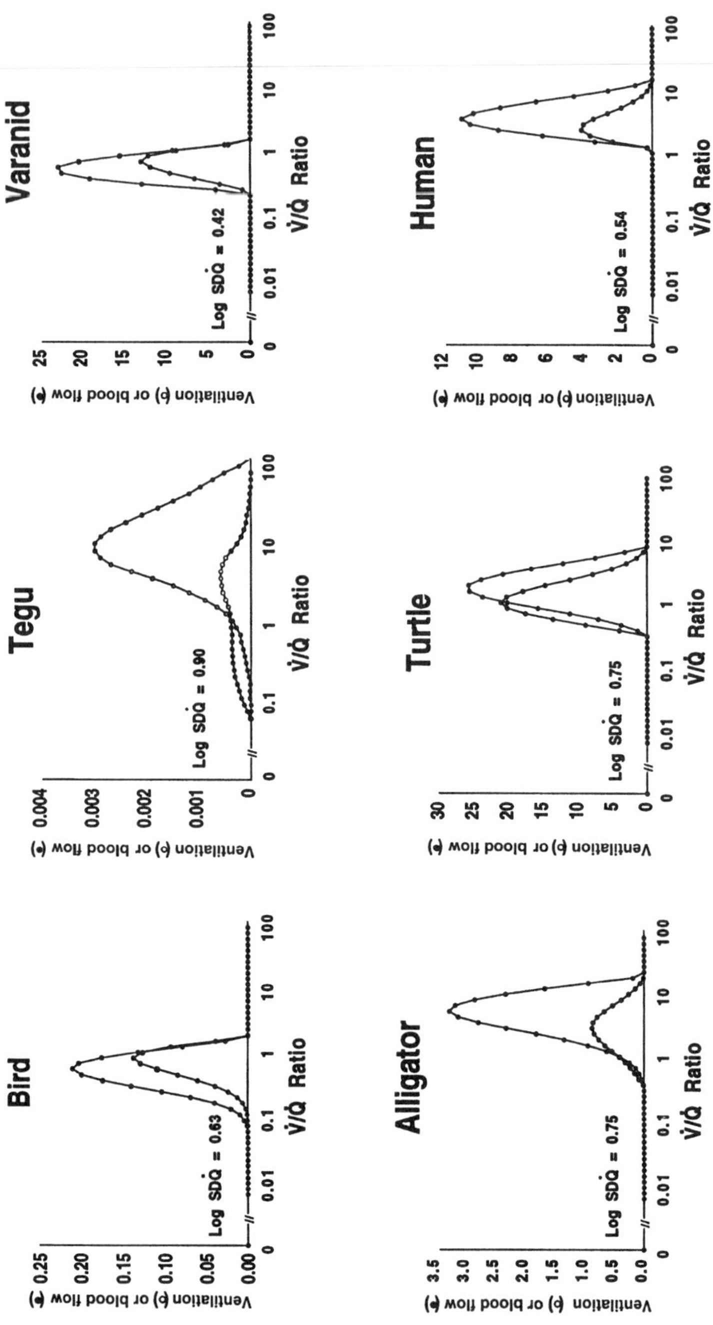

Figure 3 Ventilation–perfusion distributions in resting vertebrates obtained using the multiple inert gas elimination technique. For clarity, intrapulmonary shunting and dead space are not shown. (Data from Refs. 13,17,19,39,79,80.)

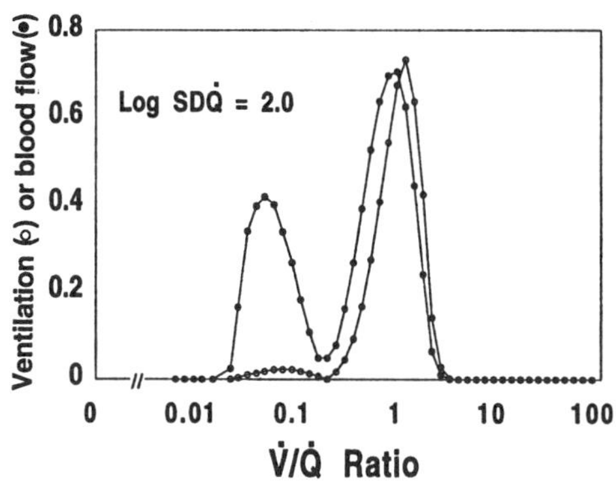

Figure 4 Ventilation-perfusion distribution from a patient with chronic obstructive pulmonary disease. Note the bimodal distribution with perfusion of areas of low $\dot{V}/\dot{Q}$ ratio. (Data supplied by Peter Wagner.)

III. Comparative Effects of $\dot{V}/\dot{Q}$ Heterogeneity on O_2 Exchange at Rest

A. Mammals

In the ideal mammalian lung at rest, the alveolar–end capillary Po_2 difference is predicted to be zero. In reality, the small amount of $\dot{V}/\dot{Q}$ heterogeneity that is present results in a Po_2 difference that is less than 10 torr. Intrapulmonary shunting in most mammalian species is so small that often it cannot be measured (12–15). Extrapulmonary shunts, such as from the bronchial circulation and thebesian veins are less than 1% of the total cardiac output and lower the arterial Po_2 only slightly from end capillary.

B. Reptiles

Reptiles, may have considerably greater differences between lung and left atrial Po_2. Although this is somewhat analogous to the A-aDO_2 in humans, we use the term lung-left atrial Po_2 difference because alveoli are not found in reptilian lungs, and cardiac shunting in all reptiles considerably lowers arterial Po_2. By using left atrial blood gases, the problem of cardiac shunts is avoided because the shunts occur in the ventricle. However, cardiac shunts can completely mask the effects of $\dot{V}/\dot{Q}$ heterogeneity on Po_2 exchange in reptiles, so it is difficult to interpret the physiological significance of such heterogeneity unless the cardiac shunt state is also known. This problem has been studied extensively in reptiles, but it is still not clear whether the active physiological control of cardiac shunts in reptiles is adaptive for O_2 transport (16). The similarity of $\dot{V}/\dot{Q}$ heterogeneity in different classes (mammals and reptiles) with different mechanisms dominating control of P_{O_2} (pulmonary and cardiac, respectively) suggests that O_2 exchange may not be the most important factor in the evolution of complexity in vertebrate lungs.

In varanids, the 14–28 torr lung-left atrial P_{O_2} difference is explained almost completely by $\dot{V}/\dot{Q}$ heterogeneity and intrapulmonary shunting (17). In these animals, the intrapulmonary shunt is more than 5% of total pulmonary blood flow (17). In these active animals, there is no evidence for resting pulmonary diffusion limitation for oxygen. Extrapulmonary right to left cardiac shunts (see below) further lower arterial P_{O_2} below left atrial P_{O_2} and are approximately 9% of cardiac output (18).

The turtle has a larger difference between lung gas and left atrial blood P_{O_2}, which varies with pulmonary blood flow (and ventilatory state). This difference is about 33 torr in resting anaesthetized animals (19). Approximately half is due to $\dot{V}/\dot{Q}$ heterogeneity and a 17% intrapulmonary shunt. However, it is possible that these animals may have some degree of resting diffusion limitation (19). A rigorous determination of diffusion limitation requires a definitive modeling of the turtle O_2 dissociation curve. The turtle has multiple hemoglobins (20), with the result being that it is difficult to model the curve within the inert gas subroutine. Another possible cause of hypoxemia in turtles is extrapulmonary shunt, but the placement of catheters in the left atrium excludes cardiac shunts in this case.

C. Birds

Whereas the ideal alveolar-end capillary P_{O_2} difference is predicted to be zero in mammals and reptiles, it is predicted to be negative in the cross-current lung of the bird (approximately −10 torr) (21). In reality, the expired-arterial difference is about +15 torr, or about 25 torr greater than the ideal expired-arterial P_{O_2} is about 25 torr (21). (We refer to "expired gas" in the bird and avoid using the term alveolar because birds have no alveoli). More than half of this discrepancy can be accounted for by $\dot{V}/\dot{Q}$ heterogeneity measured with MIGET (21). Usually, a difference between the actual Pa_{O_2} and the value predicted for measured $\dot{V}/\dot{Q}$ heterogeneity is interpreted as a diffusion impairment for O_2 (22). However, a more likely factor explaining less than ideal Pa_{O_2} values in anesthetized, artificially ventilated birds is extrapulmonary shunting. This can average 5% of cardiac output in birds under these conditions, which is much more than in mammals and is apparently explained by vertebral-pulmonary venous circulatory connections (23). Physiological estimates of D_{LO_2} corrected for $\dot{V}/\dot{Q}$ heterogeneity agree well with morphometric estimates, and diffusion equilibrium is predicted for such high diffusing capacities (4,24). Therefore, resting diffusion limitations are unlikely.

The advantage of cross-current gas exchange in a bird lung becomes apparent in hypoxia, when birds show a negative expired-arterial Po_2 (21). Although $\dot{V}/\dot{Q}$ heterogeneity is not changed by hypoxia, it increases expired-arterial Po_2 less because gas exchange takes place on the steep part of the O_2-blood dissociation curve (21). The extrapulmonary shunt described above is not seen in hypoxia. Half of the 4 torr difference between measured and ideal Pao_2 in hypoxic resting birds is explained by $\dot{V}/\dot{Q}$ heterogeneity and the other half is consistent with a small diffusion limitation from estimated DLO_2 (21).

In summarizing, similar degrees of $\dot{V}/\dot{Q}$ heterogeneity in resting normoxic birds and mammals reduce the theoretical differences in Pao_2 between these classes. $\dot{V}/\dot{Q}$ heterogeneity is also similar in reptiles but cardiac shunts are the primary determinant of Pao_2 in this class.

IV. Lesson Two: Mammals at Rest Define the Optimal Conditions for Minimizing $\dot{V}/\dot{Q}$ Heterogeneity in Ventilated Pool Lungs of Mammals and Reptiles

Most models of gas exchange assume that ventilation and blood flow are steady state (25). In reality, ventilation and blood flow are cyclic, even in birds and mammals that breathe continuously. Ectotherms add extra complexity to this analysis because their breathing patterns are not cyclic, but rather intermittent, in which one or more breaths may be separated by long periods of apnea. However, ectotherms, under some conditions, such as exercise, which elevates metabolic rate to levels observed in resting mammals (26), may adopt a more "mammalian" respiratory pattern and breathe continuously. Conversely, an intermittent breathing pattern may emerge in mammals under conditions of reduced metabolic rate, such as occurs during hibernation. Consequently, in addition to the problem of *spatial* matching of ventilation and perfusion, these animals have the challenge of *temporal* matching of ventilation to perfusion.

Temporal matching of ventilation and perfusion is well studied in the turtle. Turtles exhibit an intermittent breathing pattern in which brief ventilatory periods are interspersed with periods of apnea of varying duration. This breathing pattern is in keeping with the behavior pattern of some turtles, in which the animal may spend several hours at a time submerged, with only brief forays to the surface to breathe air. When the animal is not ventilating, there is a reduction in heart rate and increased pulmonary vascular resistance with a concomitant reduction in pulmonary blood flow. In the turtles, approximately 50% of the variable pulmonary resistance occurs proximal to the lung parenchyma and an additional site is at the *bulbus cordis*, a muscular structure at the base of the pulmonary artery. During the brief periods of ventilation, the converse happens: heart rate is increased, pulmonary vascular resistance decreases, and pulmonary blood flow may increase by five to seven times over the apneic conditions.

These changes are likely the result of adrenergic vasodilation (27–29) because stimulation of vagal afferents results in a twofold increase in pulmonary blood flow in turtles, which is attenuated following infusion of bretylium (27). This temporal matching of ventilation and perfusion is termed cardiorespiratory synchrony and acts to ensure that adequate blood flow is delivered to the lungs when ventilation occurs.

Interestingly, cardiorespiratory synchrony in the turtle may act to improve spatial matching of ventilation and perfusion. In anesthetized ventilated turtles, when pulmonary blood flow is decreased and ventilation is maintained (by applying a vascular occluder to the pulmonary artery) $\dot{V}/\dot{Q}$ heterogeneity increases such that the log$SD\dot{Q}$ is increased to about 0.95 (19). For comparison, this is greater than the degree of $\dot{V}/\dot{Q}$ heterogeneity usually seen in humans with exercise but is less than typically observed with human lung disease such as COPD. Intrapulmonary shunting may also be slightly decreased under these conditions, but it is still greater than 10% of total pulmonary blood flow. The effect of the increasing $\dot{V}/\dot{Q}$ heterogeneity is a decrease in the P_{O_2} of the blood returning from the lung of about 25 torr, which is approximately a one-to-one decrease, that is, a 1% increase in log$SD\dot{Q}$ results in a 1% decrease in P_{O_2}.

When pulmonary blood flow is increased in these animals using intracardiac infusion of epinephrine, under the same experimental set-up (19), $\dot{V}/\dot{Q}$ matching is improved such that the log$SD\dot{Q}$ is reduced to about 0.55, a value that is greater than is generally seen in humans at rest, anesthetized dogs, or monitor lizards but less than is reported for the tegu lizard. The effect of this reduction in log$SD\dot{Q}$ and decreasing $\dot{V}/\dot{Q}$ heterogeneity is an increase in P_{O_2} of about 5 torr of the blood returning from the lung. The magnitude of the increase in P_{O_2} is small relative to the change in log$SD\dot{Q}$, because the P_{O_2} is already high. In an animal that did not have such an overall high $\dot{V}_A/\dot{Q}$ ratio, the effect of this reduction in log$SD\dot{Q}$ on the P_{O_2} would be greater.

In normal awake animals during an apneic episode, it is possible that the effects of low pulmonary blood flow may be less than are seen with the above experimental preparation. It is unlikely that, in normal healthy animals, ventilation would be elevated while pulmonary blood flow remained low. However, when pulmonary blood flow is increased (e.g., during a ventilatory episode in these animals) $\dot{V}/\dot{Q}$ matching is likely improved as described, and pulmonary gas exchange is optimized. The mechanisms of decreased heterogeneity with increased flow are unknown, but they may be a general property of patterns of vascular branching in vertebrate lungs. The comparative approach could provide an interesting test of this hypothesis by examining the distribution of blood flow at different rates in amphibian lungs. This would also test the generality of this lesson for all ventilated pool lungs. Also, comparative studies of the effect of flow rate on the distribution of blood flow in the parabronchial lungs of birds and alveolar lungs of mammals could provide a strong test of this hypothesis.

V. Lesson Three: Alterations in Metabolic Rate Increase the Complexity of Pulmonary Gas Exchange, Independent of Lung Structure

A. Effect of Low Metabolic Rates: Gas Phase Diffusion Limitation

Under conditions such as hibernation (or torpor) in mammals or rest in reptiles, many animals can sustain very low metabolic rates. A consequence of low requirements for oxygen is a reduction of respiratory rate and bulk convective flow of oxygen. For example, the big brown bat (*Eptesicus fucus*) couples its ventilation to metabolic rate. Above 30°C, this animal breathes continuously (30), but, below this body temperature, intermittent apneas become more pronounced. At temperatures below 20°C, the respiratory rate is two orders of magnitude lower than at 30°C and approaches that seen in some resting reptiles (17). In these animals, blood and lung O_2 stores can account for only 21% of the metabolic requirements; much of the balance is likely supplied by diffusion and nonventilatory bulk convection down the airways past an open glottis (31). Bulk convection occurs because the high capacitance of the blood and tissues for Co_2 and the respiratory quotient CO_2 do not completely replace the volume of O_2 lost from the lungs. Because mechanical forces act on the lung to maintain volume, there is a passive influx of ambient air to replace oxygen lost from metabolism. Also, the heart may serve an important respiratory function under these circumstances, and cardiogenic mixing may provide acceleration of intrapulmonary gas mixing (31,32).

A consequence of lowered bulk convection of air into the lung is the increased potential for incomplete intraregional gas mixing in the lung (33). When gas mixing is incomplete, significant axial gradients for resident gases occur, reducing the efficiency of gas exchange. Diffusion-dependent heterogeneity or gas-phase diffusion limitation can be defined as a molecular-weight–dependent impairment of gas-phase diffusion. Although this must occur in the torpid bat, the problem has not been studied in hibernating or torpid mammals. However, the intermittent breathing described for reptiles above could also cause increased gas-phase diffusion limitation. These animals may be especially vulnerable to the development of gas-phase diffusion limitation because the lung structure of many reptiles is characterized by larger subunits and therefore larger diffusional distances. Therefore, reptiles offer a good model to study this problem, which is more likely to affect gases of high-molecular-weight and can be detected from the inert gas analysis.

Increased gas-phase diffusion limitation for inert gases is suggested by high residual sum of squares (RSS), which occurs as a result of nonrandom error. Gas-phase diffusion limitation affects the retention and excretion of each gas to a different extent depending on the solubility of the gas and its molecular weight (34). The mean RSS, the difference between the measured retention and the predicted retention for the $\dot{V}/\dot{Q}$ distribution, is expected to be about 5 for six gases given random experimental error (35). The error (ε) between the measured retention and prediction retention for enflurane, the heaviest gas, and cyclopropane, the lightest gas, is expected to increase in the presence of gas-phase diffusion limitation because the retention of the heaviest gas is increased in contrast to gases of low-molecular-weight (36). In the absence of increased gas-phase diffusion limitation, the errors, although small, may be nonzero, because of experimental error and numerical analyses. Thus, it is not enough to merely show that ε enflurane–ε cyclopropane exceeds zero to demonstrate increased gas-phase diffusion limitation. Recovered errors must be compared with a similar data set in which the data do fit the model or with a Monte-Carlo simulation set in which small random errors (simulating experimental error) are introduced to a theoretical data set for a representative $\dot{V}/\dot{Q}$ distribution (37).

Increased gas-phase diffusion limitation can be expected to distort the inert gas $\dot{V}/\dot{Q}$ distributions such that log SD$\dot{Q}$ is reduced in the main mode with increases in perfusion to areas of low and high $\dot{V}/\dot{Q}$ (34,38). Oxygen and carbon dioxide, which have molecular weights an order of magnitude smaller than enflurane, are affected much less by gas-phase diffusion limitation, and the contribution of gas-phase diffusion limitation to the overall resistance to respiratory gas transport has not been established (33).

Increased gas-phase diffusion limitation has been observed in awake, spontaneously breathing, resting varanid lizards (17), but not in the same animals during treadmill exercise. It also has been reported in anesthetized alligators that were ventilated at relatively low rates (39). Increased gas-phase diffusion limitation has not been observed in the anesthetized ventilated tegu or in anesthetized turtles ventilated at a high rate corresponding to the level of ventilation observed during a ventilatory episode (19). In the turtle, it is likely that the high ventilation that was used in these animals improved convective gas mixing within the lung and prevented incomplete intrapulmonary gas mixing. Also, the turtle may have additional mechanisms that prevent limitations of gas exchange resulting from incomplete gas mixing during periods of apnea. Spragg et al., (40) found that movement of limbs and contraction of lung smooth muscle within the lung increased displacement of gas from the posterior to the anterior parts of the lung and facilitated gas mixing.

In summary, two factors may predispose the lung to the development of increased gas-phase diffusion limitations. First, lung with large diffusional distances may accentuate the problem. Second, low bulk convective flow associated with low respiratory rates such as occurs in resting spontaneously breathing reptiles and torpid bats may be important. This later effect is another manifestation of the second lesson, that is, $\dot{V}$ and $\dot{Q}$ levels in resting mammals define the optimum conditions for ventilated pool lungs of reptiles and mammals.

B. Effect of Increasing Metabolic Rate: $\dot{V}/\dot{Q}$ Heterogeneity and Blood–Gas Diffusion Disequilibrium

Although better $\dot{V}/\dot{Q}$ matching could be advantageous for gas exchange during exercise, this is not observed in nature. Similar to the situation described above for hypometabolism, heterogeneity increases with exercise if $\dot{V}/\dot{Q}$ heterogeneity does change. In some athletic animals, such as thoroughbred race horses, heterogeneity does not markedly increase, but diffusion limitation may occur in maximal exercise (14). Therefore, animals may vary in their susceptibility to physiological mechanisms that increase heterogeneity, and comparative studies can help elucidate these mechanisms.

1. Humans

During very light levels of exertion, the alveolar-arterial difference for oxygen ($AaDo_2$) may decrease with exercise (41), possibly from redistribution of pulmonary blood flow, resulting in improved matching of ventilation and perfusion (13). During heavy and maximal exercise, the $AaDo_2$ increases (42–46) and may reach more than 40 torr in highly aerobic human athletes (45). The magnitude of the gas exchange impairment is sufficient that, in some individuals, a decrease in Pao_2 occurs, to the extent that desaturation of hemoglobin may result (43,45,47). Many studies (12,13,48–50) have shown that $\dot{V}/\dot{Q}$ heterogeneity increases with increasing exercise intensity and, in very highly aerobic subjects, $\dot{V}/\dot{Q}$ is responsible for more than 60% of the $AaDo_2$ at exercise intensities approaching $\dot{V}O_2$ max (13). At sea level, increasing $\dot{V}/\dot{Q}$ heterogeneity results in a broadening of the normally narrow $\dot{V}/\dot{Q}$ distribution without the development of areas of very low $\dot{V}/\dot{Q}$ ratios. Increased $\dot{V}/\dot{Q}$ heterogeneity with exercise is accentuated by hypoxia (49,51) and reduced by breathing 100% oxygen (12). The abnormality persists well into recovery from heavy exercise, after ventilation and cardiac output have returned to normal (50).

2. Other Gas Exchange Impairments with Exercise

In addition to $\dot{V}/\dot{Q}$ heterogeneity, pulmonary diffusion limitation has also been implicated in the increased $AaDo_2$ with exercise in humans (13,43,49). Cardiac output in human athletes may reach over 40 $L \cdot min^{-1}$ (52). Therefore, limited contact time in the pulmonary capillary bed is a potentially important determinant of pulmonary diffusion limitation. Compounding the effect of high cardiac output and a short pulmonary capillary transit time, low mixed venous Po_2 and a rightward shifted oxygen-hemoglobin equilibrium curve may contribute to the failure of end-capillary diffusion equilibrium (53). Although pulmonary diffusion limitation is thought to result from rapid pulmonary transit (54), the possibility of interstitial edema increasing the diffusional distance from the alveolus to the capillary blood cannot be eliminated. The decrease in CO diffusion capacity after exercise may reflect increased $\dot{V}/\dot{Q}$ heterogeneity as well as diffusion limitation (55).

3. Horses

Horses and humans have similar lung structure, but which differ in the pulmonary gas exchange response to exercise. In the resting horse, ventilation is very closely matched to perfusion and the logSD$\dot{Q}$ is usually less than 0.3, which is at the lower limit of the normal range for humans (14,37). Horses have significant pulmonary limitations to maximal exercise and develop arterial hypoxemia, which is associated with both a widened $AaDO_2$ and an increase in arterial PCO_2; thus, there is both a deterioration of pulmonary gas exchange and a lack of compensatory hyperventilation. During maximal exercise, approximately 70% of the $AaDO_2$ can be attributed to pulmonary diffusion limitation (14), which is much greater than is seen in humans. There is little deterioration in $\dot{V}/\dot{Q}$ relationships between rest to maximal levels of exercise in the horse and the logSD$\dot{Q}$ increases to about 0.4 with exercise, the level that is approximately the same as resting humans. This small degree of heterogeneity is sufficient to account for the balance of the increased $AaDO_2$ with maximal exercise in the horse. During prolonged submaximal exercise, the findings are similar (37). There is no progressive deterioration in pulmonary gas exchange. The logSD$\dot{Q}$ increases from rest to exercise, roughly doubling by the first 5 minutes of exercise, but it does not deteriorate further with exercise extending to 30–40 minutes' duration. The recovered distributions are unimodal and there are no areas of low $\dot{V}/\dot{Q}$ ratio. In contrast to exercise of higher intensity, there is no evidence of pulmonary diffusion limitation.

4. Varanid Lizards

To date, the varanid lizards are the only reptiles that have been studied during exercise with MIGET. These animals have one of the highest aerobic scopes (7,8), supported by one of the most mammalian-like cardiopulmonary systems. The lung surface area for gas exchange is threefold greater than for other lizards (56). However, the mass-specific gas exchanging surface area is less than 25% of that of a mammal. In addition, the oxygen diffusion capacity of the tissue barrier is an order of magnitude smaller than that of mammals. Although the lungs of these lizards are structurally different than mammalian lungs, the gas exchange response to exercise is strikingly similar to that in humans. In these animals during heavy exercise, gas exchange limitations can occur, as evidenced by lung-arterial PO_2 differences of more than 30 torr during maximal exercise.

Like those from exercising mammals, the recovered $\dot{V}/\dot{Q}$ distributions are smooth and unimodal and the logSD$\dot{Q}$ increases during heavy exercise to 0.78, only slightly greater than reported for highly trained humans (13).

The major difference between the $\dot{V}/\dot{Q}$ distributions recovered from these exercising lizards and mammals was a modest intrapulmonary shunt of less than 2% during exercise. The varanid lizard has evidence for pulmonary diffusion limitation of oxygen, which accounts for about 10 torr of the lung-arterial P_{O_2} difference, which is also similar to that reported in normal humans (44).

5. *Birds*

Exercising birds have not been studied with the inert gas technique. However, it has been used on resting birds and can be considered with studies of O_2 exchange in exercising birds to estimate the importance of heterogeneity versus diffusion limitation.

Oxygen exchange has been studied in ducks resting and running on a treadmill in hypoxia (57) and the O_2 diffusing capacity of the lung has been calculated to increase with exercise. Recruitment of diffusing capacity with elevated cardiac output and reduced $\dot{V}/\dot{Q}$ heterogeneity are the two most likely physiological mechanisms for the increased D_{LO_2}. Diffusing capacity recruitment is the most likely explanation as it is in anesthetized hypoxic ducks, when $\dot{V}O_2$ is increased by 2,4-dinitrophenol (24) and the diffusing capacity for oxygen is corrected for $\dot{V}/\dot{Q}$ heterogeneity. $\dot{V}/\dot{Q}$ heterogeneity was estimated from CO_2 exchange and did not change with increasing $\dot{V}O_2$. There is also good agreement between D_{LO_2} estimates in the two studies, indicating the effects of heterogeneity are minor.

Unfortunately, these data do not address normoxic exercise. Changes in D_{LO_2} with 2,4-dinitrophenol hypermetabolism in normoxic ducks (58) are similar increases to those reported for hypoxic ducks by Hempleman and Powell (24,59). The normoxic study did not correct for heterogeneity and the increased D_{LO_2} could have been only apparent from decreased heterogeneity. However, it seems unlikely that the same increase in D_{LO_2} would increase in normoxia and hypoxia by an apparent increase in one case and a true increase in the other.

The increased D_{LO_2} observed by Hempleman and Powell (24) is most closely correlated with increased cardiac output. It is reasonable to assume that this also explains the other increases reported, but evidence for recruitment of pulmonary capillary volume and surface area with increased cardiac output in birds is not as convincing as it is for mammals. The avian lung is relatively rigid and pulmonary vascular resistance measurements indicate limited capillary distention and recruitment (60). However, evidence of potential recruitment (i.e., folds) are observed in avian pulmonary capillaries (61) and recruitment seems to be a general feature of vertebrate gas exchange organs, also occurring in fish gills (62).

C. Possible Causes of Increased $\dot{V}/\dot{Q}$ Heterogeneity with Exercise

$\dot{V}/\dot{Q}$ heterogeneity during exercise contributes substantially to the gas exchange impairment observed with heavy or maximal exercise, but the cause of $\dot{V}/\dot{Q}$ heterogeneity is unknown. Possible mechanisms include heterogeneity of hypoxic pulmonary vasoconstriction (63), reduction of gas mixing in large airways (64), and interstitial pulmonary edema (50,65,66).

Interstitial pulmonary edema, resulting from rapid transcapillary fluid flux in excess of the lymphatic drainage capacity of the lung, is the most likely causative factor for the following reasons: 1. the relationship of $\dot{V}/\dot{Q}$ heterogeneity to hypoxia and exaggeration in extreme hypobaric hypoxia, 2. the improvement in $\dot{V}/\dot{Q}$ heterogeneity with 100% O_2 breathing, which would be expected to reduce pulmonary arterial pressure and reduce driving pressure for fluid flux, 3. the lack of evidence for bronchoconstriction, despite moderately severe $\dot{V}/\dot{Q}$ heterogeneity, 4. other indirect evidence that pulmonary edema occurs with exercise, detailed below. To date, investigators have focused on the development of $\dot{V}/\dot{Q}$ heterogeneity with very short-term, near maximal exercise. The effect of longer term exercise is not established, although a reduction in lung volumes and DLCO has been reported in runners completing a marathon (67,68).

D. Other Evidence for Pulmonary Edema

In addition to the $\dot{V}/\dot{Q}$ data previously discussed, there are several independent pieces of evidence that extravascular lung water may accumulate with exercise. In humans after exercise, there is an increase in transthoracic electrical impedance (65), a decrease in vital capacity, and an increase in residual volume (55,65,66). This suggests early airway closure secondary to subclinical pulmonary edema. Several authors have shown a reduction in diffusing capacity after exercise, which may persist for periods of up to 24 hours (67,69,70), and they have argued that this prolonged change in lung function may represent pulmonary edema. Subjects who have a history of high altitude pulmonary edema (HAPE) have an increase in exercise-induced $\dot{V}/\dot{Q}$ heterogeneity compared to normal subjects without a history of HAPE (71). This has led to speculation that the underlying mechanism of increased $\dot{V}/\dot{Q}$ heterogeneity with exercise and HAPE may be the same. Recently (72), we demonstrated that athletes exercised for short periods of time at very high intensity have increased levels of protein and leukotriene B_4 in bronchoalveolar lavage fluid, similar to those in HAPE subjects (73), indicating an increase in the permeability of the blood-gas barrier.

VI. Summary

Comparative studies of $\dot{V}/\dot{Q}$ heterogeneity provide insights about both the origins and mechanisms of complexity in vertebrate lungs. Experiments suggest that factors other than O_2 transport have been important in the evolution of lung complexity. $\dot{V}/\dot{Q}$ heterogeneity is similar in the ventilated pools of reptiles and mammals, despite the fact that the O_2 transport efficiency is dominated by cardiac shunts under most circumstances in reptiles and by pulmonary factors in mammals. $\dot{V}/\dot{Q}$ heterogeneity is also similar in mammals and birds with entirely different lung designs. Although cross-current gas exchange in the parabronchial avian lung is theoretically more efficient than alveolar O_2 exchange in mammals, Pa_{O_2} is not generally higher in birds compared to mammals. Similar amounts of $\dot{V}/\dot{Q}$ heterogeneity in birds and mammals reduced ideal P_{O_2} more in birds, so O_2 exchange is similar in resting birds and mammals.

This all suggests that a general vertebrate plan for bronchial and vascular branching in lungs may be responsible for similar degrees of $\dot{V}/\dot{Q}$ heterogeneity in different classes. Our laboratory has suggested this previously in a comparative analysis of diffusion limitations in different lung designs (59). Recently, this idea has been formalized in a mathematical model of transportation networks in living organisms such as vasculature and bronchial tree (74). This model minimizes the energy of transport in a fractal, branching network of tubes that fill the space of an organism (e.g., vasculature) or organ (e.g., lung). The model successfully predicts the three-fourths power scaling of physiological functions with body mass that is observed in nature in contrast to the more logical two-thirds power scaling expected with simple geometric constraints. The authors of this model hypothesize that, considering the model, "it is not surprising that the diversity of living and fossil organisms is based on the elaboration of only a few successful designs" (74).

In addition to comparative studies, experimental manipulations may be used to test this hypothesis soon. The gene controlling respiratory tracheole branching in fruit flies has been discovered to code for a protein that is closely related to mammalian fibroblast growth factor (FGF), and mice embryos with FGF receptor "knocked out" have reduced lung branching (76,76). The possibility to compare animals with experimentally altered lung branching would provide a strong test of the hypothesis that $\dot{V}/\dot{Q}$ heterogeneity in vertebrates depends on an evolutionarily ancient pattern of branching.

Comparative studies can also provide valuable insights to the mechanisms of $\dot{V}/\dot{Q}$ heterogeneity. Measurements of ventilation and perfusion heterogeneity in the lungs of different sized animals provided some of the first evidence that factors other than gravity were important in determining complexity. Modern microsphere data have revealed a fractal nature to perfusion heterogeneity in alveolar lungs, and it would be valuable to see whether this behavior also occurs in lungs of different designs. Such findings would provide further support for the paradigm that the vascular tree is the primary determinant of blood flow complexity in the lung (see Chapter 15). Mechanisms responsible for matching ventilation and perfusion could also be tested with comparative models that have, for example, different degrees of airway branching, or different susceptibilities to pulmonary edema (e.g., reptiles [16]).

References

1. Szewczak JM. Matching gas exchange in the bat from flight to torpor. Am Zool 1997; 37:92–100.
2. Perry SF, Duncker HR. Lung architecture volume and static mechanics in five species of lizards. Respir Physiol 1978; 34(1):61–81.
3. Gans C, Maderson PFA. Sound producing mechanisms in recent reptiles: review and comment. Am Zool 1973; 13:1195–1203.
4. Powell FL, Scheid P. Physiology of gas exchange in the avian respiratory system. In: King AS, McLelland J, eds. Form and Function in Birds. Vol. 4. San Diego: Academic Press, 1989:393–437.
5. Perry SF. Mainstreams in the evolution of vertebrate respiratory structures. In: King AS, McLelland J, eds. Form and Function in Birds. Vol. 4. San Diego: Academic Press, 1989:1–67.
6. Dunker H-R. General morphological principals of amniotic lungs. In: Piiper J, ed. Respiratory Function in Birds, Adult and Embryonic. Heidelberg: Springer-Verlag, 1978:2–15.
7. Gleeson TT, Mitchell GS, Bennett AF. Cardiovascular responses to graded activity in the lizards Varanus and Iguana. Am J Physiol 1980; 239(1):R174–R179.
8. Mitchell GS, Gleeson TT, Bennett AF. Pulmonary oxygen transport during activity in lizards. Respir Physiol 1981; 43(3):365–375.
9. Perry SF. Reptilian lungs. Functional anatomy and evolution. Adv Anat Embryol Cell Biol 1983; 79:1–81.
10. Wagner PD, Naumann PF, Laravuso RB. Simultaneous measurement of eight foreign gases in blood by gas chromatography. J Appl Physiol 1974; 36:600–605.
11. Wagner PD, Saltzman HA, West JB. Measurement of continuous distributions of ventilation-perfusion ratios: theory. J Appl Physiol 1974; 36(5):588–599.
12. Gale GE, Torre-Bueno JR, Moon RE, Saltzman HA, Wagner PD. Ventilation-perfusion inequality in normal humans during exercise at sea level and simulated altitude. J Appl Physiol 1985; 58(3):978–988.
13. Hopkins SR, McKenzie DC, Schoene RB, Glenny R, Robertson HT. Pulmonary gas exchange during exercise in athletes. I: Ventilation-perfusion mismatch and diffusion limitation. J Appl Physiol 1994; 77(2):912–917.
14. Wagner PD, Gillespie JR, Landgren GL, Fedde MR, Jones BW, de Bowes RM, Peischel RL, Erickson HH. Mechanism of exercise-induced hypoxemia in horses. J Appl Physiol 1989; 66(3):1227–1233.

15. Wagner PD, Laravuso RB, Goldzimmer E, Naumann PF, West JB. Distribution of ventilation-perfusion ratios in dogs with normal and abnormal lungs. J Appl Physiol 1975; 38(6):1099–109.
16. Hicks JW. Cardiac shunting in reptiles: mechanisms, regulation and physiological functions. In: Gaunt A, Gans C, eds. Biology of the Reptilia. (Morphology G) Vol. 19. Ithaca, NY: Soc for the Study of Amphibians and Reptiles, 1998:425–483. In press.
17. Hopkins SR, Hicks JW, Cooper TK, Powell FL. Ventilation and pulmonary gas exchange during exercise in the Savannah monitor lizard (*Varanus exanthematicus*). J Exp Biol 1995; 198:1783–1789.
18. Ishimatsu A, Hicks JW, Heisler N. Analysis of intracardiac shunting in the lizard, *Varanus Nilodicus*: a new model based on blood oxygen levels and microsphere distribution. Respir Physiol 1988; 71:83–100.
19. Hopkins SR, Wang T, Hicks JW. The effect of altering pulmonary blood flow on pulmonary gas exchange in the turtle *Trachemys (Pseudemys) scripta*. J Exp Biol 1996; 198:2207–2214.
20. Maginniss LA, Song YK, Reeves RB. Oxygen equilibria of ectotherm blood containing multiple hemoglobins. Respir Physiol 1980; 42(3):329–343.
21. Powell FL. Birds at altitude. In: Scheid P, ed. Functionanalyse biologischer systeme. Vol. 23. Stuttgart: Fischer, 1992:351–358.
22. Torre-Bueno JR, Wagner PD, Saltzman HA, Gale GE, Moon RE. Diffusion limitation in normal humans during exercise at sea level and simulated altitude. J Appl Physiol 1985; 58:989–995.
23. Bickler PE, Maginniss LA, Powell FL. Intrapulmonary and extrapulmonary shunt in ducks. Respir Physiol 1986; 63(2):151–160.
24. Hempleman SC, Powell SC. Influence of pulmonary blood flow and O_2 flux on DO_2 in avian lungs. Respir Physiol 1986; 63(3):285–292.
25. Piiper J, Scheid P. Models for a comparative functional analysis of gas exchange organs in vertebrates. J Appl Physiol 1982; 53(6):1321–1329.
26. Gleeson TT, Bennett AF. Acid-base imbalance in lizards during activity and recovery. J Exp Biol 1982; 98(439):439–453.
27. Comeau S, Lance VA, Hicks JW, Conlon JM. Purification and biological activity of alligator bradykinin. Am J Physiol 1992; 263(2):R400–404.
28. Hastings AB, White FC, Sanders TM, Bloor CM. Comparative physiological responses to exercise stress. J Appl Physiol 1982; 52(4):1077–1083.
29. Heisler N, Neumann P, Maloiy GM. The mechanism of intracardiac shunting in the lizard *Varanus exanthematicus*. J Exp Biol 1983; 105(15):15–31.
30. Szewczak JM, Jackson DC. Ventilatory response to hypoxia and hypercapnia in the torpid bat, *Eptesicus fuscus*. Respir Physiol 1992; 88(1–2):217–232.
31. Szewczak JM, Jackson DC. Apneic oxygen uptake in the torpid bat, *Eptesicus fuscus*. J Exp Biol 1992; 173(217):217–227.
32. West JB, Hugh-Jones P. Pulsatile gas flow in the bronchi caused by the heart beat. J Appl Physiol 1961; 16:697–702.
33. Engel LA. Gas mixing within the acinus of the lung. J Appl Physiol 1983; 54(3): 609–618.
34. Hlastala MP, Scheid P, Piiper J. Interpretation of inert gas retention and excre-

tion in the presence of stratified inhomogeneity. Respir Physiol 1981; 46(3): 247–259.
35. Powell FL, Wagner PD. Measurement of continuous distributions of ventilation-perfusion in non-alveolar lungs. Respir Physiol 1982; 48(2):219–232.
36. Downs D, Wagner PD. Detectability of diffusion-limited gas mixing by steady-state inert gas exchange. Fed Proc 1983; 41:4102.
37. Hopkins SR, Bayly WM, Slocombe RF, Wagner PD. Pulmonary gas exchange during prolonged strenuous exercise in the horse. J Appl Physiol 1998. In press.
38. Scheid P, Hlastala MP, Piiper J. Inert gas elimination from lungs with stratified inhomogeneity: theory. Respir Physiol 1981; 44(3):299–309.
39. Powell FL, Gray AT. Ventilation-perfusion relationships in alligators. Respir Physiol 1989; 78:83–94.
40. Spragg RG, Ackerman R, White FN. Distribution of ventilation in the turtle *Pseudemys scripta*. Respir Physiol 1980; 42:73–86.
41. Whipp BJ, Wasserman K. Alveolar arterial gas pressure differences during exercise. J Appl Physiol 1969; 27:361–365.
42. Gledhill N, Froese AB, Buick FJ, Bryan AC. $\dot{V}a/\dot{Q}$ inhomogeneity and $AaDO_2$ in man during exercise: effect of SF_6 breathing. J Appl Physiol 1978; 45(4):512–515.
43. Dempsey JA, Hanson PG, Henderson KS. Exercised-induced arterial hypoxaemia in healthy human subjects at sea level. J Physiol (Lond) 1984; 355:161–175.
44. Hammond MD, Gale GE, Kapitan S, Ries A, Wagner PD. Pulmonary gas exchange in humans during exercise at sea level. J Appl Physiol 1986; 60(5):1590–1598.
45. Hopkins SR, McKenzie DC. Hypoxic ventilatory response and arterial desaturation during heavy work. J Appl Physiol 1989; 67(3):1119–1124.
46. Thompson JM, Dempsey JA, Chosy LW, Shahidi NT, Reddan WG. Oxygen transport and oxyhemoglobin dissociation during prolonged muscular work. J Appl Physiol 1974; 37(5):658–664.
47. Powers S, Dodd S, Woodyard J, Beadle R, Church G. Alterations in hemoglobin saturation during incremental arm and leg exercise. Br J Sports Med 1984; 18: 212–216.
48. Bebout DE, Storey D, Roca J, Hogan MC, Poole DC, et al. Effects of altitude acclimatization on pulmonary gas exchange during exercise. J Appl Physiol 1989; 67(6):2286–2295.
49. Hammond MD, Gale GE, Kapitan KS, Ries A, Wagner PD. Pulmonary gas exchange in humans during normobaric hypoxic exercise. J Appl Physiol 1986; 61(5): 1749–1757.
50. Schaffartzik W, Poole DC, Derion T, Tsukimoto K, Hogan MC, et al. $\dot{V}A/\dot{Q}$ distribution during heavy exercise and recovery in humans: implications for pulmonary edema. J Appl Physiol 1992; 72(5):1657–1667.
51. Wagner PD, Sutton JR, Reeves JT, Cymerman A, Groves BM, et al. Operation Everest II: pulmonary gas exchange during a simulated ascent of Mt. Everest. J Appl Physiol 1987; 63(6):2348–2359.
52. Ekblom J, Hermansen L. Cardiac output in athletes. J Appl Physiol 1968; 25:619–625.
53. Dempsey JA. Is the lung built for exercise? Med Sci Sports Exerc 1986; 18(2): 143–155.

54. Hopkins SR, Belzberg AS, Wiggs BR, McKenzie DC. Pulmonary transit time and diffusion limitation during heavy exercise in athletes. Respir Physiol 1996; 103(1): 67–73.
55. Rasmussen BS, Elkjaer P, Juhl B. Impaired pulmonary and cardiac function after maximal exercise. J Sports Sci 1988; 6:219–228.
56. Young IH, Woolcock J. Changes in arterial blood gas tensions during unsteady-state exercise. J Appl Physiol 1978; 44(1):93–96.
57. Kiley JP, Faraci FM, Fedde MR. Gas exchange during exercise in hypoxic ducks. Respir Physiol 1985; 59(1):105–115.
58. Geiser J, Gratz RK, Hiramoto T, Scheid P. Effects of increasing metabolism by 2,4-dinitrophenol on respiration and pulmonary gas exchange in the duck. Respir Physiol 1984; 57(1):1–14.
59. Powell FL, Hempleman SC. Diffusion limitation in comparative models of gas exchange. Respir Physiol 1993; 91(1):17–29.
60. Powell FL, Hastings RH, Mazzone RW. Pulmonary vascular resistance during unilateral pulmonary arterial occlusion in ducks. Am J Physiol 1985; 249:R39–43.
61. Powell FL, Mazzone RW. Morphometrics of rapidly frozen goose lungs. Respir Physiol 1983; 51(3):319–332.
62. Farrell AP, Sobin SS, Randall DJ, Crosby S. Intralamellar blood flow patterns in fish gills. Am J Physiol 1980; 239(5):R248–436.
63. Hultgren HN. Pulmonary hypertension and pulmonary edema. In: Loeppsky JA, Reidsel ML, eds. Oxygen Transport to Human Tissues. New York: Elsevier/North Holland, 1982:243–254.
64. Tsukimoto K, Arcos JP, Schaffartzik W, Wagner PD, West JB. Effect of common dead space on $\dot{V}A/\dot{Q}$ distribution in the dog. J Appl Physiol 1990; 68:(6):2488–2493.
65. Buono MJ, Constable SH, Morton AR, Rotkis TC, Stanford PR, et al. The effects of an acute bout of exercise on selected pulmonary function measurements. Med Sci Sports Exerc 1981; 13:290–293.
66. Buono MJ, Wilmore JH, Roby FB. Indirect assessment of thoracic fluid balance following maximal exercise in man. J Sports Sci 1983; 1:217–226.
67. Manier G, Moinard J, Techoueyres P, Varene N, Guenard H. Pulmonary diffusion limitation after prolonged strenuous exercise. Respir Physiol 1991; 83(2):143–153.
68. Maron MB, Hamilton LH, Maksud MG. Alterations in pulmonary function consequent to competitive marathon running. Med Sci Sports Exerc 1979; 11(3):244–249.
69. Hanel B, Gustafsson F, Larsen HH, Secher NH. Influence of exercise intensity and duration on post-exercise pulmonary diffusion capacity. Int J Sports Med 1993; 14, Suppl 1:S11–S14.
70. Hanel B, Clifford PS, Secher NH. Restricted postexercise pulmonary diffusion capacity does not impair maximal transport for O_2. J Appl Physiol 1994; 77(5):2408–2412.
71. Podolsky A, Eldridge MW, Richardson RS, Knight DK, Johnson EC, et al. Exercise induced $\dot{V}A/\dot{Q}$ inequality in subjects with prior high-altitude pulmonary edema. J Appl Physiol 1996; 81(2):922–932.
72. Hopkins SR, Schoene RB, Martin TR, WRH Jr., West JB. Alterations in pulmonary

barrier function in competitive athletes following intense exercise. Am J Respir Crit Care Med 1995; 151(4):A619.
73. Schoene RB, Roach RC, Hackett PH, Harrison G, Mills WJ. High altitude pulmonary edema and exercise at 4,400 meters on Mount McKinley. Effect of expiratory positive airway pressure. Chest 1985; 87(3):330–333.
74. West GB, Brown JH, Enquist BJ. A general model for allometric scaling laws in biology. Science 1997; 276:122–126.
75. Peters K, Werner S, Liao X, Wert J, Whitsett, et al. Targeted expression of a dominant negative FGF receptor blocks branching morphogenesis and epithelial differentiation of the mouse lung. EMBO J 1994; 13(14):3296–3301.
76. Sutherland D, Samakovlis C, Krasnow MA. Branchless encodes a Drosophila FGF homolog that controls tracheal cell migration and the pattern of branching. Cell 1996; 87(6):1091–1101.
77. Dunker H-R. Functional morphology of the respiratory system and coelomic subdivisions in reptiles, birds and mammals. Vehr Dtsch Zool Ges 1978; 1978:99–132.
78. Perry SF. Structure and function of the reptilian respiratory system. In: Wood SC, ed. Comparative Pulmonary Physiology. Current Concepts. Vol. 39. New York: Marcel Dekker, 1989:193–236.
79. Hlastala MP, Standaert TA, Pierson DJ, Lutchel DL. The matching of ventilation and perfusion in the lung of the tegu lizard, *Turinambis nigropunctatus*. Respir Physiol 1985; 60:277–294.
80. Powell FL, Wagner PD. Ventilation-perfusion inequality in avian lungs. Respir Physiol 1982; 48(2):233–241.

19

Heterogeneity in the Lung
Concepts and Measures

ROBB W. GLENNY

University of Washington School of Medicine
Seattle, Washington

I. Introduction

When examined across space or time, biological structures and processes are complex and heterogeneous. They are not randomly heterogeneous but rather spatially or temporally correlated. Despite the wide variability in local daily temperatures over time, the nearer 2 days are in time, the more likely they are to have similar temperatures. When examined with appropriate statistical methods and at an adequate spatial or temporal resolution, all structures and processes have an organized pattern.

Biological structures are likely determined by functional needs of the organ or organism and temporal patterns are likely driven by a number of interacting physiological forces. Characterization of spatial and temporal patterns should provide insight into the structure and function of biological processes. This chapter introduces the concept of heterogeneity, highlighting the changing perspective in physiology that heterogeneity is a fundamental property of all biological processes and structures. This chapter also focuses on the importance of spatial and temporal resolution and present statistical methods used to characterize the observed heterogeneity.

II. Changing Perspectives

A common approach to scientific exploration is creation of a "model" or "concept" that is a simplified version of a complex system. While retaining the general behavior of the original system, a model can be more easily understood in part and therefore in total. A general characteristic of these models is the extraction of a few "important" features with disregard for other elements. Once a simplified model is accepted, it can restrict the peripheral vision of researchers by requiring new observations to be interpreted within the context of the prevailing model. In simplifying complex systems, deviations from the model are interpreted as statistical noise or random variation. With the recent realization that heterogeneity is a fundamental property of many biological systems, scientists are beginning to develop models that incorporate the observed variability. This new focus on the heterogeneity of biological systems has opened many new avenues of exploration in diverse areas of scientific inquiry.

Blood supply to cardiac and skeletal muscle was previously thought to be homogeneous and well matched to metabolic requirements (1). Higher spatial resolution data demonstrate that both regional myocardial perfusion (2) and local function are quite heterogeneous and poorly correlated (3). Studies measuring regional venous oxygen content in the heart have shown a large variability in regional oxygen extraction (4). The presently accepted paradigm is that the vascular branching geometry of the coronary circulation and microcirculation produces heterogeneous flows that may not be well matched to local metabolic demands.

On a smaller scale of resolution, the concentration gradient of O_2 from capillary to mitochondria is classically modeled as a monotonically decreasing function (Krogh cylinder). However, with the realization that there are local heterogeneities in red cell distribution and velocities (5,6), mitochondrial densities (7), mitochondrial function (8), and cellular O_2 consumption (9), O_2 concentrations may be heterogeneous as well. Data from micropuncture of guinea pig brain cortex (10) demonstrate a large heterogeneity of local O_2 pressures (Figure 1).

Heterogeneities of vascular regulatory mechanisms exist from one vascular bed to another and between vessels of different diameters (11–14). Pelletier et al. (15) have recently shown in horses that methacholine relaxes pulmonary arterial rings from dorsal lung regions and constricts ventral located arterial rings. Heterogeneous vasoconstriction induced by hypoxia has been documented using high-resolution angiography (16). These observations demonstrate that data obtained from isolated vessels in an organ perfusion bath may not be extrapolated to the entire vascular network.

Efficiency of gas exchange, the primary lung function, requires tight matching of ventilation and perfusion. Traditional models of ventilation and

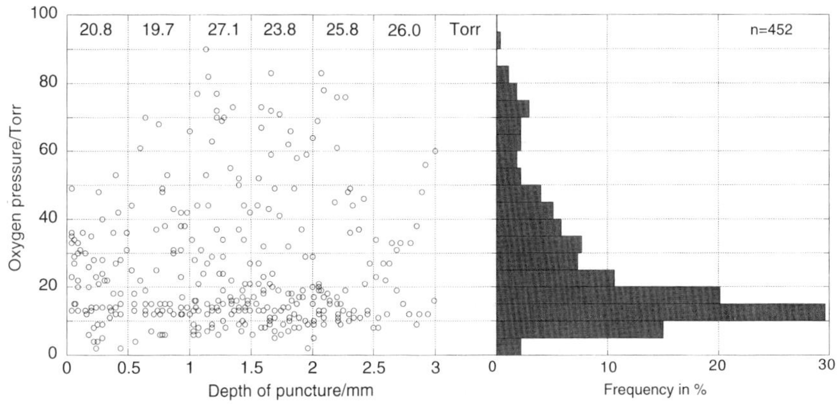

Figure 1 Heterogeneity of local PO_2 within the brain tissue of guinea pigs. The local PO_2 is measured by the polargraphic microaxial needle electrode. **Left**, Local PO_2 measurements ($n = 450$) are very heterogeneous. **Right**, PO_2 frequency histogram. (From Ref. 10.)

perfusion distribution state that the matching is due to the shared influence of gravity (17). However, studies documenting the large variability in blood flow and ventilation within isogravitational planes suggest that mechanisms other than gravity are more important in local gas exchange.

Given the great variability in lung structure and function, it is remarkable that lungs function so efficiently. Some authors (18) speculate this complexity to be a fundamental advantage. West (19) demonstrated that fractal processes or structure have the advantage of being more error tolerant than classical processes or structures. From a functional perspective, the fractal geometry of the lungs provides an optimal solution to the problem of maximizing surface area for gas exchange while minimizing the energy needed to build the structure and perfuse it with blood (18). Heterogeneity and redundancy of function also allows the lung to compensate for focal disease processes. If one lung region becomes dysfunctional, other similar lung regions can assume the function of the diseased region.

High-resolution methods demonstrate that heterogeneity in biology is the rule rather than the exception. This new awareness is causing scientist to use statistical tools that better characterize this heterogeneity and to develop models that incorporate heterogeneity as a fundamental property of the biological system. One inherent problem with this perspective is that heterogeneity measures are confounded by dependence on the scale of resolution used to make the observations (20). Fractal analysis, a new mathematical science (21), obviates this problem by providing a scale-independent measure of heterogeneity.

III. Statistical Measures of Heterogeneity

Variability within a distribution can be quantified by a number of statistical measures, such as range, variance, and standard deviation (SD). These measures can also be used to compare variability between two different groups or distributions. However, if mean values of the two distributions differ greatly, direct comparisons may be misleading. For instance, suppose distribution of blood flow to 100 lung regions is determined in two different conditions with an average flow per region of 20 and 200 mL/min. The standard deviation of flow to the 100 pieces may be 8.4 and 84.0, respectively, and blood flow heterogeneity appears greater during the high flow condition. However, the SD is proportional to the magnitude of flow in both conditions. The coefficient of variation (CV), or relative dispersion (RD), is defined as SD/mean and is commonly used to compare the relative variation between distributions. The CV and RD are the SD normalized to the mean and represented as a fraction or percentage and are used interchangeably throughout the chapter.

The CV is not necessarily the best measure of heterogeneity in most biological processes. The SD or CV adequately characterize the variability in normal distributions because they are symmetric, although most biological distributions are asymmetric. Frequency distribution of blood flow to an organ is shown in Figure 2. Note the distribution is skewed to the right or toward higher flow because blood flow cannot be less than zero. Because the SD and hence CV do not capture this quality of the distribution, it is possible for two distributions to have similar CVs but very different distributions.

The third moment of the distribution is a measure of this skewness, defined as

$$\frac{\sum_{i=1}^{n} (X_i - \mu)^3}{n} \tag{1}$$

where X_i is the value of each observation, *i*, and μ is the mean of the distribution. The skewness coefficient is positive for distributions skewed to the right and said to be significantly different from normal if it is four times greater than the SD of the distribution.

Because the CV is a general measure of blood flow distribution, it may not reflect flow changes to individual regions within that distribution. Flow to a particular organ piece can change significantly from one time to another without a change in the overall distribution. For instance, some high-flow pieces may become low-flow, and some low-flow pieces may become high-flow, while the frequency distribution of flow remains unchanged.

Observed heterogeneity in a system is composed of the true variability

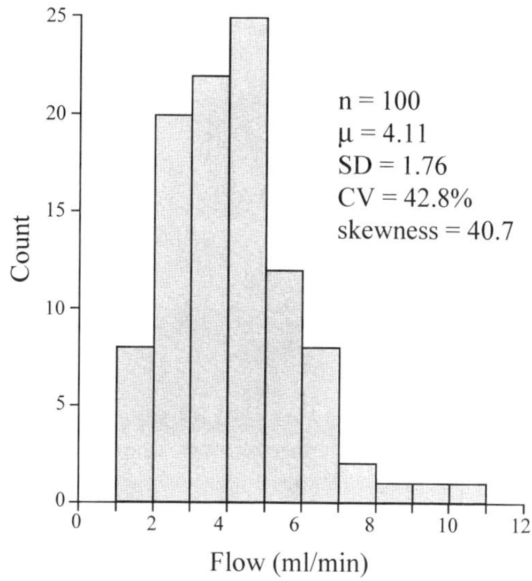

Figure 2 A typical frequency distribution of blood flow to 100 pieces of an organ. Heterogeneity of this distribution can be quantified by the coefficient of variation (CV). Note that organ blood flow distributions are skewed to the right (toward higher flows).

and any variation resulting from to measurement noise (22). Hence, any measure of heterogeneity must be corrected for the variability introduced by the experimental method. If these sources of variability can be assumed to be independent from one another and Poisson in nature, the observed heterogeneity can be expressed as

$$CV_{obs}^2 = CV_{true}^2 + CV_{method}^2 \tag{2}$$

where CV_{obs}^2 is the variability of the observed data, CV_{true}^2 is the true variability in the system, and CV_{method}^2 is the variability introduced by the method.

Another important issue when using the CV as a measure of heterogeneity is the dependence on the scale of resolution used to obtain the data. If blood flow in each of four pieces of an organ is measured, one can obtain the mean, SD, and thus RD of flow in the organ. If these same pieces are progressively subdivided, then for 16, 64, 256, or more regions, the mean remains constant but the estimated SD and RD increase (Figure 3). After appropriate corrections for experimental error, the largest estimate of RD will is from the finest subdivisions of the organ. This issue can be addressed with fractal methods described below.

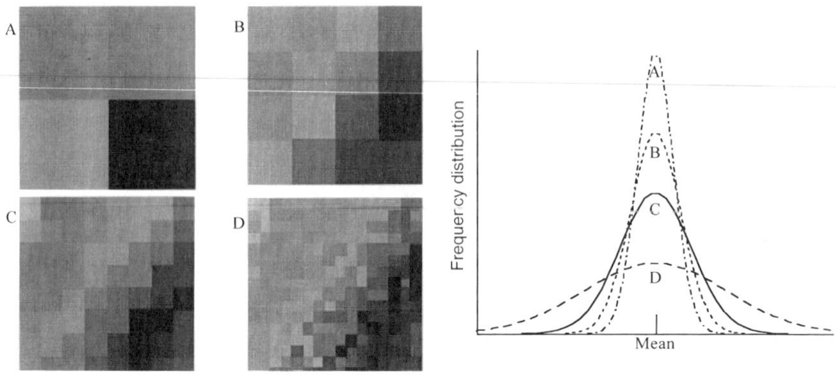

Figure 3 Observed heterogeneity increases as the scale of resolution decreases. Gray shades indicate the magnitude of an observation at different scales of resolution (**A** to **D**). The observations can be on the number of colonies in a petri dish or the amount of blood flow to organ regions. With increasing resolution from *A* to *D*, the mean of the distribution is constant but the SD and CV increase.

IV. Measurement Resolution

When a natural object is viewed from a sufficient distance, it appears smooth. On closer inspection, the surface may be quite irregular. For example, the Earth appears to be a smooth sphere from space, but the terrain is quite varied. Similarly, any biological process appears homogeneous when observed at low resolution, and irregular or heterogeneous at higher resolutions. When the whole organ is viewed, pulmonary blood flow has a smooth gravitational gradient. However, when inspected at the microvascular level, pulmonary perfusion is very heterogeneous.

At what level of resolution should we characterize biological systems? To an astronomer, the Earth is adequately modeled as a sphere; to the urban planner, all mountains and streams must be considered (Figure 4). Physiologists interested in the primary function of gas exchange in the lungs must explore function and structure across many scales of resolution (from the pulmonary artery to the microcirculation where gas exchange occurs). In an entire organ, ventilation and perfusion are relatively well matched between the right and left lungs. However, a considerable amount of V/Q heterogeneity exists at the level of gas exchange (23).

The most powerful solution to this scaling dependency is to characterize the heterogeneity of a biological system across its entire range of scales. A new mathematical science, fractal analysis, has been heralded as a language of nature, capable of describing processes that do not vary across scales of resolution. In 1623, Galileo stated that "[The] universe is written in the language of mathe-

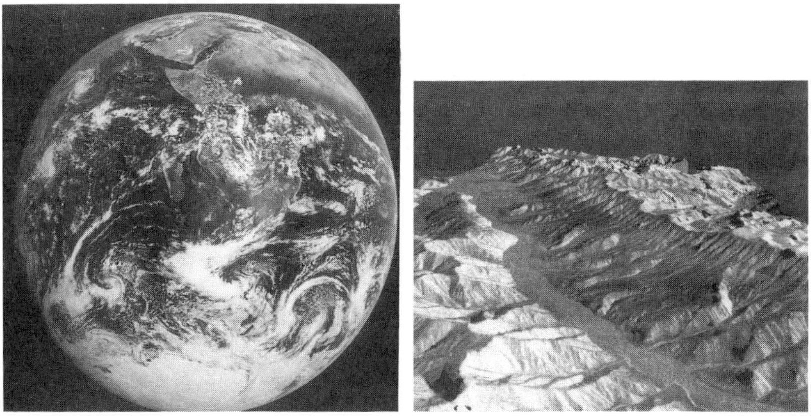

Figure 4 The scale of resolution used to obtain data is dependent on the measurements of interest. To an astronomer, the earth can be modeled as a sphere while to the geographer and urban planner, all of the mountains and streams must be considered. **Left**: Earth from Apollo 17. **Right**: Karakax Valley in the northern Tibetan Plateau of western China acquired by the Spaceborne Imaging Radar-C/X-band Synthetic Aperture Radar (SIR-C/X-SAR) aboard the space shuttle Endeavor. Permission for both pictures granted by NASA.

matics and its characters are triangles, circles, and geometrical figures" (24). In contrast, Benoit Mandelbrot claimed that "Clouds are not spheres, mountains are not cones, coastlines are not circles, and bark is not smooth, nor does lightning travel in a straight line" (21). Mandelbrot has championed the idea that nature does not necessarily adhere to man-made systems such as Euclidean geometry, but may have a simple language of its own that has the potential to create complex structures.

A fractal structure or process can be loosely defined as having a characteristic form that remains constant over a magnitude of scales. A *structure* is fractal if its small scale form is similar to its large scale form. A *process* is fractal if a variable, as a function of time, undergoes characteristic changes that are similar regardless of the time interval of the observations. In the parlance of fractal analysis, this is the quality of *self*-similarity, also termed scale-independence.

The Koch curve (Figure 5), created by Swedish mathematician Helge von Koch in 1904, is a fractal structure that introduces the concepts of self-similarity and fractal dimensions. This curve is defined by the following iterative transformations: Beginning with a straight line of length l_0 (see Figure 5, top line), the middle third of the line is replaced with two segments of length $\frac{1}{3}l_0$, forming part of an equilateral triangle (see Figure 5, second line). The next iteration repeats this procedure on each of four resultant straight line segments. Subse-

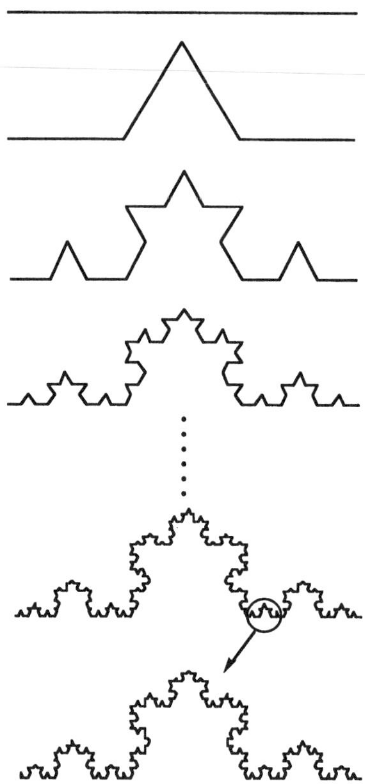

Figure 5 Generation of the Koch curve. The curve is produced by a simple iterative transformation beginning with a straight line (*top*). At each step, the middle third of each line segment is replaced with two segments, one-third the length of the line, forming part of an equilateral triangle. The completed curve has an infinite number of iterations. Regardless of magnification of scale, any part of the curve resembles the whole (*bottom*). (From Ref. 30.)

quently, identical generations are formed, and the completed figure represents the infinite expression of this iterative procedure. The completed Koch curve exemplifies properties of self-similarity because, regardless of the scale used to examine any portion of the Koch curve, it maintains its characteristic form.

Examples of self-similar structures abound in nature. A tree maintains a quality of self-similarity independent of the perspective or scale from which it is viewed. Branching angles and their proportionate diameters remain constant, whether being viewed at the main trunk or the terminal branches. Clouds are fractal, with each billowing appendage similar in form to its entirety. Without a reference scale, it is impossible to estimate the size of a cloud from a photograph

(24). The classic example of fractal structures are coastlines that appear to maintain the same degree of irregularity regardless of size or detail of the map studied (25).

V. Contour Measuring Method

A second principle of fractal structures and processes is a corollary of self-similarity. Because the underlying form of a structure or process remains similar through successive magnifications of scale, it follows that a measured length of its form cannot approach a limit. Remembering the Koch curve, the set of segments that contribute to its length can be expanded indefinitely. Although this property is a necessary requirement for a structure or process to be fractal in a strict mathematical sense, it is possible to discuss fractal properties of natural objects over a limited range of scales.

The Koch curve (Figure 6, *left*) is a good model to formally examine the characteristic of the scale-dependent length of fractal structures. Because it is jagged, the apparent length, L(l), of the curve depends on the length, l, of the measuring device chosen. If we use a stick of length l_0, equal to the straight line distance from one end of the curve to the other, none of the protruding structures is measured and the apparent length of the entire line is l_0. If the measuring stick length, l, is decreased to $(1/3)l_0$ and then $(1/9)l_0$, the apparent contour

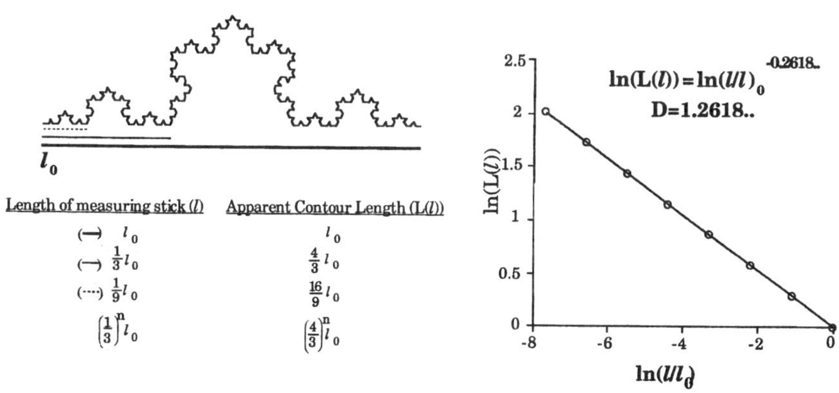

Figure 6 The apparent contour length of the Koch curve is dependent on the length of the measuring stick. **Left,** The finer the scale (greater magnification) the greater the apparent length of the curve. **Right,** Fractal (log-log) plot of apparent length, L(l), of the Koch curve as a function of the length of the measuring device, l relative to l_0. The line through the points represents the least squares linear regression fit. The relationship appears linear with a slope of –0.2618 and thus a fractal dimension, D = 1.2618. (From Ref. 34.)

length increases to $(4/3)l_0$ and $(16/9)l_0$, respectively. Generalizing this process for n iterations and a measuring stick of length $l = (1/3)^n l_0$, the corresponding measured length is $(4/3)^n l_0$. Therefore, as l becomes infinitely small, or as $n \to \infty$, the apparent contour length of the Koch curve becomes infinite. As increasing magnification reveals more detail, the overall appearance of the new segment examined remains similar to the previous segment.

Mandelbrot derived the fractal dimension to characterize the complexity of fractal figures (21). The ratio of the contour lengths can be related to the ruler lengths by the fractal dimension, D.

$$\frac{L(l)}{L(l_0)} = \left(\frac{l}{l_0}\right)^{1-D} \tag{3}$$

For the Koch curve, in which $\frac{L(l)}{L(l_0)} = \frac{4}{3}$ and $\frac{l}{l_0} = \frac{1}{3}$ for each iteration, the fractal dimension, $D = \frac{\ln(4)}{\ln(3)} = 1.2618$. Unlike the Euclidean dimension, the dimension of a fractal structure is not usually an integer, but a fractal structure always has a dimension that is equal to or less than the Euclidean dimension of space in which the structure is defined.

Taking the logarithm of both sides of Equation 3 and rearranging the terms yields the following:

$$\ln L(l) = (1 - D) \cdot \ln\left(\frac{l}{l_0}\right) + \ln L(l_0) \tag{4}$$

In this form, a log-log plot of L(l) versus l/l_0 produces a line with a slope of $(1 - D)$ and an intercept of $\ln(L(l_0))$. Figure 2, *right*, shows such a plot for the Koch curve, demonstrating a slope of -0.261 or a $D = 1.261$. Equation 3 defines a fractal process or structure. A process or object may be fractal if the logarithm of the measured value is linearly related to the logarithm of the scale of measurement. The fractal dimension, D, is 1.0 minus the slope of this linear relationship.

An intuitive grasp of the meaning of a fractal dimension can be obtained from examination of some different fractal figures. A straight line has self-similarity properties; at higher and higher resolutions, it maintains its same straight shape. It has a topological, fractal, and Euclidean dimension of one. For different fractal line algorithms generated in two space, a topological dimension of one and a Euclidean dimension of two are maintained, but the more complex line figures have progressively increasing fractal dimensions. When the line becomes so complex that it nearly fills the plane, the D_S approaches 2.0. Figure 7 illustrates some fractal curves that are produced by different iterative rules, yielding different fractal dimensions. Even at the limited level of iteration illustrated in Figure 7, it can be seen that the curves with higher fractal dimensions

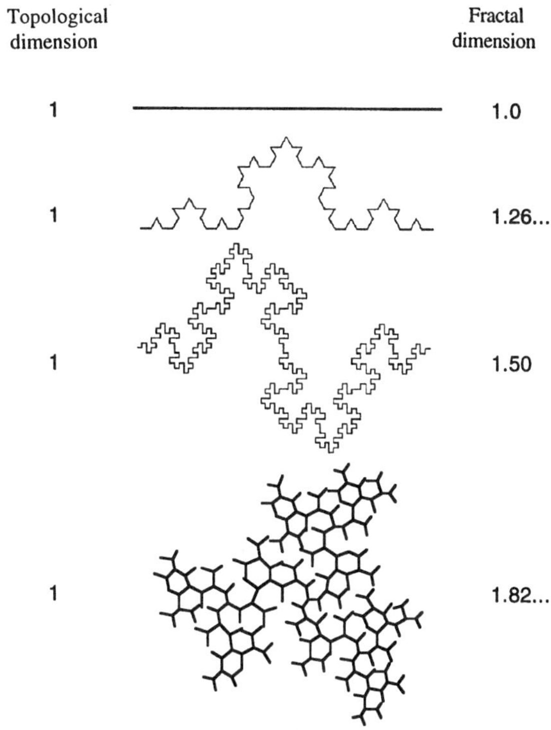

Figure 7 Lines of topological dimension 1 with different fractal dimensions. The fractal dimension is bounded by the topological dimension and the Euclidean dimension (1 and 2 in this case). The greater the irregularity of the line or the more space it fills, the greater the fractal dimension. (From Ref. 30.)

fill more space. The fractal dimension, therefore, is a measure of complexity independent of scale. As shown later, this measurement of complexity can be used to characterize biological structures and processes that have fractal properties.

VI. Box Counting Method

Other methods for determining fractal dimensions use similar iterative scaling algorithms. The box (26) or grid approach covers a fractal figure with a grid of side length l (Figure 8) and determines the number of boxes, $N_{box}(l)$, containing part of the figure. The side length, l, is decreased and a new $N_{box}(l)$ is determined. Using this technique, the fractal dimension, D, can be determined from the slope of the log-log plot of $N_{box}(l)$ as a function of side length, l. As noted with the measuring stick method, it is useful to examine as large a range of *l* as

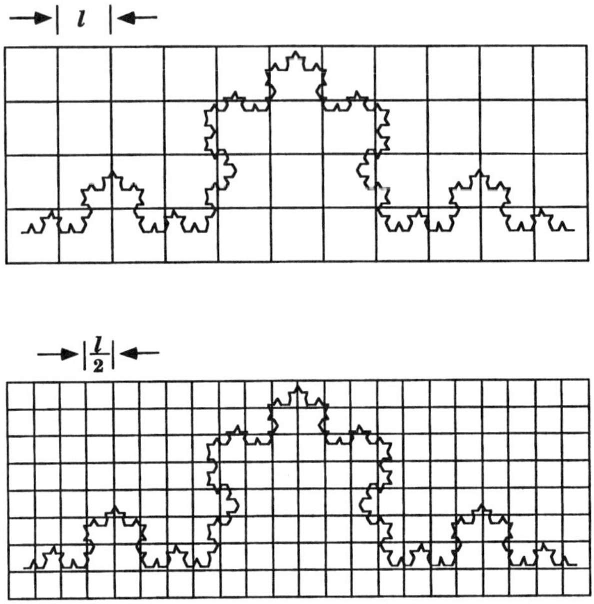

Figure 8 The box or grid approach to determining the fractal dimension of an object. The number of boxes containing a portion of the curve, $N_{box}(l)$, is determined for progressively smaller box dimensions, l. For the l of the top example, $N_{box}(l) = 23$ of the 44 boxes. When l is decreased by 1/2, $N_{box}(l/2) = 56$ of the 176 boxes. The fractal dimension, D, can be determined from the log-log plot of $N_{box}(l)$ as a function of l.

possible and to average D over a number of different placements of the grid or boxes (24). D is again determined from the slope of a log-log plot. The boxes need not be arranged on the rectangular grid, but they can be shifted to minimize the number of boxes used at each level. The position of the line shifts on the log-log plot, but does not affect the estimate of D. Using this approach to determine a fractal dimension for the Koch curve (see Figure 8) yields an estimate of D of 1.23. Although close, this estimate differs from the theoretical value of 1.2618 because only a finite number of boxes and sizes can be used to measure a line of infinite length.

The box counting method used by Boxt et al. (27) determined the fractal dimension of pulmonary arteries in both normal rats and in those with pulmonary hypertension. They found the spatial structure of the pulmonary arterial tree to be fractal in both groups and estimated the fractal dimensions to be 1.62 and 1.44 in the control and hypertensive group, respectively.

VII. Fractal Characterization of Spatial Heterogeneity Using Relative Dispersion Analysis

Whereas small scale variability in organ flow has been described as random, the branching structure of vascular anatomy suggests that regional flow is also best described by fractal measures. Heterogeneity of regional blood flow in an organ can be characterized by measuring the RD of regional flows when the organ is divided into a number of pieces. The observed relative dispersion is the sum of spatial variation and fluctuation of local flow over time (22). When the distribution of flow is measured by a single rapid injection of a deposited flow marker, there is little contribution from the temporal fluctuations to the total heterogeneity.

The heterogeneity of organ blood flow can be characterized independent of scale by employing fractal analysis (2,28–33). The fractal equation describing relative dispersion of flow for a given spatial resolution (piece size) is given by rephrasing Equation 3 using RD_S as a function of volume of size v:

$$\frac{RD_S(v)}{RD_S(v_0)} = \left(\frac{v}{v_0}\right)^{1-D_S} \tag{5}$$

Here, $RD_S(v)$ is the measured relative dispersion when the organ is partitioned into regions of volume v, $RD_S(v_0)$ is the RD_S found for an arbitrarily chosen piece size, and D_S is the derived spatial fractal dimension. Multiplying both sides of Equation 5 by $RD_S(v_0)$ and taking the logarithms, we obtain the following:

$$\ln RD_S(v) = (1 - D_S) \cdot \ln\left(\frac{v}{v_0}\right) + \ln RD_S(v_0) \tag{6}$$

If the slope of log $RD_S(v)$ versus $\log(v/v_0)$ is constant over a rangeof partitions, the system behaves fractally within that range. A greater rate of increase in observable heterogeneity with an increase in resolution yields a greater fractal dimension. The fractal dimension therefore serves as a measure of the scale independent irregularity, roughness, or variation of a system (20). This analytical approach is advantageous because it provides an estimate of D_S from easily obtained measurements of the RD_S of regional organ flow during successive subdivisions of the tissue pieces down to v_0.

Although regional blood flow to an organ is distributed in three-dimensional space, when characterized as a relative dispersion, flow heterogeneity is one dimensional (34). In RD analysis, a D_S of 1.0 indicates totally correlated magnitudes of flow between neighboring regions of the organ because flow is the same everywhere, whereas a D_S of +1.5 indicates that the magnitude of flow is not correlated or randomly distributed among neighboring pieces of the organ. D_S values above 1.5 indicate inversely or negatively correlated flows.

Pulmonary blood flow distribution can be characterized by fractal methods (30). A composite fractal plot of the $RD_S(v)$ for six supine dogs is presented in Figure 9. The fractal dimension, D_S, for these animals ranged from 1.07 to 1.12 with an average of 1.09. Note that there was appreciable variation among animals for the CV calculated at the smallest piece size, but the D_S values were quite similar. The data fit the fractal model well with an average correlation coefficient, $r = 0.98$. The observed measures of RD_S appear to oscillate about the linear regression line. As discussed earlier, this may be due to the fact that the lung pieces (measuring stick) are not the proper shape or orientation for our measurement. The appropriate sectioning of the organ would be along the vascular tree, with regions of common perfusion being grouped together. The data points shown in Figure 9 do not include the first four subdivisions of the lungs, because those measurements are disproportionately small.

The heterogeneity of myocardial (2,28) and skeletal muscle (31–33) blood flow has been characterized by fractal analysis as well. The distribution of radiolabeled microspheres in the heart was analyzed by progressively subdividing the heart into finer pieces. In this original application of the RD approach, regional

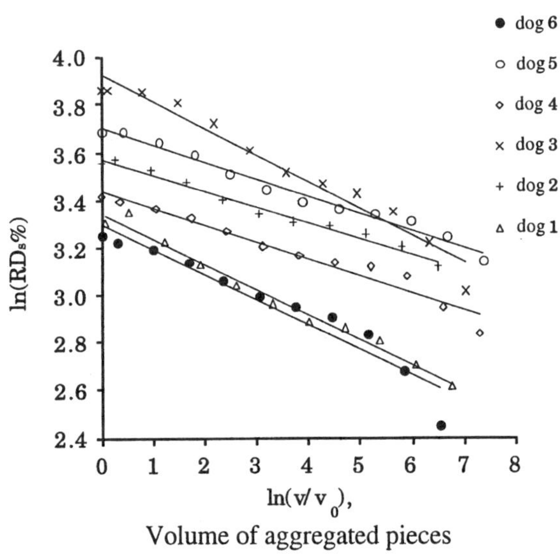

Figure 9 Relative dispersion of regional pulmonary blood flows in six dogs plotted as a function of the volume of the aggregated lung pieces. The smallest regions (v_0) are "voxels" from a planar gamma camera in which the voxels are $1.5 \times 1.5 \times 11.5$ mm or 24 mm^3. (From Ref. 30.)

flows were normalized to mass rather than to volume. The spatial heterogeneity of cardiac blood flow in baboons, sheep, and rabbits, as characterized by the fractal dimension, is shown in Table 1, along with the fractal dimensions for pulmonary blood flow in dogs. Although the number of pieces in the cardiac data sets are relatively small, the fractal dimensions are significantly different in some of the species and organs. This tells us that the spatial distribution of flow differs among these organs, suggesting either this is necessary for different functions or it is due to dissimilar morphogenesis.

An important feature of fractal analysis is that measurements from different experiments, species, and laboratories can be compared regardless of units or scales of measure. Heterogeneity of blood flow in baboon and sheep hearts measured by one technique can be compared with heterogeneity of blood flow in dog lungs measured in another laboratory using very different methods.

Iversen and Nicolaysen (31) recently used fractal analyses to characterize blood flow heterogeneity of cardiac and skeletal muscles; even though they found a range of fractal dimensions across animals, they demonstrated a strong correlation (Figure 10) between the two different muscle beds within animals. They concluded that a common mechanism may be responsible for distribution of blood flow within different organs of the same animal and speculated that the same genetic code may be responsible for development of different vascular beds.

The construction of self-similar structures reveals the potential advantage of coding for growth and development of the complex vascular, neural, and airway networks (34). Complex mathematical fractal figures can be constructed from simple recursive algorithms (24), permitting a concise description of remarkably complex structures (35). Because a complete genetic description for construction of every alveolus and capillary cannot exist, there must be elemen-

Table 1 Fractal Dimensions of Blood Flow Heterogeneity to Different Organs (2,28–33)

Animal	Number of Animals	D_s
Baboon hearts	10	1.21 ± 0.04
Sheep hearts	11	1.17 ± 0.06
Rabbit hearts	6	1.25 ± 0.07, 1.29 ± 0.05
Pig hearts	11	1.35 ± 0.14
Dog lungs	6,5	1.09 ± 0.02, 1.13 ± 0.006
Sheep lungs	8	1.14 ± 0.09
Rabbit muscle	46	1.37 ± 0.06
Sheep muscle	5	1.35 ± 0.08
Cat muscle	8	1.40 ± 0.07

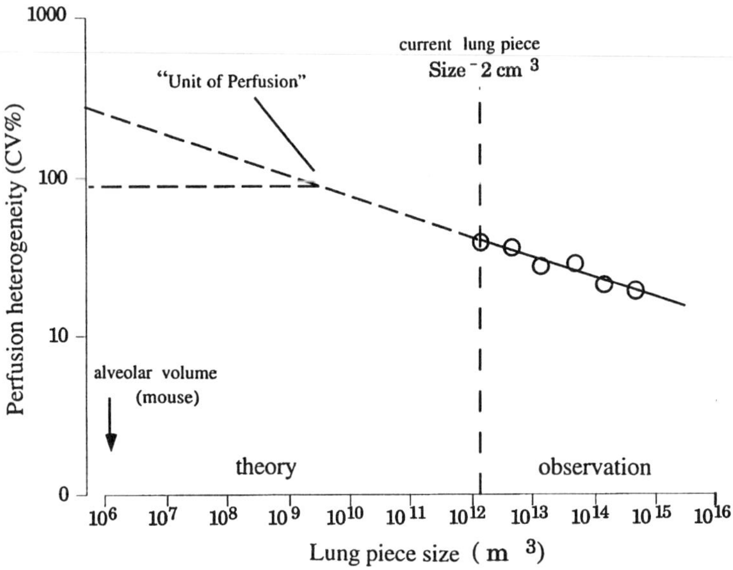

Figure 10 Relationship between the fractal dimension of blood flow to myocardial and skeletal muscles within the same animal. The high correlation suggests a common mechanism may be responsible for the distribution of blood flow within different organs of the same animal.

tary recursive rules that guide their construction. These construction codes are probably not fractal but must be deterministic rules defining basic elements that are influenced by the environment wherein the structure grows. Branching structures of the vascular system and bronchial tree represent examples wherein it is unknown whether branching angles and diameters are determined by the parent branch or by the similar environment in which they are constructed. Although mechanisms by which these rules operate are speculative, a coding for self-similar structures most efficiently and appropriately explains both order and complexity of ontogeny.

Blood flow heterogeneity can be fractal over a limited range. If increasingly smaller pieces are used to measure flow to a region of tissue, eventually flows become more similar as the anatomical limit of a capillary is reached (28). When heterogeneity is fractal, the log of RD_S remains linear with respect to the log of piece volume. However, as the functional unit of perfusion is approached with smaller piece sizes, the relative dispersion stabilizes and the fractal plot plateaus (36) (Figure 11). Theoretically, fractal analysis can determine the functional unit of flow in a lung by identifying the piece size in which an inflection in the slope of the fractal plot exists (30). The method we used to

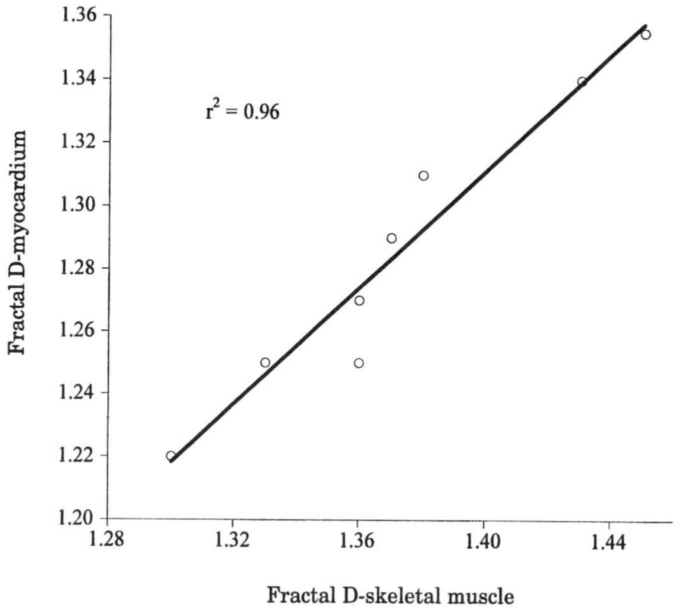

Figure 11 Fractal plot showing perfusion heterogeneity as a function of piece size. Experimental data (*open circles*) demonstrate a linear relationship across the range of piece sizes obtained with current methods. Theoretically, perfusion heterogeneity could continue down to the alveolar level or it may plateau at the "unit of perfusion." Recent data using higher resolution methods suggest that flow heterogeneity continues to increase fractally down to the gas exchange level. (From Ref. 61.)

measure regional blood flow distribution could examine pieces of lung 24 mm^3 in size. No inflection point could be detected, suggesting a unit of uniform perfusion smaller than 24 mm^3.

To explore blood flow distribution at higher resolutions, a fluorescent cryomicrotome is being developed that will allow the spatial distribution of organ blood flows to be measured at the capillary level. The system rapidly collects data from organs containing up to four different colors of fluorescent microspheres. Fluorescence images are acquired using a digital camera (2040 × 2040 pixel array). The cryomicrotome serially sections through the frozen organ at the selected slice thickness. Following each slice, five digital images of the tissue surface (en face) are obtained. Four of the images are acquired with appropriate excitation and emission filters to isolate each of the individual fluorescent colors. The X, Y, and Z (slice) locations of each microspheres are determined and saved in a text file. The fifth image of the lung cross section produces a three-dimensional binary map defining the spatial location of lung parenchyma.

In preliminary studies (37), four ~30-g mice were anesthetized with intraperitoneal injections of pentobarbital. After sonicating and vortexing the microspheres, approximately 30,000 red microspheres suspended in 300 μL of saline were injected into a tail vein of each mouse. The X, Y, and Z locations of each microsphere determined from serial sections using image recognition software. The lungs were randomly sampled at a preselected sample volume (2×10^{-4} mm^3). The number of microspheres in each sampled volume was determined and a frequency distribution obtained from the pilot mouse experiments (Figure 12).

This distribution is similar to pulmonary blood flow in larger animals (such as dogs) and is heterogeneous and skewed to the right. The sampling volume used in this distribution totaled 1884 pieces, more than normally obtained from a 25-kg dog lung (~1400, 2-cm^3 pieces).

A fractal plot of perfusion heterogeneity as a function of the sampled volume of lung can be constructed from this high-resolution data (Figure 13). The data are obtained by random sampling of the lung at increasing sample volumes, determining the number of microspheres in each sampled volume, and calculating a coefficient of variation for each sample size. The coefficient of variation is corrected for noise introduced by the small number of microspheres in the smaller sample volumes. The relationship remains linear as the piece size

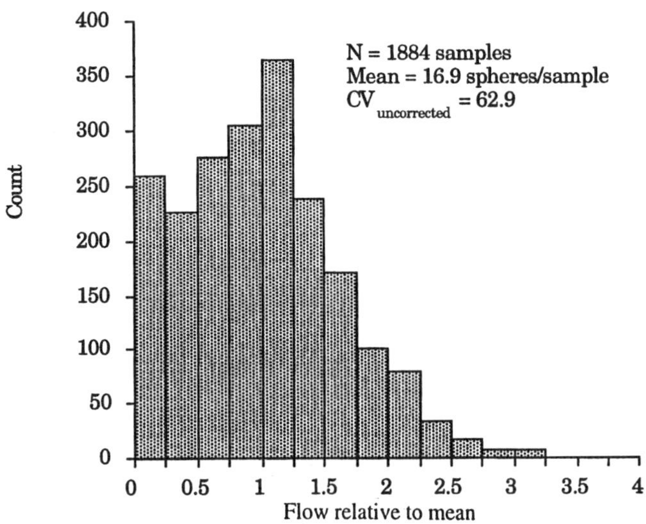

Figure 12 Frequency distribution of number of microspheres counted per sampled volume of lung. A total of 31,694 microspheres were injected with an average of 16.9 microspheres/sample volume, which was ~2×10^{-4} mm^3. Distribution is similar to that in dogs and pigs; it is heterogeneous and skewed to the right. Flows derived from number of microspheres/piece were normalized to a mean flow of 1 for this histogram.

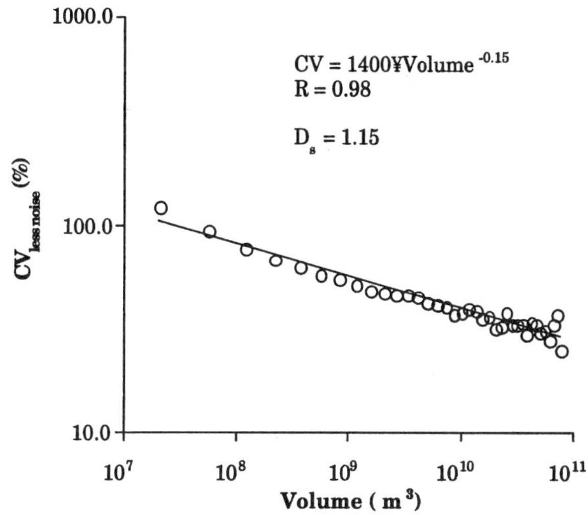

Figure 13 Plot of perfusion heterogeneity as a function of sampled volume of lung. The relationship remains linear down to a volume of ~10^7 μm^3. A mouse alveolar volume is ~10^6 μm^3. (From Ref. 61.)

decreases, demonstrating for the first time that perfusion continues to become increasingly heterogeneous down to the acinar level.

VIII. Spatial Correlation of Blood Flow and of Ventilation

Pulmonary blood flow is spatially correlated with neighboring regions of lung having similar magnitudes of flow and distant pieces exhibiting negative correlation. When regional blood flow is determined to ~2 cm^3 volumes of lung in dogs, high-flow regions are adjacent to other high-flow regions and low-flow regions are adjacent to other low-flow regions (Figure 14) (38).

This relationship can be quantified using the correlation coefficient between flows to pairs of lung pieces. Left f(i,j,k) be a process defined over the three-dimensional space. The spatial correlation, ρ(d), is the correlation between values of f at one position and a second position displaced from the first by a distance d. For example, the cubes in Figure 15 represent pieces of an organ distributed in space. The magnitude of blood flow to each piece is known. The spatial correlation between adjacent pieces, ρ(1), is determined by creating all possible pairs of cubes with a distance of one between their centers and calculating the correlation coefficient for all pairs. The spatial correlation between pieces separated by a distance of two, ρ(2), is determined by creating all possible pairs of cubes with a distance of two between their centers. The correlation

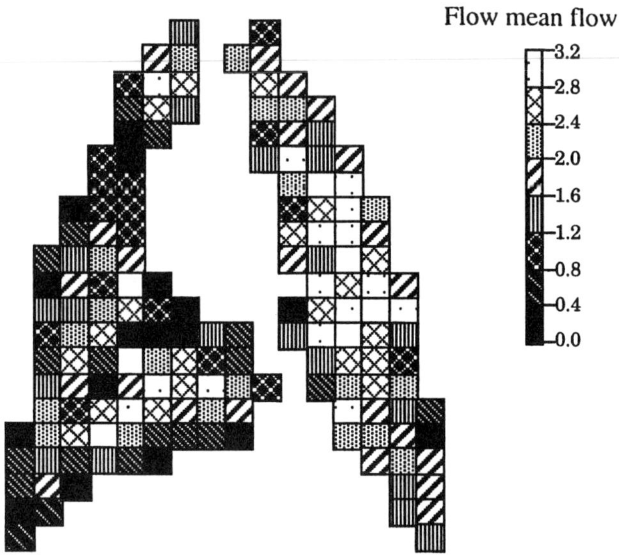

Figure 14 Distribution of regional perfusion within an isogravitational plane. The flows have been binned into eight levels to facilitate the graphical presentation. Regional perfusion is spatially correlated with high-flow regions near other areas of high-flow and low-flow regions near other areas of low flow. (From Ref. 37.)

coefficient has a range of $-1.0 \le \rho(d) \le 1.0$ where $\rho(d) = 1.0$ indicates a perfect positive correlation between all pairs, $\rho(d) = -1.0$ means a perfect negative correlation between pairs, and $\rho(d) = 0.0$ indicates a random association between all pairs.

The spatial correlation of regional pulmonary perfusion should be greatest for neighboring pieces when $d = 1$ and should decrease with increasing distance between pieces. As flow becomes uniform throughout the organ, the correlation should approach 1.0; more heterogeneous flow should reduce correlation more rapidly with distance. Observations from agriculture and geology support the empirical formula that the spatial correlation decays as a power law of distance, with the spatial correlation becoming zero at large distance but never becoming negative.

$$\rho(d) = Cd^{-\alpha} \tag{7}$$

When the spatial correlation of perfusion is determined for regional pulmonary perfusion, a strong positive correlation is noted for neighboring pieces (Figure 16). On average, $\rho(d) = 0.72$, with $d = 1.2$ cm; thus, the spatial correlation decreases with distance between pieces. The spatial correlation eventually becomes negative in all cases, an observation not predicted by empirical power

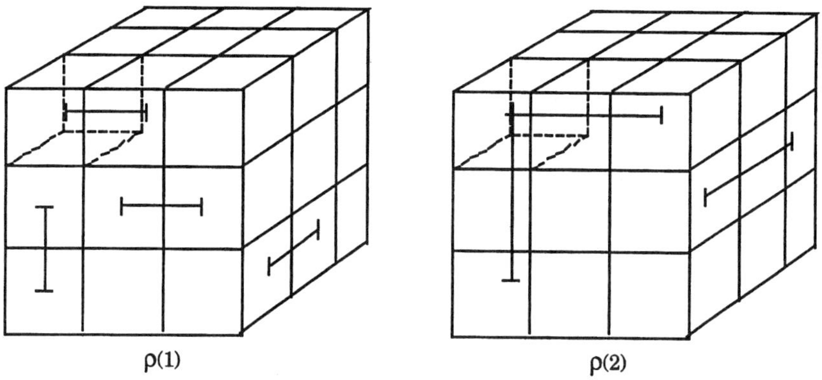

Figure 15 Concept of spatial correlation. The cubes represent pieces of an organ distributed in space. The magnitude of blood flow to each piece is known. The spatial correlation between adjacent pieces, $\rho(1)$, is determined by creating all possible pairs of cubes with a distance of one between their centers and calculating the correlation coefficient for all of these pairs. The spatial correlation between pieces separated by a distance of two, $\rho(2)$, is determined by creating all possible pairs of cubes that have a distance of two between their centers. (From Ref. 61.)

laws observed in other natural processes and is probably due to blood flow conservation within an organ (38).

Because a fixed amount of blood is distributed to a limited volume, high-flow regions can exist only at the expense of flow to low-flow regions. Regions of similar flow magnitude tend to be located near one another because of the shared heritage of the vascular tree. Other examples of negative spatial correlation have not been reported, suggesting that it is unique to organ blood flow.

The spatial correlation of pulmonary perfusion many be caused by a branching pattern in the vascular tree. To test this hypothesis, blood flow can be modeled by a dichotomously branching tree, with a fraction of flow from parent to daughter branches being γ and $1\text{-}\gamma$ at each bifurcation (Figure 17) (39). The flow asymmetry parameter, γ, is randomly chosen for each bifurcation from a normal distribution with a mean of 0.5 and a standard deviation of σ.

Flow distributions in this model are similar to those observed in experimental animals, with heterogeneous flows that are skewed to the right (Figure 18).

This two-dimensional model can be extended to three-dimensional space by requiring branches to develop along three orthogonal directions to create a space-filling structure (Figure 19) (40).

Modeled blood flow values can be calculated to each terminal branch and the spatial correlation of flow determined for a three-dimensional distribution

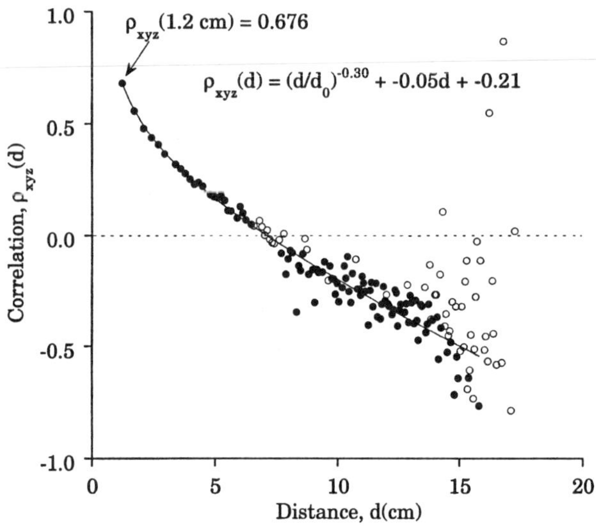

Figure 16 Spatial correlation as a function of distance. Plot of $\rho_{xyz}(d)$ for one supine dog. The curve represents the best fit to the equation $\rho_{xyz}(d) = (d/d_0)^a + b{\cdot}d + c$. The fit is weighted by the number of paired regions determining $\rho_{xyz}(d)$ at each d. The curve fits the data points quite well when d is small; there is a large amount of scatter in the data points for larger d. Filled circles indicate points with spatial correlation significantly different from 0.0 ($p < 0.05$). (From Ref. 37.)

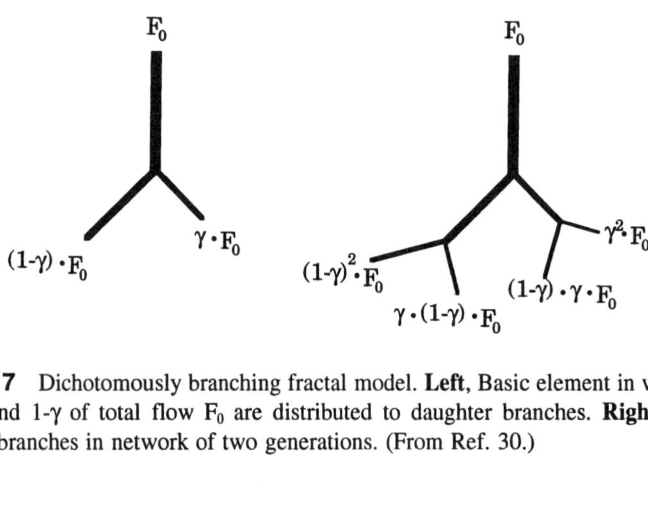

Figure 17 Dichotomously branching fractal model. **Left,** Basic element in which fractions γ and $1-\gamma$ of total flow F_0 are distributed to daughter branches. **Right,** Flow at terminal branches in network of two generations. (From Ref. 30.)

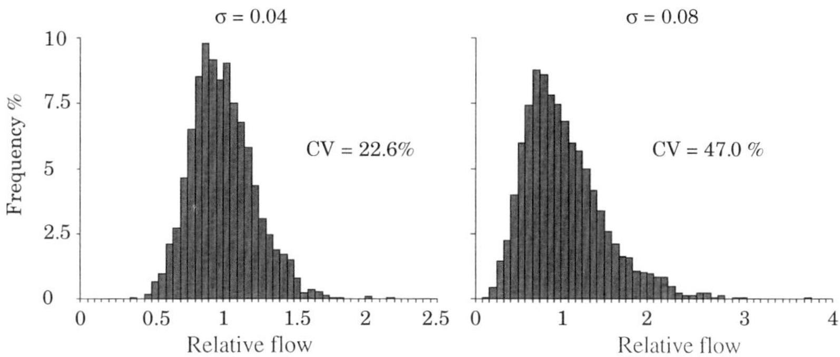

Figure 18 Heterogeneity of perfusion created by vascular branching model with different values of σ. As σ increases, the heterogeneity of perfusion increases. This degree of heterogeneity is comparable to previously reported distributions using lung pieces of similar scale. Note scale differences in the abscissa (relative flow) between the two distributions. (From Ref. 61.)

(Figure 20). These distributions are similar in experimental animals, with highly correlated flow to neighboring regions and negatively correlated flows to distant regions (40).

Spatial correlation measurements have also been applied to the regional distribution of ventilation. Rodarte and coworkers (41) explored variability in regional lung expansion using computed tomography scans of isolated dog lung lobes. Variability of parenchymal tissue density and parenchymal volume changes were determined at the scale of resolution equal to a voxel (1.5 mm per side). They reported tissue density to be variable, with neighboring voxels positively correlated; the spatial correlation of parenchymal density decreased exponentially as a function of distance with an exponential scale of 0.3 cm. The spatial correlation of regional lung expansion, related to distance by an exponential function that cannot be less than zero, differs from the spatial correlation of regional pulmonary blood flow that becomes negative at large distances. This may be due to blood flow conservation across space, whereas parenchymal density is not conserved and therefore shows no negative correlation.

IX. Statistical Analyses of Spatially Distributed Point Processes

All analyses presented so far are from continuous data associated with spatial locations. Another field of inquiry, spatial and temporal distribution of discrete objects, includes spatial locations of galaxies (42), bird nests (43), tree saplings (44), and the temporal occurrence of neuronal discharges (43). Methods for

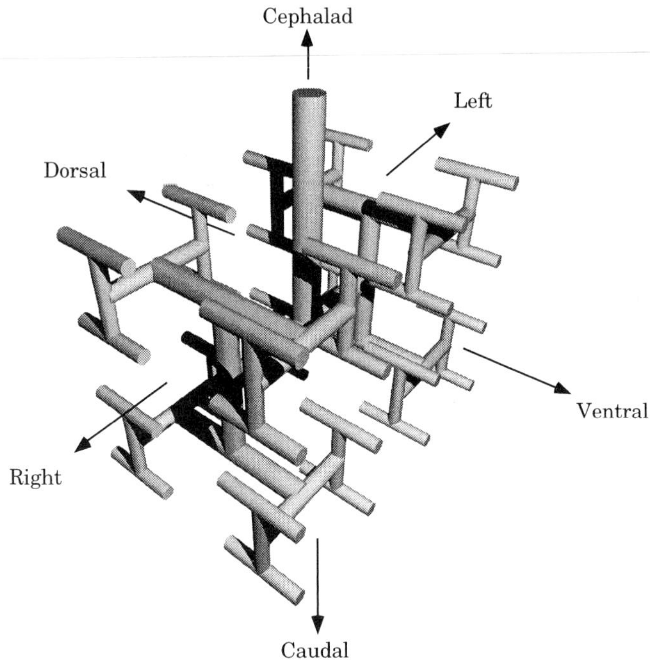

Figure 19 Three-dimensional branching model. Dichotomous branching model is extended into three dimensions by designating branching directions at each bifurcation along one of three orthogonal axes. The branching directions can be arbitrarily designated as dorsal/ventral, caudal/cephalad, and right/left. (From Ref. 39.)

analyzing these data are nicely described by Diggle (45), Ripley (46), and Brown and Rothery (43), exemplifying the role that modern computers can play to simulate random events and test statistical significance.

Brown and Rothery (43) suggest the following test for spatial and temporal patterns: 1. set up the null hypothesis of randomness, 2. select a metric to detect the features of interest, and 3. determine significance (p-value) of the observed metric by repeated simulation of random patterns and application of the chosen metric to each realization. The final step, referred to as Monte Carlo testing, uses computer simulations to construct frequency distributions of the chosen metric for a random process. If observed data are distributed in a pattern different from chance, the value of the metric from the observed data will occur outside the distribution containing 95% of the values from the random simulation.

Although any quantitative measurement can be used as a metric, Brown and Rothery (43) offer three different metrics, depending on the type of pattern to be characterized. The arithmetic mean of the nearest neighbor distances, M,

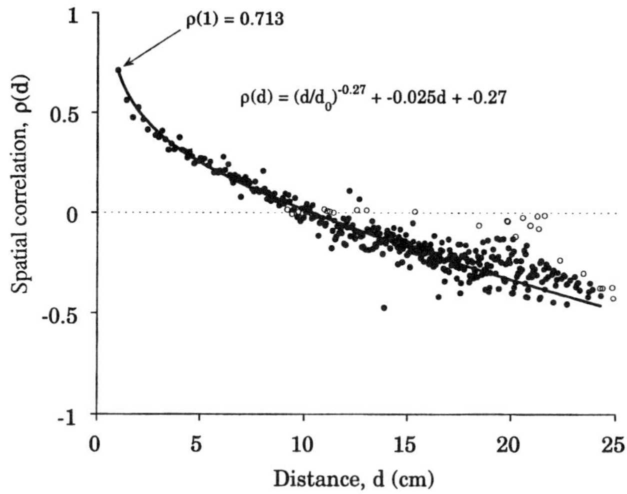

Figure 20 Spatial correlation as a function of distance. Plot of $\rho_{xyz}(d)$ for a modeled data set. The curve represents the best fit to the equation $\rho_{xyz}(d) = (d/d_0)^a + b\cdot d + c$. The spatial correlation of the modeled data is very similar to the experimental data (see Figure 16). Filled circles are points with spatial correlations significantly different from 0.0 ($p < 0.05$). (From Ref. 39.)

indicates a pattern more regular than random for large values. The square of the coefficient of variation of the squared nearest neighbor distance, S, has small values for regularly spaced events. The ratio of the geometric mean of the squared nearest neighbor distance to their arithmetic mean, G, approaches unity when events are evenly spaced. If the nearest neighbor to the ith event is at a distance d_i, the above metrics are defined as follows:

$$M = \frac{\sum_{i=1}^{n} d_i^2}{n}; S = \frac{\sum_{i=1}^{n} (d_i^2 - M)^2}{(n-1)M^2}; G = \frac{\left(\prod_{i=1}^{n} d_i^2\right)^{1/n}}{M} \tag{8}$$

where n is the number of events.

Figure 21 shows 30 points that are distributed within a fixed two-dimensional space, each point having an X and Y coordinate. The mean-squared distance to the nearest neighbor is determined for each example and compared to that expected from a random distribution. Random data are generated by selecting random numbers between 0 and 20 for the x and y coordinates for 30 different points, and the mean-squared distance to the nearest neighbor is determined for each realization. The random data are simulated and the metric calculated 1000 times to construct a probability distribution of the metric for random pat-

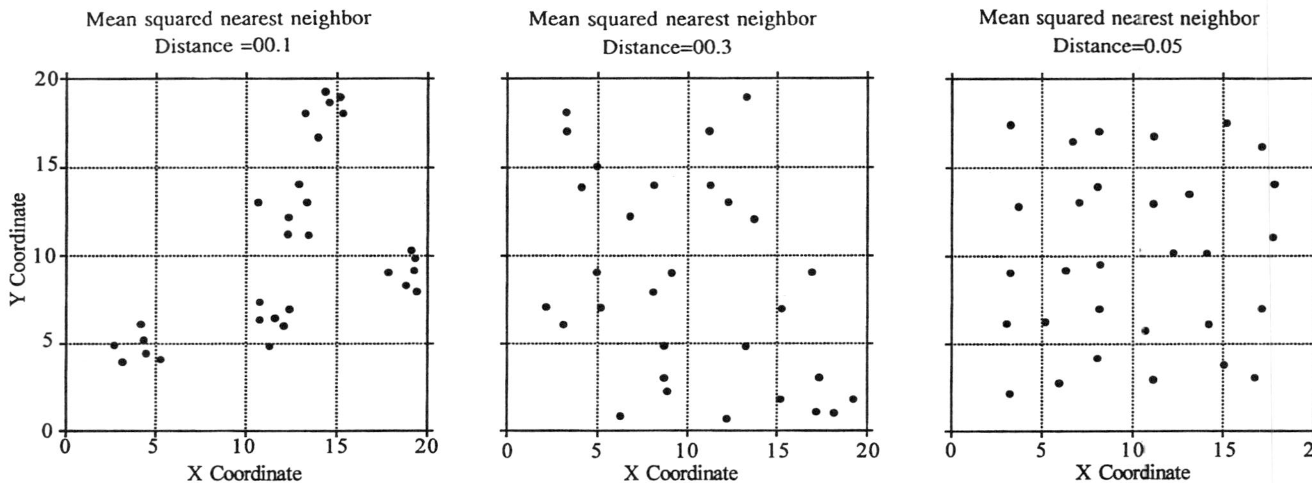

Figure 21 Three examples of 30 points distributed in two-dimensional space. The mean-squared distance to the nearest neighboring point is determined for each example. A Monte Carlo simulation is used to determined whether the points are randomly distributed across space. (See Figure 22.)

terns (Figure 22). Metrics from the observed data are compared with this distribution and deemed statistically different from random if the observed metric does not fall within the probability distribution containing 95% of the metric values. As shown in Figure 21, the spatial distribution with M = 0.01 and 0.05 are statistically different from a random pattern because they are more clustered and more regularly spaced than expected, respectively. The *p*-value is the fraction of simulations generated by chance that yielded metrics at or beyond the observed metric value.

The beauty of this approach is that statistical assumptions are not made and a normal distribution is not assumed to test the null hypothesis of chance. Because the random points are distributed within the same space as the observed data, any clustering of points resulting from spatial constraints is also applied to the Monte Carlo simulations.

In preliminary studies, four ~30-g mice were anesthetized with intraperi-

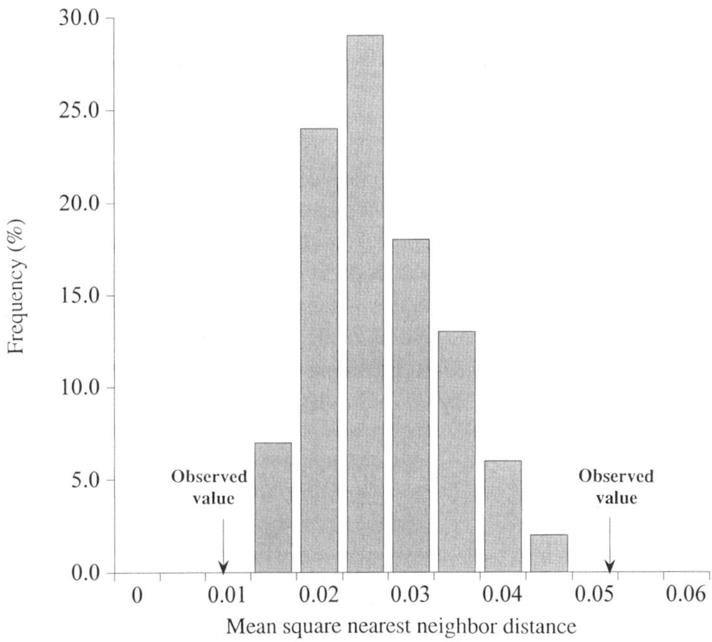

Figure 22 Monte Carlo simulation to determine the frequency distribution of the mean squared nearest neighbor distance for 30 randomly distributed points. The random data are simulated and the metric calculated 1000 times to construct a probability distribution of the metric for random patterns. The observed metric is statistically different from random when it does not fall within the probability distribution containing 95% of the random metric values.

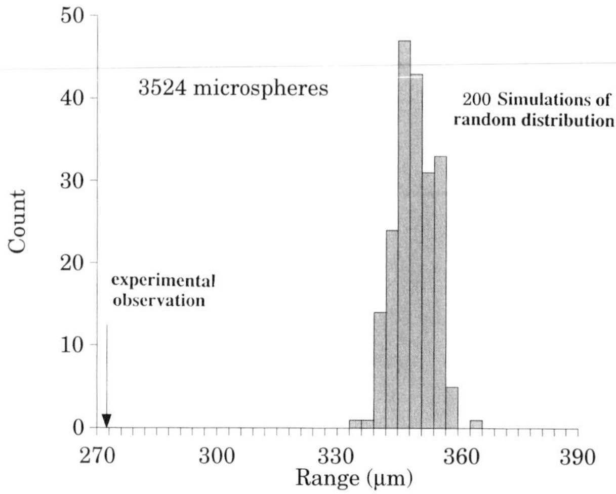

Figure 23 Mean squared distance to nearest neighboring microsphere in experimental mouse lung compared with distribution constructed from 200 simulations of randomly placed microspheres.

toneal injections of pentobarbital. After sonicating and vortexing the microspheres, approximately 30,000 red microspheres suspended in 300 μL of saline were injected into a tail vein of each mouse. The X, Y, and Z locations of each microsphere were determined from serial sections using image recognition software. Figure 24 compares the mean squared nearest neighbor distance from a mouse lung and the distribution constructed from 200 simulations of randomly placed microspheres. The observed distance is statistically less than the random distribution, showing that blood flow in mouse lungs is spatially clustered.

X. Fractal Processes, Temporal Heterogeneity, and Temporal Correlation

Many physiological processes are variable over time. With the advent of fractal analyses, the concepts of self-similarity and fractal dimensions can also be applied to observations made over time. Several methods that elicit the underlying dimensionality of such measurements have been developed for time series data. These fall into two classes: 1. dispersion analysis, which gives a measure of local correlation, and 2. minimal order analysis, which defines the minimal order of a set of differential equations that describe chaotic dynamic behavior of the system that is fluctuating unpredictably while remaining bounded and self-correlated. Although each of these approaches define fractal measures, described by a fractal dimension, they differ significantly. Dispersion analysis reduces the complexity of the system to one-dimensional, whereas the time series analysis for the dimension of a chaotic signal attempts to define the minimal degree of complexity or order of the system. For discussion of minimal order analysis, see Refs. 47 and 48.

XI. Dispersion Analysis

Three basic methods of dispersion analysis exist that can be applied to temporal observations: 1. relative dispersion, RD_τ, 2. Hurst's rescaled range, and 3. the measure of extended-range correlation. The simplest analysis is application of relative dispersions, described above for spatial variation (20). The application to a single V(t) is shown in Figure 24, in which V(t) may be any measure such as voltage, velocity, or position. A digitized signal measured at uniform intervals, τ_0, can be considered as a population of one-dimensional observations. $RD_\tau(\tau_0)$ is calculated initially for all sampled data in the upper row of Figure 24. Paired neighboring points are then (*second row*), and $RD_\tau(2\tau_0)$ is calculated. Recursive pairing to double the interval length and recalculation of the standard deviation on the combined data points gives $RD_\tau(4t_0)$, $RD_\tau(8t_0)$, . . . $RD_\tau(N\tau_0)$

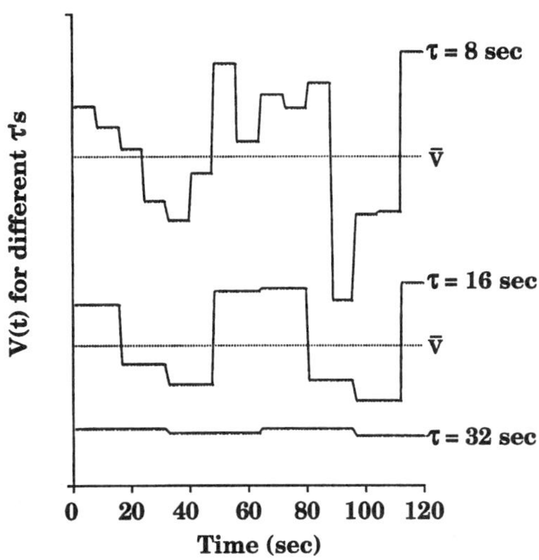

Figure 24 V(t) is a function of time at uniform intervals, $\tau = 8$ seconds, in the top curve. Successive averages over intervals (τ) of double the length are shown in the two bottom curves. Note the diminution in dispersion with successive lumpings. (From Ref. 34.)

for each row of "observations" in the figure. When $RD_\tau(N\tau_0)$ and N are plotted on logarithmic scales, they are well characterized by a fractal relationship which is a straight line:

$$RD_\tau(N\tau_0) = RD_\tau(\tau_0) \cdot N^{1-D_\tau} \tag{9}$$

The fractal D_τ for this random signal is 1.5, so the exponent of N is −0.5. Each time the averaging interval doubles to $2t_0$, $4t_0$, etc., RD_τ scales down by $1/\sqrt{2}$, i.e. to 0.707 of the RD_τ at the duration of the next smaller interval. As with the measuring stick length for the contour length method, it is not necessary to use interval doubling, because any increment yields a similar D_τ, provided enough data points are available. The D_τ of 1.5 is expected for any random signal. In this case, the random signal was Gaussian, with a mean of 1.0, an SD of 0.3, and a correlation coefficient, $r = 2^{3-2D} - 1$, of zero. The same D_τ is true for other random signals, uniform over intervals, such as Poisson or random walk. Information from this analysis is limited to the variance and does not characterize the form of the distribution or higher moments such as skewness and kurtosis.

Fractal analysis of time-dependent observations provides a means to characterize temporal correlation similar to spatial correlation. Correlation over time is also described as *memory*. If a fractal process with positive correlation is in an upward trend, adjacent observations in time also increase. Similarly, if the process is in a downward trend, neighboring observations in time decrease as well; for example, the state or position of a process, V(t), is influenced by its previous values V(t − 1). Adjacent values in time tend to move away from one another if the temporal correlation is negative.

The daily measurement of the barometric pressure in a pulmonary function laboratory can be used as an example. Figure 25 shows the barometric pressure each day over a 4-year period. The time interval of observation is analogous to the spatial resolution discussed above. Regardless of the time interval used (months or days), the pattern of variability remains similar. Despite the marked variability, some correlation or memory exists from day to day. If barometric pressure is high today, there is a good possibility that it was high yesterday and will be high tomorrow. However, even with this temporal correlation, one cannot predict the barometric pressure for the following week. There appears to be an underlying cycle every 365 days wherein the amplitude of variation increases and then decreases. When fractal analysis is applied to this data set, it becomes apparent that the system is composed of two fractal processes (Figure 26).

Daily barometric pressures are correlated positively (Dt = 1.14) over approximately 100 days and then become negatively correlated at intervals greater than this.

Zenk and colleagues (49) have used fractal analyses to characterize the temporal pattern of blood flow in alveolar capillaries. Using video microscopy,

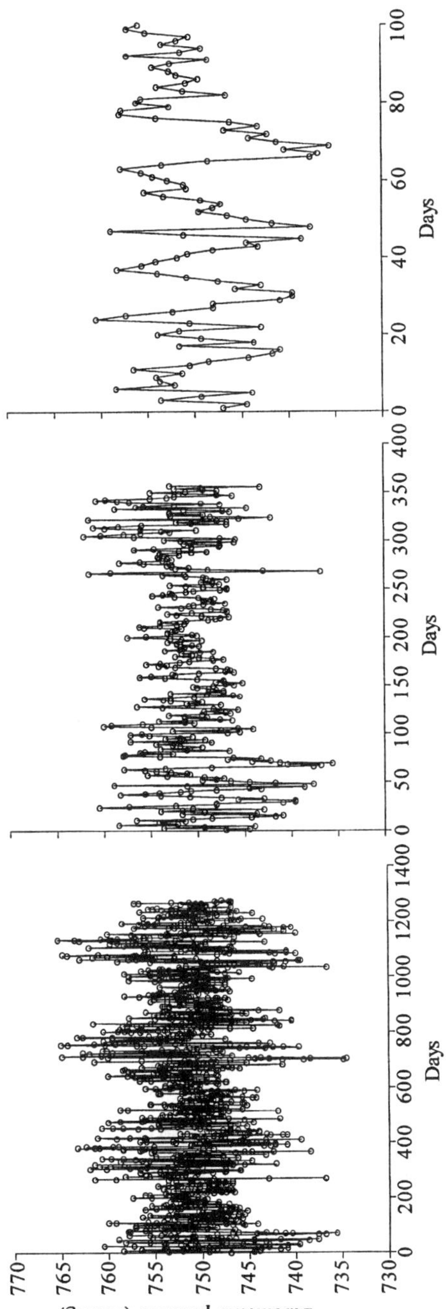

Figure 25 Variable daily barometric pressures in a pulmonary function laboratory over 4 years. Despite the wide variability over time, the nearer 2 days are in time, the more likely they are to have similar pressures. Also note that general trends over years are similar to daily trends over a few weeks.

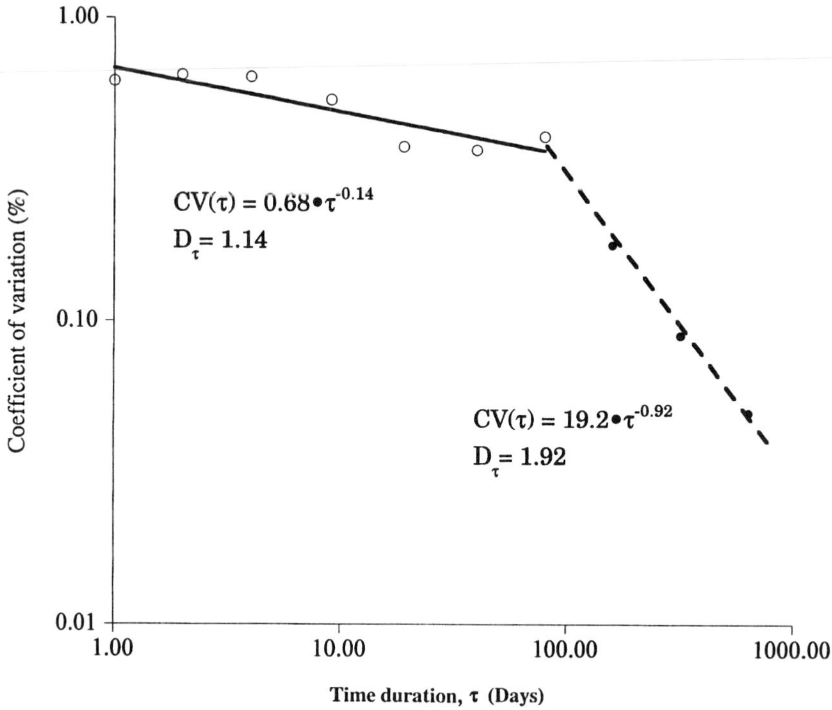

Figure 26 Fractal plot of daily barometric pressures. There appear to be two processes: 1. when pressures tend to be positively correlated over time ($D_\tau = 1.14$) and 2. when pressures are negatively correlated over time ($D_\tau = 1.92$).

fluorescent-labeled red cells passing through the subpleural capillary network were counted as a function of time. The temporal variability of red cells was fractal in nature with a fractal dimension of 1.17 ± 0.08.

Hurst's (50) "rescaled range analysis" is similar to the RD analysis and can be applied to spatial as well as temporal data. In the simplest version of this method (51), the standard deviation (SD) is normalized by dividing it into the local range, R, of the cumulative differences from the mean over the interval of length τ, rather than by the mean as in the RD analysis. R generally increases with the interval duration but SD changes little. The logarithm of R/SD is plotted versus the logarithm of τ. The slope is $H - 1$, where H is the Hurst coefficient:

$$\frac{\text{R/SD for interval } \tau}{\text{R/SD for interval } \tau_0} = \left(\frac{\tau}{\tau_0}\right)^{H-1} \tag{10}$$

The R/SD grows with the interval length τ, as expected, because the dispersion is in the denominator. When the rescaled range analysis is applied to the barometric data (Figure 27), a Hurst coefficient of 0.7 is obtained.

The values of R/SD are usually scattered for short τ or few observations, but the information is similar to that provided by the RD analysis, and H is related to the fractal D:

$$H = 2 - D \tag{11}$$

The approach is good when $H = 0.5$ (random, no correlation) and when $H > 0.5$ (correlated functions with "memory"). The coefficient of correlation between adjacent intervals is $r = 2^{2H-1} - 1$. Because the rescaled range accounts for local trends in the data, it does not identify the negative correlation observed at longer time intervals (~100 days).

Hoop and associates (52) have used rescaled range analysis to characterize the temporal variability in breathing. They have shown that tidal volumes in 4-day-old mice vary in a fractal pattern over minutes with a Hurst coefficient between 0.5 and 0.8. The Hurst coefficient changed significantly when the inhaled oxygen fraction was changed from 0.30 to 0.87.

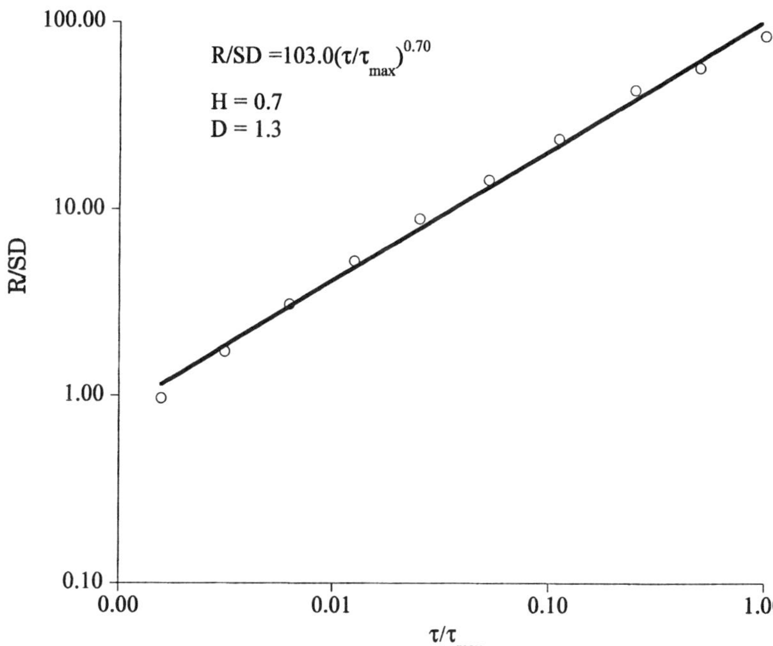

Figure 27 Rescaled range analysis of the barometric pressure data. The Hurst coefficient is 0.7, equivalent to a fractal dimension of 1.3. Compare this to Figure 26.

The extended-range correlation technique of Bassingthwaighte and Beyer (53) tests the fractal nature of a time series. The two-point autocorrelation is determined for units separated by n units, giving a statistical measure of r(n) for any n:

$$r(n) = \frac{\Sigma\, x_i(\tau) \cdot x_i(\tau + n\tau)}{\mathrm{Var}(x)} \tag{12}$$

The theoretical fractal curve for the correlation is:

$$r(n) = \frac{1}{2}\left[(n+1)^{2H} - 2n^{2H} + (n-1)^{2H^-}\right] \tag{13}$$

which, for $n > 3$, follows a simple relationship that is a straight line on a log-log plot, $\frac{r(n)}{r(n-1)} = \left[\frac{n}{n-1}\right]^{2H-2}$. Thus, H can be calculated directly from the slope, $H = \frac{\text{slope} + 2}{2}$.

Traditionally, temporal heterogeneity is characterized by statistical tools such as spectral analyses (Fourier analysis) and autocorrelation. Fourier analysis, a man-made tool, models time domain signals as composites of several periodic functions of fixed frequencies. There is no apriori reason to believe that the underlying physiology for many processes is due to multiple uniform sinusoidal processes and applying Fourier analyses to them is analogous to forcing a square peg into a round hole.

Excellent reviews are available on more traditional approaches to time series (53). This brief overview of spectral analyses is not intended to be an in-depth review, but is included to put other traditional time series analyses in the context of new fractal approaches. The intent of spectral analyses is to search for periodicity in the time series. Temporal observations are transformed into the frequency domain where new observations are transformed into a power spectrum as a function of frequency. The power spectrum is analogous to variance in traditional statistical analyses (54). The power spectrum is visually explored for frequencies that contribute proportionately more to the variability in the time series. A common application looks at parameter variations such as respiratory and heart rates (55–57).

Another traditional time-series analysis is the autocorrelation that measures dependence between two points in the same series observed at different times (54). The autocorrelation ranges from 1.0 to −1.0, indicating perfect positive and negative correlation, respectively.

When spectral and autocorrelation analyses are applied to the barometric pressure data, the power spectrum and autocorrelation plot of Figure 28 are obtained. The power spectrum suggests that most of the variability in barometric

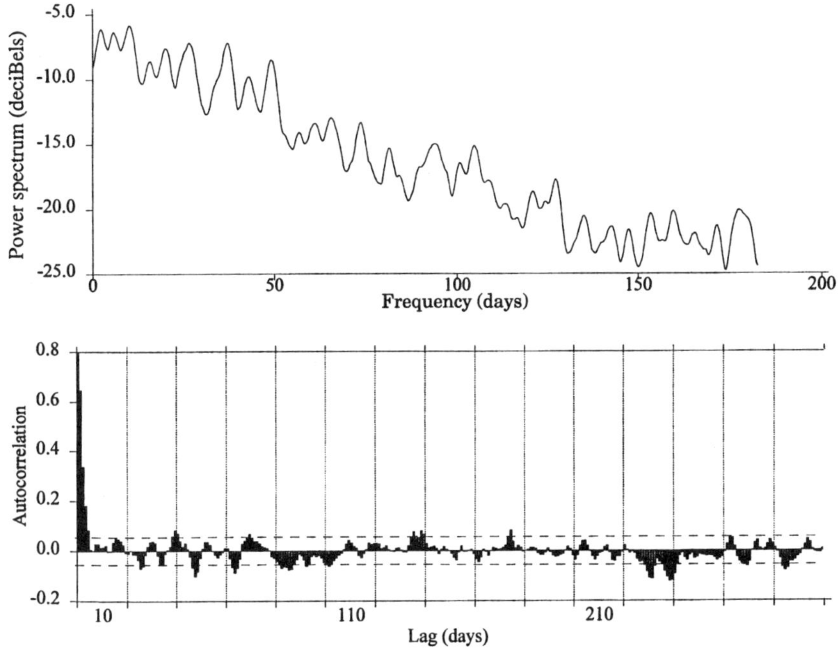

Figure 28 Spectral analysis (*top*) and autocorrelation (*bottom*) of barometric data. The power spectrum suggests that most of the variability in barometric pressures occurs at cycles lasting less than 100 days. The autocorrelation plot demonstrates both positive and negative correlation at different lag times, up to 230 days apart.

pressures occurs at cycles lasting less than 100 days. The autocorrelation plot demonstrates both positive and negative correlation at different lag times.

Fourier analysis can be used to determine the fractal dimension of a time series (58). When the logarithm of the amplitude of individual frequency components is plotted versus the logarithm of the frequency, the slope of the relationship between the two components can be a straight line with slope$-\beta$ (24). The fractal self-similarity demonstrated in this analysis is the constant ratio of power at any two frequencies, independent of the resolution (the position of the frequency scale). In this context, white random noise (all frequencies with equal power) has $\beta = 0$ and so called Brownian noise has $\beta = 2$. Noise with amplitude proportional to $f^{-\beta}$ exhibits "memory." Over this limited range:

$$\beta = 2H - 1 = 3 - 2D_\tau \quad (14)$$

Goldberger and West used frequency analysis to characterize the fractal nature of an electrocardiograph signal (59). They argued that an electrical stimulus passed through a fractal network should result in a voltage-time pulse with a power spectral density that has a linear relationship on a log-log plot. They asserted that the His-Purkinje conduction network is a fractal structure and should therefore produce a fractal process. In testing this hypothesis, they examined a single QRS complex from 21 resting subjects by using a fast Fourier transformation. When they plotted the logarithm of the mean square of the amplitude against the logarithm of the frequency for the mean data of 21 subjects, they found a linear relationship with a slope of –4.3. This corresponds to a β of 2.15 and a D_τ of 1.4, suggesting a process approaching that of Brownian motion. A more recent study (60), challenging the notion that the His-Purkinje conduction system creates a fractal power spectrum, showed that spectra from adherently conducted beats also have a fractal pattern.

It should be evident from the different approaches outlined above that a consensus does not exist on how time series data should be interpreted. Each analysis explores data from a different perspective and hence paints a different picture. No single perspective is best, and each provides more insight into the temporal process.

XII. Summary

Pulmonary gas exchange, the primary lung function, requires interactions among vascular, airway, and parenchymal components. This complex system has traditionally been studied by constructing simplified models of individual components. These "lumping" models assume that the "mean" behavior of each component adequately describes its function and that behavior of each component remains unchanged in the complete system. With the realization that heterogeneity is a fundamental characteristic of lung structure and function, new concepts incorporating the observed variability are needed.

Traditional analytical tools used by scientists are measurements of means and variances with statistical approaches based on the assumption of random error. Until recently, observed heterogeneity was interpreted as random measurement noise. The fractal revolution has brought the realization that this "error" can be analyzed as a fundamental property of a biological system. Fractal analysis permits characterization of processes or structures not easily represented by traditional analytical tools. By providing a geometric framework for the description of apparently irregular patterns, fractal analysis can capture both richness of the physiological structure and its function in a single model. The robust descriptive properties of fractal analysis to biological variability suggest that it may signal the development of a new paradigm, compelling the attention of investigators from diverse areas of scientific inquiry.

References

1. Heusch G, Schipke JD. Regional blood flow and contractile function: Are they matched in normal, ischemic and reperfused myocardium? Basic Res Cardiol 1993; 2:103–119.
2. Bassingthwaighte JB, King RB, Roger SA. Fractal nature of regional myocardial blood flow heterogeneity. Circ Res 1989; 65:578–590.
3. Franzen D, Conway RS, Zhang H, Sonnenblick EH, Eng C. Spatial heterogeneity of local blood flow and metabolite content in dog hearts. Am J Physiol 1988; 254: H344–H353.
4. Austin RE Jr, Aldea GS, Coggins DL, Flynn AE, Hoffman JI. Profound spatial heterogeneity of coronary reserve. Discordance between patterns of resting and maximal myocardial blood flow. Circ Res 1990; 67:319–331.
5. Ellis CG, Wrigley SM, Groom AC. Heterogeneity of red blood cell perfusion in capillary networks supplied by a single arteriole in resting skeletal muscle. Circ Res 1994; 75:357–368.
6. Hudetz AG, Feh'er G, Knuese DE, Kampine JP. Erythrocyte flow heterogeneity in the cerebrocortical capillary network. Adv Exp Med Biol 1994; 345:633–642.
7. Gim'enez-Amaya JM. A note upon the striatal distribution of cytochrome oxidase activity in the rat and in the cat. Acta Anat Basel 1991; 142:158–164.
8. Cossarizza A, Ceccarelli D, Masini A. Functional heterogeneity of an isolated mitochondrial population revealed by cytofluorometric analysis at the single organelle level. Exp Cell Res 1996; 222:84–94.
9. Zhu N, Weiss HR. Myocardial venous O_2 saturation becomes more heterogeneous during hypoxic and carbon monoxide hypoxia. Microvasc Res 1995; 49:253–287.
10. Lubbers DW, Baumgartl H, Zimelka W. Heterogeneity and stability of local PO2 distribution within the brain tissue. Adv Exp Med Biol 1994; 345:567–574.
11. Eichinger MR, Walker BR. Segmental heterogeneity of NO-mediated pulmonary vasodilation in rats. Am J Physiol 1994; 267:H494–H499.
12. Habazettl H, Vollmar B, Christ M, Baier H, Conzen PF, Peter K. Heterogeneous microvascular coronary vasodilation by adenosine and nitroglycerin in dogs. J Appl Physiol 1994; 76:1951–1960.
13. Kuo L, Davis MJ, Chilian WM. Longitudinal gradients for endothelium-dependent and -independent vascular responses in the coronary microcirculation. Circulation 1995; 92:518–525.
14. Zhang J, Somers M, Cobb FR. Heterogeneous effects of nitroglycerin on the conductance and resistance coronary arterial vasculature. Am J Physiol 1993; 264: H1960–H1968.
15. Pelletier N, Robinson NE, Kaiser L, Derksen FJ. Regional differences in pulmonary artery endothelial function: a role in the site of EIPH? Equine Vet J 1995; 99–103.
16. Al-Tinawi A, Krenz GS, Rickaby DA, Linehan JH, Dawson CA. Influence of hypoxia and serotonin on small pulmonary vessels. J Appl Physiol 1994; 76:56–64.
17. West JB. Regional differences in the lung. Chest 1978; 74:426–437.
18. Goldberger AL, West BJ. Fractals in physiology and medicine. Yale J Biol Med 1987; 60:421–435.

19. West BJ. Physiology in fractal dimensions: error tolerance. Ann Biomed Eng 1990; 18:135–149.
20. Bassingthwaighte JB. Physiologic heterogeneity: fractals link determinism and randomness in structures and functions. News Physiol Sci 1988; 5–10.
21. Mandelbrot BB. The Fractal Geometry of Nature. San Francisco: WH Freeman, 1983.
22. King RB, Bassingthwaighte JB, Hales JRS, Rowell LB. Stability of heterogeneity of myocardial blood flow in normal awake baboons. Circ Res 1985; 57:285–295.
23. Wagner PD, Laravuso RB, Uhl RR, West JB. Continuous distributions of ventilation-perfusion ratios in normal subjects breathing air and 100% O_2. J Clin Invest 1974; 54:54–68.
24. Voss RF. The Science of Fractal Images. Peitgen and Saupe, eds. New York: Springer-Verlag, 1988:21–70.
25. Mandelbrot B. How long is the coast of Britain? Statistical self-similarity and fractal dimension. Science 1967; 156:636–638.
26. Liebovitch LS, Toth TA. A fast algorithm to determine fractal dimensions by box counting. Phys Lett A 1989; 141:386–390.
27. Boxt LM, Katz J, Liebovitch LS, Jones R, Esser PD, Reid L. Fractal analysis of pulmonary arteries: the fractal dimension is lower in pulmonary hypertension. J Thorac Imaging 1994; 9:8–13.
28. Bassingthwaighte JB, van Beek JHGM. Lightning and the heart: fractal behavior in cardiac function. Proc IEEE 1988; 76:693–699.
29. Caruthers SD, Harris TR. Effects of pulmonary blood flow on the fractal heterogeneity in sheep lungs. J Appl Physiol 1994; 77:1474–1479.
30. Glenny RW, Robertson HT. Fractal properties of pulmonary blood flow: characterization of spatial heterogeneity. J Appl Physiol 1990; 69:532–545.
31. Iversen PO, Nicolaysen G. Fractals describe blood flow heterogeneity within skeletal muscle and within myocardium. Am J Physiol 1995; 268:H112–H116.
32. Iversen PO, Nicolaysen G. High correlation of fractals for regional blood flows among resting and exercising skeletal muscles. Am J Physiol 1995; 269:H7–H13.
33. Overholser KA, Bhatte MJ, Laughlin MH. Modeling the effect of flow heterogeneity on coronary permeability-surface area. J Appl Physiol 1991; 71:758–769.
34. Glenny RW, Robertson HT, Yamashiro S, Bassingthwaighte JB. Applications of fractal analysis to physiology. J Appl Physiol 1991; 70:2351–2367.
35. West BJ, Goldberger AL. Physiology in fractal dimensions. Am Scientist 1987; 75: 354–365.
36. Bassingthwaighte JB, van Beek JH, King RB. Fractal branchings: the basis of myocardial flow heterogeneities? Ann NY Acad Sci 1990; 591:392–401.
37. Glenny RW, Bernard S, Barlow C, Kelly J, Robertson HT. Spatial distribution of pulmonary blood flow at a microscopic scale of resolution. Am J Respir Crit Med 1995; 151:A518.
38. Glenny RW. Spatial correlation of regional pulmonary perfusion. J Appl Physiol 1992; 72:2378–2386.
39. van Beek JHGM, Roger SA, Bassingthwaighte JB. Regional myocardial flow heterogeneity explained with fractal networks. Am J Physiol 1989; 257:H1670–H1680.

40. Glenny RW, Robertson HT. A computer simulation of pulmonary perfusion in three dimensions. J Appl Physiol 1995; 79:357–369.
41. Rodarte JR, Chaniotakis M, Wilson TA. Variability of parenchymal expansion measured by computed tomography. J Appl Physiol 1989; 67:226–231.
42. Luo A, Schramm DN. Fractals and cosmological large-scale structure. Science 1992; 256:513–515.
43. Brown D, Rothery P. Models in Biology: Mathematics, Statistics and Computing. New York: John Wiley & Sons, 1993.
44. Strauss DJ. A model for clustering. Biometrika 1975; 62:467–475.
45. Diggle PJ. Statistical analysis of spatial point patterns. Mathematics in Biology 1983.
46. Ripley BD. Spatial Statistics. New York: John Wiley & Sons, 1981.
47. Glass L, Mackey MC. From Clocks to Chaos: The Rhythms of Life. Princeton, NJ: Princeton University Press, 1988.
48. Moon FC. Chaotic and Fractal Dynamics: An Introduction for Applied Scientists and Engineers. New York: John Wiley & Sons, 1992.
49. Zenk GM, Presson RGJ, et al. Temporal heterogeneity of pulmonary capillary blood flow. Am J Respir Crit Care Med 1996; 153:A817.
50. Hurst HE, Black RP, Simaika YM. Long-Term Storage: An Experimental Study. London: Constable, 1965.
51. Feder J. Fractals. New York: Plenum Press, 1988.
52. Hoop B, Burton MD, Kazemi H. Bioengineering Approaches to Pulmonary Physiology and Medicine. Khoo, ed. New York: Plenum Press, 1966:161–173.
53. Bassingthwaighte JB, Beyer RP. Fractal correlation in heterogeneous systems. Physica D 1991; 53:71–84.
54. Shumway RH. Applied Statistical Time Series Analysis. Prentice Hall Series in Statistics. Wichern, ed. Englewood Cliffs, NJ: Prentice Hall, 1988.
55. Casadei B, Cochrane S, Johnston J, Conway J. Pitfalls in the interpretation of spectral analysis of the heart rate variability during exercise in humans. Acta Physiol Scand 1995; 153:125–131.
56. Laude D, Weise F, Girard A, Elghozi JL. Spectral analysis of systolic blood pressure and heart rate oscillations related to respiration. Clin Exp Pharmacol Physiol 1995; 22:352–357.
57. van den Aardweg JG, Karemaker JM. Respiratory variability and associated cardiovascular changes in adults at rest. Clin Physiol 1991; 11:95–118.
58. Bassingthwaighte JB, Liebovitch LS, West BJ. Fractal Physiology. New York: Oxford University Press, 1994.
59. Goldberger AL, Bhargava V, West BJ, Mandell AJ. On a mechanism of cardiac electrical stability. The fractal hypothesis. Biophys J 1985; 48:525–528.
60. Berger RD, Rosenbaum DS, Cohen RJ. Is the power spectrum of the QRS complex related to a fractal His-Purkinje system? Am J Cardiol 1993; 71:430–433.
61. Glenny RW. Heterogeneity of pulmonary perfusion characterized by fractals and spatial correlations. Bioengineering Approaches to Pulmonary Physiology and Medicine 1996; 197–211.

AUTHOR INDEX

Italic numbers give the page on which the complete reference is listed.

A

C

E

H

I

M

N

O

P

Q

R

S

SUBJECT INDEX

A

D

E

F

G

H

I

K

N

O

P

R